W0227530

Lecture Notes in Medical Informatics

Lecture Notes in Medical Informatics

Edited by D. A. B. Lindberg and P. L. Reichertz

16

Medical Informatics Europe 82
Fourth Congress of the European Federation
of Medical Informatics
Proceedings, Dublin, Ireland
March 21–25, 1982

Edited by
R.R. O'Moore, B. Barber, P.L. Reichertz, and F. Roger

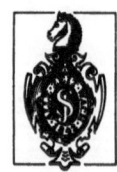

Springer-Verlag
Berlin Heidelberg New York 1982

ISBN-13:978-3-540-11208-2   e-ISBN-13:978-3-642-93201-4
DOI: 10.1007/978-3-642-93201-4

2145/3140-543210

Introduction

The European Federation for Medical Informatics is a regional coordinating body. The Congress in Dublin, MIE 82, from 21st to 25th March 1982, is the fourth in the series following MIE 78 in Cambridge, MIE 79 in Berlin. There was a break in 1980 for the World Congress - MEDINFO 80 - in Tokyo. This was followed by MIE 81 in Toulouse. The rationale behind these congresses is the scientific need to share results and ideas, and the educational need to train a wide variety of professional staff in the potential of Medical Informatics in health care delivery. All the caring professions are involved, doctors, scientists, nurses, pharmacists, paramedical staff, administrators, health care planners, community physicians, medical educationalists, epidemiologists, statisticians, operations analysts, together with specialists from the computing profession dealing with systems analysis, hardware, software, languages, data bases and marketing of systems.

The pre-publication of conference proceedings from a multi-stream conference is particularly valuable in a rapidly expanding multidisciplinary field such as Medical Informatics. It enables participants to follow work presented at sessions that they are unable to attend. More importantly, is also provides a permanent record with relevant bibliography for other workers to assess which groups are active and in which areas. All the papers have been refereed and the referees' suggestions incorporated in the final texts. Rapid publication, using camera-ready copy, reduces the time available for editing and indexing. Only a few of the most difficult papers can be retyped in the short time available. However, we have worked hard to improve the standard of communication and to reduce the number of errors.

The papers for MIE 82 Dublin are well up to our usual standard and present a broad range of topics in Medical Informatics from a wide variety of countries in Europe and many other parts of the world. In all forms of computing there has been a great upsurge of interest amongst professionals who have not previously been involved with computing. This is mainly related to reduce hardware costs, improvements in software and the advent of cheap microcomputers. This is reflected in the large number of interesting papers and posters, particularly involving clinical applications, which have been accepted for presentation in MIE 82. It is hoped that during MIE 82 there will be productive cross-fertilization of ideas between the newcomers to the profession and the older, possibly more conservative, members of the profession.

During the next decade Medical Informatics offers a key to the monitoring, evaluation and improvement of both patient care, and the administration and planning of the health services. Computer systems will proliferate in more and more areas of health care, providing specialised facilities to increasing numbers of practitioners. These papers represent another landmark in the growth of Medical Informatics and offer some insight into its current status and, hopefully, may influence its future development.

Rory O'Moore
Barry Barber
Peter Reichertz
Francis Roger   December 1981

TABLE OF CONTENTS.

       *   Paper not available.

   *   Abstract only available.

   * Paper not available.

                              *Abstract only available.

* Abstract only available.

* Abstract only available.

KEYNOTE ADDRESSES.

* Paper not available.

DESIGN IMPLICATIONS FOR DATABASE MANAGEMENT SYSTEMS

SUPPORTING HOSPITAL INFORMATION SYSTEMS

Jane B. Grimson
Department of Computer Science, Trinity College, Dublin, Ireland.

ABSTRACT

This paper examines the Hospital Information System (HIS) from the point of view of
the design of a Database Management System (DBMS) to support it. It concludes that
the HIS imposes fairly strict requirements on the DBMS, especially with respect to
flexibility, reliability and privacy. The technology, both hardware and software, is
available today to meet the demands of the HIS; the delay in the introduction of such
systems is due to problems within the application environment itself, such as the
nature of the medical record, patient record identification and user terminal devices.

1. Definitions

The term _database_ has been used to mean simply a small sequential file, at the one
extreme, and a highly complex data structure extending across several discs, at the
other. The following definitions are being used in the context of this paper:

A _Hospital Information System_ (HIS) is an interactive computer system for processing
in-patient, out-patient and administrative data for one or more hospitals. The aims
of the HIS can be summarized as follows:

  (a) to provide the medical staff with all information required in the provision
       of medical care

  (b) to provide the administrative staff with all the information required for the
       efficient management of the hospital, i.e. handling of admission procedures,
       bed census, menu planning, accounts, personnel, payroll, etc.

  (c) scheduling and resource allocation

  (d) as an offshoot, to facilitate research into the diagnosis and treatment of
       disease.

A _database_ is an integrated collection of data pertaining to several applications
without unnecessary duplication. In addition, the database includes a formal definition of the data, which exists separately from the data itself.

A _Database Management System_ (DBMS) is the name given to the software to support the
database and is assumed to provide for:

  (a) maintenance of data structures

  (b) languages for storage, retrieval and update of data

  (c) facilities for ensuring data integrity and security

  (d) reporting facilities for the Database Administrator

  (e) separation of physical and logical data structures

  (f) simultaneous access to the database by many users including those who are
       altering the data (concurrent update).

It is essential to make a very clear distinction between the HIS and the DBMS which
supports it. The HIS should always be designed first and the DBMS tailored to suit
these requirements. One of the main motivating forces behind the development of DBMSs
in the late 1960s and early 1970s was the need to provide information management systems
which would more closely reflect the natural data relationships which exist in the real
world. Traditional file processing systems forced the applications to structure their

1

data in a certain rigorous way and any changes in the file processing system had wide-spread ramifications for the applications systems. The importance of <u>data independence</u>, the separation of physical and logical data structures, cannot be over-emphasized, especially when a highly dynamic and complex application such as a HIS is being con-sidered. The introduction of a HIS requires many man-years of effort, starting with an exhaustive examination of the information flow and information processing activities of the hospital as they exist at present. The investment in terms of time and money will be enormous and it is therefore essential to ensure that the system will be able to adapt quickly and easily to the ever-changing demands of the hospital.

In the remainder of this paper, various aspects of the design of a DBMS will be exa-mined in order to determine what conditions a HIS imposes on the DBMS which affect this design. Much of the work described here was carried out in association with a survey of the information flow in the Accident and Emergency Department at the Royal Infirmary, Edinburgh, as part of research into the design of DMBSs[1].

2. General- versus special-purpose DBMS

The design of a DBMS involves vast expenditure and the hope is that a particular DBMS will be applicable in a wide variety of situations. Most of the effort today is being directed towards the design of these general-purpose DBMSs. This approach is based upon the premise that the information handling requirements of the various applications are similar. Consider, for example, airline systems; they are designed as special-purpose DBMSs and as such they could be of use only to another airline, but certainly not for a complete HIS. However, a superficial comparison between the Passenger Seat Reservation System alone and the appointment system in an out-patient department re-veals certain similarities. The patient makes an appointment (sometimes many months ahead) for a particular clinic, on a particular day, at a particular time, while a passenger usually books a seat for a specific flight, on a specific day, at a specific time. A significant difference between the two systems is that whereas the patient will generally take the first available appointment, the passenger usually wants to book a seat on a specific flight.

It would seem therefore to be a reasonable assumption that the information handling requirements of many applications are sufficiently similar for them to be supported by the same general-purpose DBMS. It should be noted, however, that given a particular application (and sufficient resources), it is always possible to design a more effi-cient special-purpose DBMS which is tailor-made for that application, than to use even the very best general-purpose system.

3. User interface

There are two different ways in which a user can interface with a DBMS. The first, and the most common for general-purpose DBMSs, is the host-language system. With this system, the user communicates with the DBMS by means of special Data Manipulation commands embedded in a high-level procedural language, such as PL/1, COBOL or FORTRAN. The second method of providing the interface with the user is chosen by the so-called self-contained DBMSs. As the name implies, the user communicates with the DBMS by means of a DBMS-supplied language. These languages are non-procedural and command-structured and are intended to be used by programmers and non-programmers alike.

There is, however, no reason why a given DBMS should provide one interface and not the other. Indeed, to support a HIS, it would be essential for the DBMS to provide both types of interface. It is well-known that in order to minimize error rates, it is preferable to capture data at source and since the main source of information in a HIS would be medical and administrative staff, i.e. non-programmers, a high-level query language interface is essential (e.g. MUMPS[2]). At the same time, there is a need to provide a host-language interface. Regular, weekly or monthly operations such as payroll and accounts, would be better written in a procedural language which could take advantage of its knowledge of the structure of the database and so make these operations run more efficiently.

4. Data structures

DBMS are classified into three main types based on the type of data structures they support; namely network, hierarchical and relational. Without going into unnecessary detail, a network structure will support m:n relationships between records while a hierarchical structure supports only a 1:n relationship. Thus, for example, a patient attending a number of different departments in a hospital would be under a number of different consultants, while a consultant would have a number of patients in his care. Such a relationship can be represented directly by a network structure, whereas in a hierarchical structure, two separate relationships would be required, PATIENT-TO-CON-SULTANT and CONSULTANT-TO-PATIENT. The relational approach is somewhat different; instead of "links" connecting two related record types, as required in both the network and hierarchical approaches, the relationships are expressed automatically in the data itself. Thus for example

PATIENT RECORDS				X-RAY REPORTS	
Name	I.D.	Location		I.D.	X-Ray No.
1. Brown, John S.	185327	Ward 32.....	1.	165329	643361...
2. Smith, Alan r.	165329	Ward 32.....	2.	165329	874432...

The fact that X-ray report record no. 1 refers to the same record as patient record no. 2 is given by the fact that they both contain the same value for the patient identification number, 165329. Effectively, this means that the relational approach can also represent m:n relationships.

A patient's medical record is a complex data structure consisting basically of 3 parts:

  (a) personal information such as name, address, date of birth (more or less fixed)
  (b) medical history (constantly growing with each episode of treatment)
  (c) current treatment (also constantly changing).

The type of information recorded in the personal information section of the medical record is common to all personnel files; its structure is known in advance and is constant for all patients. Parts (b) and (c) are much more complex when the question of computerization is posed (see also last section). Consider, for example, the recording of medical histories; should the episodes (of illness, treatment, etc.) be recorded chronologically or by problem (i.e. type of illness, symptoms, etc.)? If it could be decided once and for all which of the two approaches to adopt then a tree (hierarchical) structure would be quite sufficient. If, however, medical staff decided to switch from the chronological to the problem approach and back again, only a network or relational structure could support this without requiring a very costly structural reorganization of the database.

It is also important that the system should be able to link records for the duration of a research project. For example, all patients with disease x, admitted after date y, should be linked together, these linkages to be removed when the research has been completed.

5. Reliability

Both the hardware and software of a computer system supporting a HIS have to achieve almost 100% reliability. They have to be available 24 hours a day, 7 days a week and 52 weeks of the year. In order to do this, experience with Airline Passenger Seat Reservation Systems has shown that every item from CPU to data record must be at least duplicated; indeed many systems are triplicated. Such a dual system would be essential in a hospital which relied completely on a large central computer. With the ever-increasing use of microcomputers, it is probable that the HISs of the future will be based on networks of smaller computers each supporting its own database, located in the various departments throughout the hospital. A patient attending a number of departments in a hospital might have a number of different specialist clinical records with a central identification, history and summary section "passed round" the relevant departments. The networks could be linked together in such a way that if one computer is down, another can take on its urgent on-line work in addition to its own. Such an approach has the added advantage (apart from enhancing the reliability of the system) that each department would have direct control over its own portion of the database and it would also be cheaper than a system which required a lot of built-in redundancy.

6. Privacy

It is of the utmost importance to ensure the confidentiality of medical data. It is generally felt that records stored in a computer system are more secure, from the casual snooper, than the traditional case-notes folders[3]. VDUs can be placed in rooms to which members of the public do not have access, screens can fade rapidly and certain fields may not be displayed at all. It is not the casual snooper, however, who represents the main threat to the security of the system, but rather the professional who knows his way round. It should always be borne in mind that any security measure will cost something and the cost of providing security measures should bear some relationship to the gain to be derived from obtaining the unauthorized information.

In the eyes of the layman, it is not the fact that medical records might be stored in a computer that concerns him, but rather that the information contained in it could be disclosed to people outside the hospital. It is the potential of linking together all the records pertaining to one individual, e.g. employee, income tax, social security, medical, bank, credit rating agency, police, that is seen as the main threat of computerized data banks. It is generally accepted now and is gradually being supported by legislation in many countries, that an individual should have the right to verify the accuracy of any factual information which is stored about him. This could pose problems for the medical profession who have long held, with good justification, that it is sometimes in the patient's best interest not to see all the information stored in his medical record.

There are a number of measures which a DBMS can take to help ensure the security of the data in the database, from elaborate hardware encoding/decoding devices in a teleprocessing network to a simple password. It is doubtful whether the complex hardware security measures would be worth the expense for a HIS. However, standard software measures involving locks on individual fields in the records as well as on entire records would be essential. Alternatively, sensitive fields or records can be encoded using cryptography techniques. HISs are generally linked to District Health Board computers. Such linkage is essential for epidemiological research and for administrative purposes. Generally speaking, however, it is quite unnecessary to identify the patient as an individual, but rather to treat him simply as an anonymous statistic. Thus within the hospital, the patient is identified by name, but "higher up", he just becomes a number.

7. Conclusions

This paper has attempted to show that while a HIS imposes certain design constraints on the DBMS which supports it especially in relation to flexibility, reliability and security, these constraints are not fundamentally different from those which apply to other application systems. Thus, in principle, the technology (both hardware and software) is available today to support a full HIS. Why then is the movement towards adopting such systems by the larger hospitals so slow?

There are a number of reasons for this including patient identification, input devices and the nature of the medical record itself. There is no standard format for recording the clinical information in either the medical history or the current treatment section of the record. The doctor very often uses a personal form of shorthand together with short pieces of text and aides-de-memoires. To transfer this information directly in the form of unstructured narrative onto the computer will become cheaper with the development of optical disc memories[4]. However, the result could be that the computer would be used as a very extravagant filing system. It will be some time before really powerful Semantic Analysers are available to extract meaning from natural language. Consider, for example, a researcher who wishes to compare the treatment of a certain disease by drug A with drug B. In the manual system, he would have to examine every case notes folder to ascertain whether the patient suffered from the disease in question and, if so, whether he was given drug A or B and what the result was. Such an operation is extremely tedious. Now if the medical record was just transferred directly onto the optical disc, the same procedure would be required, although the computer could be used to assist in scanning the disc(s) for certain keywords, such as the names of the disease and the drugs in question. When a match is found, the particular record is then displayed for the researcher to examine the outcome of the treatment. This raises the question of standard medical terminology; doctors may use different names for the same drug or even the same disease. The computer has to be instructed to search for all synonyms otherwise one could be missed. There is a danger that users will know that the information is there somewhere "in the computer", but they cannot get it out easily.

The optical disc memories will probably play a major part in the development of the HISs of the future, but they do not solve the problem of how to get the information onto the disc in the first place. There is no doubt that this is one of the main difficulties which face the developers of HISs. As was stated previously, in order to achieve a low error rate, information should be captured and verified at source. Therefore, either the medical personnel themselves input the data or they are present and can verify the data as it is input by a trained terminal operator. The latter approach will be more costly and could lead to frustration as medical staff have to wait around for the data to be typed in. Many of the existing HIS adopt the former approach with data being input on a CRT and light-pen using a menu-selection system. Provided the system is carefullt designed and users do not have to "flip through" several frames before reaching the one they want, such an approach can operate efficiently and not involve highly skilled medical staff spending long periods of time at computer terminals. Obviously, when large amounts of data are being input, e.g. admission details and medical histories, doctors can dictate the information for input by a trained operator.

Another major problem associated with a medical record database is that of patient identification. The simple and most straightforward method is to use the patient's name, but it is very far from unique, is prone to mis-spelling and, in manual systems, to mis-filing. A widely used alternative to the name as the basic key to patient identification is the patient's date of birth, but it too is non-unique and patients, especially older ones, can forget their date of birth.

There is no single answer to the problem of patient identification. Assuming, however, that a patient's name, sex and approximate age are known, it would be a simple matter to devise an algorithm which could search rapidly through the indexes stored in the computer in order to identify him and extract details of his medical history. If an exact match is not found given the identification information available, a list of closest matches found could be printed. It is unlikely that a patient could be automatically and uniquely identified by the computer for it to link together different episodes of illness without any human intervention.

While the information processing requirements of the hospital environment are not vastly different from other application environments, there is one vitally important aspect which sets the HIS apart - namely, that the welfare of the individuals about whom the information is being stored is critically dependent on the efficiency and accuracy of the system. If the HIS results in a deterioration in the standard of medical care, then it is totally unacceptable, no matter how marvellous it is for the administrative and medical staffs. Great care must be taken not to decrease the quality of patient care and it would not be unreasonable to expect it to improve as a result of the more timely provision of medical data.

There can be no doubt that the benefits to be derived from a fully computerized HIS are potentially enormous for both the medical and the administrative staff and for the patients. The development of such systems must proceed slowly. For example, small laboratory systems should be developed first, following by admissions procedures and so on until gradually all aspects of the hospital's information processing activities have been integrated into the system.

REFERENCES

[1]   Grimson, J.B., <u>The design of a flexible Database Management for a virtual</u>
       <u>memory machine</u>, Ph.D. thesis, University of Edinburgh, 1980.

[2]   Greenes, R.A., Pappalardo, A.N., Marble, C.W., Barnett, G.O., <u>A system for</u>
       <u>clinical data management</u>, AFIPS, FJCC, 1969, pp. 297-305.

[3]   <u>London Hospital Computer System</u>, <u>A case study in the installation of a major</u>
       <u>real-time system</u>, Proceedings of conferences held in the London Hospital on
       Nov. 27, 1973 and April 24, 1974.

[4]   Lindberg, D.A., <u>The status of medical information technology</u>, Proceedings
       of IFIP Working Conference on Hospital Information Systems, ed. R.H. Shannon,
       North-Holland, 1979.

HOSPITAL INFORMATION SYSTEM

WITH INTERCONNECTIONS IN A DISTRICT

Dieter Schreiter, Roland Straube and Ulrich Lochmann
Medizinische Akademie "Carl Gustav Carus" Dresden
Organisations- und Rechenzentrum
GDR – 8019 Dresden, Fetscherstr.74

Abstract

The computer EC 1040, produced by Kombinat Robotron, was set
into operation in the Medical School "Carl Gustav Carus" Dresden
in May 1979 where it replaced the computer Robotron 300 which
had been working there since 1971. This paper will give a survey
of the aims, forms and present level of application of EDP
projects and computers. Priority will be devoted to their use
in the three large hospitals of the city of Dresden and the
environs. The aim of the data communication within the computer
network, the present state and the further realization stages
are presented.

1. Aims of the EDP Application in Medicine

The comprehensive social-political measures in the GDR make it
necessary to exploit all reserves in the interest of socialist
intensification also in the field of the health care service.

The general aims in this context must be:

– To maintain the health of all citizens and to ensure the speedy
recovery of the sick.

– The intensive utilization of the labour potential and
equipment of the health care service.

This gives rise to many possibilities for the use of electronic
data processing. The application of EDP in a hospital proceeds
on such a broad scale and with so many differing qualitative
demands with regard to hardware and software, including their
theoretical basis, that it is rarely matched even by large
horizontally or vertically organized combines of industry.

It follows, therefore, that the problems to be solved are
correspondingly diverse and require a new quality of work in
computing centres.

In principle, the aims of the application of EDP and computers
in the health care service, particularly in hospitals, do not
differ from those in other social fields.

Two main directions can be established in this context:

– Rationalization of the information processes and the material
processes controlled by these.

- The evaluation of algorithms for analytical, heuristic or simulation models which would be impossible to evaluate at a justifiable amount of time and work without modern computing facilities.

In detail this means:

- Effective exploitation of the facilities of the health care service for the patients. This is also a task of management, planning and administration.

- To relieve physicians and nurses of schematic processes of information processing and documentation in favour of care for the patients.

- Long-term storage of patient data.

- Medical statistics, epidemiology and medical research.

- The reduction of possible risks for the patients and their duration of hospitalization.

Favourable preconditions for the fulfilment of the listed demands in a large hospital on the basis of current computing techniques are offered by a hospital information system (1) with a high degree of integration and founded on a data bank as informational centre. MADIS is such an information system and it was conceived by the Medical School of Dresden (MAD) (2). The system architecture in seen in Figure 1.

2. Level Achieved in the Medical School of Dresden

Following the foundation of a computing centre in the Medical School of Dresden, a broad basis was established for the application of electric data processing during the years 1968 to 1971. On behalf of the Ministry of Health, a comprehensive research project in the field of "Automated Information Processing in Medicine" was launched for the first time in the GDR. Its principal purpose was the scientific preparation of the operation of electronic data processing systems to support the medical care of hospitalized and outpatients as well as for diagnostics and for the processing of measured values. The EDP projects and programs that were to be developed had to be transferable to other institutions of the GDR health care service and to medical schools after they had been successfully tested in practice.

Problem analysis resulted in the creation of the first two projects - PIV for patient-oriented information and documentation and LOL for on-line laboratory automation. Both of these projects were completed by several parts in the subsequent years, and they both formed an important basis for the current projects of the Unified Computer System and for the overall information system MADIS (3).

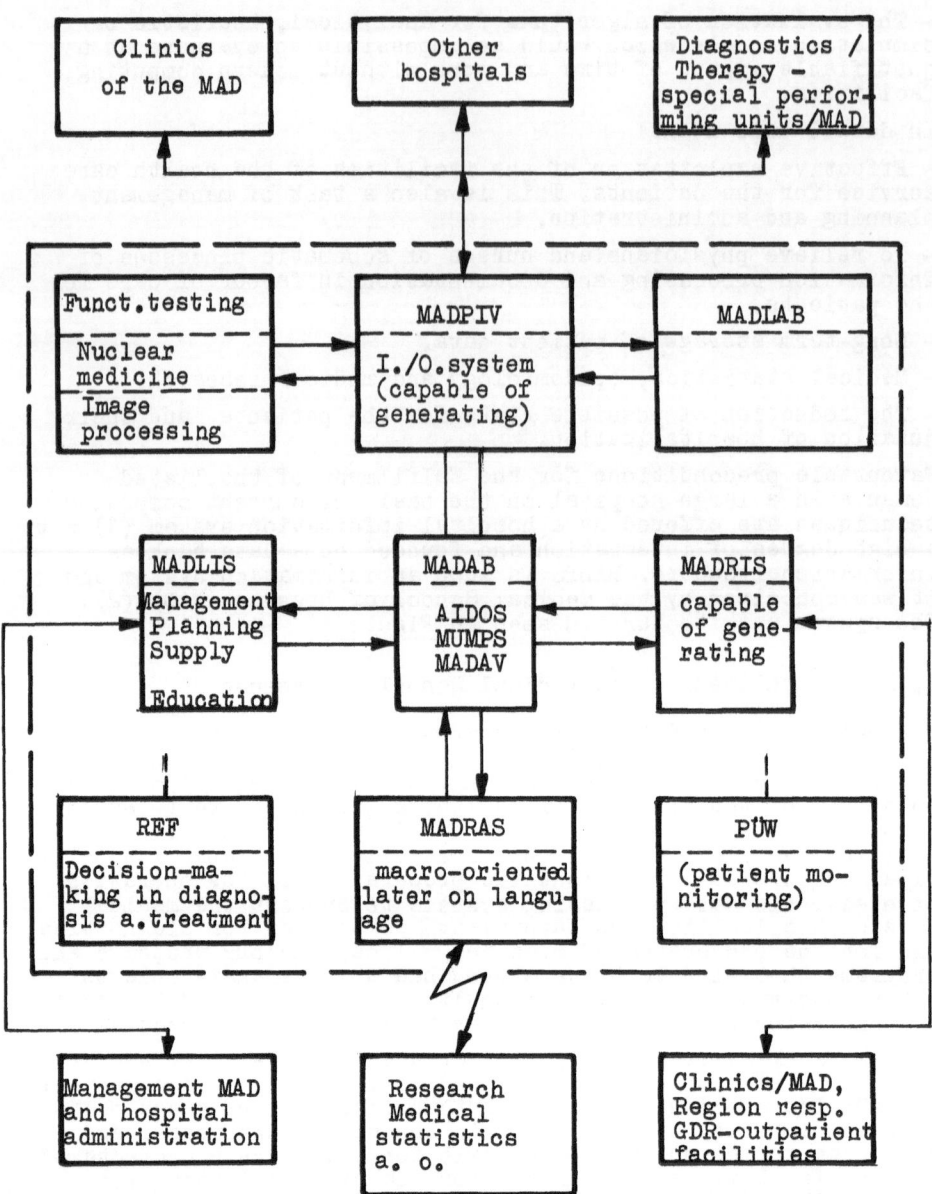

Figure 1 : Architecture of MADIS

3. The Conception of the Hospital Information System MADIS

Proceeding from past experience, and under consideration of the considerably improved possibilities obtained in the meantime (including microcomputers), the operational concept for GDR pioneer application in the Medical School of Dresden has been defined and brought up-to-date with the very latest level of development.

Development work is being concentrated on a computerized hospital information system with the following objectives, properties and conditions:

a. Backing of the activities of

- the physicians engaged in practice and research
- the other personnel, but particularly the nurses
- the hospital management and administration.

b. The hospital information system has to be designed as an open system for step-by-step implementation, i. e. the informational relations of the health care facilities of the same and superior level of management must be covered and given the required computer backing.

c. Wherever possible, data should be collected and stored only once. The data must be made available for multivalent use by the differing groups of users. Technical data safeguarding, and the confidential nature of the data, must be assured.

d. The users should have direct access to their stocks of data to the extent required. For this purpose it is necessary to implement the functions:

- Storage
- Up-dating
- Queries

Dialog processing must be applied as a mode of operation for these functions, and especially for certain processing functions.

The components are briefly described in (2).

In conformity with the progressive system architecture, all data are managed by one or a few data bank operation systems. MADAB – MAD Data Bank – is already operating with AIDOS/OS. A medical specific data management, known as MADAV – is provided for the first version. This system is based on the relational data model, it offers, however, still a number of additional functions.

MADPIV – MAD patient-oriented information/documentation – consists of an efficient input/output system.

MADRIS – MAD register information system – is used to keep a medical register with the backing of all the necessary routine processes such as supervision, ordering, etc.

MADRAS – MAD query and evaluation system – is used for (statistical) evaluation of autonomous data stocks or of data stocks of the centralized pool of the data bank.

A later version will give the researching physician direct access to the computer via a problem-defining language.

MADLIS – MAD management information system – supports management and planning, and the running of the hospital, in the fields of personnel, supplies, pharmacy, statistical reports of services rendered, etc.

MAD – MAD laboratory information system – always operates with a separate laboratory computer. The system automates the clinical-chemical and hematological laboratory.

4. Particular Aspects of the Hospital Information System under Consideration of the Target of a City and a District

The locations of the three connected hospitals of the city of Dresden are shown in <u>Figure 2</u>:

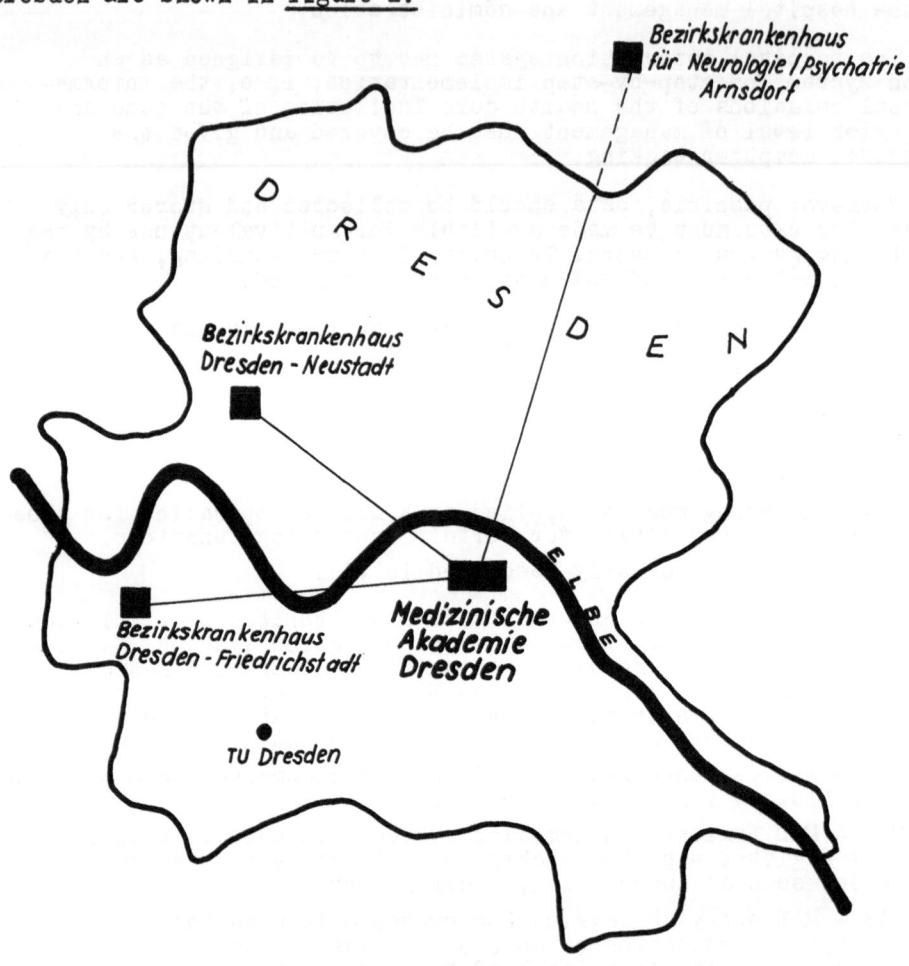

The components of our hospital information system commented in the above section are function-oriented. In other hospital information systems (1), (4) one mainly finds dedicated partial systems which orient themselves by the concerned application field. The basic conception chosen by us is very flexible and comparatively easily enables other hospitals to be linked to the original hospital information system of the Medical School. Thus a patient-oriented data communication network may be established, and novel health-political aims may be attained under utilization of planned co-operative interrelations between the linked hospitals and outpatient departments.

Moreover, more extensive data stocks are available for statistical evaluations in research, epidemiology etc. In the following some aspects of the benefits of a regional integration within the framework of a city shall be traced more in detail. By the support of the patient-oriented information exchange between the hospitals, the expenditure for multiple-examinations can be avoided. For defined patient groups underlying special health surveillance, centrally administrated patient files shall be established which can be made use of by all hospitals included in the system (for example, high risk patients, children and juveniles). Furtherly, such a regional system could contribute to an optimum utilization of the treatment capacities of the individual hospitals. This particularly concerns the emergency admission to the hospital by the "urgent medical aid" as well as tasks of the highly specialized medical care. To a hospital information system in our opinion also belong commonly useable inquiry systems (e. g. for drugs, drug side-effects, intoxications and the like).

On the basic of hitherto gathered experiences, components of a speciality-oriented medical information system for all patients of a district are being established. These experiences concern both a basic project of patient-oriented information/documentation, and the speciality-oriented medical record psychiatry and neurology which was worked out in a further stage.

The selected application item neurology/psychiatry is regarded as an appropriate model for the conservative specialties with an interdisciplinary feature. A further aspect for the selection of these specialties is that two of the four special hospitals for psychiatry in the district of Dresden already use these named projects in batch mode for several years.

A concerted establishment and use of the first developmental stage in a clinic of a Medical School (Dresden) and a special hospital, twenty-five kilometers distant, yield particularly favourable conditions for either side interesting problems under consideration of regional aspects.

This concerns, for example, epidemiologic investigations in a health care area, studies on stationary incidence resp. prevalence of disease groups which have to be under stationary treatment, planning strategies of the health care facilities and the region, optimizing diagnosis and therapy, increasing the number of patients required for the analysis of scientific problems.

References

(1) Shannon, R.H. (eds.):
     Hospital information systems –
     An international perspective on problems and prospects
     IFIP Working Conference, Capetown,
     North-Holland Publishing Company
     Amsterdam, New York, Oxford 1979

(2) Schreiter, D.:
     Elektronische Rechentechnik im Großkrankenhaus
     Rechentechnik/Datenverarbeitung Volume 15 (1978),
     No 7, pp. 10 to 13

(3) Schreiter, D.; R. Straube and D. Tölle:
     "Zur Anwendung der EDV und Rechentechnik an der Medizinischen
     Akademie Dresden in Vergangenheit, Gegenwärt und Zukunft"
     Scientific conference "Information Processing in a Large
     Hospital", 21st September, 1979, MAD

(4) Bakker, A.R.:
     Scope and limitations of a mini-based centralized
     Hospital Information Systems
     In: Proceedings MEDINFO 80 Lindberg, D.A.B., Kaihara, S.
         North-Holland Publishing Company Amsterdam, New York,
         Oxford 1980

ORGANIZATION OF A COOPERATION FOR FURTHER DEVELOPMENT AND
IMPLEMENTATION OF AN INTEGRATED HOSPITAL INFORMATION SYSTEM.

A.R. Bakker

BAZIS, University Hospital

Leyden, The Netherlands

Abstract.

At Leyden University hospital in the period 1972 - 1976 a sponsored project was
carried out for the experimental realization of an integrated HIS. The project
resulted in an operational HIS at Leyden, independent evaluation lead to very
positive conclusions. Already in 1976 other university hospitals in the Netherlands decided to implement the system and share their efforts for the further
development and maintenance of the system.
The structure of the cooperation (that at present covers in total 10.000 hospital
beds, also of general hospitals) is described. Attention is paid especially
to the organization of application software development.
Some figures on the growth of the cooperation are presented. Some remarks are
made on the further development and the questions involved.

Introduction

A project for the development and implementation of an integrated HIS was started
at Leyden University Hospital in 1972. The aim of the project, that was set-up
as a full size experiment, was to gain knowledge and experience in this field
and to check whether development of such a project was technical feasible and
whether such a system was useful for the hospital. Although the project was not
aiming at a complete HIS, sufficient parts had to be developed and implemented to
check the feasibility. This government sponsored project was planned to last
4 years. Because of delays in the approval process and because of the difficulty
to hire sufficient staff, the project was (within the approved budget) extended
with one year. At the end of the sponsored period the system was not only operational
at Leyden University Hospital, also two other Dutch university hospitals had
decided to implement the system and to cooperate with Leyden University Hospital
in the further development and implementation. A concluding report covering the
period 1972 - 1976 was produced [1]

The Dutch minister of science and education decided in 1977 to have the project
evaluated by an independent management consultant under guidance of a committee

of outside experts. This evaluation that took about 3 manyears was carried out
mainly during 1978. The report of this evaluation [2] concludes amongst that:
- the system has a positive effect on patient care and on the communication within
  the hospital,
- costs and quantifiable benefits are in equilibrium; benefits will double in 5
  years (costs will be stable),
- user satisfaction is very high,
- availability is very good; dataprotection is satisfactory,
- the system is transportable and can also be applied in general hospitals.

Based on the results of this evaluation the minister decided that university
hospitals that were going to introduce a computer based information system had
to choose the Leyden HIS. Several general hospitals were also interested in implementation of the system. The HIS however was a system under further development
and no commercial enterprise. It was decided to set-up a cooperative structure on
a non-profit base for the further development and support. This structure is
described in the sequel.

Characteristics of the Leyden HIS

Some characteristics of the Leyden HIS that are described in more detail elsewhere
[3] are summarized here. The HIS is set-up as a collection of application subsystems (packages of programs) around a central databank. Within the databank both
the patient data (both medical and administrative) and data on the facilities of
the hospital are stored. The application programs are formulated in a high level
programming language (FORTRAN); libraries of subroutines are available amongst
others for screen manipulation and record i/o. There is a formal interface between
application programs and the databank. The system is highly conversational
(at Leyden over 200 terminals). The system is aiming at the high availability
(99,5% round the clock);for that reason the computer system is duplicated. Dedicated
system software, to deal with the special requirements as to workload and dataprotection, is developed as a part of the project. Last but not least users were
involved heavily in the specification and implementation of the system; by the
projectteam this was experienced as one of the main reasons for the success of the
system.

Structure of the cooperation

It was decided to distinguish in the cooperation between:
- a central development and support group, BAZIS and
- the data processing departments of participating organizations.
BAZIS is set-up as a foundation with as members of the board representatives of

the management of the participants.

A participant is a (group of) hospitals that will implement the HIS. A participant
has its own data-processing department with its own (duplicated) computer equipment,
this department is responsible for implementation and running of the HIS.

The BAZIS group has as tasks:

- (further) development, maintenance and second line support of application software,
- (further) development, maintenance and second line support of system software,
- coordination and standardisation.

Besides the board that meets about 4 times a year, there is the coordination
meeting where the director of BAZIS and the heads of the d.p. departments of the
participants meet every three weeks to discuss plans, procedures, development and
implementation. Apart from participants that will implement the complete HIS
in their organizations, BAZIS has contracts with some other organizations (clients)
that will implement only parts on the HIS (in most cases the system-software).

Costs of BAZIS are covered by contributions of participants and clients (the number
of personnel of BAZIS amounts to about 50). There are 8 participants, six of which
are university hospitals, the others are two groups of general hospitals (in total
10 general hospitals are using the HIS, one of these is hooked up to the computer
system of a university hospital);

The main guiding document within the cooperation is the activity plan that describes
the planned activities as to development, implementation and coordination for the
coming two years. That plan that also contains statements on the policy in the
planned period is updated each year. Installation, expansion or replacement
of equipment is coordinated; an equipment plan gives planned actions for the coming
year and indications for the three following years. There is a common policy on
types of equipment to be used, this leads on one hand to standardization and on the
other hand to attractive quantity discounts.

Whereas for system software the development and the maintenance is fully centralized
within BAZIS, this is not entirely the case for application software, the next
section deals with the organization of application software development.

Application software development

Application software is organized in subsystems being packages of application
programs. Although the organization of the participating hospitals differs
(sometimes to a large extent),the majority of the applications are basically the
same for all participants. Some applications however are very specific for only
one participant. This consideration leads to the distinction between class 1 and
class 3 applications. The former applications are called class 1, the latter
class 3. Class 1 applications are developed under responsibility of BAZIS. Class 3
development is a responsibility of the related local d.p. department. The assignment
of class 1 or 3 to an application is a formal action. After discussion in the
coordination meeting, the director of BAZIS assigns a class (possibly he leaves
the decision to the board). For class 3 applications BAZIS has only a limited

16

responsibility in so far that integration aspects are checked, mainly by the central database manager. To achieve general applicability of class 1 application responsible representatives of the participants both from the users side and from the d.p. side are organized in so called contact groups. These groups have the task to come to functional and technical specifications of the subsystem to be developed.

Within the hospital at least implementation teams are formed that prepare the introduction of the subsystem. The implementationteam of the hospital where a subsystem will be implemented first has a special role. The meetings of the contact groups are shared by a BAZIS project coordinator who is responsible for integration aspects and quality of the product.

Typical examples of class 1 applications are:

-patient registration - clinical laboratories - diagnosis registration - radiology- kitchen - general ledger - invoicing - appointment scheduling - operations registrations.

Typical examples of class 3 applications are:

- eurotransplant (only present at Leyden) - anticoagulent dosage prescription (only at Leyden part of the university hospital) - ECG-registration (no common opinion yet) - patient monitoring (no common opinion yet).

The actual development of a subsystem is carried out by a project team, headed by a project leader. The size of the team depends on the size of the subsystem and the required speed of development; sizes range from 1 - 6.

Both the BAZIS group and the d.p. departments of participants are involved in development of application subsystems. Each subsystem is assigned to one location where under supervision of BAZIS the actual development is performed. Maintenance and second line support are also assigned to the same group. At present about 50% of application software development is done by BAZIS, the other 50% by d.p. departments of participants. Although there appears to be more similarity for the applications between the various hospitals than often is assumed there exists a need for the possibility to adapt the subsystem to the specific organizational environment of the participant. In the HIS there are three technical ways to achieve this:

a. within the sourceprogram certain portions can be inserted conditionally.
   This means that these portions will only be compiled for specific circumstances
   (e.g. a specific way of handling stat-tests in a laboratory). Although such
   portions of the package may be applicable for only one participant these are
   maintained by the central projectteam.

b. The program can be made parameter-driven; by setting of the right parameter
   values, the package is customized for a specific participant. The advantage
   over the technique mentioned under a. is that the programs need to be compiled only once and no recompilation is necessary when a parameter value
   has to be modified.

The disadvantage is the larger program length.

c. Within a package interfaces can be defined where class 3 program modules can be attached to. This technique turns out to be useful for organization dependent output of results (an additional list; labels, etc.) Such class 3 modules are maintained by the local d.p. department.

It should be emphasized that it is found in practice that the vast majority of the coding is applicable for all participants.

Growth of the cooperation

In fig. 1 the scope of the cooperation is shown.

In fig. 2 the total number of hospital beds within the cooperation is shown.

In spring 1978 it was defined as a policy that the cooperation should grow in 4 years to a size of about 10.000 beds to be sufficiently powerful. From the figure it is clear that the target has been achieved, this leads to some questions that will be discussed in the next section.

In figure 3 the growth of the total number of the production terminals is shown for all participants together.

In figure 4 the growth of the conversational load is shown for all participants together. As a measure is taken the average number of input messages per day during the dayshift (7.30 am. - 5.00 p.m.)

Further development

In the application area the development in the coming years will deal with:
- completion of packages and new packages to improve communication (e.g. decentral testordering, appointment scheduling).
- Support of nursing functions.
- More management information.
- Preparation of reports and storage in the databank
- Communication with the first line health care.
- On a longer term support of medical decision making.

This list is not intended to be complete, it only indicates that although a lot has still to be specified the medium term goal and the way to go is fairly clear.

Main areas for development in the system software are:
- databank facilities for more organizations partially sharing the databank [4].
- Improved logging and recovery facilities.
- Better development tools.
- Deactivation and reactivation of data.
- Application of a hierarchy of storage media (also video disk).
- Transportable version of the whole system software.

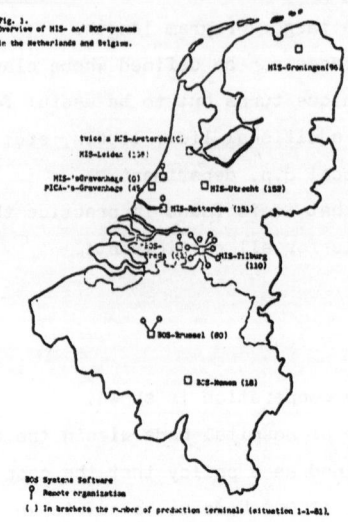

Fig. 1.
Overview of HIS- and BOS-systems
in the Netherlands and Belgium.

HIS-Groningen(96)

twice a BCB-Amsterdam(C)
HIS-Leiden (138)
HIS-'sGravenhage (0)   HIS-Utrecht (152)
PICA-'s-Gravenhage (45)
                  HIS-Rotterdam (151)
                       HIS-Tilburg
                       (110)

BOS-Brussel (80)

BCB-Ronse (18)

BOS System Software
Remote organization
( ) In brackets the number of production terminals (situation 1-1-81).

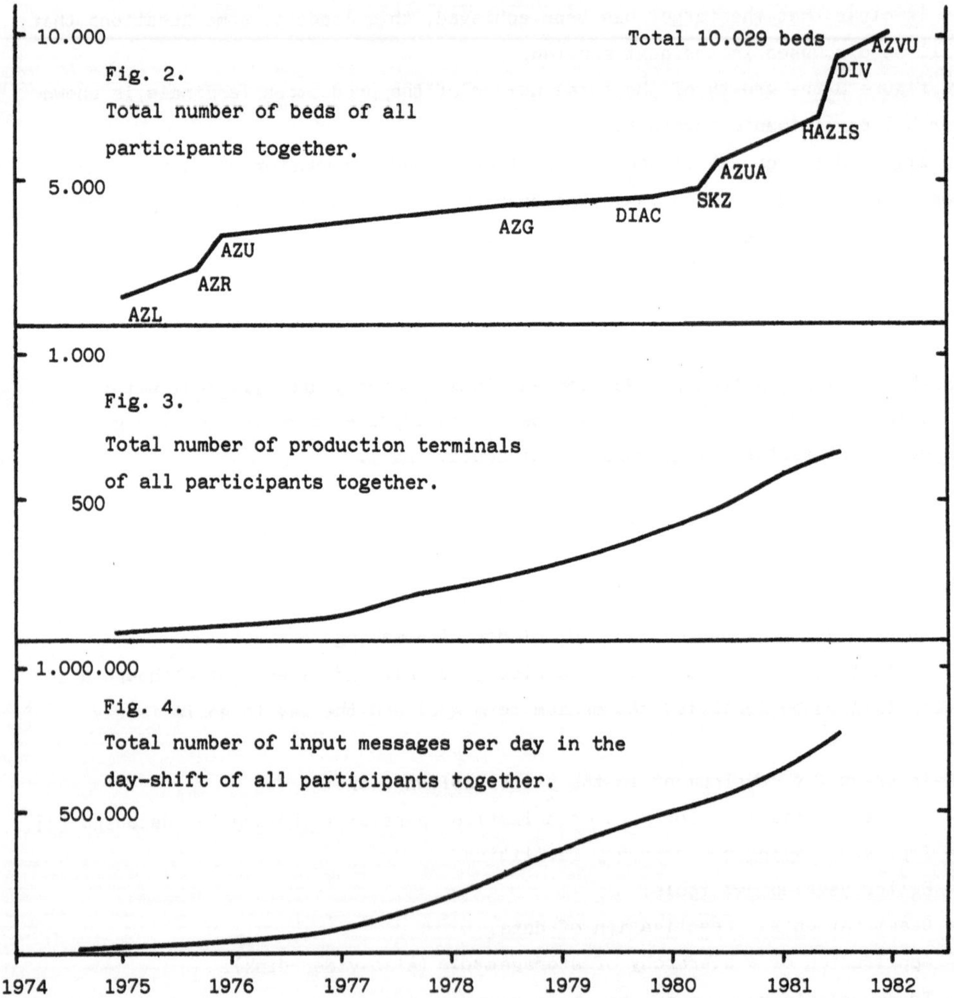

10.000   Total 10.029 beds   AZVU
                                                               DIV
     Fig. 2.
     Total number of beds of all   HAZIS
     participants together.
                                                    AZUA
5.000   SKZ
                                        DIAC
                              AZG
                AZU
           AZR
      AZL

1.000
     Fig. 3.
     Total number of production terminals
     of all participants together.
     500

1.000.000
     Fig. 4.
     Total number of input messages per day in the
     day-shift of all participants together.
     500.000

1974   1975   1976   1977   1978   1979   1980   1981   1982

19

As to the organizational structure it was stated in the BAZIS-activity plan 1981-1982 that the present structure was applicable only as long as the cooperation did not exceed 8 participants. At present this number has been reached and the question has to be answered what next? There are several options:

a. restrict the HIS-cooperation to the present participants;

b. restrict the HIS-cooperation as it is to the present participants, offer the product to new candidates via BAZIS on a real or pseudo commercial base.

c. Restrict the cooperation to the present participants, bring the HIS on the market by means of a separate commercial enterprise.

d. Restructure the cooperation to facilitate more than 8 participants.

There is a clear need now to define a new policy, success leads to new questions. Whatever solution would be chosen a close contact with the user is considered to be essential for the development of a successful system.

References

1. Concluding report on the NOBIN-ZIS project 1972 - 1976 (available from BAZIS, University Hospital Leyden, the Netherlands).

2. Evaluation of the Leyden HIS. Report (in Dutch) to the ministry of education and science made by an independent consultant (Van de Bunt), Staatsuitgeverij 's-Gravenhage, 1979. (Translation available from BAZIS, University Hospital Leyden, the Netherlands).

3. Bakker, A.R., Implementation approach and evaluation of the use of Leyden University Hospital Information System. Proc. Medinfo 77 Shires, D.H.,Wolf, eds. (1977) p.943

4. Kouwenberg, J.M.L., Bongers, A., Bakker, A.R., Storage structure in a large database. In: Lecture Notes in Medical Informatics. Berlin Proceedings 1979. Ed. B.Barber, F. Grémy, K. Uberla and G. Wagner, 1979, pp. 590-594.

The Information System of the Göttingen Hospital

Carl-Theo Ehlers, Rüdiger Klar

Abteilung Medizinische Informatik
der Universität Göttingen
Neues Klinikum
Robert-Koch-Str. 40
D - 3400 Göttingen

Summary

Die Abteilung für Medizinische Informatik an der Universität Göttingen
entwickelt und betreibt ein Informationssystem nach einem integrierten
Konzept für Krankenversorgung, Administration und Wissenschaft. Dafür
kommt ein DB/DC-System (23.000 Transaktionen/Tag, DB mit 230.000 Pati-
enten) zum Einsatz. Eine Gesamtübersicht der Anwendungen und einige
medizinorientierte Beispiele wie medizinische Dokumentation, die Integration der OP-Dokumentation in das gesamte Informationssystem, die
Befundübertragung von Laborwerten und die Führung der Fieberkurven
werden behandelt.

1. Introduction

In 1972 the University of Göttingen created the Department of Medical
Informatics. The main task of this new institution was the responsible
collaboration in the planning and realization of a computer-controlled
hospital operation for the new University Hospital facilities which
were being built at that time. The remaining structures of the old
University Clinics also had to be considered, as well as the regular
teaching and research duties of an university teaching hospital.

A few figures might enable the reader to form an idea of the size of
the medical faculty of the Göttingen University and of the new University Hospital facilities: 1,500 beds of which 1,100 are located in the
new facilities: 300,000 out-patient visits and 340,000 in-patient days
p.a.; 230 million DM operational costs in 1980; 4,000 employees; 590
beginning medical and dental students each year; 500 medical assistant
trainees.

Figure 1 shows an overview of the Göttingen Hospital Information System
with its main frame computer (IBM/370-158MP) and its applications
which have been divided into four main categories. This concept is a

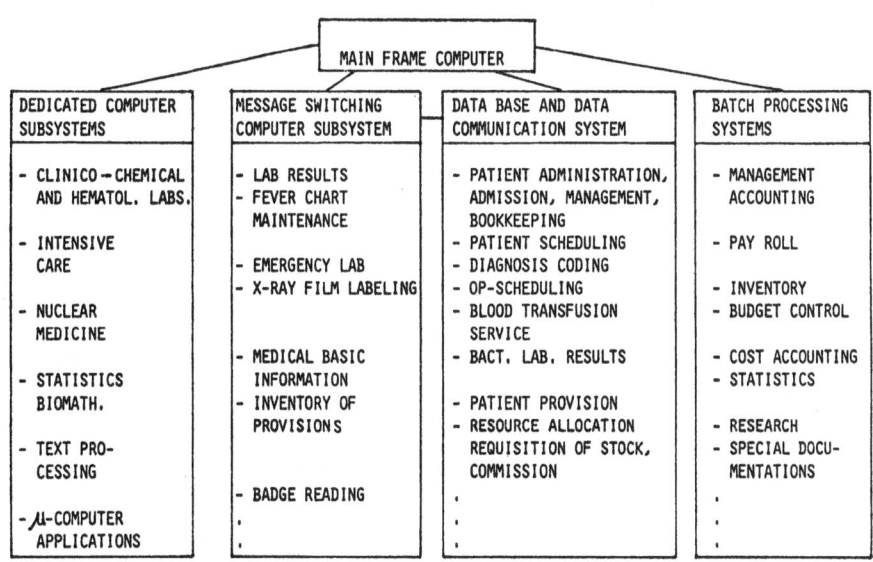

MAIN FRAME COMPUTER
DEDICATED COMPUTER SUBSYSTEMS
- CLINICO-CHEMICAL AND HEMATOL. LABS.
- INTENSIVE CARE
- NUCLEAR MEDICINE
- STATISTICS BIOMATH.
- TEXT PROCESSING
- μ-COMPUTER APPLICATIONS
MESSAGE SWITCHING COMPUTER SUBSYSTEM
- LAB RESULTS
- FEVER CHART MAINTENANCE
- EMERGENCY LAB
- X-RAY FILM LABELING
- MEDICAL BASIC INFORMATION
- INVENTORY OF PROVISIONS
- BADGE READING
DATA BASE AND DATA COMMUNICATION SYSTEM
- PATIENT ADMINISTRATION, ADMISSION, MANAGEMENT, BOOKKEEPING
- PATIENT SCHEDULING
- DIAGNOSIS CODING
- OP-SCHEDULING
- BLOOD TRANSFUSION SERVICE
- BACT. LAB. RESULTS
- PATIENT PROVISION
- RESOURCE ALLOCATION REQUISITION OF STOCK, COMMISSION
BATCH PROCESSING SYSTEMS
- MANAGEMENT ACCOUNTING
- PAY ROLL
- INVENTORY
- BUDGET CONTROL
- COST ACCOUNTING
- STATISTICS
- RESEARCH
- SPECIAL DOCUMENTATIONS

FIG. 1: The Göttingen Hospital Information System

Central patient admission
Entrance
Central archives
Care management
Computer center
Kitchen
Appointment DB
Historical patient DB
Current patient DB
Bed DB
Scheduling
Out-clinic head office
Assurance of payment
Administration
Ward food orders
Station office

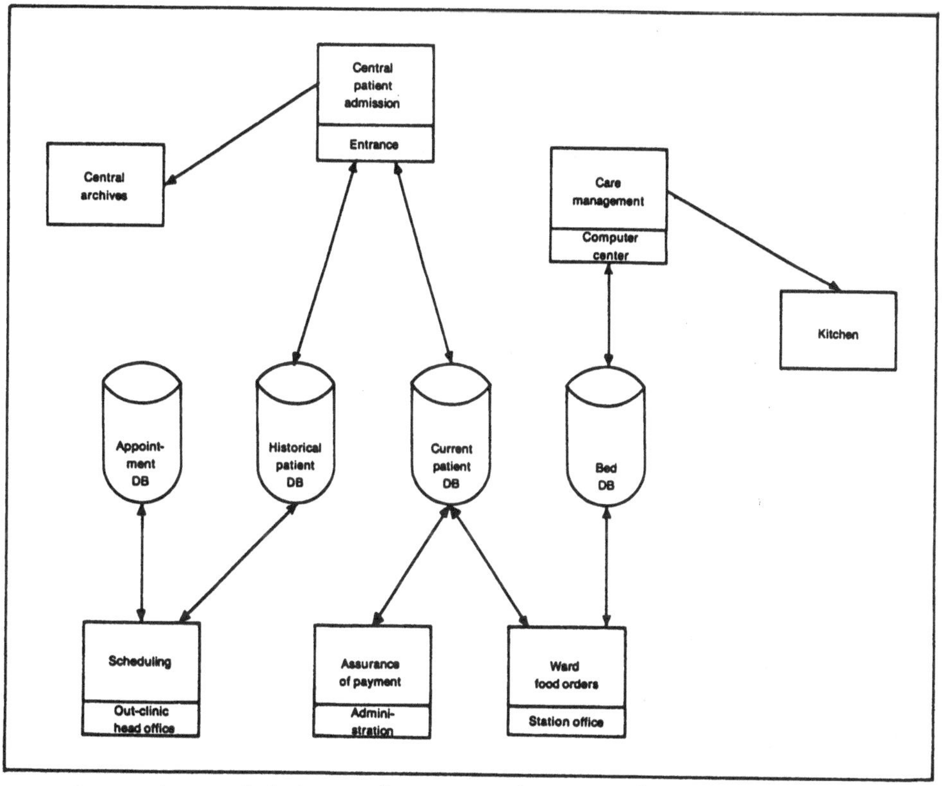

FIG. 2: Patient administration: Data bases and application areas

typical centralized Hospital Information System as described by Collen
(1) or Lindberg (2) but with an emphasis on a high integration of the
subsystems. Ehlers et al. (3) give a general description of our system.

2. The data base and data communication concept

From the very beginning, the data base and data communication system
IMS has been in use with all its important functions such as on-line
update, automatic restart, and data base recovery. This was the first
time that IMS was used in its entirety in a hospital context. In this
way the first step to an overall EDP system was rapidly in operation
from the point of view of the user. Decentralized data entry at data
source locations combined with centralized data storage enables the
user to retrieve reliable and valid data quickly. At the moment, more
than 90 terminals (dialog-oriented displays and printers), 70 telephone
terminal sets and several other on-line devices are handled by IMS. A
special data line network for local and remote terminals was developed
which is independent of the telephone lines for better privacy and
data security. In addition, process control computer projects e.g. in
the chemicoclinical laboratories, nuclear medicine and intensive care
units were realized. These computers, several microprocessors and a
special front-end-processor (IBM 3750) for controlling the telephone
terminal sets are connected on-line under IMS/VS to the main frame
computer.

Nearly all administrative and many medical fields are supported by EDP
in the new hospital facilities and the remaining structures of the old
clinics. An indicator of the high degree of EDP application is, for
example, the rising rate of on-line transactions per day - 23,000
(May 1981). The two most important hierarchically structured patient data
bases are the historical and the current data base. At the moment, data
of 250,000 patients are directly accessible from the historical data
base. Figure 2 gives a comprehensive survey of the most important data
bases and applications (including the point of acquisition and use of
the data) in the field of patient administration. Klar (4) presented
further descriptions of the data bases and a comparison with other
medical DB's.

3. Medical documentation

The medical documentation is supported by a special on-line method for
entering, encoding and displaying basic medical data such as diagnoses,
risk factors and operations (5), (6). The need is obvious: to relate all
these medically significant items about the same patient, gathered at

23

different times and locations. Our system combines the advantages of free text and coding methods and is an integrated part of the routine work of the wards. The main part of this system consists of the semi-automatic coding of diagnoses using the German KDS-classification, which we have extended and which is compatible with the ICD. The physician describes the current case by entering data in free text from the patient's problems into a computer printout of a condensed medical history of the patient. A ward clerk receives this completed printout and is able to enter the new items at a display terminal. The encoding program presents a list of selected KDS-items on the screen. The clerk finds the correct KDS-formulation of the entered diagnosis or operation text, with a high probability on one of the first lines of the screen, and selects it using a light pen. The basic medical data are stored in the patient data base and are used for such clinical routine tasks as discharge summaries, for administration and research.

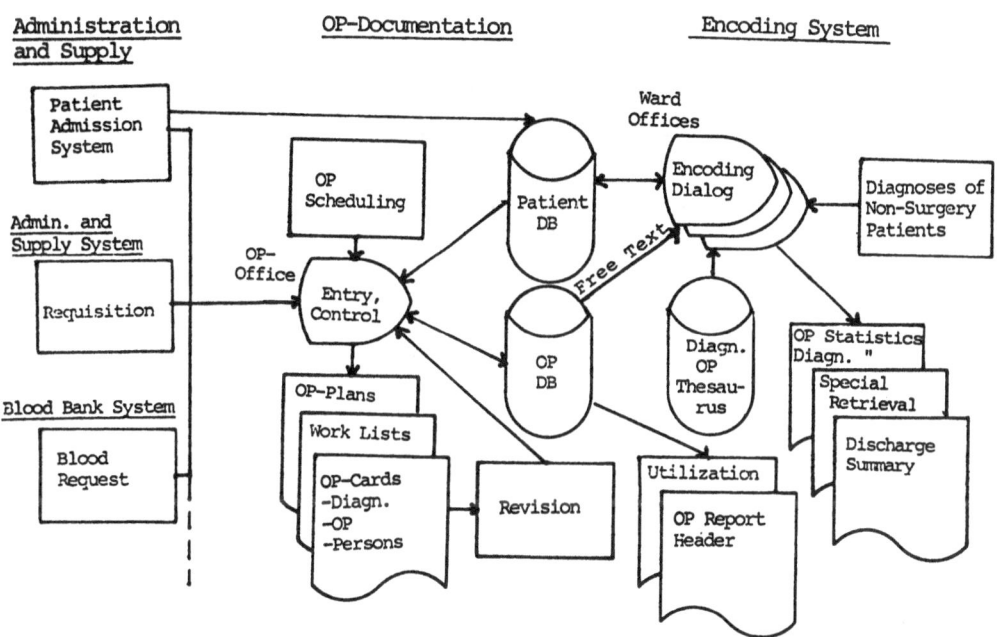

Fig. 3: The integration of the EDP-supported OP-documentation into the Göttingen University Hospital Information System (with details of the connection to the encoding subsystem).

4. OP-documentation

The EDP-supported OP-documentation is another example of the integration
of different computer applications for medical documentation (Figure 3).
All relevant data for the planning of operations are entered on-line
into the OP data base and every day several lists, sorted according to
the operating theater, surgical discipline, etc. are printed in order
to inform the surgeons, anaesthetists, blood bank, medical staff, etc.,
of the planned operations. After the operation the surgeon or the OP-
nurse receives a small print out (OP-card) with all pre-OP data. He or
she may then revise these data; the corrections and completions are
entered at the display terminal of the OP-office. The same day the
surgeon receives a printout with all OP items which is used as the
leading part of the OP-report. This service is very well accepted by
the users for it facilitates the OP-scheduling, dictation of the reports
and secretarial work. The diagnosis and operation text is automatically
transferred to the encoding system described above. In this way it is
not necessary for the physician to write the diagnosis several times
in different forms. Using these data bases, it is easy to generate
high quality evaluations. In comparision with other OP-scheduling and
documentation methods (e.g. (7), (8), (9)), our system is not isolated
from the clinical routine and from other EDP-activities, gives more
on-line support and yields more differentiated and better statistics.

5. Laboratory results and patient's chart maintenance

Another support of the medical documentation is given by the small
telephone terminal sets (telephone, monitor, mini-printer) which are
installed on each ward. For example, using a telephone terminal, the
nurse enters the medication data. Several worksheets, statistics,
printouts for the fever chart, etc. are then available. Compared to the
computerized unit dose methods, our system can provide the same medical
advantages (such as drug interaction, drug surveilance) without actually
being a single dose distribution system with all its problems in
packaging in the pharmacy.

Another printout for the patient's chart is produced for the clinico-
chemical and hematological results by the telephone terminal set. The
laboratory computer is connected to the central computer, so that the
current lab results are transmitted to the central data bases and
different reports, e.g. cumulated over 7 days, are transmitted via front-
end-processor to the ward (11), (12). This is one of our best accepted
EDP solutions; it enables reliable information to be transmitted rapidly

to the wards without incurring the disadvantages of verbal data transmission by telephone.

The bacteriological findings are stored in a separate data base and are transferred to the ward in the same above mentioned way. Evalutions of the bacteriological data base provide important insight into epidemiology, hospital hygiene, and in connection with other data bases insights into the analysis of use and efficacy of medication, as well as initial chemotherapy (13).

6. Summary

We have tried to describe some aspects of the Göttingen Hospital Information System and we have emphasized the medical record related parts. We cannot explain here the other computer applications shown in Figure 1 and we can only affirm that the continuing approach of integrating the various computer projects, the work flow and organization of the hospital is essential for the success of our hospital information system.

REFERENCES

(1) Collen MF (ed.). Hospital Computer Systems. New York London Sydney Toronto 1974.
(2) Lindberg DAB. The Growth of Medical Information Systems in the United States. Lexington Toronto 1979.
(3) Ehlers CTh et al. (eds.). Data Processing in the Hospital of the Georg-August-University Göttingen. Göttingen 1980.
(4) Klar R. Hierarchisch strukturierte Datenbanken in der Medizin. In: Reichertz PL, Schwarz S (eds.). Informationssysteme in der Medizinischen Versorgung. Proceedings Gmds Jahrestagung 1976, Stuttgart 1978; 326-339.
(5) Klar R, Haase J, Ehlers CTh. On-line Support for Basic Medical Information in a large University Hospital. In: Anderson (ed.). Medical Informatics Europe 1978, Berlin 1978; 671-677.
(6) Klar R, Prange H, Ehlers CTh. Erste Erfahrungen mit der EDV-gestützten Dokumentation klinischer Daten in einer Neurologischen Klinik. In.: Reisner H, Schnaberth G (eds.). Fortschritte der technischen Medizin in der neurologischen Diagnostik und Therapie. Proceedings Tagung der DGfN/GÖNP 1979, Wien 1980; 411-416.
(7) Bendix R, Bhargava V, Griffith w et al. Computer Scheduling for the OR. Modern Health Care, 1976; 1611-160.
(8) Greenberg AG. Computers in Emergency Systems, Surgery and Intensive Care Units: An Overview. In: Lindberg DAB, Kaihara S (eds.). Medinfo 80, Amsterdam New York Oxford 1980, Proceedings; 1184-1189
(9) Lange HJ, Thurmayr R (eds.). Klinische Datenverarbeitung in der Fakultät für Medizin der TU München, München 1979.
(10) Kühn H. The Use of the Computer to analyse Drug Prescription Habits. IFIP-TC4 Conference on Computer Aided Drug Therapy, 6-10.3.78, Bern 1978.
(11) Kühn H, Pietrzyk P. On-line Befundpräsentation von eilbedürftigen Laborwerten. Proceedings, Medizinische Informatik 1981, Wien 27-28.11.81 (in print).

(12) Maulbetsch RA. Das Diagnostik-Informationssystem (DIS) der
     Medizinischen Universität Tübingen. In: Wagner G (ed.). Laboratory
     Information Systems. Stuttgart 1978; 17-25.
(13) Klar R, Ehlers CTh, Wegener U, Ansorg R: EDV-Einsatz für die
     bakteriologische Verlaufs- und Befunddokumentation. In: Horbach L,
     Duhse P (eds.). Nachsorge und Krankheitsverlaufsanalyse. Proceedings
     Gmds Jahrestagung 1980, Stuttgart 1981.

The Extension of the MSH Basic Medical Documentation System to Allow for Interactive Data Acquisition

Hoffmann,W.D., Pocklington,P.R., Lehtomies,T.

Institute for Medical Informatics
(Director: Prof. Dr.med. P.L.Reichertz)
Medical School Hannover
D-3000 Hannover, W.Germany

1. SUMMARY

Within the Hannover Medical School (MSH)   a central facility (1) for the documentation of summarizing medical record data was developed in 1970, functioning under the responsibility of the department for medical informatics.

In 1975 the initial processing system for these data was re-designed (2) to solve problems that had resulted from the limited acceptance from the clinical side that the documentation procedures had encountered. The main characteristics of this re-designed system were: the use of OCR techniques for data acquisition (to improve turnaround for the incorporation of data into the system) and the implementation of error-checking routines and data correction and verification cycles (to improve confidence in the overall reliability of the stored data). At the same time an interactive dialogue for data acquisition was developed, which, however did not gain acceptance in routine use.

This paper reflects the developments and strategies subsequently used which eventually achieved acceptance of interactive data acquisition.

2. SYSTEM LOGISTICS

The purpose of the system is the documentation of medical data (risk factors, diagnoses, surgery, therapies, complications, and modifiers). While the physician dictates the discharge summary he documents the medical items considered of importance to be typed on a specially designed face sheet of the medical record.   The complete medical record is later passed to the central documentation facility where documented items are transformed to numerical codes.

The data can be input to the processing cycle by means of either OCR-forms or by means of a dialogue at a display terminal.   The data collected during a day are processed the following morning, undergoing plausibility checking and producing hardcopies of the data recorded. The hardcopy is then checked by a physician for medical-logical errors and he can then either validate the data or return the protocol to the documentation unit with appropriate information causing the necessary corrections of the data to be carried out. The plausibility check routine also prints easily understandable messages to describe the located errors and prepares error-correction cards so that the documenting personnel has merely to punch the corrections. After another inspection and subsequent validation the data then are inserted into the permanent MSH-patient data base.

Over the last five years (1976-1980) 91613 medical records have been documented using this system. Documented was a total of 485115 diagnosis, therapy- complication- or modifier-codes. The number of records processed yearly has increased from 14000 in 1976 to nearly 24000 in 1980.

3. CONVERSION STRATEGY

The general re-design of the basic medical documentation system in 1975 also introduced the option of interactive data acquisition. At this time however, this did not meet the requirements for routine usage mainly due to hardware reasons leading to frequent breakdowns of the CPU and unacceptable response-times during the interactive dialogue.

The carrier-system DIES (3) under which the basic documentation system is implemented has been extended to incorporate a number of error-recovery features, which reduces the effect of system breakdowns (which are also considerably less frequent with a new CPU).

It was therefore decided to re-introduce the possibility for interactive data acquisition, taking into consideration both the negative experiences from the previous aborted attempt, and the experiences with the use of OCR acquisition. In June 1980 a new interactive dialogue was developed, making use of the improved display facilities, with the major emphasis being on the provision of low response-times (i.e. minimal error checking upon initial acquisition).

4. ERROR ANALYSIS

In addition to these conversion activities an error analysis was carried out (4) to see if the conversion from OCR to interactive data acquisition has advantages for the documentation process and the data quality.

This analysis was devided into three phases covering 3 weeks each. In the first phase (time1) the documenting staff knew about the analysis, in the second phases (time2) the staff was not informed and from the results of these parts some improvements were implemented into the online dialogue which were tested in a third phase (time3).

For the purpose of this analysis, two basic categories of error were determined, the 'formal-logical' errors (i.e. those that could be detected automatically by the error-checking algorithm - corresponding to WAGNER's definition (5) of formal errors as those 'which can be ascertained without any knowledge of the true facts or are incompatible with other data'), and 'medical-logical' errors (i.e. those located during the inspection by the physician in the verification cycle of the records processed with regard to their medico-semantic consistency).

The formal errors were defined as follows:

- the number of items documented did not correspond to the number specified,
- incorrect identification of physician-in-charge,
- incorrect admission or discharge code,
- incorrect patient identification,
- incorrect date of surgery,
- incorrect date of admission,
- incorrect specifier for diagnosis, therapy, complication or modifier codes, or the use of a non-existent MSH-KDS code,
- incorrect clinical department/ward identification,
- invalid code of documentalist, and
- incorrect date of documentation.

The medical-logical errors were classified into the following categories:

- the code chosen for diagnosis, therapy, complication or modifier did not sufficiently correspond to the particular finding,
- the logical connections between items were incorrectly specified,
- documentation of redundant information,
- missing data,
- the documented text did not correspond semantically with that specified by the physician, and
- the risk-factor codes were not given.

5. EXTENSION OF INTERACTIVE DATA ACQUISITION TO INCORPORATE ERROR CHECKING

Based on the results of the error analysis it seemed appropriate to incorporate error check procedures directly into the interactive acquisition routine. It is obvious that only formal errors can thus be detected. So it was decided to build in checks for the most severe and frequent errors as seen from the results of the error analysis.

In Figure 1 the frequency of formal errors is shown, with some of the main errors being: number of items, physician-in-charge, patient identification, and the MSH-KDS-code which together account for more than 50% of all formal errors detected.

A new release of the acquisition system was developed incorporating checking for the above errors and inserting the date of documentation and documentalist code into the stored record (covering a further 16 to 20% of errors) by automatic error-free insertion of the data. The addition of these verification procedures did not lead to any noticable deterioration of the response times. Consequently this has now been accepted for routine use, with also the possibility for selective echo-verification of codes entered, intended to reduce also the number of medical-logical errors.

6. DISCUSSION

The average amount of errors in the investigated documentation system seem to be amazingly constant, the error rate was 10% at three different time points (Table 1), and there were no significant differences between OCR or interactive input techniques.

Regarding the formal errors (Figure 1) the results of the first two phases lead to some improvements in the input dialogue. This way the error type 'date of documentation' and 'documenter code' did not appear in the third evaluation, other errors could be reduced 'number of items'. But surprisingly some types of error were more frequent e.g. 'date of surgery' which could be explained by greater amounts of records from the surgical disciplines at the evaluation time and the 'specifier of the MSH-KDS-code' which in future can be avoided by more plausibility checks during the input process.

Within the medical-logical errors (Figure 2) only slightly alterations can be stated which is not very suprising because the improvements in the dialogue could not influence this type of errors.

Another way to reduce the error rate could be the automatic or semi-automatic coding of diagnoses like it is used for example in Goettingen (6). At present some disciplines are under investigation in the MSH to implement such an attempt.

Apart from the error analysis some other aspects have been pointed out by the documenting personnel as improvements, among which are:

- easier and faster handling of the keyboards
- lower noise-levels
- no OCR-reading-errors to be corrected
- automatic field and frame selection
- no preparation and extra-archiving of OCR-forms

Since interactive input is only possible where a terminal is installed it is intended to continue to offer both possibilities. In the central documentation facility and those peripheral departments where a terminal is installed the interactive dialogue is clearly prefered, while for data acquisition OCR-techniques will remain of value for back-up purposes and in cases of external documentation without terminal-connection with the MSH.

Documented protocols	Time 1				Time 2				Time 3	
	OCR		online		OCR		online		online	
	Abs.	%	Abs.	%	Abs.	%	Abs.	%	Abs.	%
correctly documented	501	91.8	912	89.4	482	89.6	732	88.9	1397	89.3
incorrectly documented	45	8.2	108	10.6	56	10.4	123	11.1	167	10.7
	546	100.0	1020	100.0	538	100.0	855	100.0	1564	100.0

Table 1: Frequency distribution of correctly and incorrectly documented protocols in influence on the input medium.

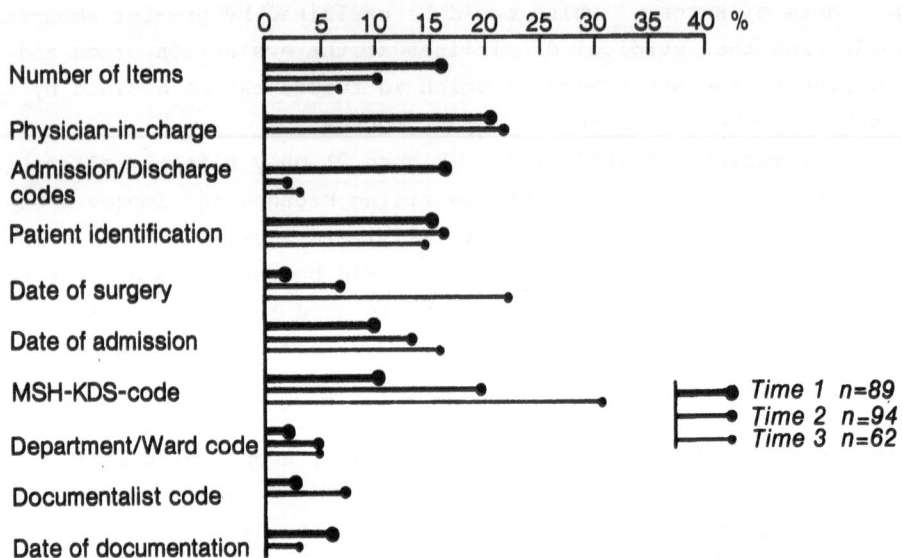

Figure 1: Relative Frequency distribution of Formal Errors analysed at three different time points. (Time 1, Time 2, Time 3)

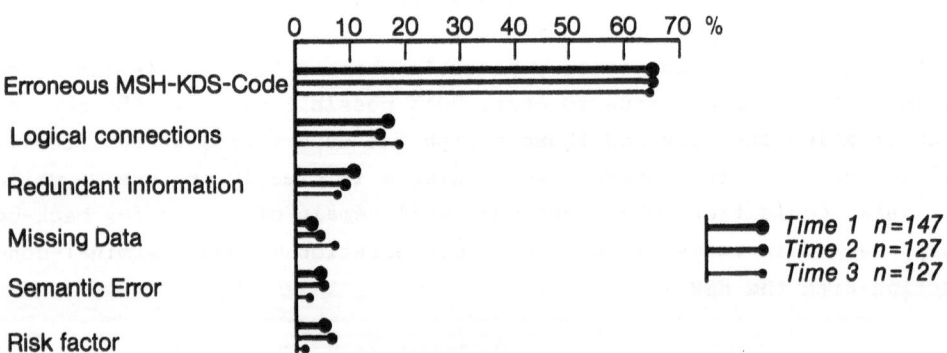

Figure 2: Relative Frequencies of medical logical Errors at three different time points. (Time 1, Time 2, Time 3)

7. REFERENCES

(1) Holthoff G.:   Aufbau einer multidiziplinaeren, zentralisierten Medizinischen Basisdokumentation.   Dissertation,   Tieraertzliche Hochschule Hannover, 1976

(2) Holthoff G. Pocklington PR.:   An analysis of 3 years experience with the re-designed system for basic medical documentation within the MSH In: Anderson,J.   Medical Informatics Europe 78, Berlin, Springer Verlag 1978; 19-28

(3) Pocklington PR.:   The Necessity for Requirements and Basic Design of a General Data Interpretation and Evaluation System In: Anderson J, Forsythe JF. (eds.): Medinfo '74, Amsterdam, North Holland Publishing Co. 1975; 411 - 418

(4) Lehtomies T. Hoffmann WD. Pocklington PR.: Error Analysis within the Central Basic Documentation System of the Hannover Medical School, Paper to be presented at the 5th European Conference on Health Records Brighton, April 1982

(5) Wagner G.:   Quality Control and Error Checking In: Anderson J, Forsythe JM.:   Information Processing of Medical Records Amsterdam, North-Holland Publishing Co. 1970; 222-236

(6) Ehlers CT. et al.: Data Processing in the Hospital of the Georg-August-University, Goettingen 1980

A COMPUTER ASSISTED RADIOLOGY REPORTING AND RETRIEVAL SYSTEM

P. Allegaert [*], E. Kint [**], J.L. Willems [*], E. Ponette [**] and A. Baert [**]

[*]   Department of Medical Informatics and

[**]   Department of Radiology, Univ. Hospital St. Rafaël, 3000 Leuven, Belgium

SUMMARY

In the first half of 1979 a market study was made of various existing radiology reporting systems. Since no existing system was acceptable or available in Dutch, the
decision was taken to develop our own system and to tackle the problem in a progressive
way. Use is made of a dedicated HP minicomputer which is linked with other HP computers in a star-network. The reporting subsystem is developed with the following main
features : report entry is done by the radiologist on standard CRT terminals in a conversational manner with predefined and user-determined branching. Entry is done through
a menu-selection method. By means of subsequent menu's the radiologist is guided in a
systematic way to select preassembled, standard statements for normal and also for
abnormal findings. The menu selected computer report codes are stored in an IMAGE
data base and are accessible via a query language.

1. INTRODUCTION

The radiology department of the University Hospitals of Leuven with 1683 beds is managing at present 28 X-ray rooms, remotely dispersed over 7 units. Half of these are
centrally located. A total of 263.000 diagnostic procedures have been performed in
1978. The personnel of the diagnostic radiology department consists of 115 people,
of which 34 are medical doctors, full-time staff and residents included.

Until recently all functions except for billing were performed with conventional manual techniques. In view of the increasing complexity of managing the radiology services and the success of other applications in the hospital information system (laboratory, pharmacy, dietetics, outpatient services ...) it was decided to provide computer support to several X-ray departmental operations.

Early in 1979 we made an evaluation of various commercially available computer systems
designed for use in radiology, such as MARS (1), MEDELA (2), DRIS (3), RAPORT (4),
SIREP (5), ... Several of these systems appeared to have had a rather short life time,
or did not attract sufficient users outside the developmental or promotional hospitals,
especially not in Europe. None of the existing systems did respond to the particular
needs of our hospital. We therefore decided to design and develop our own computerized
radiology subsystem. (6)

Over the last eight years a computer network has been elaborated by the medical informatics division at Leuven University, which has a team of 24 analists and programmers.
The main administrative hospital information applications using a central patient

data base are implemented on a dual IBM 4341 system. For specialized medical applications, such as on-line laboratory automation, computer ECG analysis, nuclear medicine, patient monitoring, dedicated Hewlett Packard minicomputer systems are used. These systems are linked together in a star-network. They are also coupled to the IBM-systems by means of a RJE-link. The administrative and management applications of the radiology system at Leuven University have been implemented on the central IBM computer system. An HP 1000 minicomputer is used for the reporting functions.

2. HARDWARE AND SYSTEM SOFTWARE

The present hardware of the dedicated radiology reporting system consists of
- a minicomputer, model HP 21 MX-E with 256 K bytes core memory (350 nanoseconds basic cycle time) ;
- 2 hard disks with a capacity of 120 megabytes each ;
- 11 CRT's model HP 2621 A, to be expanded in the near future ;
- 1 console model HP 2645 with cassette reader ;
- 5 daisy-wheel printers ;
- a hardware link to the center node of the HP minicomputer network.

The present hardware allows the attachment of 50 CRT or printer p eripherals. The 265 K bytes of core memory is segmented into 8 partitions for running all system and user programs. Use is made of the HP RTE IV B operating system, IMAGE and DS 1000 software. All user programs are written in FORTRAN IV.

3. REPORTING SUBSYSTEM

3.1. General description and main features

The reporting subsystem is developed with the following main features : report entry is done by the radiologist on standard CRT terminals in a conversational manner with predefined and user-determined branching. Entry is done through a menuselection method. The report consists out of 3 parts : the heading with the patient identification, next the descriptive findings and finally a diagnostic conclusion.

By logging on the radiologist is presented first with a screen on which a total of 10 different organ systems or groups of X-ray procedures are listed (see fig. 1). In the next two frames specific procedures are listed from which he selects the examination of current interest (see fig. 1). At present a total of 181 different X-ray procedures can be reported through the system. By means of subsequent menu's (see fig. 2a and 2b) the radiologist is guided in a systematic way to select preassembled, standard statements for normal and also for significant abnormal findings as far as possible. On a high level of the tree staff members and experienced residents can key in whole strings in order to speed up the process. Entry of free text is possible at each level but kept to a minimum. This is especially reserved for the concluding remarks section.

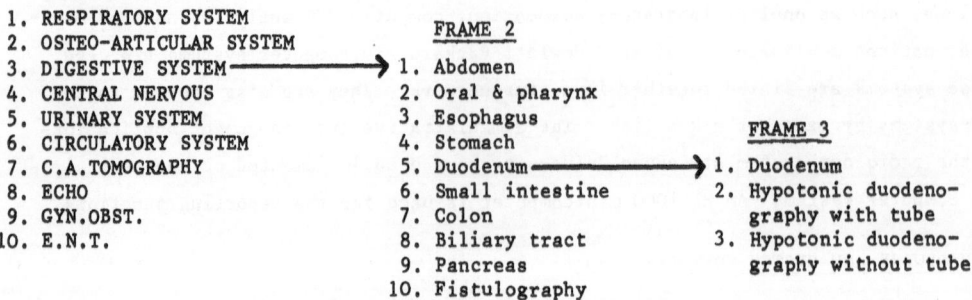

```
     MAIN FRAME

1.  RESPIRATORY SYSTEM
2.  OSTEO-ARTICULAR SYSTEM
3.  DIGESTIVE SYSTEM ─────────────▶  FRAME 2
4.  CENTRAL NERVOUS                  1. Abdomen
5.  URINARY SYSTEM                   2. Oral & pharynx
6.  CIRCULATORY SYSTEM               3. Esophagus
7.  C.A.TOMOGRAPHY                   4. Stomach                    FRAME 3
8.  ECHO                             5. Duodenum ───────────────▶  1. Duodenum
9.  GYN.OBST.                        6. Small intestine            2. Hypotonic duodeno-
10. E.N.T.                           7. Colon                         graphy with tube
                                     8. Biliary tract              3. Hypotonic duodeno-
                                     9. Pancreas                      graphy without tube
                                    10. Fistulography
```

Figure 1 : Main frame and selected frames 2 and 3


```
     FRAME 4                              FRAME 5

1.  Bulbar expansion ───────────────▶  1. Normal bulbar expansion
2.  Deformity                          2. () decreased expansion at
3.  Mucosal changes                    3. A stenosis is seen with () filling at
4.  Filling defects                    4. A narrowing is () located at
5.  Stenosis                           5. () dilatation of
6.  Filling grade
7.  Emptying
```

Figure 2a and 2b : Selected frames used for reporting of X-ray of the duodenum

3.2. Encoding of normal findings

The most important task in the reporting subsystem is the encoding of the descriptive
statements. The various sentences in the data base are being accessed through codes,
which will function as IMAGE key search items. The codes are formed by making a string
of the different item numbers selected by the radiologist on his way through the various frames of the menu. The string is composed out of 2 bytes of the main frame and
one byte generated by each of the next successive frames, modifiers or localisation
descriptions. Since the code so obtained is a key item for the data base, immediate access is achieved to the predefined statements or parts of the stored sentences.

The first four bytes of the code uniquely define a specific X-ray examination, out of
the present total of 181 procedures. When all findings are normal, a zero is stored
in position 5 of the code and no further information is needed to retrieve the canned-
normal-report for this examination.

3.3. Encoding of pathological findings

The structure of the statement codes for a patient with pathologic or aberrant findings
is more complex. Encoding will be done for each descriptive statement and various
descriptive findings (fig. 2a and 2b). Provisions have been made for the insertion

of quantitative terms, describing for example the size in diameter (in cm) of certain lesions or the percentage of a stenosis. By means of qualitative modifiers other features can be described e.g. the extent of tumor infiltration, etc. The detailed localization of an abnormality can also be added in various statements.

In order to construct a "pathologic" statement code, use is made of files containing various modifiers (e.g. slight, moderate or severe ; increased or decreased ; upper, median or lower) and segments in the syntax data base containing localization and size descriptors.

The statement codes, referring to pathologic findings, have a variable record length. They may contain up to 20 bytes of information (fig. 3). Bytes 1 to 4 of the statement codes always refer to the specific X-ray procedure. This is formed through the selections made out of the main frame and out of frames 2 and 3 (see example in fig. 1). Item numbers selected in frame 4 (fig. 2a) are stored in bytes 5 and 6. These six bytes are sufficient to identify so-called standard abnormal statements or so-called "variant" normal findings.

1	4	5	6	7	8	9	14	15	20

Byte

```
 1 -  4 : specific X-ray procedure
 5 -  6 : descriptive statement
 7 -  8 : qualitative modifiers
 9 - 14 : quantitative terms
15 - 20 : localisation descriptors
```

Figure 3 : Structure of the code used for accessing pre-assembled statements

In case qualitative modifiers need to be added, they will be stored in bytes 7 and 8 (fig. 3). Quantitative terms if any, are stored in bytes 9 to 14 of the statement codes. Pointers to localization descriptors (up to a maximum of 3) will be stored in bytes 15 to 20 (see fig. 3). Parentheses indicate when modifiers can be added to certain statements (see fig. 2b). They are automatically displayed on the screen for selection by the radiologist. Modifiers are very useful in order to differentiate and qualify certain descriptive findings. The use of modifiers, quantitative terms and localisation descriptors also saves disk space, since repeating the same sentence with only subtle differences in terminology would have required much more disk capacity.

Each statement code, defined in this way, refers to one specific sentence. The descriptive section of the report of a patient with pathologic or aberrant findings, will be composed out of several of these statement codes. These codes are also stored in the X-ray report data base for subsequent retrieval.

3.4. Concluding remarks and final X-ray diagnosis

Until now, concise concluding remarks and final X-ray diagnoses are entered as free formatted text. In general this is not more than 3 lines of up to 72 characters.

4. RETRIEVAL SUBSYSTEM

The menu selected computer report codes are stored in a daily temporary and a permanent data base. It is possible to review material by any key word such as identification number and name of the patient, the radiologist number and even pathological terms of the concluding remarks. Provisions are being made for the retrieval of coded reports for research and teaching purposes as well.

5. CONCLUSION

With the development of a computer assisted radiology reporting system we aimed at the following objectives :
1. to enhance the readability of the X-ray reports ;
2. to reduce secretarial and related costs ;
3. possibly to decrease and not to increase the workload of the radiologist ;
4. to promote a systematic approach in radiology reading and reporting (educational objective) ;
5. possibly to shorten turnaround time between the radiological examination and the delivery of the report.

Although the system is by far not completed, we feel that we are achieving these objectives. The system is in daily use since December 1980, for the reporting of normal X-ray results of the digestive, urinary and the central nervous system and for several computer axial tomography procedures. The reporting of pathological findings of other organ systems is gradually implemented. Canned-normal-reports can be produced for 181 different X-ray procedures accessible via the main frame and frames 2 and 3.

The system proves to be user-friendly. The operating instructions are easy to comprehend and the required training for new radiology residents is very limited. The radiologists in general are satisfied with the system. One of the keys to the present success is the involvement of the radiology staff in the development of the system. However, in the coming months the real test still has to come, when reporting of abnormal findings will be requested also from less motivated radiologists.

In the literature on automated reporting one inviolate rule is often quoted : "Never slow down the radiologist". Radiologists will not tolerate a system which impedes their speed of interpretation and reporting. This apparently is not the case with our system and may be another reason for its acceptance. A major reason, however, lies in the fact that the radiology department in our hospital has a limited secretarial staff. Up to 70 % of the radiology reporting in certain units, had to be done manually in handwriting by the radiology residents. In the past this has led to several problems of readability, which the computer assisted system now has cured. Keying in findings through the item-menu selection method does not require more time from the radiologist than in the old manual system. These are probably the major reasons for the present success of the computer assisted radiology system which we continue to implement at the University of Leuven.

ACKNOWLEDGMENT

Development of the system has been supported by grants from the Belgian Ministry of Science, through Project 26/63 of the "Impulsprogramma voor Informatica".

BIBLIOGRAPHY

(1) Lehr J.L., Lodwick G.S., Nicholson B.F. and Birznicks F.B. : Experience with MARS (Missouri Automated Radiology System). Radiology 106 : 289-294, 1973.

(2) Brolin I. : Erfahrungen mit dem MEDELA-System. Radiologe 14 : 297-305, 1974.

(3) Barnhard H.J., Jacobson H.G. and Nance J.W. : Diagnostic Radiologic Information System (DRIS). Radiologe 14 : 314-319, 1974.

(4) Irwin G.A.L. and Tillitt Jr.R. : A computer assisted radiological reporting system. Radiology 118 : 329-331, Feb, 1976.

(5) Wheeler P.S. and Gitlin J.N., Computers in Radiology : A viewpoint of pitfalls and payoffs in Proc.Sixth.Conf. on Computer Applications in Radiology. June 18-21, 1979, IEEE pp 1-4.

(6) Allegaert P., Kint E., Willems J.L., Baert A. : Automatisatie van de verslaggeving en archivering in de radiologie in Proc. MIC '80. March 26, 1980, pp 171-175

(7) Willems J.L., Govaerts H., Huygens W., Allegaert P., Kint E., Daneels F., Baert A. : A radiology subsystem in a hospital information computer system in Proc.Second Symposium Computers in Diagnostic Radiology. Amsterdam June 4-6, 1980, pp 357-361.

A COMPUTER-ASSISTED PATIENT RECORD SYSTEM

J.C. Petrie, O.J. Robb, D.J. Taylor, T.A. Jeffers.
Department of Therapeutics and Clinical Pharmacology,
University of Aberdeen.
G. McLeod, K.F. Allen, G.M. Dawson, P. Murphy,
Computing Department, Grampian Health Board.
G. Innes, R.D. Weir,
Department of Community Medicine, University of Aberdeen.

1.   SUMMARY

A computer-assisted patient record system which holds information about patient and
drug factors on over 6000 patients is described.   The system has been developed
using a CODASYL type database management system and maintained on a medium configuration mini-computer.   The principal aim of the system is to improve and facilitate
the transfer between doctors of clinically important information about high-risk
patients.

2.   INTRODUCTION

Unintentional and preventable iatrogenous disease is common in clinical practice (1,2).
There are many pressures on medical staff and important patient and drug factors
are overlooked because of the difficulty, and time involved, in attempting to retrieve
information from hospital and general practice case record folders which often contain a bulky, chaotic and disordered array of notes and investigation results (3).
We believe that important patient and drug factors should be readily available to
clinical staff and easily assimilated by the users of the medical record.

We describe a computer-assisted patient record system (PRS) which at present holds
information on over 6000 patients.   The principal aim of PRS is to improve and facilitate the transfer between doctors, both in hospital and general practice, of clinically important information about high-risk patients.

3.   THE PATIENT RECORD SYSTEM

3.1 Clinical aspects

The record is stored and processed by a mini-computer.   The printed output from PRS
is part of and complementary to the main Grampian hospitals manual medical records
system (3).   The summarised clinically important information which is held on PRS
includes:
- patient identification data (name, date of birth, age, address, marital status,
  maiden name, mother's maiden name).
- practitioner identification data (name, address, practice code).
- consultant/clinic/ward identification/specialty date.

- problem/diagnoses listing (active, inactive, date of onset).
- drug listing (start date, related problem, name, dose, route, frequency, cessation date).
- drug information notes (including warnings).
- selected additional information (see section 3.1.1.1).
- dates of previous patient contacts with PRS.
- follow-up plans.

3.1.1   Entry of clinical information to PRS

3.1.1.1   Initial Input

Two main categories of patients have been defined for inclusion in PRS. The first includes all patients discharged from a general medical unit at Aberdeen Royal Infirmary and selected patients discharged from two other general medical wards. Information about these patients is entered using the Discharge Summary program. The second category of patients consists of a limited number of high-risk and high hospital user patients who are selected for inclusion in PRS by the consultants in charge of their care. Information about these patients is added to the PRS database using a Registration program.

The input of clinical information is by the secretarial staff of the consultant in charge of the patient. Both the discharge summary and registration programs follow a sequence of prompts on visual display units (VDU). The clinical information is obtained from the problem list and drug list in the patient's manual case record(4,5). Both lists are audited by a clinician before input to PRS. Additional defined clinical information specific to a specialty group, for example selected patients with asthma or renal disease, may be provided to the secretary on a proforma and added to PRS using the VDU, again following a sequence of prompts. The registration program includes the facility to allocate patients into sub-groups belonging to an individual clinician or selected specialty group.

Input of problem titles/diagnoses or drug names (approved or proprietary) is unrestricted although suggested guidelines for clinical users are provided. Entries which do not exactly match existing titles in PRS are held on a temporary problem or drug dictionary. Auditing of the temporary dictionaries is carried out by a member of the clinical team using the VDU and the Dictionary Edit program. Up to 150 problem titles can be audited per hour. The approved dictionary of problem titles contains 8000 entries. These are being matched with International Classification of Disease Coding (ICD9). The average number of problem titles relating to each patient is eight with a maximum to date of 29.

3.1.1.2   Output of information

The clinical information entered in PRS through the registration and discharge summary programs is available to the clinician using a Database Interrogation program.

This allows approved users to find patients by unit number or name, and can display or print out any information held for that patient. The program also can find all patients with a given problem title, or treated with a particular drug (current or past), or in a specific at-risk group, or belonging to an individual practitioner or practice. Patients with a given combination of the above criteria can also be identified.

A computer-generated printout of information about patients in PRS (identification data, problem list, drug list and warnings, follow-up plans) is provided for planned patient-doctor contacts at outpatient clinics, in wards or in general practice. The format is a patient profile.

Drug information warnings linked to selected high-risk drugs are added automatically to patient profiles and to output for clinical users. The drug warnings contain information about drug-drug and drug-host interactions. The drug notes are restricted to two lines to prevent a flood of information diluting the impact of clinically important information (6).

Further output of information includes:
- listings of patients with appointments at clinics or in general practice.
- listing of patients with overdue follow-up appointments, together with standard follow-up letters addressed to the patients concerned.
- letters to practitioners including production of clinical information about patients, with individually addressed, headed letters (see also section 3.1.1.3).

All letters produced through PRS are printed in upper and lower case on trimmed NCR paper, with copies for practitioner and hospital notes.

3.1.1.3 Updating of information.

Secretarial staff update the information on the PRS database using either the registration or update programs. Additions, amendments, deletions are notified to the secretarial staff by the return of the encounter document - the patient profile (see section 3.1.1.2) - completed at the time of, or following the clinical interview and examination. The update program prompts the user of the VDU with questions which follow the order of presentation of the data in the patient profile. Dictated clinical comment can also be added, using the VDU. No duplication of correct information already in PRS is required, for example identification data, problem lists and drug lists. Secretarial time is saved because the output from PRS following the update program includes all current identification details and clinical information about the patient. Copies of all computer-generated clinically relevant output are filed within the Grampian medical records manual system.

3.1.2 Clinical users.

The benefits of the system accrue from the ability to gather information about patients from different sources and present this data to the clinician in a form which is pertinent and readily assimilated.

PRS extends beyond the acute general medical unit where it was developed to include two other medical units, their associated outpatient clinics, and a large hypertension clinic.   Clinical information about 6000 patients is held on the PRS database. PRS is also used by clinicians to facilitate the management of selected groups of high-risk out-patients in the Grampian Area, including patients with renal disease, asthma and mucoviscidosis.   Selected patients with good clinical histories and physical signs, who are willing to participate in undergraduate teaching are also included in PRS.

The principal input of patients to PRS has been through the discharge summary program. This was the natural evolution as the computer-assisted patient records project pro-gressed through the early development phase while programs were developed and while a limited number of staff in these units became involved with PRS.   The processing capacity and facilities of PRS were thus restricted to a limited number of users, and to patients who might not be reviewed regularly or at all at out-patient clinics. Analysis of the PRS database showed that half the patients had an in-patient episode only, without subsequent follow-up through PRS.

The favourable reception by clinical users to the facilities available from PRS has now led to a change of emphasis towards the registration of selected groups of high-risk high-hospital user patients.   Much clinical and paramedical activity, resource and follow-up, is directed at such patients.   The clear presentation of clinical data, together with the savings of secretarial time achieved with the facilities of updating and follow-up of PRS outlined in section 3.1, has proved very attractive to clinical users.

The hypertension clinic, for example, has over 1000 at-risk patients in PRS.   The benefits of achieving satisfactory control of elevated levels of blood pressure by monitoring progress of such patients through follow-up are clearly established. Those patients with a principal diagnosis of hypertension attending the hospital hypertension clinic have been classified into three principal categories as follows:
a)   borderline need for treatment of elevated levels of blood pressure.
b)   blood pressure controlled with conventional doses of standard therapy.
c)   blood pressure control difficult because of resistance to treatment or other
     special factors.
Patients in categories a) and b) have been discharged from regular follow-up at the hospital clinics to a shared-care computer-assisted follow-up in collaboration with the general practitioners.   Patients in category c) continue to attend the hospital hypertension clinics until the elevated levels of blood pressure are satisfactorily reduced.   The shared-care scheme for patients in the first two categories operates as follows:
1) A computer-generated letter is sent to patients at regular intervals (6 or 12

monthly) asking them to visit their practitioner within 1-4 weeks.

2) At the same time the encounter document – the <u>patient profile</u> specific to that
patient – is sent to the practitioner with a request to return it to the specialists
of the clinic for review, audit and comment.   Depending on the clinical progress of
the patient, and the occurrence of unintentional initiation of drug-drug or drug-
host interactions, a further appointment is planned and a letter containing appropriate clinical comment is produced for the practitioner using the facilities of PRS.

Two hundred local practitioners are now cooperating fully with this shared-care
scheme which will be described in detail elsewhere.

The exchange of information between hospital and general practice in the shared-care
scheme has been most instructive.   Numerous clinically important new patient and
drug factors have been identified and notified to practitioners.   The reduction in
hospital follow-up, together with the provision of a back-up check and follow-up
scheme for defaulters allows more attention to be paid to the particular management
problems of patients with resistant hypertension.

Clinicians from the asthma clinic, mucoviscidosis clinic and medical renal unit are
also using the facilities of PRS.   Patients are entered using the registration program described in section 3.1.1.1.   These clinicians are also entering carefully
defined additional data clinically relevant to the follow-up and research aspects of
the group of patients under long-term surveillance.   For example, the additional
data for renal transplant patients includes chemical pathology data, blood group,
blood transfusions and HLA status.

Clinicians from the Diabetic Clinic are preparing problem and drug lists from the
manual case records and defining the type of selected additional data to be entered
to PRS for diabetic patients.   It is also proposed to register the high-risk patients
in Grampian Area on the anticoagulant warfarin, and on the toxic antirheumatoid arth-
ritic agent penicillamine.   Further high-risk groups are under discussion.

The PRS register of patients of special interest for undergraduate and postgraduate
teaching is being used increasingly as the pressures on severely ill hospitalised
patients from exposure to successive groups of students are better appreciated.   The
availability of selected and cooperative patients who are invited to the wards, or
are even seen at home (Rehabilitation teaching), at a date relevant to the clinical
undergraduate curriculum has obvious advantages to student and teacher.   The facilities
of PRS are used to invite the patient to the ward, to update the record and to thank
the patient for attending.

3.2   Computer aspects.

A computing network project was formed in 1972 in Grampian with the aim of working
towards a campus network of computers.   Emphasis was placed on the transferability
of applications to other machines with a CODASYL compatible database management

system (DBMS). A CTL Modular One computer was made available in 1973. The configuration included 224 Kbytes of store, four 28 Mbytes exchangeable disc drives, two tape decks and a number of input/output peripherals. The programs were written in FORTRAN using in-house software for database management, screen handling, transaction update and recovery (7,8).

Funding for the Grampian network project ceased in 1977. A successful application was then made for support to attempt to develop aspects of the network project in the direction of the present patient record system. The CTL Modular One has recently been replaced by a CTL 8046.

4. DISCUSSION

The computer-assisted patient record system is now integral to the process of care of several thousand patients in the Grampian Area and is in routine use by clinicians involved in a variety of specialty interests, and secretarial staff working in different clinical units.

The discharge procedures are well established and there is considerable potential for extension of PRS to take on patients discharged from further clinical units. However, this seems a less desirable development than extension of the facilities provided by PRS to include at-risk patients suffering for example from diabetes mellitus, or on high-risk drugs such as warfarin or penicillamine. An approach has also been made by members of a local general practice to have elderly at-risk patients in their practice registered on PRS. The implications of such developments could have considerable influence on the prevention of predictable complications of disease, and on the prevention of the unintentional initiation by doctors of iatrogenous disease (9, 10).

Extension of PRS to new local users has been carefully explained and introduced gradually as a pilot scheme so that misuse and misunderstandings do not unnecessarily prejudice the attitudes of newcomers to the facilities of PRS. Our experience in the introduction and implementation of the manual problem orientated medical record in hospitals has been helpful (5). Gradual extension to new users is more successful, in our opinion, than sudden 'across the board' introduction, without adequate explanation, of new systems to a group of poorly informed users.

The next phase in the development of PRS is to take on further groups of at-risk patients. The commitment of the clinicians of the Diabetic Clinic to undertake a major review and preparation of their manual case records is a clear indication of their willingness to join PRS. An augmentation of the patient profile will be developed to cope with the special requirements (laboratory results, risk factors) of diabetic patients and their clinicians. A similar exercise will be undertaken for clinicians supervising groups of patients on high-risk drugs. This high level of activity in PRS now requires the development of a multi-access facility, and an archiving policy. A link to the Grampian hospitals and community index of patients has also been suggested once the replacement ICL 2966 machine is available. A re-write of PRS, using commercially supported database management systems, to permit operation of PRS on non-CTL equipment is also under discussion.

5. ACKNOWLEDGEMENTS

We wish to acknowledge financial support from the Scottish Health Service Common Services Agency. OJR and DJT were in receipt of junior fellowships in Community Medicine sponsored by the Scottish Home and Health Department.

We also wish to thank all clinical, computer and secretarial staff who have con-tributed to the implementation of the patient record system.

6. REFERENCES

(1) Starr KJ, Petrie JC. Drug interactions in patients on long-term oral anti-coagulant and antihypertensive adrenergic neuron-blocking drugs. Br med J. 1972; 4: 133-35.

(2) Logie AW, Galloway DB, Petrie JC. Drug interactions and long-term anti-diabetic therapy. Br J clin Pharmac. 1976; 3: 1027-32.

(3) Wilson LA, Petrie JC, Dawson AA, Marron AC. The new Aberdeen medical record. Br med J. 1978; 2: 414-16.

(4) Weed LL. Medical records, medical education and patient care. Chicago. Year Book Medical Publishers. 1969.

(5) Petrie JC, McIntyre N. (eds). The problem orientated medical record - its use in hospitals, general practice and medical education. Edinburgh, Churchill Livingstone. 1979.

(6) Howie JGR, Jeffers TA, Millar HR, Petrie JC. Prevention of drug interactions. Br J clin Pharmac. 1977; 4: 611-14.

(7) Lindsey DC, Meredith AL, Petrie JC. An experimental database for clinical and administrative use. Medcomp. 1977; 725-39.

(8) Allen KF, McLeod G, Petrie JC. Does a database really help health care? Ann World Assoc of Med Informatics. 1980; 207-212.

(9) Cluff LE, Petrie JC. (eds). Clinical effects of interaction between drugs. Amsterdam, Elsevier, North Holland Biomedical Press. 1975.

(10) Petrie JC. (ed). Clinically important adverse drug interactions - volume 1 - cardiovascular and respiratory disease therapy. Amsterdam, Elsevier, North Holland Biomedical Press. 1980.

A MEAL-DISTRIBUTION SYSTEM IN AN INTEGRATED HIS

Kees Byl and Bob van Spengen

BAZIS, University Hospital Leiden
Rynsburgerweg 10 , 2333 AA Leiden
The Netherlands

INTRODUCTION

Besides nursing and medical care the supply of healthy food is probably one of the factors that is most benificial to the healing proces.
In a hospital, particularly in a University Hospital, there is a
special aspect regarding the supply of meals, namely the great number of exceptions, such as the many different diets (or diet-combi-
nations) , meals needing a seperate preparation, special supplies
which are not in the standard assortment, etc. Thus, the exceptions
threaten to exceed the rule. Three times a day approx. 700 meals have
to be served in one hour, from which ca. 50 % with a dietprescription.
Our hospital uses for the distribution a CENTRAL-SERVING system
(by means of conveyor belt), instead of a so called BULK system.
In the past, hand-made MEALCARDS were used, on which coloured labels
were fixed to indicate the patients diet. This system was responsible
for delays and errors, because the people who served the meals
had to decide which course matched the patients diet.
Furthermore, hand counts of the number of requested components had to
be made.
These problems were the reason for automating the distribution system.
The objectives were : The translation of a patient request and patient
diet into a component ; More choice possibilities for the patient ;
The making of production-lists at the earliest possible moment and of
mutation-production lists at the last possible moment; late mutations have to be possible. The realised meal-distribution system shares
the facilities of the integrated Hospital Information System (HIS) of
Leiden University Hospital [1].

PROBLEM DEFINITION AND SOLVING

With the above mentioned objectives in mind a system was developed
and built, and has been in use since 1978. In figure 1. the meal-distribution system is represented in a very simplified form. It shows
in brief which data is needed to serve a meal.

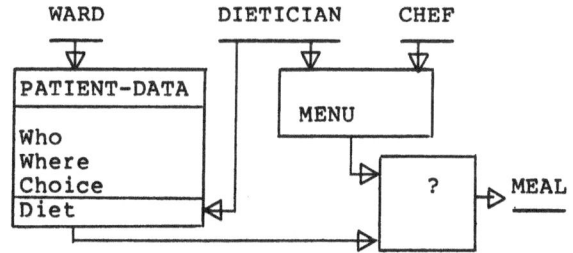

figure 1. The meal-distibu-
tion model in its most sym-
plified form. The question
mark must be solved.

The coding-problems are solved as follows. For every patient a REQUEST
-FORM is filled in only once (figure 2), with per assortmentgroup the
choice and the desired quantity. If necessary a DIET-FORM is filled in.

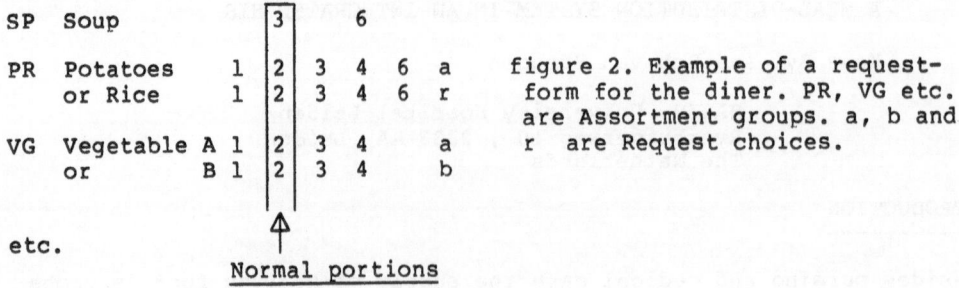

```
SP  Soup            │3│   6
PR  Potatoes    1  │2│ 3  4  6  a      figure 2. Example of a request-
    or Rice     1  │2│ 3  4  6  r      form for the diner. PR, VG etc.
                   │ │                 are Assortment groups. a, b and
VG  Vegetable A 1  │2│ 3  4     a      r  are Request choices.
    or        B 1  │2│ 3  4     b
                    ⇑
etc.              Normal portions
```

On the coded mealcard (figure 3) is for each post along the conveyer
(= a partition on the card) printed how much from which 'food-container' has to be served. In other words, the system translates per assortment-group, a REQUESTED-CHOICE and the desired quantity to a POST-
INDICATION and a FOOD-CONTAINER-CODE with portion-magnitude, naturally
taking the patients diet into account.(e.q: a request for vegetable
,choice A and portionsize 2 is translated to a partition and food-
container code P)
   Alterations in choice can now be made daily without problems (decentral) by changing e.g. VG A (=Vegetable choice A) into VG B.
The system makes a new mealcard with the right foodcontainer code.
Furthermore it has to take into account the many other alterations per
patient, such as wardtransfer, change of diet ,etc., up to the last
possible moment. Because of the time-critical nature, the system must
have high availability and reliability. The availability is achieved by the use of a duplicated computer system. The reliability is
achieved by a great effort in development, training and extensive
RESTART-PROCEDURES. Practice is of course the best test. In three years
it has never been necessary to switch back to a manual system. The
system has been developed as flexibly as possible by using parameters
and reference-files in order to intercept alterations in organisation,
menu-composition and dietetics.

```
                                    KK  K          BBBB   RRRR
                                    KK K           BB  B  RR  R
DINER FRIDAY        02-10-1981      KKK            BBBB   RRRR
                                    KK K           BB  B  RR  R
PATIENT K.     1.312.545 M 26-02-23 THIC (  5)     KK  K           BBBB  RR   R

DIET  : NA-

   3 CHICKEN SOUP  NA-
   2 RICE
   2 FRENCH BEANS   NA-
   2 STEAK  NA-             AAA  IIII   AAA     BBBB  PPPP   CCCC
   2 BEEF GRAVY  NA-        AA  A  II    AA  A   BB  B PP  P  CC
   2 APPLE SAUCE           AAAAA   II   AAAAA    BBBB  PPPP   CC
   1 NUTMEG                AA  A  II    AA  A    RB  B PP     CC
   1 STEWED MUSHROOMS      AA  A IIII   AA  A    BBBB  PP     CCCC
   2 SPOON, KNIFE AND FORK
                           22222
                               2
                           22222
                           22
                           22222
```

figure 3 .A coded mealcard for the diner.On the right the part for the
serving-out is shown. When no number below the code is printed than it
is a standard portion.On the left the part for the patient is shown.

REALISED DISTRUBUTION SYSTEM

The realised distribution system consists of the following files and programs.

A. The assortment

With the help of the Assortment-programme the ASSORTMENT can be built up (including all courses which,up till now, have been supplied). In the assortment is per course,the name, DIET-SUITABILITY, etc. defined.

B. The menu-cycle

The MENU-CYCLE is the total number of courses available for a fixed period(e.g. during the summertime). Within such a cycle a ´repeating Menu´ is defined, e.g. every two weeks. In other words the Menu-file contains all the courses that can be supplied during those fourteen days. Per course the following items are stored: Daynumber (1-14), Mealsort(breakfast,etc.), Request-code, Diet suitability, Postnumber Food-container code(this code is printed in the card partition for a post), etc.

C. The patient location system (clinically active patient-file)

This system is used by many other applications in the HIS in order to know in which ward the patient lies. This data is useful e.g. for controlling who should receive a meal (management). There is a similar file for out-patients, visitors or personnel.

E. Meal-orders

As mentioned above , there is a request per assortment-group, a choice and a quantity. This data is input centrally with the help of a program.

F. Production

The manager can make a worklist per course. After that he can always update the worklist by printing the differences. At the last possible moment the meal cards are printed.

CONCLUSIONS

The automated meal-distribution system has proved its usefulness during the last 3 years without breakdown. For the patients the system has created the possibility to choose a number of course alternatives.

Thanks to an extensive authorisation control, decentral input is already possible at this moment. In the past three years there has been an increase in decentral, instead of central data-input. However, decentral input runs up against organisational problems. Although the system has great advantages it will probably only pay for itself when the development and maintenance costs are shared over more hospital organisations. Several implementations of the meal-distribution system are planned in other hospitals, which use the same HIS-system.

Besides this growth in breadth it is now after 3 years experience possible to develop in depth too, for example a complete course choice by the patients themselves.

REFERENCES

1. Bakker, A.R. (1977) Implementation approach and evaluation of the use of Leiden University Hospital Information System, in: Medinfo 77 eds. D.B. Shires and H. Wolf (North Holland, Amsterdam) p.p. 943-947

INFORMATION ABOUT PATIENTS IN HOSPITAL
ENGLISH RECOMMENDATIONS FOR A NATIONAL MINIMUM DATA SET

Alastair Mason, Secretary to the NHS/DHSS Health Services
Information Steering Group.

Patricia Annesley, Statistician, Department of Health and
Social Security, London.

John Ashley, Senior Medical Officer, Office of Population
Censuses and Surveys, London.

Kevin Cottrell, Regional Statistician, North Western
Regional Health Authority, Manchester.

Lorna Wainwright, Co-ordinator of Training and Pilot
Studies for NHS/DHSS Health Services
Information Steering Group.

SUMMARY

In England recommendations are currently being considered for a
new national minimum basic data set for all patients using a
hospital bed, covering all clinical specialties and including
day case admissions. For each data item recommended, standard
definitions and classifications have been developed. By March
1982, consultation with health authorities and the testing of
the recommendations will have been completed and a final report
will be issued to the Department of Health in Spring 1982.
It is hoped to start implementing the proposals in 1983.

THE NHS/DHSS HEALTH SERVICES INFORMATION STEERING GROUP

In February 1980 the Secretary of State for Health and Social
Security set up a national steering group to carry out a
comprehensive review of the information and informations systems
available for the management of health services in England.

The Steering Group has adopted the following philosophies:

a. In developing data set for health services management, the
needs of operational managers at hospital and health
authority levels should be identified first, and for the most
part the information needs of managers at a strategic level
should be served by the data used for operational management
and planning.

b. In developing data sets to be implemented nationally, a
philosophy of the minimum data set which is desirable, feasible
and affordable has been pursued; thus allowing individual
health authorities to collect further data which are relevant
to their own particular circumstances. The minimum data set with
associated standard definitions and classifications will permit
realistic comparison between clinical activity in different
health authorities.

At an early stage in its work, the Steering Group identified the urgent need to review the information systems
concerned with hospital clinical activity and in particular
information about patients who have used a hospital bed.
Recommendations about a minimum basic data set for hospital
patients were published in July 1981. The report has been
widely circulated for comment and the proposals have been
field tested in four of the 200 health authorities in
England. A final report incorporating the results of the
consultation process and the field trials will be
available in Spring 1982.

GENERAL PRINCIPLES

In considering the minimum data set about patients using
a hospital bed the following general principles guided
the work.

a. Relevance. Data items, classifications and definitions
    must reflect clinical reality and the information
    system must take into account the ways medical care
    is currently provided. In England this includes
    taking account of the flexible ways in which wards are
    used by specialties, and the frequency of transfer
    between wards and consultants during the same stay in
    hospital.

b. Comparability of data outputs. Health services manage-
    ment has few hard and fast indicators of good or bad
    performance. Comparison with similar organisations
    is an important of information use.

c. Linkage of activity data with financial and manpower
    data systems. Experience has shown that data about
    patient activity is more useful to decision making
    when it can be linked to financial and manpower
    information.

d. Simplicity of the system. To assist data collection
    and processing an attempt has been made to include
    all patients regardless of specialty in the system.
    At present in England data about patients using psych-
    iatric beds and those using maternity beds are collected
    and processed in systems separate from that for
    general specialties.

THE RECOMMENDATIONS

The Steering Group has recommended that a minimum set of
data items should be completed on all patients who use a
hospital bed. The same items should be collected for all
specialties and standard definitions and classifications
have been developed for each data item.

The data is input to a computer at different stages namely:

a. Details on admission
b. Details on transfer between wards
c. Details on transfer between consultants
d. Non-clinical details on discharge
e. Clinical details on discharge

The items in the admission data set are:-

a. District patient number. All the contacts with hospitals in a defined geographical area (the health district) made by one patient should be identified by a single unique number.

b. Sex.

c. Geographical code of usual residence recorded as a post code.

d. Date of birth.

e. Marital status recorded in a way compatible with that used for national population censuses.

f. Code of primary care practitioner usually responsible for the patient's care.

g. Category of patient: the classification is a mixture of fee paying category and legal status which denotes whether the patient's admission is voluntary or compulsory.

h. Date of admission.

i. Source of admission which identifies whether the patient was admitted from his usual domestic residence or from another institution.

j. Method of admission which distinguishes patients admitted electively from those admitted as emergencies.

k. Date of clinical decision about need for elective admission. This allows the calculation of the time patients spend waiting for elective hospital admission after it has been decided that they should be admitted.

l. Management intention is a data item which identifies the intended pattern of bed use of a patient. Patients have been classified as:-

   i)   Intention to stay at least one night in hospital.

   ii) Intention to have no overnight stay in hospital.

   iii) Intention to be admitted regularly for a planned sequence of days or nights but returning home for the remainder of the 24 hour period.

If intentions are fulfilled as shown by the actual length of stay, category 2 are designated day case admissions and category 3 are regular day or night admissions. All other patients are designated as ordinary admissions.

    m. Initial consultant code.

    n. Initial ward code.

The items in the <u>ward transfer set</u> are:-

    a. Linking/merging numbers.

    b. Date of transfer.

    c. New ward code.

The items in the <u>consultant transfer set</u> are:-

    a. Linking/merging numbers.

    b. Date of transfer.

    c. New consultant code.

    d. Diagnosis codes. A change of consultant is frequently associated with a change of diagnosis so main diagnosis is identified after each consultant episode.

The items in the <u>non-clinical details discharge set</u> are:-

    a. Linking/merging numbers.

    b. Method of discharge; the classification used is the same as for source of admission.

The items in the <u>clinical details discharge set</u> are:-

    a. Linking/merging numbers.

    b. Diagnostic codes using ICD 9 classification with the capability of recording up to four diagnoses.

    c. Operation/operative procedures codes using a revised classification to be produced by the Office for Population Censuses and Surveys.

MATERNITY

The minimum data set described above is applicable to both the general specialties and psychiatry. However in maternity there is a need for more data because the record of a maternity event involves at least two patients (mother and one baby) and information is required about the delivery.

The minimum data set for maternity events has been developed using the same principles as used for other specialties. Thus for each pregnancy resulting in a registrable birth there should be:

a. A minimum data set (as set out above) for the mother.

b. A minimum data set (as set out above) for each baby.

c. A delivery/notification data set for each baby.
The collection of these data is statutory in England.

Data about mother and each baby should be brought together by means of the delivery/notification record and linked by computer to give a complete maternity record.

The delivery/notification data set should contain the following items:

a. Data about mother: parity.

b. Data about baby: birth order, live/still birth, birth weight, resuscitation.

c. Data about delivery: place, original intention for place, reason for change.
Length of gestation, number of babies.
Method of labour onset, method of delivery.

d. Identifiers: Mother's number and date of birth
Baby's number and date and time of birth.

DISCUSSION

The work of developing a new minimum data set for patients using a hospital bed included a review of current European Systems. The Roger Report (2) which summarises the situation in the EEC countries was an invaluable source document. The 13 data items recommended in this Report have been included in the proposed English data set. This would permit the exchange of English data with that from other EEC countries on a comparable basis.

REFERENCES

1. NHS/DHSS Steering Group of Health Services Information. The Report of Working Groups A on hospital clinical activity statistics. Available from the Department of Health, London.

2. Roger, F. H. The minimum basic data set for hospital statistics in the EEC, a review of availability and comparability. Published by Office for Official Publications of the European Community, Luxembourg, in 1981.

CLINICAL EXPERIENCE WITH RADOS

H.E.Riemann,
Dept.of Roentgendiagnostic,
Radiological Center,
J.W.Goethe-University,
Frankfurt/M, Western Germany.

Two years ago we introduced RADOS (= Radiological Dokumentation System) consisting of hardware (e.g. P 857) from PHILIPS-MUELLER and software developed by this factory.

The system takes care of patient registration and appointment distribution in the radiology department. It also registers the dates necessary for patient identification.

Patient identification, needed for the different working areas, the wards and the management of the department are printed out together. The system registers the type of roentgen examination, the number of examinations and films per patient and thus supplies the hospital with useful statistics for management and personal planning. It also registers all dates necessary for calculation of patient x-ray dose in order with German law.

One part of RADOS is a reporting system. It is helpful for the radiologist and the clinician having soon the report examination. The radiologist has the possibility to choose between preformed texts or individual texts.

A FUNDAMENTAL DATA BASE DESIGN FOR CLINICAL LABORATORY INFORMATION SYSTEMS

A.J. Porth, C. Badke, I. Mieth
Institute for Clinical Chemistry
Laboratory Data Processing
Medical School Hanover
Germany

SUMMARY

In the following we describe a data base design allowing the changement of data structures without touching the programs, an essential feature for portable systems. Any file or input/output data set has a clearly defined structure description, which may change due to any project specific purposes. The concept is allready realized and proved in different laboratories.

1. INTRODUCTION

During the MIE 78 congress in Cambridge we presented some theoretical aspects of the "data structures and data base problems in Clinical Chemistry Information Systems" (1). Today we are able to present the result of the realization of our concept and of about three years full of experience in large and small laboratories.

With the regard of their use we have to distinguish the following types of data to be handled within a Laboratory Information System (LIS):
- data for system control and structure description
- fixed user data that must be permanent available
- variable user data for current use
- variable user data for long term filing.

Fixed user data are all parameters which describe a certain test (analysis), the corresponding result handling and check values (eg test names, test codes, measurement units, reference limits, etc.).

Variable user data concern the patient, the sample with the corresponding request, the results for the different report and retrieval purposes.

The main goals of our design for portable data base systems are:
- to warrant flexible data structures for files and input/output lists
- to make the data structures independent from programs, that means any changement of data structures has not to touch any program of the system and vice versa.

In the following we describe how to realize the management of the four
types of data within our Laboratory Information System, which we called
QUADROLAB (Quality directed, universally applicable data base and real
time oriented Laboratory Information System).

2. SYSTEM CONTROL AND STRUCTURE DESCRIPTION DATA

This data type is the most important one for the flexibility of a data
handling and data base system. Using the extensive support of our operating system MAX IV for MODCOMP-computers we installed an own dialog processor system (DIA) as one nucleus of the LIS serving to the simultanous
use of as many terminals by one task as the hardware allows. This processor guarantees immediate response ($\ll$ 1 sec) - an absolute need for any
LIS. The corresponding table set - concerning the LIS purpose - is installed within a global common array of the central memory - figure 1.
The LIS - control parameters direct:
- the program sequences and
- the program behaviour in the various situations of LIS.

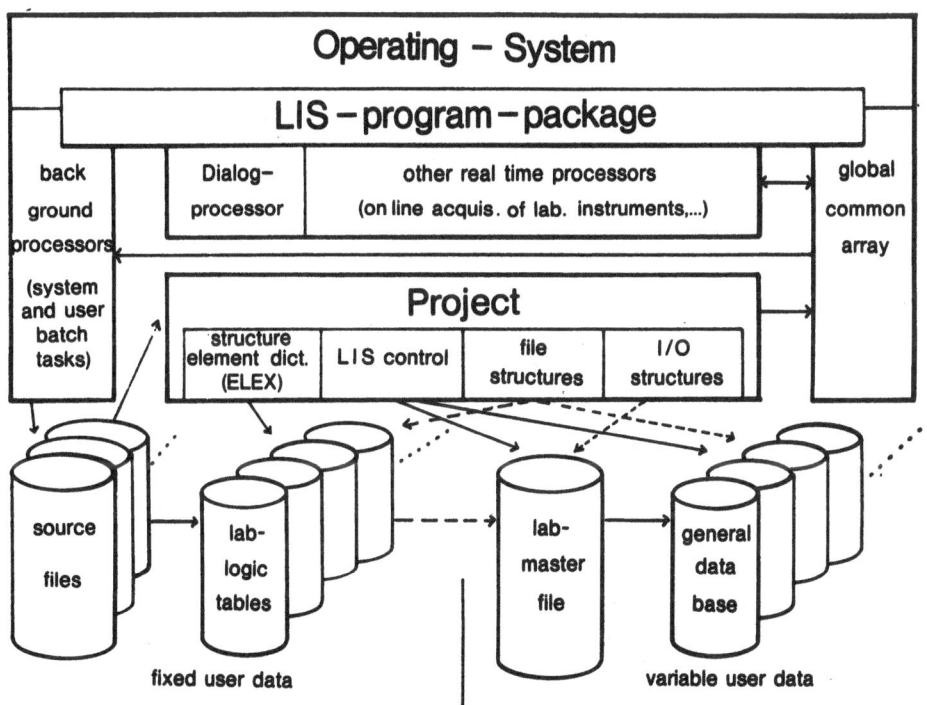

Figure 1: Overview of the QUADROLAB-System design.

2.1 The elements of structure description

All structure elements concerning the laboratory system and other project specific work are defined within a dictionary containing the element name (eg patient name), its mnemotechnic abbreviation (eg PANA, the data type (eg ASCII=A) and an indicator word for project specific data handling (eg default length in bytes, dummy content).

This dictionary of the project specific structure elements - we call it ELEX - is the fundamental bases for each laboratory information system we have to generate - figure 1. Each task, file, list or form has to use its specific subset of these elements in an autonomic way. To facilitate the use of these structure elements during all the real time procedures there is installed a table with the mnemotechnic codes and the "global" information (indicators and data type signs) within the memory. Any structure element not found in this table will be ignored by the programs. There is only the exeption concerning the output lists: any item will be printed or displayed.

2.2 The structure of files

Each data file - using a subset of elements as mentioned - has a well defined structure description with a standard set of information:
- The header of each file contains:
  -- file name, record length, start and end record number for data
  -- directory y/n, directory record length, start and end of directory
  -- security key.
- The directory contains the following information for the content of each data record:
  -- code of mnemotechnic structure element
  -- start byte within the data record
  -- number of bytes or bits to be used.
- The supplementary directories are, if needed, for problem specific information as the case may be, they will be handled by the programs themselves.
- The data will be stored in the following records according to the structure defined in the main directory.

During project generation all files are installed with their own structure and the directory. A new file configuration may cause a new generation of the project specific system.
This concept of file structures leads to the flexibility which is needed for the portability of systems with no program adaption. A set of standard read/write routines, list, sort-programs and other useful sub-

routines help to work with any individual record length and structure.

We have installed a text base system analog to the data base system.
This special problem will be published an another paper.

3. FIXED USER DATA

These must be permanent available and comprehend the project specific
information, which have to be codified at the commencement of the installation according to the laboratory needs and the structure description (lab-logic tables in figure 1). These data have relatively seldom
to be changed, replaced or complemented.

3.1 Primary tables (source level)

The primary tables contain the data on source resp. user level. The primary tables may be updated and tested independently from the LIS-routine
and they may contain any comment for their use. The table set comprehend
the following subjects:
- table of test specific data
- table of reference limits according to age and sex of patient
- quality control sample data
- billing data
- list and report handling data
- text data
- others

The amount of tables and the detailed information is project specific.
All elements and indicators which are used, have to be defined in the
system element dictionary (ELEX).

3.2 Secondary tables (LIS level), pointers and indicators (in-memory-
level)

The secondary tables extract the data from the primary tables to task
specific subsets available to run the daily routine work. The data are
stored in files which are structured according to the features described
above. For debugging we may install an auxiliary system with the place-
ment of the secondary tables in question on the work storage on disc.
This helps to check the updated primary tables before they will be introduced into the system by a new project generation.
The programs use the same package of subroutines for the general handling of structured data. A special QUADROLAB project builder generates
the integration of the LIS-control structure and of all secondary tables
to an actual working system within about 10 minutes. Usual is work some

month until the situation will cause a new generation.

Such a large table set, as we are used to handle, needs a pointer and indicator system to avoid time consuming search procedures and useless programsteps.

- The <u>pointers</u> serve to pick up the test specific information directly from disc.
- The <u>indicators</u> tell the system what steps of a certain task the test has to be undergone.

The project builder generates the corresponding global common table like a secondary table on disc, from which it will be picked up after system start to be transferred into memory.

4. VARIABLE USER DATA FOR CURRENT USE

This kind of data must be available to the system over a well defined period of time and it must be updated continously (eg request, measurement values, patient data, laboratory results etc).

4.1 The <u>laboratory master file</u> concept

The data for immediate use are stored in a big transient pool on disc until the processing is carried out and the data will be stored in the general data base system. We call this big data pool our lab-master file, it forms the heart of the laboratory internal data handling and report system. All laboratory data which may be input, handled or printed will go through this file.

The lab-master file is organized in slices of variable size and structures. Each slice of the file starts with a header and a directory as it is described above. The management of the lab-master file is done by a set of reentrant subroutines, which guarantee the simultaneous use of this file by various programs and terminals at the same time. A copy of the file management table is stored in the global common table set - figure 1.

The lab-master file contains all requests, work lists, acquisition minutes, quality control data and so on during their immediate processing through the various steps of data handling. A slice is rubbed out when the work is terminated and the data are transferred to the general data base system. The data may remain in the lab-master file as many time as they need to be processed, even for weeks in the case of requests of seldom tests needing accumulation or external treatment.

4.2 The <u>general laboratory data base</u> system

The structure description of the files is the same as presented above. There are patient, sample and result oriented files, quality control result files and special files for cross over pointers to match patient, sample and result data together. To make extensive use of the available space, the sample and result file is organized in six result packages matched to the sample data.

The updating of the data base files will be managed in a patient resp. sample oriented way. Correction of any variable data in the system has to be realized via the lav-master file and input of the new data.

While the internal report system comprehend the lab-master file work and the dialog between laboratory routine and computer, the external report system generates the final product of the laboratory from the general data base. We may produce single reports, cumulative reports, quality control reports and others.

5. LONG TERM FILING AND INTER-SYSTEM COMMUNICATION

While the data for current use is organized in separate files for patient and sample (result) handling, the data base for long term filing combines both forming a data record of variable length. This data has to be used in a sequential way as a magnetic tape.

5.1 Structure of data set

The file management for the long term filing remains the same as for any other file described above. Each patient has a record that means a slice of memory on disc or tape. A header informs that a new patient starts, a directory describes the structure of the following data block. Usually the result are multiple. This will be indicated within the directory using a code for repetition.

While a changement of file structure and configuration will cause a complete transfer of the former data to the new situation within the general data base system, the long term file concept is competely independent from any changement of structures.

5.2 Communication between systems

The consequent realization of the data base management leads to a flexible and suitable communication between computer systems. Both computers need only the same structure element dictionary or a conversion table. Each message will start with a header and a directory. The header tell the length (bytes) of the given information, the directory describes the structure of the transferred data block.

With this minimum of directives we gain a maximum of flexibility. The efforts of programming are shurely more delicate than for the structures of fixed blocks. But in the end these efforts are less high than the time consumed by correction of transfer errors.

6. <u>CONCLUSION</u>

This concept of data handling guarantees a high flexibility against changement of data structures and of the structure elements themselves. For instance a changement of the length of patient name touches only the directory builder resp. its table set. The only restriction may be caused by hardware or operating system limits.

The system we gave a short description of, is now installed in three laboratories. It is to mention that these laboratories are quite different in size and organization. The adaption of three further laboratories runs in the test phase. The integration of on line connection to various apparatus and the data transfer to a central hospital computer system is just in the phase of beeing concluded.

The programs are mainly written in FORTRAN. There is a rich library of assembler subroutines for the more delicate procedures which mainly touch the real time processing.

The experience of about two years in full charged routine of about 1000 samples a day for clinical chemistry, haematology, bacteriology, blood serology, immunology and other requests shows that we started a suitable way. The experience to adapt further laboratories with complete different configuration and demands show that we are able to build a portable Laboratory Information System.

7. <u>REFERENCES</u>

(1) PORTH, A.J., MIETH, I.: Data structure and data base problems in clinical chemistry information systems: J. Anderson (ed): Medical Informatics Europe 78, Proceedings, Cambridge, England 1978, p 489 - 496. Springer, Berlin - Heidelberg - New York 1978

COMPUTER AIDED EVALUATION OF HPLC (HIGH PRESSURE LIQUID CHROMATOGRAPHY)

WITH FLUOROMETRIC DETECTION

H.K. Biesalski, U.Wellner and G. Hafner
Institute of Physiology
Johannes Gutenberg-University

Saarstr. 21; D-6500 Mainz/W.-Germany

SUMMARY

A program system for automated HPLC measurements of vitamin A concentration is reported. This system provides for guidance of operators, for control of apparatus and for supervision of quality measurements.
This system enables serial measurements of up to 100 per operator per day as well as a high sensitivity of 1 ng vitamin A compound/ml extract.

COMMON ASPECTS

Many physiological functions in man are affected by vitamin A and a large number of pathological lesions appear in patients with vitamin A deficiency. Vitamin A plays an essential role in the function of the retina and its apparently important for growth and differentiation of epithelial tissue.
In addition the vitamin A is required for reproduction, embryonic development and normal bone formation. With the development of sophisticated methods in clinical chemistry for the estimation of vitamin A and its derivates some unknown interactions of the vitamin with several diseases (M.Crohn, Diseases of the Thyroidea, Cancer, etc.) were found.
For the investigation of the effects of vitamin A on a cellular level as well as for the realization of epidemiological studies a method is necessary which on one hand has high selectivity and sensitivity and on the other hand allows a great number of analyses a day. These demands are met by HPLC in conjunction with a fluorescence detector and a procedure of analysis we developed (1,2,3).
In series analyses a large number of measurements are carried out that produce a large amount of data. Since high degree of precision must also be achieved for trace analyses, the coupling of HPLC measuring equipment with a computer presents itself (Fig. 1) (4-6).

To achieve reproducible and reliable data the following features of LC have to be taken into account: Scott and Reese (7) demands:
"The precision of measurement can only be achieved under the following controlled conditions:
1. A pump is employed that controlls the column flow rate to $\pm$ 0.07 %
2. The solvent composition is maintained constant to $\pm$ 0.02 % (w/v)
3. The temperature of the mobile phase and column is maintained constant to $\pm 0.02°C$
4. The ambient temperature or the temperature of the pump and mobile phase supply must be maintained constant to $\pm$ 0.4°C
5. The charge on the column for any one solute must be less than 0.1 µg
6. The rate of data aquisition must be greater than 10 samples per sec and appropriate noise elimination procedures must be employed that do no distort the peak or produce band dispersion of an unacceptable level."

Substantial interference of one of these parameters can lead to changes in the qualitative and/or quantitative analysis (Table 1).

Deviation of solvent composition as well as temperature deviations can be prevented by the special construction of our measuring place (see illustration).
Inaccuracies can be detected by the computer with the help of sensors (temperature, flow, pressure) and either eliminated directly or reported.
The determination of concentration of certain substances in the substance mixture cannot be performed directly. The fluorescence detector only delivers the chromatogram which contains the concentrations of interest as signal parameters. These have to be

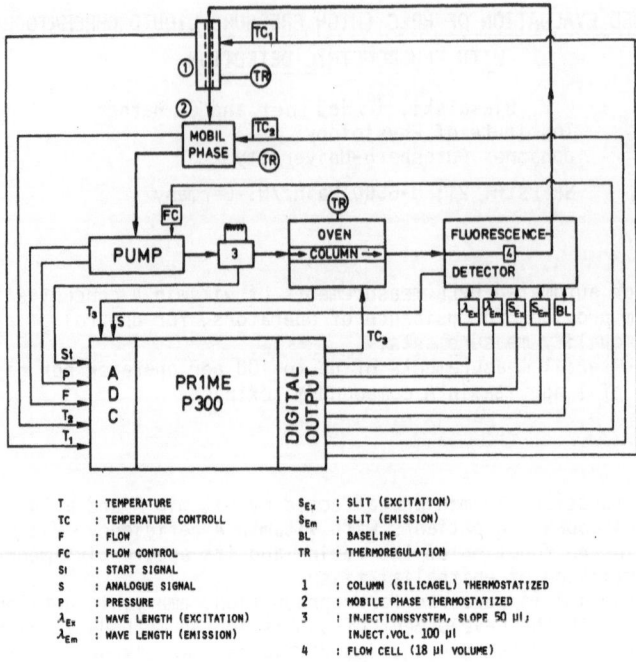

Fig. 1:   Computer coupled HPLC experimental devices.

derived from the signal by special mathematical procedures. The computer also does this task by leading the signal by way of an ADC to digital processing.
A number of different analytical procedures exist for chromatograms (8-11). The exactness of the quantitative analysis depends especially on the form of the chromatograms (sum of all substances to be analyzed). This form can be influenced by the choice of processing procedures of the substance to be analyzed (quantitative extraction in defined volumes) as well as by the choice of the mobile and stationary phase. In addition such parameters as temperature, pressure and flow have a crucial influence (12,13). Also the characteristics of the substance are naturally important if the k' values are disadvantageous and since they cannot always be optimized by the above parameters an optimal separation may not be possible and the interpretation very difficult or impossible.
If the form of the chromatography is adequate peaks can be assigned to single substances (assignment through the position in the chromatogram = retention time).
The concentration of each substance can be calculated using the parameters area or amplitude of the peaks. The choice of a suitable parameter in dependence of the chromatogram is discussed in length in the literature (14-16).

For our purpose the amplitude of the peak is a suitable measure. The amplitude is given preference to the area since it can hardly be influenced by deviations in flow, noise or baseline drift (7,13,17-19). The factors which have an influence on the amplitude, such as temperature deviations and the constancy of solvent composition can be controlled more by easily suitable measuring place than flow, noise or baseline drift. By establishing a suitable form of the chromatogram - separation of peaks down to the baseline, avoidance of shoulders - a linear relationship between concentration and amplitude was found by comparison with the amplitude or external standards.

Table 1: Effects of different problems and their prevention.

Problem	Qualitative	Quantitative	Prevention
Solvent:			
Change of composition	Change of retention time	Form changes: height > area	Recycling (closed system)
Change of H_2O content	Change of k'-values	Between substances the baseline is not reached Evaluation difficult	Recycling system with humidity control
<u>Injection volume not constant</u>		Results false + or -	Injections volume > loop
<u>Concentration to high</u>	Not in the linear range of the isotherme → Change of ret.-time	By fluorescence detection → cancellation	Conc. < 0.1 mg/g adsorbens
<u>Flow not constant</u>	Change of retention time (small)	Change of area	
Change of temperature			
1. Column	Change of retention time	Poorer separation	Column heater Temperature control
2. Solvent	Change of retention time	Change of fluorescence intensity	Temperature control
Column			
Stability	Change of retention time	Tailing: area > hight <	Control by computer
Overload		Pressure ↑ → Flow change	Rinsing steps

For each problem of analysis the conditions which affect
 - instrument dependent parameter (flow, detector-adjustment, etc.)
 - instrument independent parameters (temperature, mobile and stationary phase, etc.)
 - external standards (individually for each substance)
have to be established or empirically determined.

For each of our problems we determined whether the procedures outlined are permissible, that is to say, if
1. the peakform of the standard or standard mixture corresponds to the biological substrate;
2. the increase with a corresponding standard of different concentrations leads to a linear increase of the amplitude (exclusion of mutual amplitude interference of single derivatives); and,
3. the precision in the series has a VK of below 2 % from day to day.

PROGRAM

To complete the measurement system outlined above a computer program must be written which will comply to the stated conditions. The program system incorporates, in addition to aquisition and evaluation of the chromatographic data, control of the entire measurement process as well as database functions.

According to the mentioned theoretical considerations the measurement process has to be devided into three distinct tasks.

A. Calibration

Individual calibration functions are calculated using linear approximation. Standard deviations are estimated.

This program task will be seen for substances in consideration about every six weeks (durability of stock standard solution).

The task features the following supervisory actions:
1. Rejection of distorted analogue signals
2. Rejection of measurements which are not plausible
3. Rejection of measurements yielding high standard deviations.

All calibration functions obtained are filed in a data base.

B. Checking

1. Check of hardware-functions, e.g. temperature control, control of flow and pressure. Preceeding this test, the boundary conditions are adjusted according the kind of material to be used.
2. The quality of the chromatographic signal is judged. This includes the determination of signal parameters such as noise as well as parameters concerning the chromatographic pattern itself.
3. Test of day to day precision. Here the program will walk along a decision tree in several stages. At each stage a special dialogue will be established between operator and program. The aim of this procedure is not only to determine the mentioned precision but also to trap any faults in operator or hardware function and to trace them down to the possible causes.

This task is mandatory to the run at least each day; it is also required to be executed whenever the boundary conditions have to be changed.

C. Measurement

This task will determine the unknown concentration of a chosen substance in the samples to be analyzed. Three steps are programmed:
1. Test of quality of the chromatographic signal and of plausibility of signal parameters (such as retention time). If this check fails the program tries to track the possible cause of malfunction; it may about the measurement task and demand for execution of task B or even task A.
2. Actual measurement of concentration. Here plausibility is checked too.
3. Filing of the results. All accepted measurements are stored together with additional information (such as source of sample, way of preparation of sample, hardware parameters) in a data base.

This task may be repeated a given times, then task B has to be executed again.

The program-system has to be designed in such a way that it will guide the operator by giving commands on how to proceed. Furthermore, all detectable fault conditions have to be trapped and reported. The operator will to instructed to correct these faults. If fault conditions cannot corrected further measurements must be inhibited. The operator only has a limited influence on the sequence of the program tasks, that sequence essentially is determined by the supervisor of the program itself. For example the execution of task C is inhibited as long as task B has not been completed in a satisfactory way. Bacause of the sensitivity of the HPLC process, extensive checking has to be done in order to prevent the acceptance of faulty measurements. The program has the power to force the execution of special checks and readjustment procedures as they are described in task A and B. In general, the operator cannot override the demands of the supervisor task. He may only change the sequence of tasks in a conservative way, e.g. the A-task may be executed at any time. It has to be mentioned that the criteria will lead to a programmed change in sequence will have to be determined separately for trace measurements and serial measurements.

DISCUSSION

The procedure we described differs from automated HPLC measurement procedures already discussed in literature (4-6, 20,21). It takes into consideration the organizational aspects of the measurement by limitation to a priori determined selection of biolog- ical substances for analysis as well as the individual treatment of the single pro- blems of analysis.

The necessity for such a procedure results from the fact that we want to observe metabolic changes of vitamin A metabolism which take place in the lower ranges of detection limits and that we want to conduct longitudinal epidemiological studies with large samples. This necessitates demands a limitation of the analysis time to time units which allow a great many reliable measurements a day.

By chosing the corresponding side conditions more than 100 measurements a day can be performed and evaluated with our measuring place. However, our system of analysis allows an expansion to other questions if the choice of the corresponding conditions is adjusted to the respective object of analysis taking into account the constancy of the instrument parameters.

Furthermore, as a result of the modular construction of our program it is possible to exchange algorithms for each other, the determination of concentration could be executed by determining the area under the peak by changing the corresponding algorithm in the program modul pattern recognition.

REFERENCES:

(1) Biesalski HK, Ehrenthal W, Hafner G, Harth O. Eine neue Methode zur Bestimmung von Vitamin A und seinen Derivaten in biologischem Material. I. Bestimmung von Reti- nol im Serum. Z f Lab Suppl 5. 1981; 4-11.
(2) Biesalski HK, Hafner G, Harth O. Eine neue Methode zur Bestimmung von Vitamin A und seinen Derivaten in biologischem Material. II. Bestimmung von Vitamin A und sei- nen Derivaten in Organen. Z f Labormedizin. 1981 (in press).
(3) Biesalski HK, Harth O, Hafner G. Determination of retinol and retinyl esters in the spiral ligament, vascular stria, and basilar membrane in the cochlea of guinea pig. (submitted for publication).
(4) Chilcote DD, Scott CD. Use of a small dedicated computer with a high resolution liquid chromatograph. Chemical Inst. 1971; 3 : 113-124.
(5) Barth H, Dallmeier E, Courtois G, Keller HE, Karger BL. A study of precision in modern liquid chromatography using a dedicated computer. J Chromatogr. 1973; 83: 289-311.
(6) Kaiser RE. Vergleich von HPLC unter dem Aspekt der Automatisierung. Chromatographia. 1979; 12: 338-344.
(7) Scott RPW, Reese CE. Precision of contemporary liquid chromatographic measure- ments. J Chromatogr. 1977; 138: 283-307.
(8) Malczewski ML, Grushka E. Multiple peak recognition in high performance liquid chromatography by fast fourier transformation. J Chrom Sci. 1981; 19: 187-194.
(9) Stockwell PB, Telford I. Automatic data processing in chromatography - a mixed blessing. Chromatographia. 1980; 13: 665-668.
(10) Leitch RE. Precise quantitative analysis with a stable high speed liquid- liquid chromatography column. J Chrom Sci. 1971; 9: 531-535.
(11) ASTM (American Society for Testing and Materials). An evaluation of quantitative precision in high performance liquid chromatography. J Chrom Sci. 1981; 19: 338-348.
(12) Bakalyar SR, Henry RA. Variables affecting precision and accuracy in high per- formance liquid chromatography. J Chromatogr. 1976; 126: 327-345.
(13) Engelhardt H. Hochdruck-Flüssigkeits-Chromatographie. Berlin-Heidelberg-New York: Springer Verlag 1977
(14) Brown PR. High Pressure Liquid Chromatography. New York: Academic Press, 1973

(15) Wasserfallen K, Rinderknecht F, Baumgartner E. Qualitativer und quantitativer Vergleich von Chromatogrammen unter Verwendung eines Rechners. Chromatographia. 1977; 10: 176-180.

(16) Delley R. Effizienz der Chromatographie. Chromatographia. 1976; 9: 10-16.

(17) Kipiniak W. A basic problem - the measurement of height and area. J Chrom Sci. 1981; 19: 332-337

(18) Fleischer J. Eich- und Standardisierungsprobleme in der HPLC. Chromatographia. 1979; 12: 386-389.

(19) Goedert M, Guiochon G. A study of sources of error in quantitative gas chromatography: Reproducibility of the response of the catharometer. J Chrom Sci. 1969; 7: 323-339.

(20) Mikkelsen L, Poole J, Stefanski A, Biesel HT. The use of new computer technology in chromatography. Chromatographia. 1974; 7: 447-451.

(21) Hegedus LL, Petersen EE. Integration of chromatographic signals by digital computers: an approach for the small chromatographic laboratory where digital computer services are available. J Chrom Sci. 1971; 9: 551-553.

STRUCTURED ANALYSIS, A METHOD TO DOCUMENT
CLINICAL LABORATORY SYSTEMS

C. SEVENS

Dept. of Clinical Chemistry

Akademisch Ziekenhuis V.U.B.

1090 Brussels, BELGIUM

M. THEYS

Fac. Sc. Sociales, Politiques et Economiques

U.L.B., 1050 Brussels, BELGIUM

SUMMARY

Structured analysis is a powerful tool to describe and document complex
systems involving automated, computerized and human elements.
It structures the data onto three hierarchical levels. The retrospective study of a clinical laboratory system has been achieved
with this method.

1. Introduction

Without definite statistical data but with a good approximation one
can admit that between 30 to 50 % of the clinical chemistry laboratories
in most western European contries, eg (1), are computerized. It is
well known from the great amount of literature about this subject and
the tremendous investments made in this field for the last fifteen
years, that choosing and introducing a computer system into the
clinical laboratory remain very controversial subjects. It is therefore
rather surprising that modelling or analysis techniques have not been
used more frequently to try to outline this complex problem (2,3).

Structured analysis enables a description of events and through an
abstraction process to distinguish between components, actions and
relationships. It takes human, automated and computerized factors
into account and seems particulary adapted to the man/machine
interface existing in laboratory computer systems. The method has
been used to retrospectively document a clinical chemistry laboratory
system developed in the mid 70's.

2. Description of the method and its use in the clinical chemistry laboratory.

The method is based on the principle that all computerized functions can be considered as sequences of <u>discrete transitions</u>. The logic sequence <u>data/activation/transformation</u> serves as a <u>basic block</u>. Data can be all variables that are to be found in the system. These data undergo transition processes able to change state. However these transformations necessitate activation processes which control the transformation of the data. To get to a coherent model of complex systems one should, next to the computer, take automated (machines) and human factors into account. Any human action can be considered as a an infinite number of discrete transitions. A symbolism similar to that used for computer systems but surely distinguishing the elements is used (figure 1). A man can read, write, decode messages (data). The control processes he is using are decision, choices, thinking. These enable him to act equalling the transformation processes of computer systems. As such he will encode messages, write instructions, transport things. In automated systems examples of data are potentials, fluid levels, resistances, speeds. The transformation and control processes of these data can happen through human or computerized mechanisms.

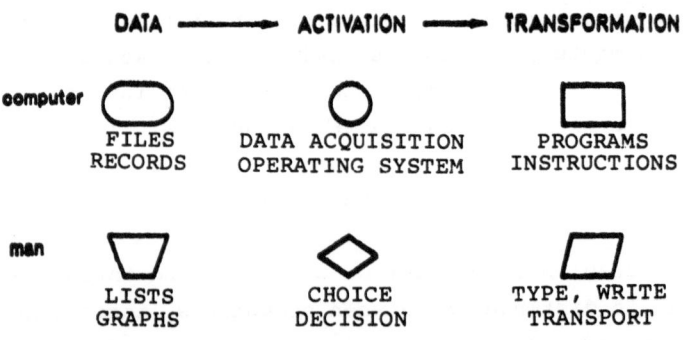

Figure 1 Dedicated language

Such combination makes the description of complex systems possible, in particular the clinical laboratory systems. The degree of detailed informations one can get to is according to one's needs. For computer information it stops at the bit level. For human elements one could ultimately get to (sub)cellular functions.

2.1. Description of occurences

The facts are described sequentially in terms of tasks to be performed, for example the chain of events between blood drawing and the clinical analysis. However the amount of data as such is not usable and need to be structured.

2.2. Logical transition diagrams

At this level of abstraction things are described in the way they logically happen in terms of **types of tasks**. Relationships between the three constituents of the basic block are structured into types of data, types of activations and types of transformations. Timely aspects of the initial sequential description and analytical details are levelled off (figure 2).

2.3. Physical transition diagrams

The second abstraction step enables one to consider any system **in terms of workcenters**, whatever their nature, human, automated or computerized, unrelated to sequence nor time. Keystones are easily made apparent, their role and their relationship with other components being depicted in an understandable and functional approach. This last step enhances the understanding of the fundamental aspects of a system (figure 3).

2.4. The **aggregation process** is an additional facility that can be used at any level of the analysis. A chain of processes is replaced by a block. Considering a number of relationships as a whole clears the model of less relevant or detailed data that otherwise would unnecessarily bear on the description and at the higher levels of abstraction considerably decrease the efficiency of the method.

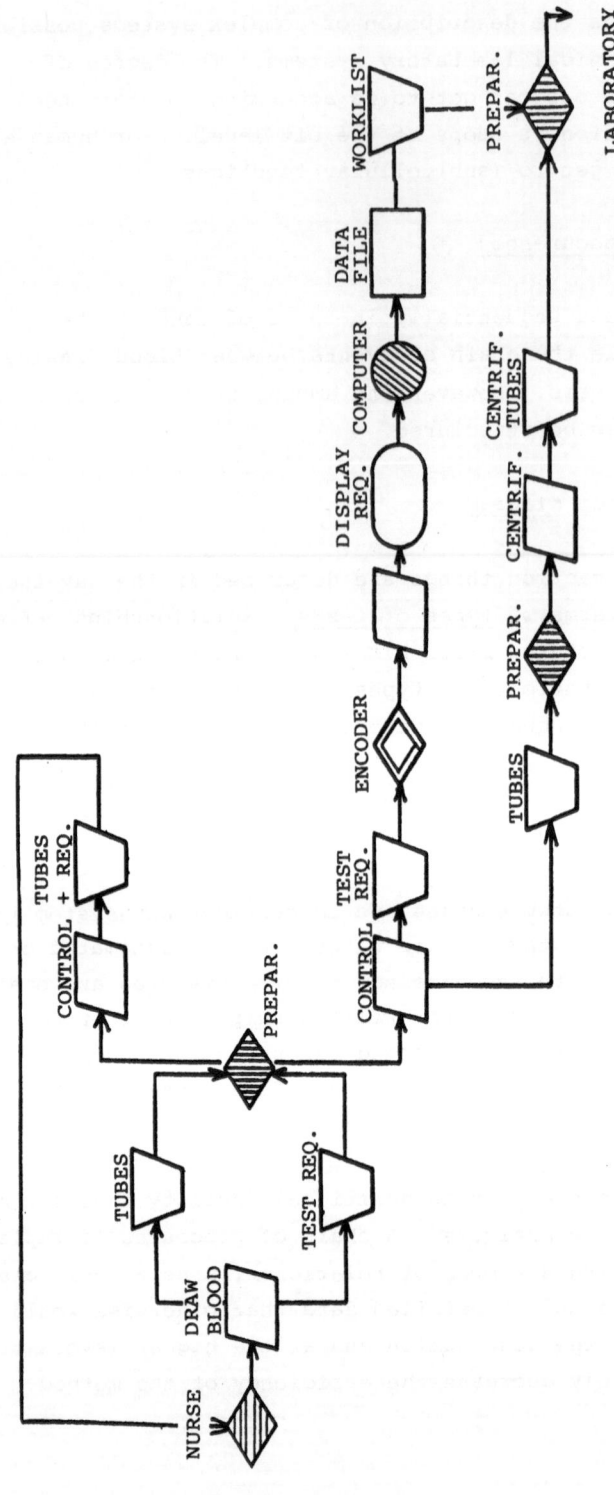

Figure 2 Logical transition diagram

73

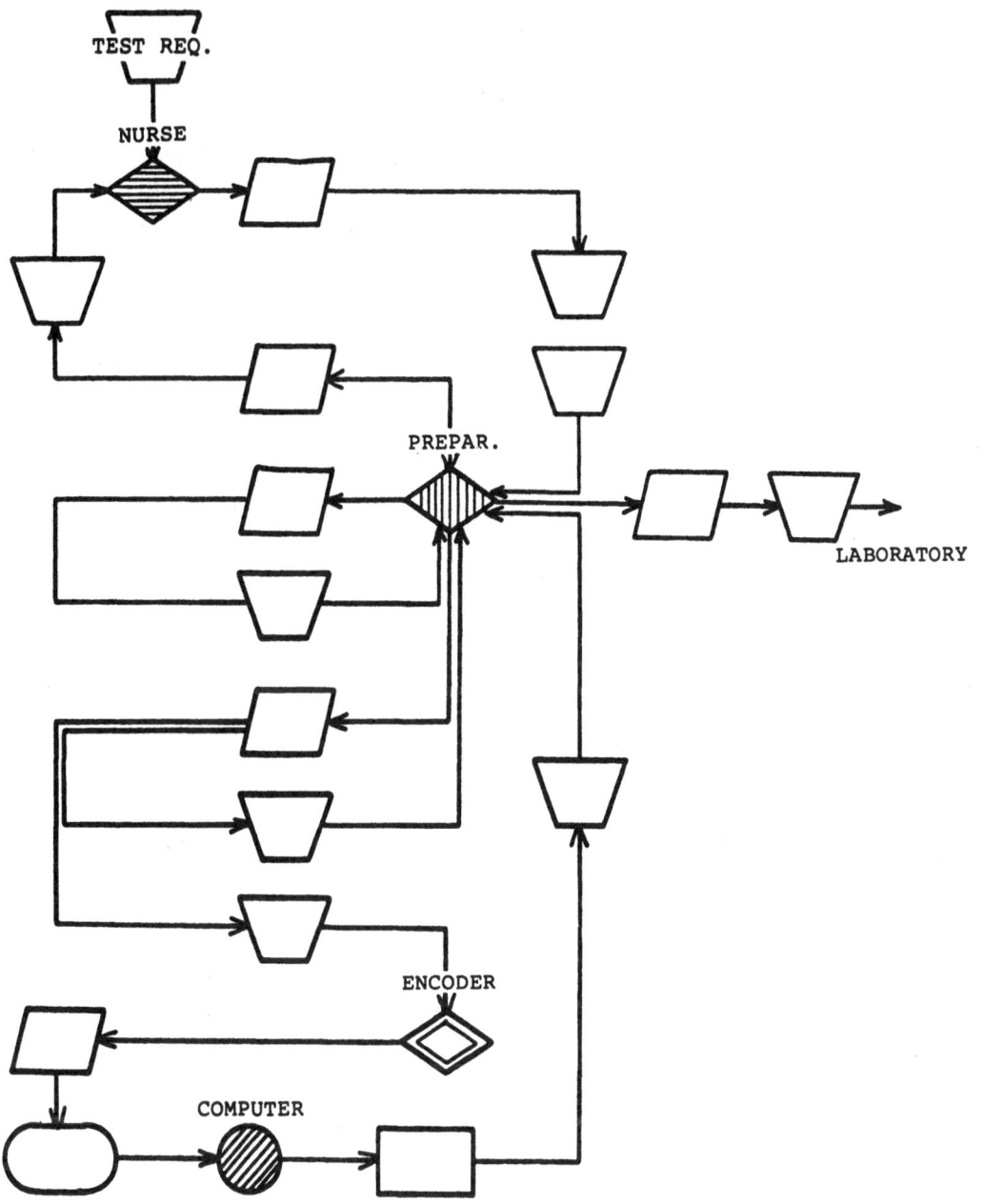

Figure 3 Physical transition diagram

74

3. Discussion and conclusion

A description language of discrete systems is used to reduce the complexity of the model of description. It integrates specifications coming from different origins using a dedicated language for exchange of informations between various specialists and also between man and computer. It improves robustness and flexibility through modularization. Structured analysis can be used at design time to verify coherence and exhaustiveness. At documentation time it proves to be man usable and hierarchical and at operation time it serves as an interface between man and computer. From the examples shown structured analysis can undoubtedbly be considered as an efficient tool to improve the design of complex systems. This approach has taught us that the complexity of clinical laboratory systems has been largely underestimated and that the human contributions to the organizational aspects of the problems have been neglected.
In recent years vendors of turnkey systems seem to have solved part of the problems inasmuch they can offer more adaptable software. However there still exists a need for real transferability of systems between laboratories. Slight but important differences between organizational structures, types and number of tests, type and degree of emergencies could play a negative role into finding an adequate solution.

References

(1) Assicot M., Valdiguié P., Report on the use of computers in the French clinical laboratory Computers in clinical laboratory. R.S. First Inc., Dusseldorf 1979.
(2) Huet B., Martin J., Evaluation d'un système informatique de laboratoire à partir de la simulation d'une journée de travail au laboratoire. Lecture notes in medical informatics, Third Congress of the European Federation, Toulouse 1981, Edited by F. Grémy, P. Degoulet, B. Barber and R. Salamon, Springer-Verlag, 1981.
(3) Spiegel K., Network model for scheduling workflow. 3rd Internat. Conference on Computing in Clinical Laboratories, Birmingham 1980.

AUTOMATION OF A NUMBER OF SIMILAR LABORATORIES WITHIN A SINGLE HOSPITAL

W. Heijser

BAZIS, University Hospital

Leyden, The Netherlands

ABSTRACT

In order to computerize clinical chemistry and haematology laboratories a large number of laboratory information systems is available at this moment. Generally these systems are designed for use by one laboratory. The existence of more similar laboratories within a single hospital is a complicating factor for the lab-automation, certainly when interactions between those laboratories are present.

The problems which may arise as a consequence of the existence of a number of similar laboratories within one hospital are treated in this paper. On the basis of the objectives of laboratory automation it is discussed which additional demands are made upon (a) labsystem(s) when more laboratories want to use it. Some models to handle this situation pass in review. Attention is given to the influence which the presence of a total hospital information system may have.
Finally, the approach which has been realized in our laboratory system LABZIS is discussed.

INTRODUCTION

During the past decade a large number of information systems for chemistry and haematology laboratories has been developed.
In the scope of this paper we want to divide the objectives of laboratory systems into three classes :
A. Improving the course of things within the laboratory, like enlarging the production-capacity with the available physical and human resources, and increasing the quality.
B. Support of the laboratory management, by providing better, more extensive, faster information.
C. Improved presentation of the laboratory to the (poli)clinics : faster service, fast retrieval of historical results. This is especially true if the laboratory system has been coupled to, or is part of, a Hospital Information System (HIS).

At first the need for automation arose at the larger laboratories (1965-70).
In order to be able to make head against the growing work-load, automation was absolutely necessary. Later on (1975-80), as a result of the decreasing hardware-prices, automation also became interesting to the medium-sized laboratories.

For this category many systems are available at this moment.

Often automation is hardly interesting to the smaller laboratories.
Sometimes even the opposite is true.
At small laboratories ($<$ 100 samples per day) everything can be looked over well, and manual systems often satisfy excellently.
In this situation automation can take time instead of yield time.

MORE LABORATORIES WITHIN ONE ORGANIZATION/HOSPITAL

These introductory remarks referred to the situation of (a hospital with) one independent laboratory. The hospitals for which we are working, mainly large university hospitals, generally have more than one laboratory, e.g. separate laboratories for chemistry, haematology, stat-tests, endocrinology, tests in cerebral spinal fluid, the children ward, etc. We also know hospitals which do not have one large central routine-lab, but in which (groups of) wards have their own laboratory (these hospitals are spread over a large number of buildings).

In such circumstances some things change with respect to the automation.
We want to comment on this situation in the light of the groups of objectives, mentioned in the preceding section.
(N.B. The following holds too, or even stronger, for one laboratory, divided into a number of more or less independent sub-laboratories).

Ad. A. When the laboratories concerned are fully independent of each other, every laboratory can determine for itself whether it introduces automation, and, if so, it can choose a system with an optimal fit to the procedures in this laboratory. However, often there will be some form of interaction between the various laboratories. Some examples of interaction are :

- joint sample collection
- some laboratories will have certain tests done by other labs
- as a result of this, some sight on each others progress is desired
- joint reporting (this also concerns B and C)
- joint invoicing (this also concerns B)
- exchange of staff

The existence of such interactions may have a large influence on the choice/design of a laboratory system.

Ad. B. The hospital- and the (overall) laboratory-management will prefer the information of the various laboratories to be presented as uniform as possible (insight into the progress, quality reports, surveys, possibly an overall-picture, etc.).

Ad. C. The presentation of the various laboratories to the (poli)clinics should
preferably have some uniformity too. Actually joint reporting is required.
Furthermore it is important that all historical test-results of a patient can be
retrieved at one go.
You may safely say that this is even essèntial if the lab system(s) is part of a
hospital information system.

All these considerations argue for a joint, or at least coordinated approach of the
automation of all laboratories within the hospital.

FORMS OF AUTOMATION OF MORE LABORATORIES

We mention some possibilities for the approach of automation in a number of
laboratories within one hospital :
(1) Every laboratory chooses completely independently its own system. It will be
    obvious that, in the light of the considerations in the previous section, this
    will cause a lot of problems.
    Furthermore, within this approach it will be difficult to bring the smaller
    laboratories to automation.
    An important advantage is that every laboratory can choose the most optimal
    system in this way.

(2) Each laboratory chooses a system (both hardware and software) from the same
    series, from the same manufacturer. A number of objections which apply in (1)
    is eliminated (e.g. interaction/coupling will be less complicated, uniform
    presentation).

(2') Like (2) but not with a separate computer for each lab system, but all systems
    running on one computer.
    Interaction between laboratories is now further simplified.

    Both for 1, 2 and 2' a combined database is an important advantage.

(3) One laboratory system, used by all laboratories.
    The system recognizes to which laboratory a user of the lab system belongs, and
    takes it into account in the (joint) programs and files.
These forms of automation in more laboratories vary from no cooperation (1) to a
fully integrated system (3). Of course all sorts of intermediate forms are possible.

We have chosen for the highest form of integration, viz. model (3).
In this framework we can meet the demands, mentioned ad A, B and C in the best way.
Before going further into the motives for this choice, and into the system itself,
three more remarks :

Firstly, model (1) provides each laboratory that wants to computerize, with the system most suited for this laboratory. If you want to use one system on more laboratories (3), this should be a very flexible system, usable under different circumstances (large and small labs, chemistry and haematology, etc.).

Secondly, whereas for (1) certain (small) laboratories would surely not computerize, for (3) automation of these labs is much more obvious :
introduction of a lab system now only requires adjusting of a number of system-parameters, filling (up) of files and installation of the necessary terminals.

This may be very useful, because it is expected that, for the sake of completeness (especially in the case of a total hospital information system, see also remarks ad B and C) there will be put pressure on such small laboratories by the hospital management to computerize too.

Thirdly, we have not yet brought up the cost-aspect. We will not deal with this subject extensively, we only remark that in our opinion model (3) is the most economical one.

APPLICATION IN LABZIS

Our laboratory system LABZIS is part of the Hospital Information System, which is used in the Netherlands in 8 (groups of) hospitals, with a total number of 10.000 beds. Each of these (groups of) hospitals has its own computer system (a double PDP 11/70 configuration). We refer to ref. (1) - (3) for further details about this HIS (its history, development, nature, the hospitals concerned, etc.).

The hospitals in question are big, for the greater part university hospitals, with 700-1200 beds. These hospitals have, without exception, not one but more laboratories, sometimes going up till 10-15 per hospital (examples are given in a previous section). The existence of so many laboratories is closely bound up with the university character of these hospitals. This situation is opposite to the one in the mostly smaller general hospitals (usually <600 beds), which generally have only one laboratory and which have the rare tests done by other specialized (external) laboratories.

LABZIS is a comprehensive laboratory system. A wide range of programs is available, including programs for
- order entry/sample registration
- sample-collection lists
- label printing
- work lists

- result entry, both manual and via a data-acquisition system
- authorization
- reporting, stat, daily, cumulatively and/or on request
- archiving
- invoicing
- management support, like reporting of the progress, day-, week-, month- and
  year-surveys
- quality control, among which a so called "delta-check" program

LABZIS is restricted in its capacity by only a few practical limits. The system
consists of about 60 start programs, 170 modules, 90.000 (FORTRAN) statements.

LABZIS was designed for and first employed in the Leyden University Hospital, in the
(large) Central Chemistry Laboratory (1972-1975). On behalf of the automation in a
second large laboratory in the same hospital, the Central Haematology Laboratory,
the lab system (programs and files) was almost completely duplicated. However, for
both laboratories the same (HIS) computer was used (so this was model (2') in the
previous section).
Consequently, from automation's point of view these laboratories were fully
independent, no interaction took place. Actually this was in agreement with the
working-method of both laboratories.

Afterwards a number of smaller laboratories in the Leyden Hospital has "moved in"
into one of both lab systems, but for these labs some functions of LABZIS could not
be performed independently. When e.g. the large laboratory authorized, or reported,
this was automatically done for the small labs too.

The same solution, duplicating of the lab system, was chosen one more time, in the
Rotterdam University Hospital Dijkzigt, again for the Central Chemistry and
Haematology laboratories.

Of course the question arose, what to do when a third and a fourth laboratory would
want to computerize, more or less independently of the other ones. Going on
duplicating programs and files ?

At this point we must mention that (till 1978) LABZIS had a serious restriction :
The maximum number of different tests in files and programs was limited at 254.
During the design of the system it was not foreseen that this maximum would ever
be reached. Actually this maximum turned out to be even too small for one large
laboratory, not to mention for a number of laboratories. This restriction of LABZIS
greatly affected our choice for the way of automation of the second laboratory.

In 1978-79 we removed the limit of 254 different tests, now the "limit" is 16.000.
After this action it became possible to switch over to model (3) : one laboratory
system for all labs, with a differentiation per lab within the programs. We have
performed this as follows :
- the labsystem consists of one set of programs and one set of files (one requests-
  file, one tests-reference file, etc.), which are jointly used by all laboratories.
- the laboratories concerned are numbered 1,2,3,... (till the maximum of 32)
- for each user of the labsystem a permission-matrix is defined.
  The size of this matrix is the maximum number of laboratories (32) x the number
  of LABZIS-functions for which a separate permission is required (e.g. order entry,
  worklists, authorization, reporting). Therefore it is possible to indicate for
  each user of the labsystem for each function for each laboratory :
  permitted / not permitted
- for each test in the tests-reference file it is indicated in which laboratory this
  test is done
- with each request in the requests-file it is stored in which laboratory the
  request was entered. When a request has been finished, this item is also stored
  in the database.
- the file with all sorts of system-parameters has a general part, and a part for
  each of the laboratories concerned. If e.g. differences in the execution of
  programs are desired between the laboratories, this can be indicated in this file.

With this framework we are able to offer an "own" lab system to each laboratory, in
which the desired interaction/cooperation with other laboratories can easily be
adjusted, and in which individual wishes of certain laboratories can in principle
be met.
We can "create" fully isolated laboratories (system-users of these laboratories
only have permissions for their own requests and tests), whereas all kinds of
cross-permissions are also possible (e.g. sight on the progress / results of
other labs, joint reporting of some / all labs, combined surveys, combined
retrieval of historical results, etc.).

REFERENCES :

(1) Bakker, A.R., Scope and limitations of a mini-based centralized hospital
    information system. Proc. MEDINFO 80, 505.
(2) Bakker, A.R., Costers, L., Mol, J.L., Concluding report on the NOBIN-ZIS
    project 1972-1976 (available from BAZIS, University Hospital Leyden, the
    Netherlands).
(3) Bunt, v.d., Evaluation of the hospital information system (HIS), Leyden
    (available from BAZIS, University Hospital Leyden, the Netherlands).

EXPERIENCE WITH A MUMPS BASED SYSTEM FOR CLINICAL CHEMISTRY.

R.R.O'Moore*, Wm.Clayton Love*, J.Ryan+, J.Ratcliffe+, J.McSweeney*,
A.Cranny* and L.Field*.
* Federated Dublin Voluntary Hospital, James's Street, Dublin 8.
+ Health Computing Ireland Limited.

Summary.

A MUMPS based laboratory system is described which has been implemented
during the merging of two large clinical biochemical departments within
new premises. The success of the project to date is attributed to the
versatility of the software and the speed with which it was altered to
suit a rapidly changing working environment.

Introduction.

The Federated Dublin Voluntary Hospitals comprises seven general
hospitals of between 150-350 beds each with a total of 1,200 beds.
Between them they provide a complete range of medical and surgical specialities. The hospitals are sited in a ring within a radius of two
miles around the centre of the increasingly traffic congested centre of
Dublin (Fig.1). Until early 1980 the laboratory services had been
provided by centralization of single specialities in three of the Federated Hospitals and one specialty in the nearby University Medical
School. In late 1980 the relocation and merging of the F.D.V.H. Laboratory Medicine Services with those of the St. James's Hospital (1000
beds) in a new central laboratory on the St. James's site commenced.
Small emergency satellite laboratories were to remain in each of the
Federated Hospitals. It was apparent that this enforced centralization
would place an increased strain on the already inadequate inter-hospital
communications network. In mid 1980 the Central Biochemistry Department
computer system was reviewed to determine whether further computerization
might provide a solution.

The Problem.

The Central Biochemistry Department has a full range of automated
equipment. The annual workload is 140,000 tests per annum, giving a
yearly output of over 750,000 results. There is also a specialist
endocrinology division with an output of over 50,000 tests per year,
which provides a service to a large number of hospitals throughout the
country. An IBM System 3 Model 4 was introduced in 1977. The

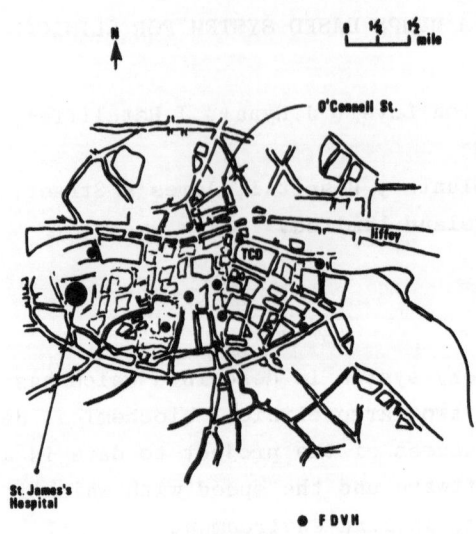

FIG.1   CENTRAL DUBLIN.

implementation was partially successful, some of the problems encountered have been reported [1].   In the endocrinology department the computer became the'linchpin' being most useful in replacing the onerous data processing tasks in radioimmunoassay and in providing reports and basic patient enquiry facilities for specialized clinics.   Its presence enabled the endocrinology division to increase efficiency, expand the workload by a factor of four with no increase in staff.

Following an extensive review of the system it was clear that because of limitations in both hardware and software it was unlikely to solve the problem.   The available turnkey systems were then surveyed during which time several agreed constraints and conditions emerged:-
1) No additional funding was available - the present system being leased.
2) The proposed replacement should fulfil all the performance criteria of computers for large laboratories.[2]
3) High quality local maintenance of both hardware and software should be guaranteed.
4) The system should be capable of providing simultaneous multi task activities for at least seven remote sites.
5) It should be designed to form the nucleus of a proposed total path-ology system.
6) Endocrinology packages would have to be implemented first and also over a very short time.
7) The computer should be capable of taking on the additional workload

and instrumentation of St. James's Hospital Laboratory - 250,000 additional tests.

8) The system should be versatile.   It would have to be partially implemented before the merger.   Due to trade union negotiations this date was unknown.

The market survey revealed that several available systems could meet the requirements of 2, 3, 4, 5 and 7 but not the other requirements. One company, Health Care Ireland Ltd., offered a MUMPS based 'Lab 55' package with the configuration shown in Figure 2.   The cost of this system was well in excess of our present budget.   However, the problem was solved by replacing the expensive data acquisition modules, necessary because of the unsuitability of MUMPS for complex arithmetic manipulations, with low cost microprocessors and standard interfaces designed for our IBM system.[3]

Several other reasons led us to accept this solution.   For example, the operating software was written in MUMPS which, being non compiled, allows for the necessary rapid programme changes.   It was also agreed that endocrinology (potentially the most difficult task) would be implemented first and that the most useful facilities from our IBM system would be incorporated.   The hardware manufacturers had a strong base in Ireland.   The vendors had several ex-members of the F.D.V.H. computer department on their staff.   We believed this would save both systems analysis and implementation time.   Finally, HCIL were in the process of installing a MUMPS based patient administration system in three of the Federated Dublin Voluntary Hospitals.   A future link with our laboratory system seemed probable.

The Hardware Configuration.
This is shown in Figure 3.

Software.
The system is run on Digital Standard MUMPS (DSM11) a multi user time sharing system which has several improved facilities over earlier versions of MUMPS.

General Design.
The system provides the features found in most biochemical laboratory computers.   However it has several important advantages:
- It was designed as a transferable package.   Most of the individual laboratory characteristics are 'system' table driven.   The tables are created and maintained by a suite of interactive programmes which allow amendment at anytime.

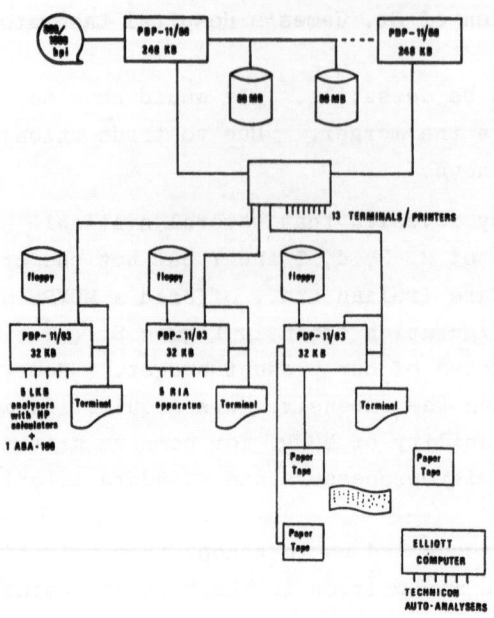

FIG.2. A LAB 55 SYSTEM.

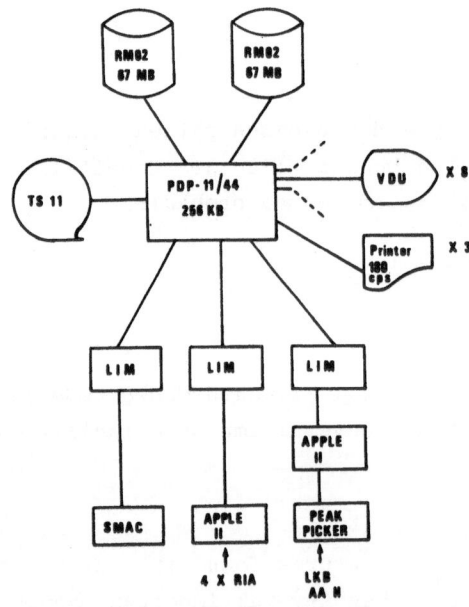

FIG.3. THE PROPOSED SYSTEM.

- It has the ability to smooth out the large peaks and troughs in the laboratory work patterns. Heavy processing and file updating tasks are effectively buffered from the operator by foreground VDU tasks linking to a background executive.
- The system allows data processing to progress automatically as far as possible through the system. In conjunction with the operation of the background executive the design aims to set up file entries, valid-date result data and prepare report data as early as possible. This creates the minimum delay when the next stage of the process is carried out by the operator.
- The ability to schedule and print all types of reports, worklists, etc. at any specified location. The print scheduler initiates prints in priority order at any local or remote terminal.

File Design.
The design is based on five main groups of files (Globals).
(1) The main patient identity global is indexed by other globals allow-ing access by name, hospital number, laboratory number, date of birth, consultant sode or location code.
(2) The work in progress global is subdivided by type of worklist – these are divided into pages designed to serve as a plate loading list for automated analytical equipment or as a convenient worklist format for manual tests.
(3) Result data is held in a form which assists the efficiency in both printing reports and retrieving data for patient enquiry.
(4) There are various dynamic work queues associated with functions such as background tasks, worklist printing and report printing.
(5) There are several system table globals which relate to core data. For example, test characteristics, groups of tests (profiles), worklist formats, result comment codes, clinical details codes, location codes and consultant codes. Each of these globals are under the control of interactive programmes. They may be altered at any time during the operation of the system.

Principal Operation Facilities.

(1) Patient Registration	:	Either before or after test requesting and processing.
(2) Test Requesting	:	With or without prior patient registrat-ion
(3) Worklist Management	:	Preview-Print-status display,modification.

(4) Result Input	:	Manual - via worklist by sample or test.
	:	On line (SMAC,LKB-Rack Gamma-RIA)
	:	Via paper tape (LKB Wallach RIA)
	:	By 'Peak Picker" (LKB AAII).
(5) Quality Control	:	On line/Off line
	:	Batch/Daily/Term Reports.
(6) Result Authorization	:	Selective by patient
	:	Out of range results
	:	Enter comments
	:	Beyond credibility limits.
(7) Reports	:	Daily and cumulative.
(8) Workload Statistics	:	Histograms - Work flow patterns.
(9) Administrative	:	End of day listings by hospital ward or consultant
	:	List daily requests alphabetical/sequential
	:	List tests outstanding.
(10) Patient enquiry	:	Patient Hospital Number.
	:	Name or part of name.
	:	Laboratory number
	:	Date of birth.
	:	Location code Hospital/Ward
	:	Consultant code.
(11) Remote printing	:	Via Modem any of above reports.
(12) Back-up/Security	:	Standard MUMPS back-up at end of day.
	:	Journaling during day.
(13) Archiving	:	Inactive data held on demountable discs.

Progress.

The computer was installed in March 1981.   The endocrinology system was
implemented in June.   This took longer than expected, partly due to
local circumstances and partly to the frequent problem of the vendor
overestimating the similarity of bench level laboratory procedures. All
are agreed it is superior to the IBM system and compares very favourably
with a recently described system without on-line data acquisition.[4]

The main laboratory system has had a difficult implementation.
This was largely due to uncertainty in the timing of the move.   Initially
implementation of the Technicon SMA 12/60 commenced .   This was dropped
before completion when trade union agreement to the merger was reached
unexpectedly early.   The move took place in September and the computerization of the Technicon SMAC commenced in early November.   Following
a few delays it is now running successfully in parallel with the manual

system.   It is intended to take on an increasing proportion of the
laboratory workload (700 samples/day) each day until the system is
fully 'live' early in 1982.   The ability to print reports and end of
day listings via a modem in peripheral hospitals has also been demonstrated.

Conclusions and Future Development.
The project to date has been successful.   When one considers the
pressures engendered by the rapidly changing environment the speed with
which software changes have been made is impressive.   It is intended
to introduce remote reporting of laboratory reports as soon as possible.
The system will then link with the Haematology department to form the
nucleus of the projected total Pathology system.

The successful exchange of computers under difficult circumstances
has been due to several factors:
- The previous system was being leased.
- Hardware costs have reduced rapidly.
- Implementation problems were simplified by the presence of ex-members
  of our computer departmental staff in the implementation term.
- The MUMPS package has proved to be versatile.

It would seem that with such rapid changes in computer technology
it may be wiser to pay high rental charges rather than purchase.

References.

1.   Ryan J.   Proceedings of the A.C.B.I., 2, 23-24 (1979).

2.   Porth A. J.   What about turnkey systems. Medical Informatics Europe,
                   Berlin (1979). Lecture Notes in Medical Informatics,
                   Vol. 5. Ed.: B. Barber, F. Grêmy, K. Überla and G.
                   Wagner, p. 303-311, Springer-Verlag Berlin Heidelberg
                   New York 1979.

3.   Ryan J.   The development of a low cost laboratory interface unit.
               Medical Informatics Europe, Dublin (1982). Lecture Notes
               in Medical Informatics, Vol. 16. Ed.: R. R. O'Moore,
               B. Barber, P.L. Reichertz and F. Roger, p. 762-766,
               Springer-Verlag Berlin Heidelberg New York 1982

4.   Mosley J.   A computer based laboratory record system in an endocrin-
                 ology laboratory. Annals of Clinical Biochemistry (1981),
                 18, 169-176.

Monitoring Antibiotic Sensitivity and Bacterial Infections in a Hospital

K.F. Trespe, E. Wolters, I. Tripatzis

Department of Biometrics and Medical Informatics
Department Microbiology and Hygiene
Medical School Hannover
Karl-Wiechert-Allee 9
3000 Hannover 61
F.R. Germany

Abstract

Data collected during the interactive reporting process in a microbiology laboratory opens up the possibility to monitor continuously the development of resistance of microorganisms to antibiotics and occurrences of infectious hospitalism in early stages. After installing a reporting system in the laboratory all reports are evaluated under these aspects. This paper discusses the first results obtained.

Kurzfassung

Die interaktive Datenerfassung im Mikrobiologischen Laboratorium ermoeglicht die kontinuierliche Auswertung der Resistenzentwicklung von Bakterien gegen Antibiotika und die Frueherkennung des infektioesen Hospitalismus. Alle mikrobiologischen Befunde werden routinemaessig ausgewertet. Diese Arbeit berichtet ueber die ersten Ergebnisse des Auswertungssystems.

Introduction

Important clinical problems such as the control of infectious hospitalism and resistance developments of bacteria against antibiotics can only be solved by data processing facilities in the microbiological laboratory. Conventional methods for comparison and evaluation of data from hundreds of patients have had only limited results. Consequently it is necessary to apply data processing techniques to reduce the burden of the laboratory personnel and to achieve better results for patient care in a hospital (1,6).

Description of the System

Since 1977 reporting in microbiology at the Medical School Hannover is carried out by the interactive carrier system DADIMOPS (DAta DIrected Medically Oriented Processing System, 7). The goal of the implemented reporting system is a complete EDP-support for the laboratory. The main functional areas are

- report data acquisition,
- report storage for direct access from every authorized terminal within the hospital,
- transmission of printed reports to the requesting ward,
- result documentation in the laboratory,
- administrative support.

Approximately 60,000 reports are processed each year. Report data are acquired online directly in each laboratory as soon as the data are available. Thus an error prone transscription process is avoided. Immediately upon acquisition physicians and nurses at the wards have online access to the reports by the Patient Information Display System within the Medical System Hannover (MSH, 2). In addition printed reports are sent daily to the requesting wards by pneumatic tube. All reports remain in direct access for a time period of about six months. After that time they are usually transferred to magnetic tape for further evaluation (4).

Report Evaluation

Besides the patient oriented daily routine report processing all bacteriological data are evaluated under the aspects of

- continuous antibiotic sensitivity control
  and
- early detection of infectious hospitalism.

The analysis of bacterial resistance to antibiotics is essential for a successful therapy and an effective solution of bacterial problems in a hospital (5). Every three months the actual bacterial situation for all units is traced. Fig. 1 shows the evaluated data of the intensive care units of the Medical Scool Hannover in 1980. Resistance analyses of other hospital units, especially outpatient clinics, show different profiles. These differences are certainly based on the specimen tested (e. g. surgical intensive care unit vs. urology ward) and on different medication habits of physicians. Therefore the evaluations have to be made separately for each unit or ward (3).

Fig. 1: Antibiotic resistance of the most frequent bacteria in intensive care units

gram—negative rods	n=	Ampi-cillin	Azlo-cillin	Mezlo-cillin	Ticar-cillin	Cefa-zolin	Cefo-xitin	Cefu-roxim	Cefo-taxim	Genta-micin	Tobra-micin	Co-Tri-moxazol
Pseudomonas aeruginosa	384	100	32	62	44	100	100	100	61	NT	9	90
Escherichia coli	251	22	17	14	14	14	11	10	0	4	2	4
Enterobacter cloacae	224	96	60	52	58	94	94	52	25	30	15	4
Klebsiella pneumoniae	164	96	61	46	77	18	3	5	0	14	5	6
Proteus mirabilis	113	33	9	7	9	26	5	23	0	0	3	12
Proteus indol +	52	94	16	19	8	93	21	64	2	1	0	7
Serratia marcescens	21	78	9	9	17	93	27	87	0	9	4	9

n = number of infected patients
Antibiotic resistance in percent

This information may serve as a medication guideline if patient specific data are not available and therapy with antibiotics has to be started immediately. The continuation of this therapy can then be based on the first laboratory results. The therapy is especially monitored for intensive care unit patients by condensed weekly printouts of the reports.

At the Medical School Hannover the following developments are continuously monitored:

■ changes (increase) in the frequency of isolated microorganism on wards
■ accumulation of bacterial strains with similar resistance patterns
■ resistance (changes) of certain bacterial species to specific antibiotics.

Observations covering several years serve as a basis for the valuation of these incidents. Seasonal relationships are taken into consideration.

Regular surveillance of these events enables the early detection of infections hospitalism and of developments of bacterial resistance to antibiotics thus leading to appropriate countermeasures.

For example in October 1980 the number of patients infected with Pseudomonas aeruginosa in an intensive care unit increased from an average of 15 per month to 32. Suitable precautions were taken and the number of infected patients dropped during the next month (Fig. 2).

Fig. 2: Infection rates within an intensive care unit of the Medical School Hannover in 1980

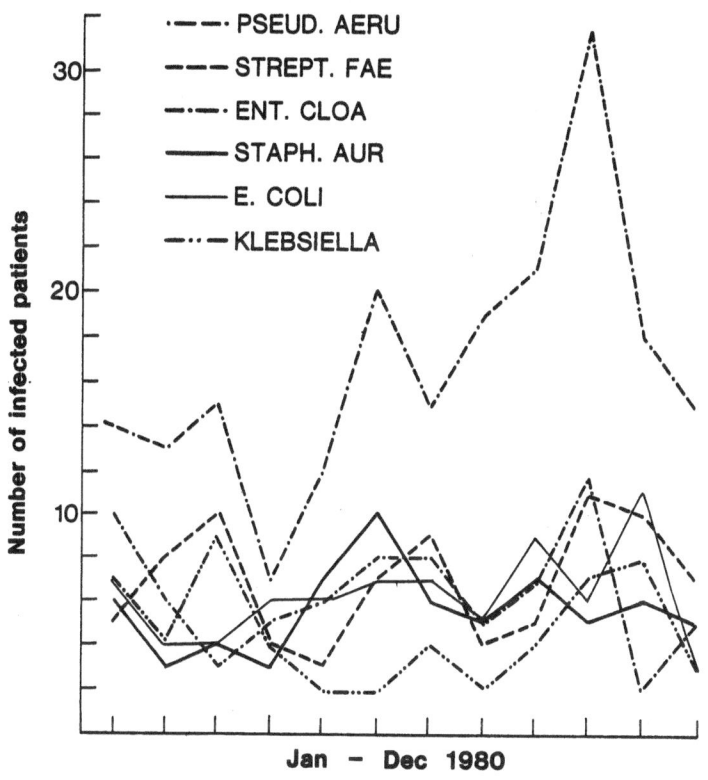

An additional benefit of these evaluations is an improved quality control of the laboratory and of therapeutical actions. From January 1979 to February 1980 evaluations indicated a rapidly increasing resistance of bacteria to Amicacin (Fig. 3). The investigation of this development led to a technical error in the laboratory process. After correction of this error the resistance to Amicacin returned to normal rates.

Fig. 3: Development of antibiotic susceptibility to Amikacin

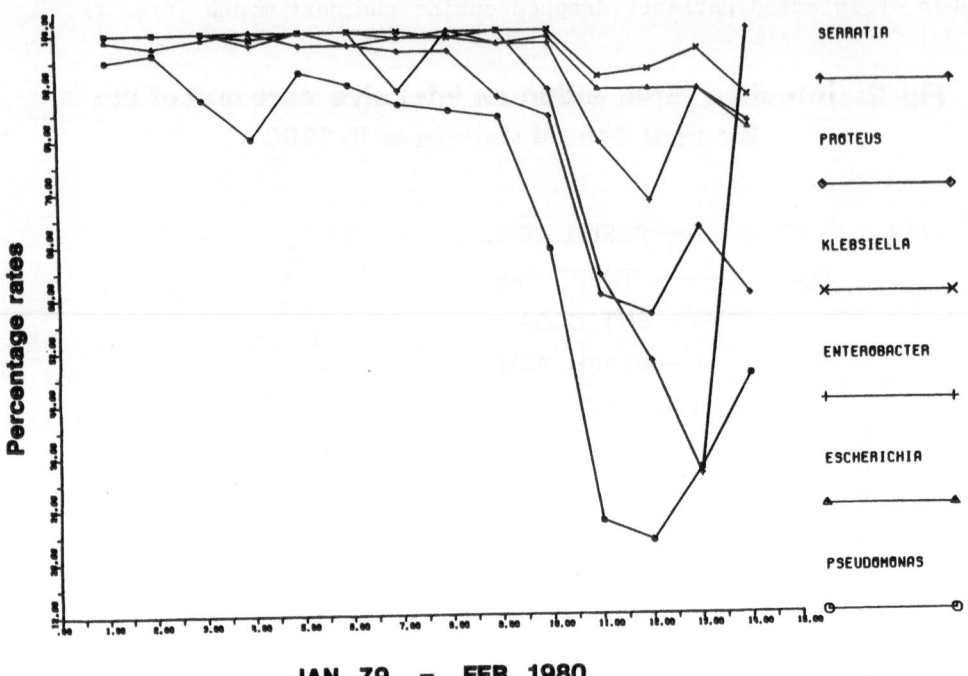

JAN 79 — FEB 1980

Conclusion

The long term analysis of resistance of bacteria to antibiotics and accumulated report listings combined with the experiences of clinical and laboratory personnel are being used to develop a long term strategy for the therapy with antibiotics in the hospital. In addition the evaluation of microbiologic reports has proven to be useful in clinical practice, since attitude changes in bacterial infections are recognized immediately and appropriate actions can be taken.

References

(1) BERGQVIST, F., BENGTSSON, S.: The BACTLAB System - A Data System for Bacteriological Routine. Computer Programs in Biomedicine, 4 (3), 1975, 144-157

(2) REICHERTZ, P.L.: The Medical System Hannover (MSH). In: COLLEN, M.F.(Ed.). Hospital Computer Systems, New York, 1974, 598-661

(3) Trespe, K.F., Malottke, R.: Keim und Resistenzkontrolle in einem Klinikum. Vortrag 26.GMDS - Jahrestagung, Giessen, 21.-23.9.1981

(4) TRESPE, K.F., TRIPATZIS, I., WOLTERS, E., POTEL,J.: Interaktive Keim- und Resistenzueberwachung im Krankenhaus - Modell Medizinische Hochschule Hannover. Hyg. + Med., 6, 1981, 100-104

(5) TRIPATZIS, I.: Zur Frueherkennung des infektioesen Hospitalismus mit Hilfe der Datenverarbeitung in der Mikrobiologie. Fortschritte der Medizin, 89 (12), 1971, 526/527

(6) TRIPATZIS, I., FREIESLEBEN, H., HENKEL, W.: Laufende Ermittlung des Resistenzspektrums durch Datenverarbeitung in der bakteriologischen Routinediagnostik. Zbl. Bakt. Hyg., I. Abt. Orig. A 220, 1972, 217-223

(7) WOLTERS, E.: Generalized Communication Tools in Medical Systems. In: LINDBERG, D.A.B., KAIHARA, S. (Eds.). MEDINFO 80, Proc. of the Third World Conference on Medical Informatics, Amsterdam, 1980, 744-748

DISTRIBUTED INFORMATION PROCESSING IN HISTOPATHOLOGY

Volker Loy, Ulrich Gross
Institut für Pathologie

Hartmut Enke
Wissenschaftliche Einrichtung für Medizinische Informatik

Klinikum Steglitz, Freie Universität Berlin
Hindenburgdamm 30, D 1000 Berlin 45, Germany

1. SUMMARY:

In recent years more and more small computers are used in pathology. The main purpose of these dedicated systems is to assist with clerical tasks. They are mostly too small to be integrated into hospital information systems and do not allow information retrieval on a large scale. The hitherto often proposed centralized systems for data acquisition, data processing and information retrieval use central computer facilities very effectively but are not flexible enough to meet the needs of the pathologists. To avoid these disadvantages, we decided to run a medium sized dedicated systems in the Department of Pathology. It offers many possibilities of larger systems and is conveniently connected to the central medical computer via teleprocessing. Data collected centrally are used in routine work on the "department computer" and need not be collected twice. Mass data to be archived can be transmitted to the central facilities; print files either go to the slow but pretty printing wheel printers in the Department of Pathology or are shifted to the quick but less refined line printers of the central computer. On the other hand, design and availability of the peripheral facilities are completely managed by the pathologists themselves, thus bringing the computer as close as possible to the location where it is needed.

2. INTRODUCTION

Efforts have been made in the last few years (3) to run mini computers in histopathology. These systems are now mostly used in order to assist with clerical functions. The Departments of Pathology and Neuropathology at the Steglitz Hospital of
the Free University in Berlin have been using a medium-sized dedicated system connected to the central medical computer since 1980. We think this new approach to the
old problem of data processing in histopathology avoids the pitfall of pure information retrieval systems or pure clerical systems.

3. PURPOSE:

a) Data acquisition from the various departments (1400 surgical, 800 autopsy reports per year). Printing the reports in a typewriter-like style without delay.

b) Processing collected reports in the Department of Pathology in order to get the
   input for an already existing natural language retrieval system.

c) Updated lists of diagnoses and patients should be printed at least once a day in
   the order of the laboratory accession number. An alphabetical list of the patients
   should be also provided once a day.

d) Easy interactive access to all reports, at least of the past 6 months.

e) At least some assistance in handling texts.

f) A data structure applicable to different problems.

g) Communication and sharing of the workload with the central computer of the hospital, i.e., access to the centrally stored files of the patient data and use of
   the central printers, disks and tapes processing mass data.

h) Management of the computer by the Departments of Pathology and Neurpathology.

i) Easy access to the computer for unskilled users.

4. METHODS

Hardware: The computer used is a Wang 2200 VS with a maximum store of 512 KB, actually we use 192 KB. Exchangeable disc: 75 MB. 1 magnetic tape unit (1600 bpi). 7 visual display units (vdu). 2 wheel printers. 1 diskette drive. 3 lines for teleprocessing. 2 of the vdus are located near the cpu, 2 in the library of the Department of Pathology, 2 at a distance of about 300 m, the last in the Department of Neuropathology as remote workstation. One of the teleprocessing lines connects the Wang 2200 VS with the central computer of the hospital (Siemens 7738), another connects the vdu of the Department of Neuropathology and the third is for planned extensions.

Software: The Wang 2200 VS is supplied with a "virtual memory" and provides each user with 1 MB. It supports multiple workstations. The logic sections of identical programs are automatically shared by different users, thus eliminating unnecessary duplicating. The overall design was established in close collaboration between the Department of Pathology and the Central Computer Department of the hospital. Application programs have been written in COBOL.

Data: Primary subject of the whole system is the biopsy report. It is stored completely in one master file. Primary key is the laboratory accession number, be it for biopsy reports, autopsy reports or the Department of Pathology or Neuropathology. The most recent report of a patient refers to all prior examinations.

The master file has several sources:

a) Patient identification data: they are collected manually (outpatients) or copied from the file in the central medical computer (inpatients). b) Contributor's address: file of contributors. c) Pathologist: user file which includes additional information for the print program (e.g., full academic degree, etc.). d) Specimen: file of specimens containing information on topography and operation. e) Prior examinations: they are supplied by the master file itself. f) "New" data: workstations.

All information concerning one case flows into the master file. From it, all or part of the information comes back to the pathologist. When data has been collected and the examination terminated, all further processing starts with this file. In order to get the different information in one file the structure has to be quite flexible: any department should have the opportunity to collect its data according to different formats. It should be possible to change formats or to collect new sorts of data at any time without changing the whole system. The record of the master file is divided into four parts: 6 bytes: used temporarely, e.g., current user of the record. 15 bytes: primary key. 4 bytes: length. 1975 bytes: variable data.

Primary key:

Byte 1:   Department and area (e.g. "A" Department of Pathology, autopsy; "O"
            Department of Neuropathology, biopsies).

Byte 2-4:   year including century, e.g. "981"

Byte 5-9:   laboratory accession number.

Byte 2-3:   number of additional reports concerning one laboratory accession number.

Byte 4-13: type of record, e.g., "AA" patient identification data, "EA" diagnosis
            of biopsy report.

Byte 14-15: subsequent number for one record type.

There are 4 alternate keys in the patient identification data: name, identification number, admission number of the hospital, maiden name.

5. ORGANIZATION:

a) Patient care: Patient identification data are collected centrally for all inpatients and provided for distributed systems via teleprocessing once a day. Identification data of inpatients can be copied from the file received from the central medical computer; outpatient data are collected manually. New data are printed once a day as the updated part of a list containing identification data and diagnosis. The list from the Department of Pathology is printed on the central printer, since it is considerably longer than the updated parts of the Department of Neuropathology, which is printed in the Department of Pathology. Furthermore once a day an alphabetical list of all patients is provided for members of the staff who are not acquainted with the computer. This list is also sent to the central printer. As soon as the pathologists have dictated the reports, the typists add the text to the patient identification data and the reports are printed on the wheel printers in the Department of Pathology.

b) Management, science, teaching: For the management of the department the system provides different information: examined material with reference to contributors, examined material with reference to different pathologists, completion of reports. The system is not a word processing system, nevertheless the usual editor provides a lot of opportunities to rationalize the typing of all sorts of texts. E.g., there are now several pathologists who are typing their drafts of scientific papers using the proceduralized system editor. In addition, we have generated a small system of collecting scientific references, which can be printed according to different criteria. The scientific purpose of the system is natural language retrieval, which is not discussed here. In the teaching area, we have collected multiple choice questions for the students.

6. DISCUSSION:

Many papers dealing with data processing in pathology regarded documentation, i.e. data retrieval, as the most important problem. This too was the sole purpose of the magnetic tape cassette system we used formerly (2). In recent years, mini computers have been discussed more and more as a tool for supporting essentially clerical tasks in histopathology (3). We think there is an unnoticed gap between these two modes of application, both of which offer certain advantages but neglect new application possibilities of data processing. Retrieval systems require good data collecting systems and large computer facilities. This means considerable expense, which can be covered only by central computer departments. But their only purpose is data retrieval. Though pathologists accept the possibilities and the importance of data retrieval, they often do not accept the consequences of a system run by another department. One solution seemed to be separating the pathologist from data processing: the routine work is done in a conventional manner without interference of a computer, and documentation is linked in a secondary step. This is certainly not practicable, because, once data processing is separated from routine work one will always find good arguments showing that it is less important than other things at any given time. The other way, i.e., using mini computers, offers interesting possibilities for the pathologist (3). He can be supplied by the manufacturer with a simple and rather inexpensive system which solves more or less all clerical problems. Moreover word processing systems are now used more and more in order to save typists. The disadvantage of mini computers is that they are strongly bound to a particular purpose: clerical tasks. Apart from that, the small computers offer little support, or they have to be enlarged at a considerable expense. Communication with larger systems is impossible or difficult. After disappointing experiences with a centralized system and increasing knowledge about the possibilities of data processing in pathology, we decided in 1978 to use a medium sized system. Tasks exceeding its scope are transfered to the central medical computer, e.g., data retrieval is done by the combined use of a commercial retrieval system and a natural language system (1,4), whereas preparing data and updating the thesaurus can be done in the Department of Pathology at any time. If large resources like line printers are needed, data are switched to the central computer. If a pretty printed output is needed, we use our own wheel printer, as for all reports. On the other hand, archiving, sorting and merging is done on the central system. A very important development is the growing use of the computer by unexperienced doctors for personal purposes, like typing darfts or maintaining their personal files of scientific references. Thus perhaps a point will eventually be reached, where the computer is no longer a foreign body but a simple tool as any other in pathology. We think the first step on this way was the decision to bring the computer to the pathologist and not the pathologist to the computer.

7. CONCLUSIONS:

a) Running a medium sized dedicated system now offers many facilities of larger computers, a prerequisite of getting familiar with data processing for unskilled users.

b) It can be operated by pathologists themselves.

c) Integration into the central computer system makes available the central facilities to the pathologists without disturbing their routine work by the well-known disadvantages of large centralized systems. Both components can be optimized to the benefit of the other.

d) Distributed system design leads to flexible solutions which suit the needs of the user as close as possible.

8. REFERENCES:

(1) Loy,V., Fabricius, W., Gross, U.: Retrieval and processing of biopsiy findings in pathology. Fifth Congress of the European Society of Pathology, Wien, October 6-3, 1975.

(2) Loy, V., Gross, U.: Erfassung von bioptischen Befunden im Institut für Pathologie. In: Reichertz, Holthoff: Methoden der Informatik in der Medizin (Springer, Berlin 1975).

(3) Ries,P., Küsel, W.: EDV-System auf Mikroprozessor-Basis im Pathologischen Institut Hameln. Verh.Dtsch.Ges.Path. 1979, 63: 552

(4) Röttger,P., Reul,H., Klein, I., Sunkel, H.: The automatic handling and statistical evaluation of pathologic-anatomical findings. Meth.Inform.Med.1969, 8:19-26.

COMPUTERISATION OF A NON-INVASIVE METHOD FOR THE DETERMINATION OF CARDIAC OUTPUT

Richard B Richardson* MSc
Keith J Sawdon   * BSc
Owen C Finnegan   **MRCP
Geoffrey T R Lewis **MSc

Correspondence : G T R Lewis
Respiratory Department
Bristol Royal Infirmary
Bristol   BS2 8HW

1.0 SUMMARY

Previous determination of cardiac output, using indirect Fick carbon dioxide (CO_2) rebreathing methods, have required graphical analyses derived from multi-channel polygraph recordings. This technique is time consuming and prone to transcription errors, repeated measurements become inappropriate and the results are not immediately available. A computer program written in MINC-BASIC (V 1.1) has been developed using a DEC-MINC 11/03 system, incorporating both data acquisition and real time analysis. The Program is flexible, allowing operator interaction in both controlling the experiment and reviewing the collected data for any experimental or physiological artefact prior to final analysis. The Computer system now enables this previously impractical, theoretical method to be used routinely in a clinical environment as a simple, non-invasive determination of cardiac output.

2.0 INTRODUCTION

To determine cardiac output by direct methods, invasive arterial catheterisation is required. However, the less hazardous and technically less demanding non-invasive methods are preferable. The CO_2 rebreathing method of Winsborough (1) to determine cardiac output is one application of the Fick principle, which states that flow can be calculated from the uptake or removal of a component of blood and its veno-arterial content difference. Considering CO_2 and blood flow through the lungs (equivalent to cardiac output) the Fick principle can be written:

$$\dot{Q} = \frac{\dot{V}CO_2}{C_{\bar{v}}CO_2 - C_aCO_2}$$

$\dot{Q}$ = Cardiac output

$\dot{V}CO_2$ = Carbon dioxide output

$C_{\bar{v}}CO_2$ = Mixed venous CO_2 content

C_aCO_2 = Arterial CO_2 content

---

*   Department of Medical Physics, Bristol Royal Infirmary, Bristol BS2 8HW
** Department of Respiratory Physiology, Bristol Royal Infirmary, Bristol BS2 8HW

The Winsborough method uses a simple differential mass flow equation to describe the rate of change of alveolar gas concentrations by the addition of CO_2 from the pulmonary blood flow. This implies a mono-exponential rise of alveolar CO_2 concentration asymptotically towards the mixed venous CO_2 concentration.

The rate of rise of alveolar CO_2 is measured during an "Oxygen rebreathe" (2) and the mixed venous CO_2 concentration is measured during a "Carbon Dioxide rebreathe" (3); both measurements are made while the subject is exercising on the cycle ergometer with the apparatus shown in Figure 1.

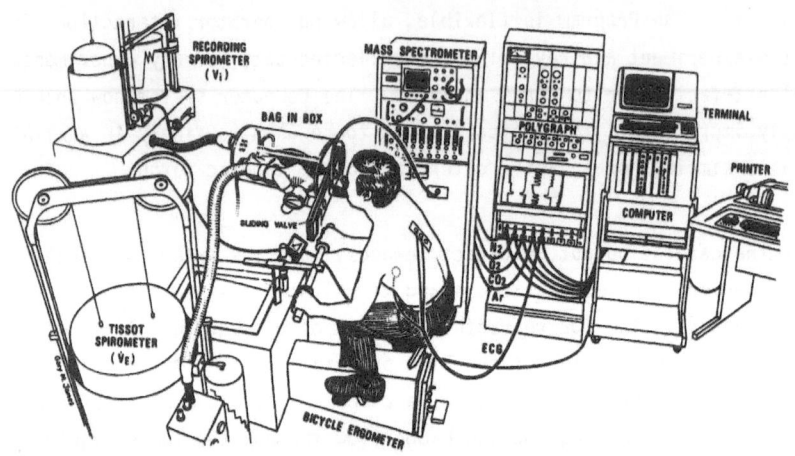

Figure 1
Apparatus and experimental layout used to obtain computerised non-invasive determination of caridac output.

3.0 METHOD

3.1 "Oxygen - Rebreathe" At the end of a normal expiration the subject inspired a carbon dioxide- free gas mixture (40% O_2, 60% N_2) and then rebreathed (45 breaths/ min) for 10-15 seconds. The fractional alveolar CO_2 concentration was monitored at the lips by a respiratory mass spectrometer (Centronics Q806) and recorded by the computer system sampling at 20Hz.

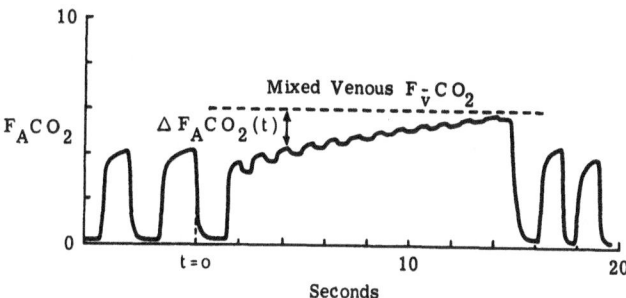

Figure 2

Alveolar CO2 concentraiton during the O2-rebreathe, where:-
$\Delta FACO2$ = $FVCO2$ - $FACO2$ (t)
FVCO2 = Estimated mixed venous carbon dioxide concentration derived from the CO2 rebreathe.

3.2 "Carbon Dioxide - Rebreathe" At the end of a normal expiration the subject inspired a gas mixture (40% O_2, balance N_2) primed with a CO_2 concentration which was slightly higher than the expected FVCO2, and then rebreathed (45 breaths/min) until a classical (3) 'plateau' had been achieved.

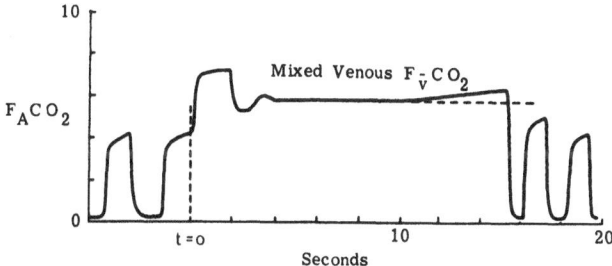

Figure 3

Alveolar CO2 concentration reaching a plateau during the CO2 rebreathe.

The operator was now able to review the data obtained during these two rebreathing manoeuvres by displaying the mass spectrometer recordings shown in Figures 2 and 3 using the full graphics facilities of the MINC system's VT105 terminal.

Having selected the relevant data from the two displayed recordings by interactive programming, a semi-logarithmic graph of

$\ln \Delta FCO2 = \ln (FVCO2 - FACO2(t))$ against time was plotted

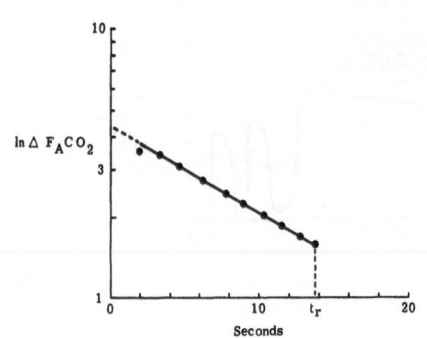

$$\text{Intercept} = \ln\{F_{\bar{V}}CO_2 - F_ACO_2(t_0)\}$$

$$\text{Slope} = \ln \{\frac{F_{\bar{V}}CO_2 - F_ACO_2(t_0)}{F_{\bar{V}}CO_2 - F_ACO_2(t_r)}\} \frac{1}{t_r}$$

where t_r = rebreathing time

Figure 4

Semi-logarithmic graph of $\ln \Delta FCO2 = \ln (FVCO2 - FACO2(t))$ against time (t).

The best straight line (least squares linear regression) drawn through the data points was extrapolated back to the intercept on the ordinate at time t = 0. The values derived from the intercept and slope of this line were then used to calculate cardiac output.

$$\dot{Q} = \frac{V_A \cdot \lambda \cdot \text{Slope}}{\alpha_{b\ell} \ (P_b - 47)}$$

$\dot{Q}$ = Cardiac output

V_A = Alveolar volume

$\alpha_{b\ell}$ = Solubility coefficient of CO_2 in blood

P_b = Barometric pressure

47 = SVP of H_2O at $37^{\circ}C$

λ is a correction for the CO_2 binding power of 'lung tissue and static pulmonary blood' and is a function of the intercept of this semi-logarithmic graph (1).

105

4.0 THE PROGRAM

The program was written in MINC-BASIC (V1.1), it is built up from five inter-linked modules (Figure 5) for calibration, data acquisition and final calculations.

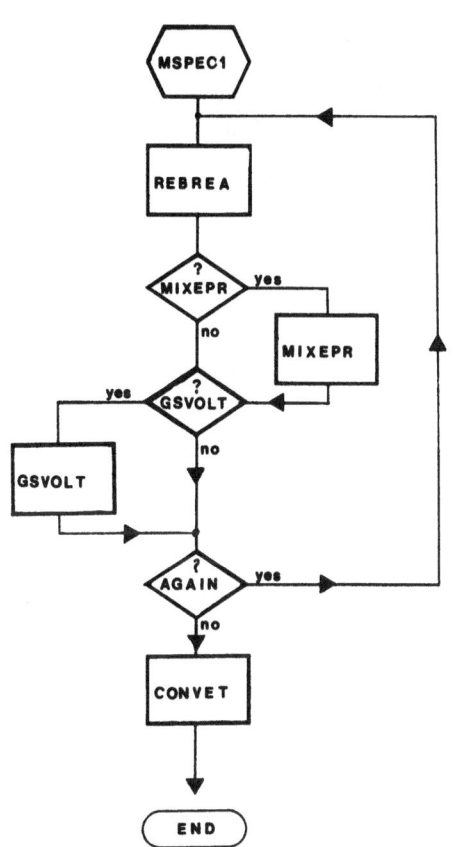

MSPEC1 is an initialisation process for input of patient data and other experimental parameters e.g. workload, barometric pressure.

REBREA is used for the collection of experimental data at 20Hz from each analogue input. It also enables the operator to review the data using the graphics terminal to record all the relevant points from the two rebreathing manouevres.

MIXEPR is an optional routine for the collection of mixed expired gas analysis (used for other metabolic studies and as a comparative method for cardiac output determinations).

GSVOLT is used for the calibration of the mass spectrometer. Simple linear regression is performed to obtain calibration lines for the mass spectrometer outputs and known gas mixtures.

CONVET calculates cardiac output and prints the results as a report form on the line printer.

Figure 5

Flow chart of the program for the non-invasive determination of cardiac output.

5.0 DISCUSSION

Cardiac output determined by this computer system compares favourably with results obtained from the graphical analyses derived from simultaneous polygraph recordings. Repeatability is better and accuracy is improved because the system does not rely on manually reading from the polygraph and subsequent transcription of data. The computer system is quicker, therefore enabling more tests to be performed by fewer people with less effort. The immediate reporting of results is a further considerable advantage in this type of clinical situation.

BASIC, although well known as being a slow programming language, is acceptable in this situation since the rebreathing manouevres were only performed every few minutes when the subject had achieved a metabolic "steady-state" at any particular workload.

This computerised method now enables the non-invasive determination of cardiac output during exercise to be performed routinely in any well equipped pulmonary function laboratory.

6.0 ACKNOWLEDGEMENTS

The authors acknowledge the help and advice of Dr. G. Laszlo and Dr. P. N. T. Wells. G. T. R. Lewis was supported by a research grant from the South Western Regional Health Authority.

7.0 REFERENCES

(1) Winsborough M M, Miller J N, Burgess D W, Laszlo G. Estimation of cardiac output from the rate of rise of alveolar carbon dioxide during rebreathing. Clin Sci. 1980 : 58 : 263-270.

(2) Lewis G T R. Pulmonary haemodynamics during rebreathing. MSc Thesis Bath University : 1979.

(3) Collier C R. Determination of mixed venous carbon dioxide tensions by rebreathing. J Appl Physiol. 1956 : 1 : 159-164.

PORTABLE MICROCOMPUTERS IN PATHOLOGY:
SURGICAL PATHOLOGY IN THE ELECTRONIC LABORATORY

RICHARD A. MACDONALD, M.D.
NORWOOD HOSPITAL & BOSTON UNIV. SCHOOL MEDICINE
NORWOOD, MASS., USA, 02062
AND
GISELLE S. PECHET, M.D.
NORWOOD HOSPITAL & BOSTON UNIV. SCHOOL MEDICINE

SUMMARY. THREE FACTORS FAVOR THE USE OF MICROCOMPUTERS IN THE HOSPITAL:
(1) THE DEVELOPMENT OF THE ELECTRONIC LABORATORY: (2) COST CONSTRAINTS IN
HEALTH CARE: (3) INCREASING SCARCITY OF TRAINED PERSONNEL, ESPECIALLY CLERICAL
AND SECRETARIAL PERSONS WHO MUST HANDLE INFORMATION. IN THIS PAPER WE DESCRIBE
A MICROCOMPUTER SYSTEM FOR SURGICAL (ANATOMIC) PATHOLOGY REPORTING AND INFORMATION
HANDLING THAT IS LOW IN COST; AND WHICH DOES NOT REQUIRE A SPECIAL COMPUTER WORK
FORCE FOR OPERATION OR MAINTENANCE. IT USES COMMERCIALLY AVAILABLE SOFTWARE,
WHICH IS INEXPENSIVE AND DOES NOT REQUIRE KNOWLEDGE OF COMPUTER PROGRAMMING.
STANDARDIZED FORMATTING OF REPORTS REDUCES PATHOLOGIST TIME, REDUCES REQUIREMENTS
FOR CLERICAL PERSONNEL, AND PERMITS READY INCORPORATION INTO HOSPITAL AND OTHER
COMPUTER INFORMATION SYSTEMS. IT IS FLEXIBLE FOR EACH PATIENT, AND IT IS
EXPANDABLE.

THE ELECTRONIC LABORATORY IS ONE THAT EMPLOYS THE NEW TECHNOLOGIES THAT
HAVE BECOME WIDELY AVAILABLE IN THE PAST 2 DECADES. A DEDICATED LABORATORY
COMPUTER FOR INFORMATION HANDLING; AUTOMATED TESTING EQUIPMENT THAT CONTAINS
MICROPROCESSORS; ELECTRONIC EXCHANGE OF INFORMATION WITH OTHER DEPARTMENTS: WORD
PROCESSING; PAPER COPIERS WITH MICROPROCESSORS:; TELEVISION AND AUDIO-VISUAL
EQUIPMENT; TELEPHONE SYSTEMS WITH MICROPROCESSORS; RADIO AND CABLE COMMUNICATION;
TELECOMMUNICATIONS AND MODEMS; REMOTE STATUS PRINTERS; NUCLEAR MEDICINE; ELECTRON
MICROSCOPY; MICROCOMPUTERS; MICROCOMPUTER NETWORKING; AND OTHER SPECIAL EQUIPMENT.

THESE TECHNOLOGIES ARE IMPRESSIVE WHEN THEY ARE OPERATING PROPERLY, BUT THERE
IS A WEAK LINK IN THE SYSTEMS. THAT IS A SCARCITY OF TRAINED WORKERS, ESPECIALLY
CLERICAL AND SECRETARIAL PERSONNEL WHO MUST HANDLE INFORMATION. THE PROBLEM IS
NOT UNIQUE TO THE HEALTH FIELD, AND IT IS PREDICTED TO INCREASINGLY BECOME A
PROBLEM BOTH IN INDUSTRIALIZED COUNTRIES (1,2) AND IN LESS WELL DEVELOPED
NATIONS.(3)

THE SUBDIVISION OF THE MEDICAL LABORATORY IN WHICH IT IS MOST DIFFICULT TO
IMPROVE PRODUCTIVITY USING COMPUTERS IS SURGICAL (ANATOMIC) PATHOLOGY. THE
PRINCIPAL OBSTACLE HAS BEEN INDIVIDUALISTIC VARIABILITY BETWEEN DIFFERENT
PROFESSIONALS. AMONG 6,000 US HOSPITALS IN 1980, ONLY APPROXIMATELY 42 USED A
COMPUTER IN SURGICAL PATHOLOGY.(4)

METHODS. TWO PROFESSIONAL STEPS IN PREPARING THE PRESENT SYSTEM ARE SETTING
UP GROSS PATHOLOGY PREFORMATTED FORMS, AND WRITING A DICTIONARY OF PRE-FORMATTED

MICROSCOPIC DIAGNOSES EMPLOYING THE TERMINOLOGY THAT WILL BE USED FOR OUTPUTTING
REPORTS TO CLINICIANS AND PATIENT RECORDS.

1. FOR GROSS PATHOLOGY DESCRIPTIONS, A FORM CONTAINS 20 TO 30 LINES TO BE
COMPLETED WITH SPECIFIC INFORMATION FOR EACH TYPE OF CASE. EACH FORM CONTAINS
THE GROSS AND MICROSCOPIC REPORT ON A SINGLE OR AT MOST 2 PAGES. INFORMATION
TO BE COMPLETED INCLUDES SIZE, SHAPE, COLOR, CONSISTENCY, GROWTHS, VESSELS, LYMPH
NODES, ET CETERA. THE PATHOLOGIST DICTATES INFORMATION IN THE ORDER IN WHICH IT
IS TO BE TYPED. PREPRINTING OF FORMS MAKES POSSIBLE A SINGLE TAB SETTING TO
BRING THE TYPEWRITER CARRIAGE TO THE STARTING POINT FOR EACH LINE. EACH REPORT
FORM HAS MULTIPLE COLOR CODED COPIES.

2. A DATA BASE OF MICROSCOPIC DIAGNOSES IS WRITTEN, ENTERED INTO THE
SOFTWARE PROGRAM, AND STORED ON FLOPPY OR HARD DISK. DIAGNOSES ARE ARRANGED
ALPHABETICALLY BY ORGAN UNDER 12 ORGAN SYSTEMS. EACH DIAGNOSIS IS ASSIGNED A
UNIQUE IDENTIFIER NUMBER. PROVISION IS LEFT FOR THE ADDITION OF NEW DIAGNOSES.
ORGAN SYSTEMS INCLUDE CONNECTIVE TISSUE, ENDOCRINE, GASTROINTESTINAL, ET CETERA.
THE KEY DIAGNOSTIC WORD IS ON THE FIRST LINE. ALPHABETIZATION IS DONE ACCORDING
TO THIS KEY WORD. EXAMPLE: CARCINOMA, FOLLOWED BY QUALIFYING INFORMATION SUCH
AS ADENOCARCINOMA, WELL DIFFERENTIATED. EACH PREFORMATTED DIAGNOSIS INCLUDES
CLASSIFICATION USING A SIX LETTER DESIGNATION AND ALSO THE SNOMED CLASSIFICATION.(5)

3. USE OF DIAGNOSES. AN ALPHABETICAL LIST OF DIAGNOSES IS POSTED AT THE
WORK STATION OF EACH PATHOLOGIST. AFTER MICROSCOPIC STUDY OF A CASE, A DIAGNOSIS
IS SELECTED FROM THE LIST. ITS NUMBER AND ANY EDITING CHANGES THAT ARE NEEDED ARE
WRITTEN ON A FORM WHICH ACCOMPANIES EACH CASE. A SECRETARY WORKS FROM THIS FORM.
THE DIAGNOSIS NUMBER IS ENTERED ON THE MICROCOMPUTER KEYBOARD AND THE SEARCH KEY
IS PRESSED. THE PREFORMATTED DIAGNOSIS IMMEDIATELY APPEARS ON THE CRT SCREEN.
TO EDIT A LINE, DATA IS TYPED OVER FROM THE KEYBOARD. WHEN EDITING IS COMPLETE,
THE DIAGNOSIS FOR A PATIENT IS SAVED ON STORAGE DISK. A REPORT FORM IS POSITIONED
IN A PRINTER, AND THE KEY FOR PRINTING IS PRESSED. THE REPORT IS PRINTED AS IT
APPEARS ON THE CRT SCREEN.

4. THE MICROCOMPUTER WE USE IS AN APPLE II PLUS WITH 64 K MEMORY, FOUR 5¼"
DIAMETER FLOPPY DISKS DRIVES, A VIDEX CARD FOR WORD PROCESSING, AND A Z-80 CARD
FOR THE CPM OPERATING SYSTEM. THE PRINTERS USED HAVE BEEN AN NEC SPINWRITER AND
AN INTEGRAL DATA SYSTEM PAPER TIGER. FOR A SYSTEM WITH LARGER STORAGE AND
RETRIEVAL CAPACITY, CORVUS 5 AND 20 MEGABYTE HARD DISK DRIVES HAVE BEEN ADDED. TWO
COMMERCIALLY AVAILABLE SOFTWARE PACKAGES FOR DATA BASE MANAGEMENT HAVE BEEN USED:
DB MASTER, (STONWARE MICROCOMPUTER PRODUCTS, SAN RAFAEL, CAL, USA); AND DBASE II
(ASHTON-TATE CO, LOS ANGELES, CAL).

5. SHOULD A DIAGNOSIS NOT BE ON THE DICTIONARY OF PREFORMATTED DIAGNOSES,
ONE CAN BE CONSTRUCTED AT ANY TIME, ASSIGNED A NUMBER, PRINTED, AND SAVED ON
STORAGE DISK FOR FURTHER USE. USE OF A PRINTER RESULTS IN A CONSISTENT QUALITY
OF TYPING. PREFORMATTED DIAGNOSES INCLUDE MEDICAL TERMINOLOGY, SO THAT THE

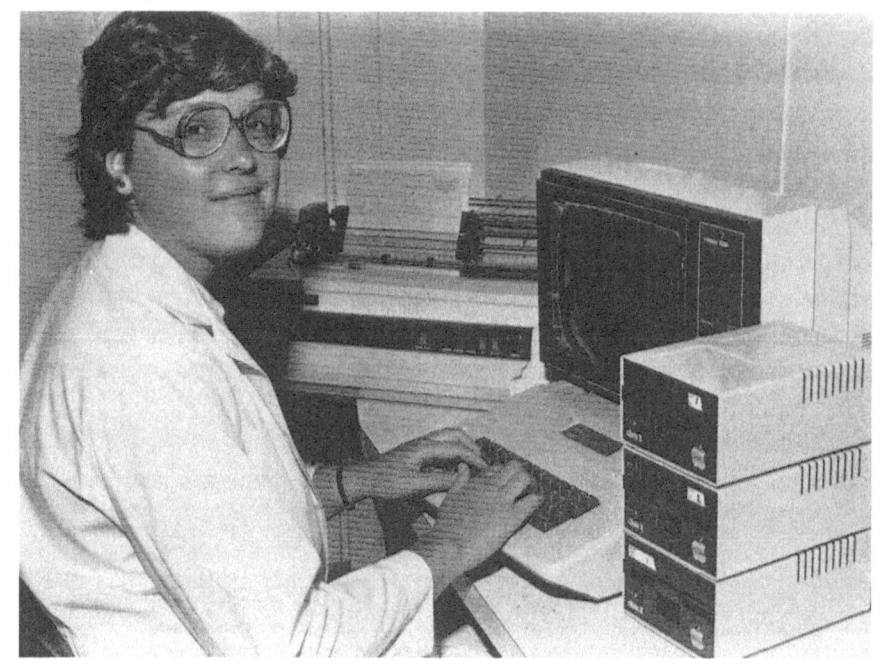

FIGURE 1 ABOVE

FIGURE 2 ABOVE

110

SYSTEM IS OPERATED BY SECRETARIES WITHOUT PREVIOUS MEDICAL TERMINOLOGY OR
PATHOLOGY EXPERIENCE.

6. FILING AND RETRIEVAL: EACH PATIENT DIAGNOSIS IS STORED ON DISK, SO THAT
SPECIFIC CASES OR CATEGORIES OF CASES CAN BE RETRIEVED BY ENTERING SEARCH
CRITERIA OR CASE NUMBERS ON THE MICROCOMPUTER KEYBOARD.

THE MICROCOMPUTERS ARE USED FOR OTHER TASKS WHEN NOT IN USE FOR SURGICAL
PATHOLOGY, SUCH AS WORD PROCESSING, MATHEMATICAL AND FINANCIAL CALCULATIONS,
TELECOMMUNICATIONS, AND PERSONNEL TRAINING.(6) THE SYSTEM HAS BEEN IN USE IN OUR
LABORATORY FOR SEVERAL MONTHS. IT HAS PAID FOR ITSELF IN SAVINGS IN PATHOLOGISTS
TIME, AND IN REDUCTION OF SECRETARIAL REQUIREMENTS.

REFERENCES

1. DRUCKER PF. MANAGING IN TURBULENT TIMES. NEW YORK, HARPER & ROW, 1980.
2. TOFFLER A. THE THIRD WAVE. NEW YORK, BANTAM BOOKS, 1981.
3. SERVAN-SCHREIBER J-J. THE WORLD CHALLENGE. NEW YORK, SIMON AND SCHUSTER,
   1980.
4. WERTMAN B, MARQUARDT VC, KRIEG AF, HOSTY TA, WERTY RK, LUNDBERG GD. THE
   CURRENT STATUS OF LABORATORY DATA PROCESSING. PATHOLOGIST, COLL AMER PATHOL
   1980; 34:461-4.
5. ROTHWELL, D.J., EDITOR. SNOMED. SYSTEMATIZED NOMENCLATURE OF MEDICINE.
   MICROGLOSSARY FOR SURGICAL PATHOLOGY. 1980. SKOKIE, ILLINOIS, COLL AMER
   PATHOL.
6. MACDONALD RA: PERSONAL MICROCOMPUTERS LINKED TO A HOSPITAL LABORATORY COMPUTER.
   PATHOLOGIST, COLL AMER PATHOL. 1982; 35: IN PRESS.

LEGENDS FOR ILLUSTRATIONS:
    FIG. 1: THE SURGICAL PATHOLOGY REPORTING SYSTEM IN USE. THE MICROCOMPUTER,
VIDEO MONITOR, 3 DISK DRIVES, AND PRINTER ARE SHOWN. NOT SHOWN IS THE HARD DISK.
TO ILLUSTRATE THE SIMPLICITY OF USING THE SYSTEM, THIS OPERATOR LEARNED TYPING IN
HIGH SCHOOL, THEN WORKED AS A WAITRESS IN A FAST FOOD RESTAURANT PRIOR TO PATHOLOGY
WORK.

    FIG. 2: A REPORT PRODUCED BY THE SYSTEM. THE MICROSCOPIC DIAGNOSIS COMPRISES
THE UPPER PORTION OF A REPORT. NOTE UNIQUE NUMBERS (6004.3 AND S-814590) ASSIGNED
EACH DIAGNOSIS AND EACH PATIENT. OTHER INFORMATION INCLUDES PATHOLOGIST, CLINICIAN,
CODED INFORMATION FOR DATE, AGE, SEX, CLASSIFICATION, SNOMED, TISSUE RETENTION
TIME. PREFORMATTED GROSS DESCRIPTION LINES ARE ON THE LOWER HALF OF A PAGE.
(NOT SHOWN).

Interdependence of Information Processing between EDP-System, Blood Bank Organization, and Blood Recipient

KLUGE Arpad (Institute for Immunology and Serology)
MANNES Hans, VONIER Joerg, WOLF Gerhard K. (Institute
for Medical Documentation, Statistics and Data Processing)

University of Heidelberg, FRG

The main fields of EDP application in blood banking are:

(1) blood donor : registration
    ----
(2) blood sample : laboratory data processing
    ----
(3) blood unit : stock supervision
    ----
(4) blood order : accounting and billing.

The blood delivery of regional blood banks usually stop at
the hospital blood depots. Hospital blood banks at the
patient's level have to meet the requirements of blood
component therapy [1]. EDP-systems of patient-oriented blood
banks therefore have to be expanded to the

(5) blood recipient : supervision of transfusion orders.

In a patient-oriented blood bank there are manifold movements of persons and materials, namely those of

- b l o o d   d o n o r s , who have to be examined for their
  state of health and identified before giving blood,

- p a t i e n t s   in the wards - and to a minor degree in
  the blood bank - requiring blood therapy, resulting
  in orders, which are often modified due to the current
  medical state of the recipient,

- p h y s i c i a n s , who examine blood donors or patients,
  decide on their state of health, and supervise blood production,

- b l o o d   u n i t s , which are drawn from donors, stored,
  and processed into a number of various products according
  to the actual demand and the stock policy,

- b l o o d   s a m p l e s from donors or patients to be
  examined in the laboratories,

- various   f o r m s , serving as data carriers for results
  and for comparison of a number of items.

The poster shows a scheme of our external data carriers' flow
in connection with the peripheral EDP devices within donor
service, product depot, and transfusion service as three sections
of the blood bank [2].
It was never our intention to handle the various organizational
movements of materials and persons by EDP, but merely to monitor
them at several check points (interfaces) for comparison and processing of data, thereby optimizing blood bank organization.

```
                                  *
The main check points of the      *  The monitoring will determine
following 3 STAGES are:           *  the following data or documents:
**********************************************************************
                                  *
BLOOD DONATION                    *
  - donor data subset             *  - product data set incl.
  - sequential donation number    *    blood unit number,
  - additional technical data     *  - lists for manual data
                                  *    processing.
                                  *
BLOOD STOCK ENTRY                 *
  - blood unit number             *  - state of product,
  - product code                  *  - lists for stock control,
  - laboratory test results       *  - accounting.
                                  *
BLOOD ORDER                       *
  - recipient data                *  - assignment(s) of blood unit
  - ordering type                 *    number(s) to a recipient,
  - blood unit number             *  - changed product state
                                  *  - special lists : "trans-
                                  *    fusion report".
                                  *
```

Some aspects of the information interdependence between EDP-system,
blood bank organization and the blood therapy are illustrated
in the poster by use of HIPO-technique.

The data input at the check points (interfaces) is facilitated by several machine- (and eye-)readable OCR-B codes and identification numbers for blood donors, blood products, blood samples, and orders for blood recipients. We decided to use OCR hand readers, because delivery of blood units is not made to those blood banks using a bar code system. On the other hand we expect (off-line) exchange of OCR-B coded data within the information system planned for our university hospital including patient administration, clinical laboratory and accounting. If the proposed standardization [3, 4] of blood unit data will be implemented, a single CODABAR reader at blood stock entry will be sufficient for reading the labels on foreign (Red Cross) blood units.

REFERENCES:

[1] Kluse A. Functions of Patient-oriented Blood Transfusion
    Services. In: Moehr J R and Kluse A. The Computer and Blood
    Banking (EDP Applications in Transfusion Medicine). Proceedings
    of the GMDS Spring Conference, Tuebingen April 1981. Lecture
    Notes in Med Inform 1981; 13:6-13.

[2] Vonier J, Kluse A, Wolf G K. ADP-supported System for Blood
    Donor Service, Blood Unit Depot, and Blood Transfusion Service
    (BluBB). (1) Organizational Concept for the Data Transmission
    with External Data Media. loc.cit.pg. 210-211.

[3] Brodheim E. Experience with machine readable labels at the
    New York Blood Center. In: Jenkins J. Machine readable labels
    in the blood transfusion service. Proc Codabar Meeting, Broad-
    way,Worcs. June 13th 1979. 1980; Lancaster,England,(MTP Press
    Ltd) pg. 20-40.

[4] Thatcher R K. Recommendations of Task Force on Codes and
    Machine-Readable Symbols. Vox Sang (Bale) 1981; 40:144-155.

COMPUTER ASSISTED REAL-TIME QUALITY CONTROL IN A HOSPITAL BLOOD BANK.

Paul T. Kelly,
Dept. of Microbiology,
Mater Misericordiae Hospital,
Dublin 7,
Ireland.

INTRODUCTION

DENIS is a software package which forms a screen based real-time, interactive hospital blood bank computer system. This system has been designed to be simple to use ; requiring a minimum of knowledge of computers or how they work. Almost all data which the operator supplies to the software are subjected to a greater or lesser degree of validation depending on the nature of the particular field. Strict adherence to standard blood banking methodologies is enforced ; the sequence of data input has been designed to ensure that specific groups of input operations are completed before exit is permitted.

The system includes a database management component written using KFAM-5, a WANG software utility which is a system permitting random access to data stored on disk . Within each record in the user file is a unique 'key' consisting of Surname, Hospital chart number and Laboratory serial number.

THE SYSTEM EXECUTIVE MENU :

FN'Key	OPERATION	FN'Key	OPERATION
00	PATIENT ID ENTRY	07	STEP-FORWARD
01	REQUEST ENTRY	08	STEP-BACKWARD
02	GROUP ENTRY	09	OLD ID+Gp. PRINT
03	X-MATCH ENTRY	10	OLD REQUEST PRINT
04	COMMENT ENTRY	11	OLD X-MATCH PRINT
05	FILE ANY DATA	12	CLOSE ALL FILES
06	FIND-OLD RECORD		

DATA INPUT

1. PATIENT I.D. ENTRY

The Patient identification (PID) entry forms the core of a logical record. The record key is constructed from it. The PID must be the first input operation to be executed before a new record can be created. The PID section of a record consists of eleven fields , which are validated variously as numeric or within a given set or check-digit. After input of these data the program exits to the executive menu.

2. REQUEST ENTRY

This routine accepts, after validation, those data which constitute the request to the laboratory (from the clinician) for blood. The REQUEST section of a record consists of four fields .These are Product , Number of units, Time required and Date required . All fields are validated, the date being finally validated by issuing the "day-of-the-week" as a prompt.

3. GROUP ENTRY

A patient's blood group is determined by interpretation of the pattern of results obtained from a battery of agglutination tests. The patient's red blood cells and serum are tested against a standard set of anti-sera and red cells. Agglutination of the red cells is a 'positive' reaction and non-agglutination is a 'negative' reaction.

This section of the record consists of twelve input fields. Eleven of these inputs are '+' or '-' characters (all other keys are disabled during this phase) ,and are written to file as a single field. For input the following mask is displayed .The cursor is moved across the mask under software control.

ANTI A	ANTI B	ANTI A+B	ANTI D	ANTI CDE	Rh Ctrl	A1-Cell	B-Cell	O+Cell	A.S. I.C.	A.S. Enz.	
+	+	+	+	+	-	-	-	-	-	-	<-- INPUT

All O.K. (Y/N) ?

At this stage the operator should re-check the results. A negative response
will force a re-entry of all reactions. The pattern of reactions must be
interpreted to determine the actual ABO & Rhesus group of the patient. The
last two fields on the mask, i.e. A.S.I.C. & A.S.Enz. are not part of the
blood group proper. However it is standard practice to include them at this
stage.There are fifteen possible combinations of the ABO & Rhesus groups.
These are displayed in two columns in a sixteen element screen menu. The
operator selects one group from the menu ,the selection directed by the
information gained above.This is done by keying the subscript of the menu
item required.

3.1.   BLOOD GROUP VALIDATION
Input is checked for,   a)Two characters maximum.
                           b)Numeric.
                           c)Falls within range >=1 & <=16
                           d)Special validation (see below).

3.2.   BLOOD GROUP , SPECIAL VALIDATION PROCEDURE.
There is a possibility that the blood group reactions may be misread or
that the pattern may be misinterpreted .An error of this magnitude could
have grave consequences for the patient. Such errors are prevented by a
special routine which reads an accessory file named "BDATA" which contains
miscellaneous information used throughout the system. During this particular access it reads-in a validation table containing the known
correct pattern for the fifteen possible blood groups. The pattern of '+'
and '-' reactions keyed-in by the operator is compared with the pattern
corresponding to the blood group chosen from the screen menu. If these two
patterns are not identical the following error message is displayed and
re-input of the entire group is forced.

          GROUP REACTION MISREAD, OR INTERPRETATION ERROR !
          GOING BACK TO RE-ENTER ENTIRE GROUP.

If the input data passes all of the validation tests, the technologist
doing the group enters his initials; control is returned to the executive.

4.   CROSS-MATCH DATA ENTRY.
A cross-match (compatibility test) is a series of tests designed to
demonstrate any incompatibility between the recipient's serum and donor
blood. This procedure is limited to detection of incompatibility due to
red cell antibodies. However , these antibodies are responsible for the
majority of significant transfusion reactions.
The cross-match section of the patient record consists of a max. of 31
fields. Each unit cross-matched will have a three field 'slot' in the
record comprising Pack Group, Pack Number & Cross match reactions, to a
maximum number of ten units.The last field contains the initials of the
person performing the cross-match.
The program will iterate to accept these data for the total number of
units specified in the REQUEST section of the record.

4.1.   CROSS-MATCH,SPECIAL VALIDATION PROCEDURE.
The groups of each of the packs to be transfused are entered by making the
appropriate selection from an eight item menu containing the groups of the
packs provided for transfusion.It is a common occurrence for a transfusion
to be carried out with blood which is not of the same ABO or Rh group as
the recipient.These transfusions are only performed when blood of the same
group as the recipient is unavailable.

A decision table has been constructed which describes the intercompatib-
ility of the various blood groups. Compatibility is considered to be at 5
'levels' for the purposes of this system.

TABLE CODE	COMPATIBILITY LEVEL	COMMENT
1	Primary	e.g. A+ to A+ , O- to O- etc.
2	Secondary	e.g. O+ to A+,B+ or AB+ etc.
3	Tertiary	e.g. A+ to A- ,Rh incompatibility, AVOID!
4	INCOMPATIBLE	ABO incompatibility,DO NOT TRANSFUSE !!!
5	Emergency	Group unknown, no compatibility checks.

4.2. COMPATIBILITY DECISION TABLE

<---------- DONOR GROUP ---------->

| Pack Group -> | | O+ | O- | A+ | A- | B+ | B- | AB+ | AB- |
Menu code ->		1	2	3	4	5	6	7	8
↑ O+	1	1	2	4	4	4	4	4	4
O-	2	3	1	4	4	4	4	4	4
R A+	3	2	2	1	1	4	4	4	4
E A-	4	3	2	3	1	4	4	4	4
C B+	5	2	2	4	4	1	1	4	4
I B-	6	3	2	4	4	3	1	4	4
P AB+	7	2	2	2	2	2	2	1	1
I AB+	8	3	2	3	2	3	2	3	1
E O'D'-	9	3	1	4	4	4	4	4	4
N A'D'-	10	3	2	3	1	4	4	4	4
T B'D'-	11	3	2	4	4	3	1	4	4
AB'D'-	12	3	2	3	2	3	2	3	1
Oh+	13	4	4	4	4	4	4	4	4
Oh-	14	4	4	4	4	4	4	4	4
↓ Oh'D'-	15	4	4	4	4	4	4	4	4
Emerg.	16	5	5	5	5	5	5	5	5

This decision table is held on disk file.When required it is read into
core and used to perform the final compatibility check. Various screen
messages are displayed depending on the code returned from the table.
These messages are roughly along the lines of the 'comments' above.

After the technologist signs his initials to the cross-match the system
will automatically print self-adhesive blood pack labels. A label is
printed for each pack ,plus two labels for the two parts of the form.
Control is returned to the system executive.

5. COMMENT ENTRY.
A freetext comment of <= 40 characters is permitted. A typical comment
would be " PATIENT'S SERUM CONTAINS Anti-KELL ". In general the comment
will contain either advice or a warning to the clinician about possible
problems with the transfusion. Note that the comment may be inserted at
any time during the processing of a particular Group and Crossmatch
once the PID has been entered.

The remaining operations are merely file-handling functions and have no
special features. Records are recalled by executing 'FIND-OLD RECORD' ;the
key is entered and the old record is displayed.The record may be updated at
this point. There is a facility to step forward or backward through the
logical records in the user file to find a particular record if the complete
key is unknown. Complete system shut-down is achieved when 'CLOSE ALL FILES'
is executed.

ON THE PECULIAR DISTRIBUTION PATTERN OF HEALTH SERVICES

OR

CLINICAL CHEMISTRY IN PRIMARY HEALTH CARE

1. AUTHOR   Ole Wilhelm Bøe

Dept. of Clinical Chemistry

Lillehammer County Hospital

N-2600 Lillehammer

NORWAY

2.SUMMARY

It is reported upon large variations in the use of laboratory tests by doctors in primary health care in Oppland County of Norway. Large differences is demonstrated between municipalities. No medical reasons have been found to explain the observations.
The doctors claimed unaware of the variability in requisitioning pattern, but when informed about it, a noticeable interest in evaluation of own work emerged. Demonstration of differences in health services may be a means of introducing medical audit.
A medical information system may seem a necessity to provide the doctor with parameters for how he works in relation to colleagues.

3. INTRODUCTION

Norwegian health authorities have announced a new plan for financing, making each
county and municipality responsible to provide its health services within an economical frame. No records,however, have been made the last 10 years on analyses requested
by primary health care. Being in charge of clinical chemistry in Oppland, the author
felt the need for such information - the tests being analysed in different laboratories all over South Norway.

4. METHODS

Doctors in primary health care in Oppland were visited in their surgery by the author.
Information was given on the reasons to perform the study and the doctor was asked to
make a record of the tests being requested over a 4 week time period. Tests performed
in the surgery were not to be included in the study, but the kind of analyses done by
the doctor was registered.   The reports from the doctors were written on floppy
discs with a Mycron microcomputer and the data treated by Mycron software program to
provide cumulative reports for each municipality. This poster report has been limited
to the data from municipalities where all doctors had delivered reports. The number
of tests per 4 weeks was multiplied by eleven to obtain an estimate for a year (44
weeks of work). Tests for the whole county was estimated by multiplying the numbers
from the examined area with a factor 1.6, i.e. the quotient between the population
in the county total - and in the examined municipalities. (179 000 inhab: 112 000)

5. RESULTS

Reports from 55 of a total of 110 doctors (65 visited) in 20 of the 26 municipali-

118

RESULTS CONTINUED -

ties were used for calculations. The large variations in tests used by different municipalities add uncertainty to the figures calculated for the whole county. The reports
were mainly made in the first and last 3 months of the year. As the professional activity will vary through the year - the reports cannot display a true picture of the
year. The available data, however, do not allow estimation of the magnitude of uncertainty.

TESTS ORDERED BY PRIMARY HEALTH CARE FROM DIFFERENT LAB SPECIALITIES

Speciality	Tests per year	Tests per inhab. year
Clinical chemistry	71 ooo	o.4o
Serology	9 5oo	o.o5
Microbiology	5 3oo	o.o3
Patholog. anat.	6 8oo	o.o4

The table above gives the numbers for annual requisitioning of different types of laboratory tests.

Figure 1 relates the 71 ooo
tests ordered in clinical
chemistry in primary health care
to tests ordered by hospital
and hospital outpatient clinics
in terms of tests per inhabitant per year.
Other institutions comprises
some smaller hospitals and nursing homes for elderly.
2 county hospitals have approx.
imately 7oo beds and 2o ooo
admissions per year.

Figure 2 next page - indicates
the annual number of tests of different kind requested from primary
health care . Few hematological
tests because the doctor performs
Hb and SR himself. But 2 doctors
do glucose and creatinine also.

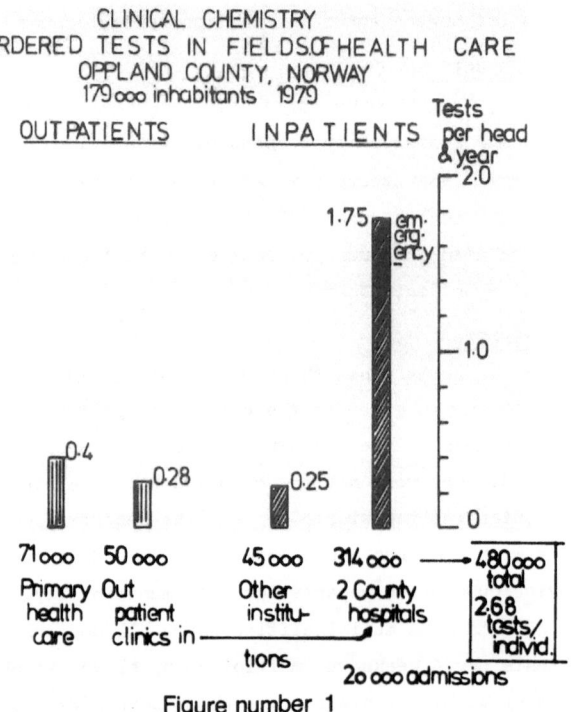

Figure number 1

Figure 3 next page - shows the number of test requested in each municipality - compared to the population, in 2o of the municipalities. Municipality 538 uses 28 % of
tests for 6 % of population, whilst 5ol only need 4 % of tests for 2o % inhabitants.

119

CLINICAL CHEMISTRY

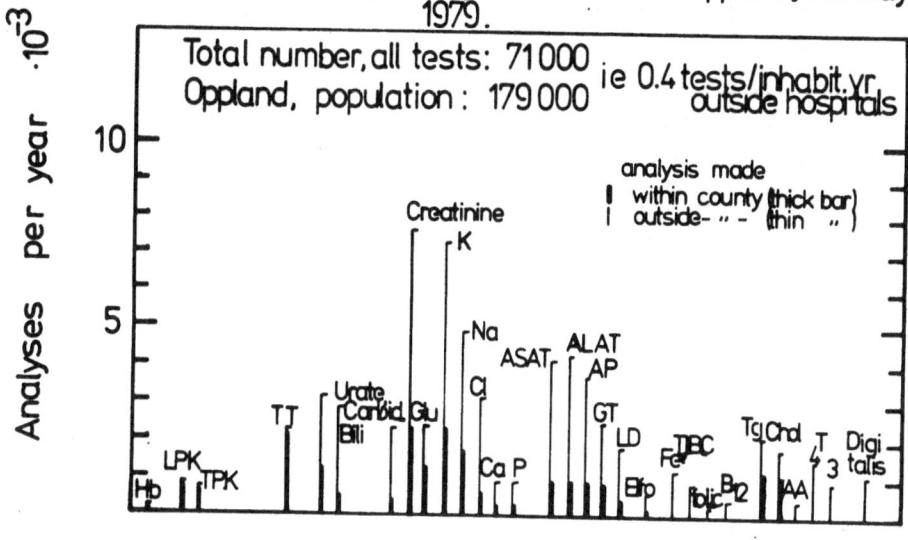

ANNUAL NUMBER AND SPECTRUM OF TESTS
ordered by primary health care. Oppland, Norway.
1979.

Figure number 2

A large variation exists in the use of clinical chemistry tests in primary health care. The results were demonstrated for the doctors. They stated that they were unaware of such a requisitioning pattern, and expressed wishes for examining these matters in the future.

6.DISCUSSION The large differences reported in usage of tests in Oppland have not been registered before. No medical explanation has to now been givenby the doctors, nor have patterns of disease or age distribution rendered cluesto the question. The distance from hospital may be of importance in 5ol where primary healthcare may be given by hospital present. Inequalities between the municipalities as to hospital admissions per capita has been demonstrated by authorities, varying from 6o to 13o around a mean of loo.%
Demonstration of inequalities in services may

Primary health care

CLINICAL CHEMISTRY TESTS VERSUS POPULATION in municipalities of Oppland Norway.

Figure number 3

NUMBERS 501-545 IDENTIFY MUNICIPALITIES

initiate medical audit. A reporting system is needed to inform doctors on requisitioning habits.

120

IRISH EXTERNAL QUALITY ASSESSMENT SCHEME IN CLINICAL BIOCHEMISTRY

F.M. McSweeney*[+], E.J. Barrett[+], J. Brady[+], P.F. Duggan[+], J.R. McSweeney[+], R.O'Moore[+]

In June 1981 the Irish Assessment Scheme was introduced. Each month a stabilised sample of blood serum is distributed and participants are requested to perform certain analyses. Sera from different manufacturers of human and animal based origin are distributed. Sera are usually lyophilised but a stabilised liquid sample has been distributed. Individual report forms are returned to the participants within two days of the closing date for receipt of results. The Scheme is operated on a confidential basis. Each participant is assigned a code number - identity of laboratory is known only to the organiser. The Scheme is based on the routine analysis of sodium, potassium, chloride, urea, glucose, calcium, phosphate, iron, urate, creatinine, bilirubin, total protein, albumin, cholesterol, LDH and AST. The Scheme is flexible and on certain months the regular list of sixteen constituents will be replaced by some less commonly analysed constituents.

The operation of the Scheme is guided by a multidisciplinary Working Party - the Scheme is financed and operated by The National Board for Science and Technology - a Government Advisory Body. Participation in the Scheme is on a voluntary basis and free of charge. Ireland has a population of 3.4 million and fifty-four publicly funded laboratories attached to hospitals service 95% (approx.) of clinical biochemical testing requirements. Many multidisciplinary small laboratories exist which prior to the inauguration of this Scheme were non-participaters in external quality assessment. The principal aim of the Working Group is to stimulate the participation of these laboratories by designing a scheme which would be interesting, useful and simple to understand.

Presently fifty three out of the fifty four laboratories participate in the Scheme. It is believed that this is the highest European level of participation seen in external voluntary assessment schemes.

* Organiser of Scheme. National Board for Science & Technology, Shelbourne House, Shelbourne Road, Dublin 4.

+ Members of National Working Party in Clinical Biochemistry.

The Scheme is based on the comparison of a participant's results with an all-laboratory, all-method result. Methods with known positive or negative bias are excluded in the calculation of the all-method mean. In the case of the enzymes the all-method mean is derived from the results of a defined optimised procedure performed at $37^{\circ}C$. Outliers, results which depart from expectation to an improbable extent, are first removed using a non-parametric elimination procedure. This approach rather than the usual parametric method of outlier elimination used in most schemes was favoured by the Working Party due to the small number of participants (53) and the likelyhood of non-Gaussian distribution of results. The non-parametric test chosen was the Reed et al (1) modification of <u>Dixons r_{10} statistic</u> in which the extreme value of observations be eliminated if the distance between it and its closest neighbour is more than one third the range.

The formulae $r = \dfrac{X_n - X_{n-1}}{X_n - X_1} > 1/3$ Or $r = \dfrac{X_2 - X_1}{X_n - X_1} > 1/3$

summarises the technique where X = lowest value, X_2 = next to lowest value, X_n = highest value and X_{n-1} = next to highest value.

Each month participants receive a two-page confidential report which contains information relating their results to the all-lab mean. The report also lists the number of participants for each constituent and details precision characteristics of each constituent after outlier elimination. Each participant is informed of their current three best and three worst methods as adjudicated by a constituent variance index score. This score is the difference between the result obtained by a participant and the recalculated constituent (all-method, all-lab) mean expressed as a percentage of the mean, divided by a chosen coefficient of variation for that determination and again expressed as a percentage. All scores over 400 are recorded as 400. Therefore each participants method-bias is compared to target precision characteristics which vary relative to the degree of complexity of the constituent and this allows the relative performance of a laboratory's methods to be compared. Examples of target coefficient of variation are - Sodium = 1.6%, LDH = 10.0% This system also allows between laboratory comparisons for each constituent to be performed. The average variance index score of all constituents analysed is calculated each month for participants. This average score for the individual participant is then compared to the scores of the best, average and worst laboratories in the country. Each constituent score is then ranked against all participants' score for that constituent. There are five possible ranks, each containing 20% of laboratory scores. A cumulative constituent score and rank is also generated so that participants can easily judge how their current months results compares to their usual level of performance.

A participant in this scheme can easily monitor within-lab analytical performance and is presented with a clear and simple method of current and cumulative between laboratory comparison. The Scheme has been well received and currently 90% of participants submit results for processing each month.

(1)   Reed, A., Henry, R., and Mason, W., Clin. Chem. 1971, 17, 275.

ON-LINE QUALITY CONTROL IN CLINICAL CHEMISTRY

Roy Baker,John Upham,Joseph Schroeder and W.B.Stewart
Department of Pathology, School of Medicine
University of Missouri,Columbia 65212.

Summary:

An on-line system for quality control in Clinical Chemistry has been developed to overcome certain problems which emerged during the replacement of a Technicon SMA 12/60 with a Technicon SMAC. The system which has been running successfully for over a year is described and the various problems and their solutions represented.

The clinical laboratory at the Harry S.Truman Memorial Veterans Administration Hospital has used a Clinical Lab-12 System for laboratory reporting and data collection since the hospital opened in 1972. This system allows real-time data collection from analog instruments and a limited quality control system. When the laboratory replaced its Technicon SMA 12/60 with a Technicon SMAC, it was faced with the problem of interfacing the SMAC with the laboratory computer system for reporting of patient results, and with the problem of maintaining adequate quality control due the number of controls run every day on the 20 SMAC determinations.

Requirements for a system to interface the SMAC included:
1) The ability to collect data output from the SMAC over a RS232 Serial ASC11 line.
2) Ability to perform real-time limits and quality control checks on the data collected from the SMAC.
3) Presenting limits and real-time error messages back to the technologist running the SMAC.
4) The ability to allow technologist to examine and modify data collected from the SMAC, without interrupting the data collection process.
5) The capability to file acceptable SMAC results into the laboratory reporting system, using existing programs available in the Clinical Lab-12 System.
6) The ability to keep track of controls run on the SMAC and calibrations performed on the instrument during the day.
7) The capability to produce control summaries at the end of the day giving means, standard deviations, and coefficient of

variations for the 20 determinations performed on the SMAC.

8) The capability to produce control summaries giving means, standard deviations for a specified period of time, usually a month at a time.

After examining the requirements for this interface computer, a DEC PDP 11/34 running the RSX11M operating system was used to develop the applications needed. Based on specifications, developed by the laboratory staff programs were written on-site in FORTRAN and MACRO.

Interfacing the SMAC to a laboratory computer system presents a number of interesting problems. The data presented to the laboratory computer from the SMAC consists of 237 characters of data formatted into six lines of data separated by carriage return and line-feed control characters. The data include some identification data entered into the SMAC computer and results for up to 20 determinations performed.

Each of the 20 test results is transmitted by the SMAC as four characters separated by a delimiter or an error code. Error codes are used to flag results that may be questionable and must be repeated, or to indicate reasons why the SMAC has not calculated or printed a given test result. The interface computer must have the capability to keep track of these flagged results and provide a mechanism to allow the laboratory staff to display and edit these flagged results before they are transmitted to the laboratory reporting system or printed on a final laboratory report.

Additionally, the data from the SMAC does not include the four calculated results which are normally available on the report from the SMAC printer. In our case, these include BUN/CREATININE RATIO, ANION GAP, INDIRECT BILIRUBIN, and CALCULATED OSMOLALITY. The interface computer must recalculate these, and also provide for recalculation of the results if one of the values is changed during the editing process.

A third problem area that must be considered is the sample identification information provided by the SMAC. Identification is provided by the SMAC IDee system which optically reads a pre-marked 6 character number from a card inserted into the sample rack. Our convention has been to use the first 3 positions of the IDee marker to identify basic sample types, and the last 3 numbers to identify sequence numbers.

An IDee number of '∅∅∅nnn' indicates a patient sample, an IDee number of '999nnn' indicates a urine or dilution (essentially "other" categories), and other 3 digit prefixes are available for control samples. Currently we are using '111nnn' to identify Level I controls, and '222nnn' to identify Level II controls.

Other combinations of IDee numbers are available for future use

125

for controls or special patient types, etc.

The SMAC links the pre-entered identification information to the sample by the IDee card, which is optically scanned as the rack passes through the SMAC sampler.   Under normal conditions this works well, but occasionally the optical reader will not read all characters and will insert a '*' character in place of the missing sample ID numbers. In this case, the SMAC prints the message "CHECK SAMPLE ID" since it cannot identify the proper pre-entered data.

A final major problem in dealing with the SMAC from the viewpoint of data collection is in handling "repeat" samples.   When a problem is detected with results from a channel on the SMAC, the technologist corrects the problem and all of the samples with bad results are repeated. The SMAC instrument detects many error conditions relating to the quality of analytical curves and errors relating to sample quality (turbidity, blank errors, substrate depletion, etc.), but the SMAC cannot check control values to make sure the tests are staying within pre-established limits.   We felt that rapid detection of out-of-control situations by the interface computer would help spot trends and possibly help reduce the number of repeat samples.

DESCRIPTION OF SOFTWARE COMPONENTS OF SYSTEM.
The system as developed contains the following software modules:
1. A User Control module which gives the laboratory staff the capability to start, stop, and display the current status of the data collection system.
2. Instrument Monitoring programs that actually interface with the instrument to collect the data.
3. Real-Time Quality Control modules which check the validity of data collected from the instrument.
4. User Editing modules to allow changes or corrections to data collected.
5. Result Filing modules which transfer edited data to the laboratory reporting system.
6. Quality Control Reporting modules which provide capabilities to maintain control information and produce control summary reports.

USER CONTROL.
The User Control features of this system allow the lab technologist to start up the monitoring system, to stop the monitoring process and to display the current status of the data collection activities.   The status display includes the current state of the monitoring program (active, suspended), the number of samples collected, number edited,

number filed, the number of calibrations, and other statistics of use
to the laboratory staff.

INSTRUMENT MONITORING PROGRAM.
The Instrument Monitoring program is activated in the morning by a
user at the CRT terminal.   The monitoring task then waits for output
from the SMAC.   After receiving the 237 characters that make up a
SMAC report, this task reformats the SMAC report, does the needed
calculations, and stores the data on disk.   This task then checks
the sample identification information in this report to determine if
the sample is a control or a patient sample and activates the appropriate real-time quality control task.   The SMAC Data Collection task
then waits for the next report to be output from the SMAC instrument.

REAL-TIME QUALITY CONTROL PROCESSING.
Patient Samples.   All results in a patient sample are checked for
extreme value limits.   Any results exceeding these limits are printed
on a hard copy printer next to the SMAC instrument.   This information
is also stored in a transaction file for end-of-day printing.   Any
result exceeding limits is flagged and the technologist must override
this flag or correct the value when editing.
Control Samples.   All results are checked against a table of expected
values.   Results exceeding -2 S.D. of the expected value are flagged
with a warning message printed to the technologist;   results exceeding
$\pm$3 S.D. are flagged as an error.   This allows rapid and positive
checking of control limits.

EDITING FUNCTIONS.
Preparing raw sample data from the SMAC for entry into our laboratory
reporting system is done by the laboratory technologists at a CRT
located near the SMAC.   The editing program has been designed for the
convenience of the user and with the intent of reducing the number of
entries to be made by the user at the CRT.   Three main functions are
provided: 1) a display mode which is used to view collected data,
2) an edit mode which allows the user to change data items as desired,
and 3) a verify mode which is used to release results for transmission
to the laboratory reporting system.   Verify mode allows the user to
enter a range of sequence numbers to be verified, then the program
scans the data looking for error conditions or result error flags.   If
one is found, the program allows the user to immediately correct the
problem.   This provides an efficient mechanism for verification of

results without using a great deal of technologist time.

RESULT FILING.

The transfer of results to the laboratory reporting system is started by the lab technician after completion of a verification session. This program runs as a background task and transfers only results that have been requested in the laboratory reporting system. After filing results, a report is printed on the hard copy terminal giving a recap of results filed.

QUALITY CONTROL REPORTING.

End-of-Day Summary.
This report is produced automatically at the end of the day when the SMAC monitoring process is shut down. This report is printed for each control that is flagged as in use in the control file. It is printed in sequence number order and includes a calibration number to indicate which controls were done with the SMAC standards during the day. Outliers are excluded by checking each result against the target value. Currently we are using ± 4 S.D. as the limit for exclusion. Any value excluded is flagged on the report. If more than 4 results on a control are outside ± 4 S.D. then the entire control is excluded from the summary totals. Totals for each determination printed at the bottom of the report include the number of control values collected, the day's mean, the day's standard deviation and coefficient of variation, and the target mean and standard deviation.

This report is used to note QC changes and is retained as the permanent QC log for the SMAC.

Cumulative Control Summary.
This feature uses the cumulative end-of-day data to allow calculation of overall means and standard deviations for a user specified date range (usually 1 month). The user may ask for all determinations or may ask for a report for a single determination. This report is used to calculate the acceptable target value for the controls in use on the SMAC.

CONCLUSIONS AND FUTURE DEVELOPMENT EFFORTS.

This system was developed to allow automated entry of result data from the SMAC into our laboratory reporting system. In the year (since August 1980) that this system has been operational, it has proved to be a reliable and productive tool for the laboratory. This system's capability to print SMAC reports as they are transmitted from the SMAC allowed us to continue operating through a two-week period when the SMAC printer was out of service.

A COMPUTERIZED OBSTETRICAL MEDICAL RECORD AND DATA BASE SYSTEM

A. Boel [*], F. Van der Voort [**], K. Verhaest [*], A. Van Assche [**] and J.L. Willems [*]

[*] Department of Medical Informatics and

[**] Department of Gynecology and Obstetrics, University Hospital St. Rafaël,

   3000 Leuven, Belgium.

SUMMARY

Over the last two years we have implemented a rather extensive computer oriented obstetrical medical record and data base system at Leuven University. A total of 404
different items can be coded, covering information mainly on the pregnant women, but
also on the husband and newborn(s). The items can be divided into 3 main categories :
data collected at the first visit, information gathered at each follow-up examination
in the prenatal period and data collected at the time of delivery and during the post-
partum period.

HP IMAGE-1000 software has been used to construct the data base on an HP minicomputersystem. Twenty six different data sets have been created which are linked with the
record number and time as the most important key items. Programs have been written
to optimize reliability and speed of data entry and to insure security and recovery
of the data. Coding is done by physicians using multiple choice lists and squares
preprinted throughout the record.

A tool has thereby been created which will be of great help to future clinical research projects.

1. INTRODUCTION

Over the last two years we have developed at Leuven University, a computer oriented
medical record and data base system for storage and retrieval of detailed obstetrical information. The main aims were

1. to improve the reliability and completeness of the recorded data, in the hope of
   providing better clinical care (patient-oriented goal)
2. to provide computer assistance in support of organizational planning, evaluation
   of obstetrical care and scientific clinical research (management and scientific
   oriented goal).

This paper will mainly focus on the contents of the medical record and on the design
and implementation of the data base system. Emphasis will be given on some of the
encountered problems and on the given or proposed solutions.

2. CONTENTS OF THE OBSTETRICAL MEDICAL RECORD AND DATA BASE

The obstetric data are recorded into three main parts of the medical record, as de-

determined by the time and sequence of the data collection : data collected at the first visit, information gathered at each of the follow-up examinations in the prenatal period and data collected at the time of delivery and during the post-partum period.

2.1. Data collected at the first visit

During the first visit anamnestic data are gathered from the patient and her husband, if applicable. This covers the following main categories :
- patient and spouse identification : name, birth date, address, telephone, unique hospital and departmental ID number, as well as name and address of the referring physician ;
- demographic, social and educational data ;
- family medical history ;
- personal general medical history, with special attention for diabetes, hypertension, smoking habits, pelvis traumata or abdominal surgery and other general obstetrical risk factors ;
- gynecological history : age of menarche, menstrual cycle history, past fertility problems, previous gynecological operations, ... ;
- obstetrical history : data and mode if previous deliveries, weight gain, eventual complications and medication taken during previous pregnancies. Information is also gathered on the sex, weight at birth, eventual congenital abnormalities, fetal distress, intensive care and survival for each of the respective children ;
- anamnestic data with respect to the present pregnancy : among which information on anticonceptive therapy, eventual fertility problems, date of last normal period, expected delivery date, smoking habits, alcohol and drug consumption, ...

	items	bytes
- Identification and demographic data		
- of patient	45	370
- of husband (+ also some medical data)	12	72
- Family and personal medical history	11	144
- Gynecological history	10	36
- Obstetrical history	25	144
- Anamnestic data with respect to present pregnancy	32	196

Table 1 : Data items recorded at first visit.

All this information is gathered from the patient's interview or from previous medical records for women which have already been treated in the hospital. Coding is done directly by the examining physician in the squares and using the minicodes, which are preprinted throughout the medical record. Data entry can thereby be performed later

by a medical secretary without recoding. One or more (if applicable) answers are
requested for each item. Table 1 provides a summary of the number of bytes which are
reserved in the data base for this part of the obstetrical record. In total this
amounts to 962 bytes, not taken into account the overhead needed for key items and
linkages.

2.2. Information gathered at each follow-up examination in the prenatal period

At each follow-up visit during the prenatal period, a number of data items may be gathered. Results are stored sequentially according to the date of follow-up. The re-
cordable data can be classified into the following categories :
- date and place of the examination (out- or in-patient department, ...) ;
- anamnestic data : questions with regard to the general subjective feeling of the
  patient, the presence or absence of peripheral oedema in the preceding period,
  fetal movements, ... ;
- clinical findings : weight, fundus, perimeter, blood pressure, heart rate, data
  from the vaginal (cervical) examination if performed, ... ;
- laboratory data : results of urine and blood tests grouped into different subsets :
  hematological, thyroid, renal, liver and pancreas function tests, oestrogen levels,
  urine,bacteriologic and certain serological findings ;
- results from technical examinations : ultrasound, fetal heart rate (FHR) recording,
  amniocentesis or amnioscopy, ... ;
- diet, medication and other therapy.

	items	bytes
- Anamnestic follow-up prenatal data	36	168
- Clinical findings	51	128
- Laboratory results	34	74
- Results from technical examinations	47	132
- Diet, medication and other therapy	4	14

Table 2 : Maximal number of items codable at the each follow-up visit in the prenatal
period

The date of the examination, some anamnestic and clinical items should always be filled in. In order to shorten the coding and data entry time, it has been decided to
leave the contents of the non-requested or non-relevant items blank. The maximum
amount of coded information, which can be stored in the data base for each follow-
up examination in the prenatal period, is listed in Table 2. This amounts to a total
of 516 bytes. The effective stored number is much lower, since only a low percentage
of all the items are filled in at each follow-up visit, especially in case of a normal
pregnancy.

2.3. Data collected at the time of delivery, during the post-partum and postnatal period

The items collected at the time of delivery and in the post-partum period can be classified into the following categories :

- data on labor : induction, spontaneous labor, progression, type of analgoanesthesia, FHR recording, details on rupture of membranes, fetal presentation, color of amniotic fluid, ... ;
- information on delivery : mode of delivery (normal, instrumental, ...), duration of second stage, complications, ... ;
- data on placenta : time of placenta delivery, macroscopic and microscopic findings of placenta and umbilical cord ;
- findings of the newborn(s) : sex, weight, Apgar score, neurological age, congenital anomalies and other perinatal morbidity or mortality findings if any, intensive care, blood grouping, type of feeding ;
- post-partum items : complications, information on iso-immunization and gammaglobulin prophylaxis, discharge date and diagnoses (ICD-9CM) ;
- postnatal visit : t°, menses, feeding, contraception, clinical findings, ...

The total number of items and bytes reserved in the data base for this part of the obstetrical record is listed in Table 3.

	items	bytes
- Data on labor period	27	128
- Information on delivery and findings of newborn	31	122
- Placenta and umbilical cord	8	18
- Post-partum data	12	72
- Final discharge diagnoses	19	50

Table 3 : Data items reserved for the delivery and post-partum findings

Comments can be added as free text, in a limited amount (40 bytes), to some of the main categories listed in Tables 1 to 3. The obstetric record and the data base have been so designed that several diagnoses or findings can be stored in certain, so-called compound or plural multiple choice items. For most items however only one numerical result or one answer out of a multiple-choice list, should be filled in.

3. OBSTETRICAL DATA BASE SYSTEM

3.1. General requirements and features

The structure of the data organisation must fulfill two main objectives : retrieval of the medical record of a single patient and selecting subgroups of patients according to a combination of selection criteria for research purposes. A data base management system can provide a solution to link logically related files containing both data and structured information. Pointers within the data base allow a user to gain access to related data and to index data across files. The HP IMAGE network data base management system is used and structured under the premise that only when one logical group of data is related to another logical group of data, a direct linkage will be constructed between them. When logical data sets are considered as nodes with direct accessing paths connecting them, a network data base is formed.

3.2. Implementation of the obstetrical data base

3.2.1. Data sets : HP IMAGE software provides the possibility of setting up a complex data organisation structure. Linking between different files is restricted to 16 relations. IMAGE data files have a fixed length record size. The total number of different item names is restricted to 255. This posed some problems to us. The high number of registered variables obliged us to use the same item names in different data sets although they have a different meaning. A cross-reference table however identifies each variable. Each file as shown in Figure 1 corresponds to a data set. All data sets are linked to a master data set containing the unique patient identification number and one with an obstetrical departmental number. Time dependent data are linked with the date as a key. Multiple follow-up examinations can thereby be sorted in chronological order. The above mentioned restriction on the number of data items was not the only reason why 14 different data sets have been created. Since not all items of the follow-up visit are encoded, this would have resulted in too much empty disc space,

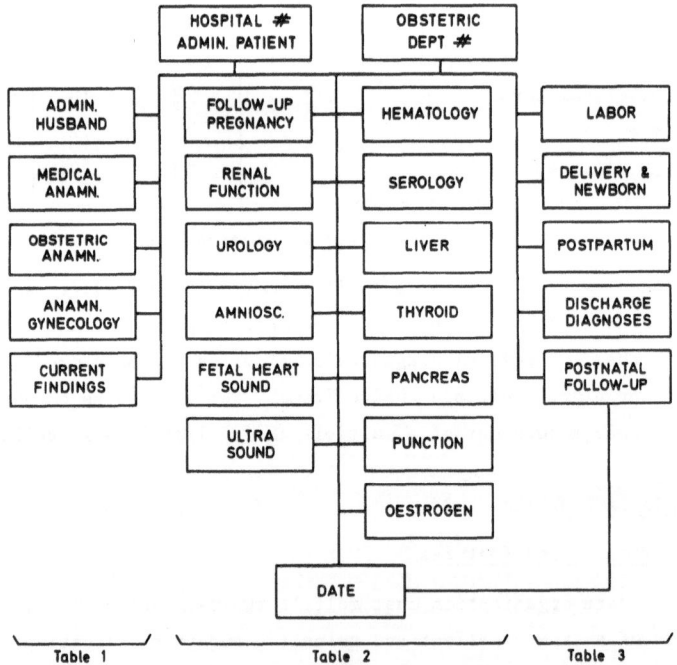

Figure 1 : Data files corresponding with the categories listed in Tables 1, 2 and 3

if all results would have been grouped into a few large data sets.

3.2.2. Data_items_ : The same item name in a different file can have a different meaning but should have the same characteristics concerning format and privacy level. Three format types are available : integer, floating point and ASCII character format. Most of the variables are stored in binary format in order to save disc space. Each of the items has two privacy levels, one for read and one for write accesses. A small number of the items are compound. A compound item accepts a vector of values, with the same characteristics. The physician for example has a choice of 99 treatment possibilities . If the compound item has 5 replicates, he can enter at most 5 different treatments out of the total of 99.

4. DATA ENTRY, VALIDATION, SECURITY AND RECOVERY

4.1. Data_entry_and_validation

The data encoded by the physician, are entered interactively by a medical secretary in a multipurpose HP 1000 minicomputer system, with 416 K bytes of core memory and 2 x 50 Megabyte of disc storage. A program has been written that enables each missing information within a data set to generate a missing value code. Relevant information is tested on minimum and maximum values. By adjusting these ranges the reliability of the data can markedly be increased (1). Although outliers are detected on-line, the user can still force the system to accept extreme values.

4.2. Security

Accessing the data base can only be performed if one has logged on to the computer system with a password and identification, has the capability of running programs of a certain level and knows the security word of the data base. Reading the data can be performed by all admitted users. Writing or updating however is restricted.

4.3. Recovery

Some supplementary programs had to be written in order to compensate for a certain lack in recovery possibilities of the HP-IMAGE data base software. Every record entered in the data base is duplicated in a sequential disc file, so that in case of troubles the last valid data base can be updated.
When the data base capacity is attained, long term storage is needed for later statistical analysis. Programs performing this offload on magnetic tape are available.

5. CONCLUSION

At Leuven University we have implemented a rather extensive computer-oriented obstetrical medical record and data base system. A total of 404 items can be coded. Results from multiple examinations performed in the prenatal, delivery, post-partum and postnatal period are being linked by means of the date of examination. The aims of the project have been stated in rather general terms in the introduction. It is still too early to forecast whether concrete objectives will be reached. First experiences in the clinic however, indicate that coding and logistic problems can be handled. A high number of problem pregnancies are being referred to our Department of Gynecology and Obstetrics. With the aid of the computerized obstetric record we hope to study certain subgroups of these patients. Emphasis will be laid on an evaluation of clinical care decisions. The design and contents of the obstetrical record have been amply discussed and carefully analysed. The record has been structured into well defined segments and is highly systematized. Multiple-choice lists and coding squares have been preprinted throughout the medical record. The analysis and construction of the data base resulted in an unexpected but positive experience for the physicians. The data base has been designed in such a way that interactive data entry and retrieval of any single or compound item is possible over a certain data collection period. A total of 20 Mega-bytes are at present on-line available for the obstetric user. It has been estimated that this can accomodate the findings of about 2500 patients. For periodic statistical analysis this size will be increased five fold by using the resources from another node of the minicomputernetwork (2). Online interactive statistical analysis will be performed with ISPAHAN (3). Further offline analysis will be made with the SPSS package. The HP IMAGE-1000 data base management software has certain limitations. Nevertheless with the aid of this package a solution could be given to some intricate linkage problems. User programs have been developed to optimize the reliability, security and recovery of the data. A tool has thereby been developed which will be of great assistance to future clinical research projects at our department of Gynecology and Obstetrics.

6. REFERENCES

1. Van Hemel, O.J.S. : An obstetric data base. Human factors, design and reliability. Thesis V.U. Amsterdam, Publ. VAM-Voorschoten, 1977, pp. 1-279.

2. Boel, A., Willems, J.L., Eelen, L., Pardaens, J., Theunissen, W. : Beschikbaarheid van gegevens en hulpmiddelen door een computernetwerk. In Proc. Impact van de Gedistribueerde Informatica, (Ed. R. De Caluwe), Publ. FBVI-Ceuterick, Leuven, 1980, pp. 105-111.

3. Lesaffre, M., Boel, A. and Willems, J.L. : Implementation of ISPAHAN on an HP minicomputersystem. In "Pattern Recognition in Practice" (Eds. E. Gelsema and L.N. Kanal), North Holland Publ., Amsterdam, 1980, pp. 527-534.

7. ACKNOWLEDGMENT

This project has been supported by a grant to the project "Mother and Child" from the Belgian "National Fund for Child Welfare". The programming assistance of M. Van de Woestijne and the secretarial help of Sonia Symens are gratefully acknowledged.

CONTINUOUS INTRAPARTUM FETAL ELECTROCARDIOGRAPHY USING A REAL-TIME COMPUTER

HML JENKINS   MB   MRCOG
Medical Research Fellow

DL KIRK   PhD   ARCS
Lecturer

EM SYMONDS   MD   MRCOG
Professor

Department of Obstetrics & Gynaecology,
and
Department of Electrical & Electronic Engineering,
University of Nottingham.

1. SUMMARY

The design of a system which continuously monitors the fetal electrocardiogram [FECG] is outlined. The system consists of two main hardware components; a data acquisition system based on a modified fetal monitor, and a data processing system based on a modern high-speed minicomputer. The system operates in real time, and is currently employed to continuously assess the various parameters of the FECG during the course of labour.

2. INTRODUCTION

Continuous fetal heart rate (FHR) monitoring in labour has become a standard technique in the modern management of labour. The source of the signal for FHR monitoring most commonly used is the fetal electrocardiogram (FECG) and the triggering signal is the fetal QRS complex.

The measurement of heart rate alone uses only a single parameter from the data provided by the fetal electrocardiogram, yet attempts to monitor other intrapartum changes in the configuration of the fetal complex have been met with limited success. The practical difficulties of monitoring these changes, particularly in a situation of continuous monitoring, are considerable. The signal to noise ratio of the fetal ECG is poor; the noise component arises from a number of fetal and maternal sources.   Thus, whilst it is a relatively simple problem to identify heart rate by measuring and recording the time intervals between consecutive R waves, the measurement of other time intervals is dependent on a technique that detects the remaining lower amplitude waves within the ECG complex.

Previous workers have analysed short samples of the FECG, but this paper describes a computer-based method for the continuous assessment of the FECG throughout labour.

3.   HARDWARE AND SOFTWARE

A schematic drawing of the facility employed in the analysis of the intrapartum FECG is presented in Figure I.   The system may be divided into two hardware sections, the data acquisition system and the data processing computer system. Within the latter, the software is divided into three subsystems: FECG complex recognition;   FECG complex averaging and enhancement;   and FECG evaluation.

3.1.   Data acquisition system

The FECG is obtained in the normal manner from a conventional stainless steel spiral scalp electrode.   The intrauterine pressure (IUP) is measured simultaneously using a flexible polythene intrauterine catheter and a Gould-Statham pressure transducer.   Both the FECG lead and pressure transducer leads are connected to a Sonicaid FM3R fetal monitor.   Internal modifications to the monitor are required as the incoming FECG signal normally undergoes several phases of filtering which reduce the bandwidth to approximately 5 to 30 Hz and considerably distort the FECG complex.   The Sonicaid ECG module has therefore been modified to give a bandwidth of 5 to 500 Hz.The machine continues to operate as a conventional fetal monitor.   The FECG and intrauterine pressure are continuously recorded by a Racal F.M. tape recorder running at 15/16 inches per second to ensure economic tape usage, one 7 inch spool of tape lasting approximately 12 hours.

The computer system performs on-line, real time processing of the FECG and IUP signals, with simultaneous recording of the latter.   Alternatively, signals may be recorded off line and processed at a later date.   In either event, the use of magnetic tape provides a permanent record of the whole labour.

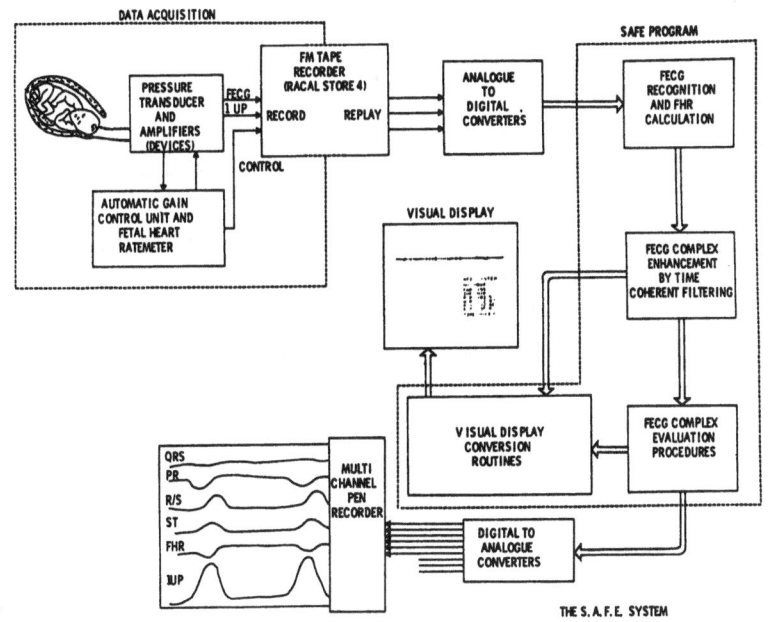

Figure 1:   Schematic drawing of computer system.

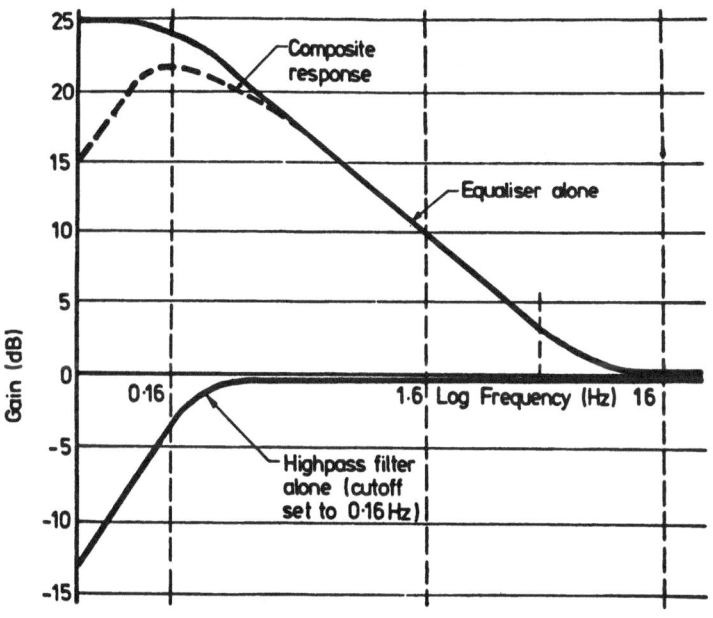

Figure 2:   Frequency response of equaliser.

3.2. Data processing system

The data processing of the FECG and IUP is performed on a DEC 11/23 minicomputer equipped with twin hard discs, line printer and terminal.   The data output is further processed by an Apple microcomputer acting as an intelligent terminal.

The analogue signals of FECG and IUP are digitised at a sampling rate of 500 Hz and input to the computer system via a 64 word buffer.   In order to compensate for the loss of low frequency components occurring in the data acquisition process, it is necessary to boost the low frequency components by a software equalisation routine.   The equaliser used is combined with a two pole high pass filter; the frequency response of the equaliser, and the composite response is shown in Figure 2.   The equaliser restores frequency components above 0.16 Hz and the high pass filter provides additional attenuation of low frequency noise below 0.16 Hz.

3.2.1. FECG complex recognition

Before the FECG waveform can be evaluated, it is necessary to recover the complexes from the incoming signal and noise.   Because of the poor signal to noise ratio of the FECG signal, the QRS complex is frequently the only recognisable feature of the waveform.

Of the several methods of QRS detection previously described, it has been found that using a matched filter gave the best results.   The frequency content of the fetal QRS complex is mainly confined to the 20-40 Hz band.   A filter has been designed which will have a passband exactly matching this spectral content and has been implemented in the software (Figure 3).

3.2.2. FECG complex averaging and enhancement

Once the FECG complex has been recognised and its time alignment precisely fixed, it is possible to enhance the signal to noise ratio of the waveform by adding the newly detected complex to a stored average of the complex made from combining previous occurrences of the waveform. This methodology was established in principle by Hon and Lee (1), who used a method of averaged transients.   In practice their technique of digital integration is limited because processing must be interrupted to reset the accumulators when they overflow.   This method has therefore been called "group averaging".   If, however, the available data

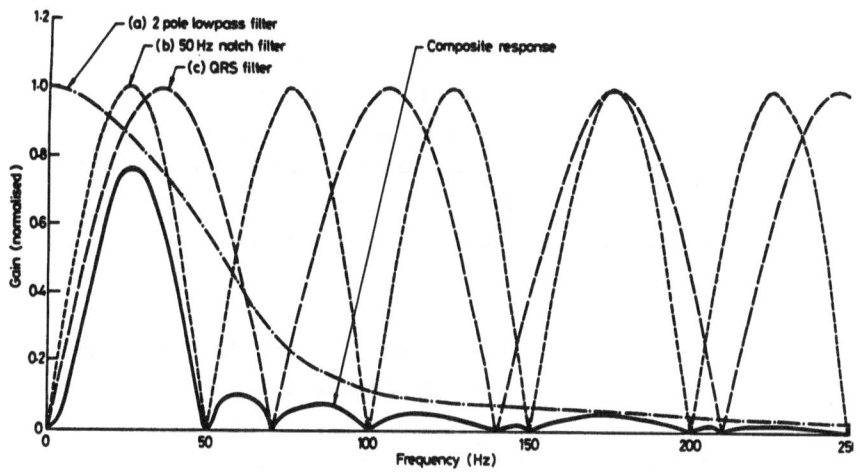

Figure 3:   Frequency response of QRS matched filter.

storage is very large, a running average may be formed by summing the waveforms within the store each time a new complex enters and the oldest leaves. This method is often referred to as the "sliding window average". Rhyne (2) improved the method considerably and overcame the problem of the large storage requirement by using a recursive hardware filter on a dedicated computer system which employed only one data storage register. He also introduced the concept of weighting the running average to give better transient responses to changes in the incoming waveform.

The method of a "weighted sliding window average" has now been implemented as a software digital filter (3). Once the QRS complex of a new beat is precisely located in time, the sampled values representing the 200 ms of signal preceding the R peak, and the 300 ms immediately following this reference point, are transferred to the input of a time coherent filter. Shield and Kirk have shown that the algorithm which generates this filter (in a time domain) is equivalent to a digital filter operating in the frequency domain, for example a Butterworth filter.

Time coherent filtering has been found to provide an excellent method of enhancing the FECG waveform. Non-repetitive transient features are filtered out, thus attenuating the noise components considerably.

3.2.3. FECG evaluation

A new method has been developed which defines the time location of wave components by calculating the intersection of two straight lines representing their rising and falling edges. The lines are calculated by a method of linear regression to obtain the least square fits of a straight line through the data points comprising the rising and falling voltage levels of a component of the ECG (4). This method has the added advantage of interpolating wave onsets and peaks to a greater resolution than the 2 ms interval used for processing the waveform.

Once the timing points of the waveform have been established, up to 11 parameters are measured by the software. During the course of a labour lasting 8 hours some 72,000 complexes will be processed. Since the sliding window technique effectively processes each complex, a very large amount of data is output by the system.

3.3. Labour profiles

Because of the difficulties of interpreting the data output, a graphical method of data display has been devised (5). Each parameter is plotted by the computer as two graphs, which show long term and short term trends respectively.

The behaviour of the FECG during the course of normal labours has been defined (6) and the system is currently employed in the study of the FECG in abnormal cases.

4. ACKNOWLEDGEMENTS

This work is supported by the Medical Research Council, Grant Number G979/462/C, and also by the Benjamin Hall Trust.

5. REFERENCES

1.   Hon, E.H. and Lee, S.T.:   Noise reduction in fetal electro-cardiography II Average technics. Am.J.Obstet.Gynecol. 1963; 87:1086.

2.   Rhyne, V.T.: A digital system for enhancing the fetal electrocardiogram. I.E.E.E. Transactions on Bio-medical Engineering 1969; 16:80-86.

3.   Sheild, J.E.A. and Kirk, D.L.: The use of digital filters in enhancing the fetal electrocardiogram. J.Biomed.Engng. 1981; 3:44-48.

4.   Marvell, C.J. and Kirk, D.L.: A simple software routine for the reproducible processing of the electrocardiogram. J.Biomed.Engng. 1980; 2:216-220.

5.   Marvell, C.J., Kirk, D.L., Jenkins, H.M.L. and Symonds, E.M. [a]: The use of labour profiles in assessing the behaviour of the fetal electrocardiogram. J.Biomed.Engng. 1980; 2:221-223.

6.   Marvell, C.J., Kirk, D.L., Jenkins, H.M.L. and Symonds, E.M. [b]: The normal condition of the fetal electrocardiogram during labour. Br.J.Obstet.Gynaecol. 1980; 87:786-796.

A UNIQUE REAL-TIME COMPUTERISED METHOD OF OBSTETRIC DATA COLLECTION

Madeleine Saunders, Stuart Campbell, Howard White
and Percy Coats

Department of Obstetrics and Gynaecology
King's College Hospital Medical School
Denmark Hill, London SE5 8RX

1. SUMMARY

The system is unique in that patient notes are created by the computer from data entered directly by the midwife during history taking. The information is entered from bar-coded questionnaires read with a light pen.

The system:-

1. Is quick, easy to use, ensures completeness and avoids duplication of data collection.
2. Improves communication and aids patient management by complete identification of antenatal risk factors.
3. Provides well designed case-notes.
4. Creates an obstetric data base for departmental analysis and review.
5. Ensures confidentiality as it is a dedicated system.
6. Can be developed to correlate paediatric developmental information with the obstetric data base.

2. AIMS AND OBJECTIVES

King's College Hospital, which is a teaching hospital of the University of London serving the deprived inner city community of Lambeth, was awarded a grant for a project aimed at reducing perinatal mortality and infant handicap in the district. The objectives were to improve antenatal care through better identification of risk factors at booking[1,2,3] and improved education of midwifery and medical staff in the management of these problems. The second initial objective was the collection of accurate departmental figures to provide statistics for analysis and discussion at regular staff meetings.

3. BACKGROUND

At the outset visits were made to several of the existing obstetric data collection projects in the British Isles. Most of these systems were of the retrospective archival type utilising documents coded by medical staff or clerks and entered into the computer by punch cards or optical mark reader forms. The main problems of these systems were incomplete data collection due to inadequate recording in medical case records, incorrect form coding and, frequently, a large back log of case records for analysis[4,5]. Another practical problem was the use of case notes which were designed more for computer compatibility than for patient management. A recent study visit to perinatal networks in the United States highlighted similar problems of incomplete and untimely data collection[6]. Thus the need for a real-time computer system was obvious from our own observations and the comments of Stead[6] "if the physician were to enter data directly into the computer data collection would be more accurate and complete" and Rosen[7] "an ideal obstetric computer-based data management system would begin with the assessment of risk from the patient's past history, pregnancy course and labor progress as a basis for analysing the condition of the fetus during labor".

4. HARDWARE AND SOFTWARE

The computer used is a Digital PDP 11/34 minicomputer with a 67 megabyte disc and a magnetic tape unit. This computer can support 10-12 terminals with a good response time and allows for simultaneous programme development. At present the computer is connected to 7 outlet points (4 ante-natal clinic, 1 ultrasound department, 2 labour ward) and 3 VDU and bar-code readers are available.

The bar-code reader used is the Telepen made by SB electronics. The light pen is of robust design with a rounded tip which does not damage the questionaire books used. It is able to read relatively poor quality print, thus we can print and photocopy our own bar-codes. A Qume daisy wheel printer is used in the clinic to print the patient's notes.   This gives an excellent quality print in red and black (see Figure 2) and the precise carriage control allows us to print out our own bar-code labels.

Programmes are written in a compiled Basic. The software system is DEC RSX 11-M which is a flexible operating system permitting multi-user operation and simultaneous programme development. The system design is very flexible and, within limits, allows alteration of questions and answers without re-programming. Although if data validation is necessary some routines may need amending.

A multi-key indexed filing system is used and records can be accessed by unit number, bar-code number, surname or maiden name. Access time to retrieve a patient's record is currently less than half a second. Data is stored in the patient file in the form of bar-code numbers, thus only a few hundred bytes of disc are needed to store an entire medical and obstetric history.

Regular copies of the disc are made onto magnetic tape and onto a back-up disc. Each time patient data is entered onto the disc a simultaneous copy is made onto magnetic tape to provide a back-up in the event of disc failure. If the computer goes down then histories can be taken using the questionaire books and entered manually onto case records. Data can then be entered to the computer using the bar-coded questionaires once the computer is running again.

Medical data files and patient's personal data files are stored separately on disc
with differing access codes. Thus by assigning limited access pass words confidentiality is ensured. As the computer is dedicated exclusively to departmental data
collection, outside access is not possible.

5. SYSTEM DEVELOPMENT

Our initial work was to develop a system utilising a keyboard and VDU mode of data
entry. However, the disadvantages of this method were that staff were unfamiliar
with the typewriter keyboard and that the operator was concentrating on the VDU screen
rather than the patient. As an alternative, a system utilising bar-coded data entry
was designed. Questionnaires were developed to cover all aspects of the antenatal
booking interview and clinical examination. Midwifery and medical staff were consulted at all stages of the questionnaire design and many revisions were made. The
bar-coded question and answer sheets (Figure 1) are photocopied from the originals
and enclosed in plastic folders for use in the clinic.

Are there any tablets,
medicines or injections to
which you have an allergy
or special sensitivity and
which you have been advised
not to take again?

Mark correct group/s

Penicillin

Other antibiotics

NO

Elastoplast

Other allergy

Figure 1. A multiple answer question.

As the history is taken the appropriate bar-coded answer is read with the light pen
and an audible signal is given. Single or multiple answers must be given to each
question in sequence. If an error is made, eg by missing a question or giving multiple answers to a single answer question, an audible signal is given and a set of
instructions appears on the VDU screen. Validation checks are built in at various
points to improve reliability of data. At the completion of each portion of the
questionnaire, the data entered is displayed on the VDU screen, this can then be
checked with the patient and any necessary corrections made. This system ensures
simple, complete and uniform data entry. There is also improved communication with

the patient as the only equipment used by the midwife is the light pen.

On completion of history taking the patient's notes are printed out on the clinic printer. Good quality paper used with the daisy wheel printer gives an excellent hard copy with important facts displayed in red or capital letters. Figure 2 is an actual set of notes printed in the clinic. A great deal of time was spent in designing a print-out which would be acceptable to all users. When the patient is seen by the doctor specific details can be hand-written onto the print-out to aid management. However, these details are not entered into the computer.

KING'S HEALTH DISTRICT (TEACHING)   OBSTETRIC DEPARTMENT

AB123456
Jean SMITH

d.o.b.: 07/12/62

booked: 09-Nov-81
age: 18
status: single
Caucasian

Past MEDICAL and SURGICAL History	FAMILY History
Recurrent UTI	Diabetes
Ulcerative colitis	Hypertension - No
No other medical problems	Cong. abnormality - No
Rubella ? (Recent contact)	
No surgical problems	

DRUGS TAKEN during pregnancy:-	smokes - 1 - 5 a day (previously 6 - 10 a day)
	Alcohol most days a week
NO allergies	Social worker referral requested

Past OBSTETRIC History   GRAVIDA 2   para 1 + 0

date	place	gest wks	pregnancy	labour	puerperium	infant
JAN 1980	King's	Term	normal	Spont. labour Forceps	normal	2.980Kg male Breast Child alive & well

Figure 2. Antenatal record print-out.

A bar-coded questionnaire has been developed for entry of data from the labour ward and a print-out for the labour and delivery data is being designed.

6. RESULTS

Tests during system development show that the bar-code reader is easy to use with the minimum of training and midwives accept it as a method of data collection and feel comfortable using it. The average time taken to obtain a standardised past medical and family history is 8 minutes 39 seconds with a range of 12 minutes 20 seconds to 6 minutes 5 seconds. A trial is in progress to compare the booking history taken with the bar-coded questionnaire with that previously obtained in the manual fashion. Full analysis of results will be presented; initial data indicate that many important pieces of information were missed in the previous non directive mode of data collection. During the trial the response of patients to the new system has been encouraging, several of them have expressed an increased confidence compared with the more haphazard manual history taking.

7. DISCUSSION

Partly due to delays in obtaining hardware, the system has taken much longer to develop than was anticipated. However, this time has enabled us to spend longer on questionnaire development and print-out design. The concentration of our efforts on ease of operation, avoidance of duplication of effort and the high quality of the print-out has aided the acceptance of the system. In fact we are now continually being asked by the midwifery staff when the computer will be available for general use!

Although we chose to start with the antenatal data collection, in retrospect a labour ward summary would have been much quicker to design and implement. This would have fulfilled our second objective, data collection, but would not have helped in patient management.

When the antenatal system is implemented we will incorporate a second print-out for each patient containing suggestions for her obstetric management based on her past history. This print-out will be used for medical staff education.

Once the labour data is entered it will be possible to design a print-out to be used as a general practitioner discharge summary[5,8]. This summary can also be placed in the infant's case-notes.

Future developments will include direct data entry from the ultrasound department and the neonatal unit. In the long-term we hope to link the paediatric developmental information with the obstetric data base.

8. REFERENCES

1. Goodwin JW, Dunne JT, Thomas BW. Ante partum identification of the fetus at risk. Can Med Assoc J. 1969; 101: 458: 57-67.
2. Sokol RJ, Rosen MG, Stojkov J et al. Clinical application of high risk scoring on an obstetric service. Am J Obstet Gynecol. 1977; 128: 652-661.
3. Hobel CJ. Risk assessment in perinatal medicine. Clin Obstet Gynecol. 1978; 21 (2): 287-295.
4. South J, Rhodes P. Computer service for obstetric records. Br Med J. 1971; 4: 32-35.

5. Tuck CS, Cundy A, Wasman H et al. The use of a computer in an obstetric depart-
    ment. Br J Obstet Gynaecol. 1976; 83,2: 97-104.
6. Stead WW, Brame RG, Hammond WE et al. A computerised obstetric medical record.
    Obstet Gynecol. 1977; 49,4:502-509.
7. Rosen MG, Sokol RJ, Chik L. Use of computers in the labor and delivery suite.
    Am J Obstet Gynecol. 1978; 132:589-594.
8. South J. A computer summary used as a discharge letter. J R Coll Gen Pract.
    1972; 22:28-32.

INTRAPARTUM MONITORING AND ITS EFFECTS ON PREGNANCY OUTCOME

J. Stack
A. R. Unwin
R. F. Harrison

Departments of Statistics and Obstetrics & Gynaecology
Trinity College Dublin,
Ireland

SUMMARY

13,112 patients were delivered at the Rotunda Hospital, Dublin, from
1st January, 1979 to 31st December, 1980.   Full data was collected
from 12,946 of which 47% received intra-partum fetal monitoring.

After necessary exclusions, the relevant parameters on 8,246 of these
deliveries were analysed, divided for comparative purposes as to whether
or not they received intra-partum mechanical fetal monitoring.

This retrospective study fails to show significant benefits attributable
to intra-partum monitoring although it appears that more of those
patients with meconium, more who had non-routine deliveries and more of
the high-risk pregnancies were monitored.

We suggest that instead of the routine monitoring of the majority of
patients that it should be concentrated on the 'at risk' patient.

INTRODUCTION

Labour is perhaps the greatest time of stress for the fetus.   The fetal
heart activity shows how well the fetus is coping with this stress.
This is noted either by stethoscope auscultation at regular intervals
or by continuous direct electrocardiographic monitor measurements (FHR)
where fetal distress is suggested by changes in the fetal heart, which
the monitor detects, allowing early corrective action.

There is disagreement about the relative merits of these two approaches
to fetal heart recordings and many studies have been carried out to
compare them[1-4].   There is also controversy amongst those who use
monitors as to whether all patients or only those at risk should be
placed on the machines.   In a large retrospective study, Mueller-Meubach
et al (1980)[1] compared 6,740 births in 1970 (none of which were monitored) with 8,174 births in 1977 (73% of which were monitored).   After
correcting for other changes in obstetric practice over the period covered
by the study, and also for changes in the patient population, they con-

cluded that monitoring significantly reduced the incidence of severe birth asphyxia but that the neonatal death rate was not significantly changed.

Neutra et al (1978)[2] studied 15,846 live-born infants to assess the effect of monitoring on neonatal deaths. No other outcomes were considered and the data was collected over a period of seven years. They stratified the patients into five categories of risk and concluded that monitoring might make a difference in the highest risk category (which only included 120 of the patients) but would have little or no effect on the much larger low-risk categories.

Prospective randomized studies have also been carried out (Haverkamp et al, 1976[3] and Kelso et al, 1978[4]) but both failed to find any benefits for monitoring. Monitored and auscultated groups were matched for age, gravidity, gestation and other variables. Both these studies were small and, since the conditions which monitoring might benefit are rare, very large populations would be needed in order to establish significant differences in these conditions between monitored and auscultated patients.

Objectives

The objectives of the study reported in this paper were to assess the diagnostic performance of monitoring and to compare monitoring and auscultation over a short period of time for large numbers of patients. The effects of monitoring on all relevant outcomes were to be assessed and the two groups of patients (those monitored and those auscultated) were to be as similar as possible.

Population Studied

All mothers who delivered at the Rotunda Hospital Dublin, Ireland, between 1st January, 1979 and 31st December, 1980 were included in the study. For these patients there is a data bank available on their general identification, obstetric history, antenatal care, labour, delivery and outcome of pregnancy. These data have been collected for research studies in the prevention of perinatal mortality and morbidity. They include of relevance to this study:

    a)   whether a mother was monitored;
    b)   the main indication for monitoring;
    c)   abnormal monitor scores;
    d)   the passing of meconium;
    e)   morbidity (using the ICD coding);
    f)   mortality.

This data set was ideal for a retrospective study of monitoring because it was collected over a short period and because approximately half the births were monitored.

METHODOLOGY

(1) Outcomes
A frequent flaw in previous studies was to assess monitoring on the basis of all neonatal deaths or all morbid conditions without regard to outcomes that monitoring could not possibly have affected. To avoid this the deaths were separated into two groups, those related to fetal distress and others. A death was classified in the former group if the main or second cause of death was recorded as any of the following:

a)	Cerebral symptoms	(ICD 7790-2)
b)	Respiratory distress syndrome	(ICD 7690)
c)	Other respiratory	(ICD 7700-8)
d)	Subdural and cerebral haemorrhage	(ICD 7670)
e)	Intrauterine death (during labour)	(ICD 7681)

A similar division of morbid outcomes into fetal distress and others was also made and included feeding problems (ICD 7800) and blue asphyxia (ICD 7686).

(2) Exclusions
Initial descriptive analyses were carried out on all 13,112 patients but to make proper comparisons between monitored and auscultated groups certain exclusions had to be made. Patients who could not have been monitored were not included. Thus late abortion deaths, macerated stillbirths, pre-labour caesarean sections and short labours were excluded from further analysis as were cases of maternal diabetes because of differences in the management of these pregnancies since the start of data collection. Private and semi-private patients were also excluded as they were socio-economically different from the public patients and were on average monitored less frequently. The effect of these exclusions (and of some due to incomplete data) was to reduce the study population to 8,246 cases.

(3) Controlling for differences in the monitored and auscultated groups
As this was a retrospective study it is not surprising that the two groups differed considerably on several factors that could possibly influence outcome. In particular the monitored group contained more high-risk patients which is probably a reflection of the policy for monitoring in the Rotunda Labour Ward. The following factors were controlled for in our analyses:

a) passing of meconium,
b) gestational age,

c) length of labour,
d) 'high-risk' mother.

A mother was defined as 'high-risk' in the event of one or more of the following applying:

a) age less than 20 years
b) pre-eclamptic toxemia
c) primigravid

Other items might have been included in the definition of risk but we found no evidence to suggest that the two groups differed on other factors. Our aim was to make the groups comparable, not to provide a global definition of pregnancies at risk.

RESULTS

(1) Differences between monitored and non-monitored groups

(a) Meconium (Table I)   The passage of meconium is a frequent indicator of fetal distress and monitoring is often carried out when this phenomenon is present. The monitored group therefore contained a higher proportion of meconium cases than the group not monitored.

Table I

Incidence of meconium in patients monitored and not monitored

| | Number of Babies | | |
	Meconium	No Meconium	Totals
Monitored	1408 (22.9%)	4741	6149
Not Monitored	722 (10.4%)	6241	6963
			13112

(b) Type of delivery (Table II) Monitoring was also associated with more difficult deliveries:

Table II

Incidence of monitoring in routine and non-routine deliveries

	Routine delivery	Other
Monitored	933 (15.2%)	5216
Not Monitored	2047 (29.4%)	4916

(2) Sensitivity and specificity of monitoring (Table III)

This table shows the monitoring scores and morbidity of monitored babies:

Table III
Assessment of monitor trace related to morbidity

		Monitor Score		
		Normal	Abnormal	Pathological
	None	2251	636	70
Morbidity	Fetal Distress	228	110	19
	Other	1400	429	51

χ^2_4 = 28.99 showing a highly significant association between monitor output and morbidity.

Nevertheless monitoring is not sensitive (64% of fetal distress cases had a normal score) nor specific (90% of abnormal or pathological scores did not indicate fetal distress).

(3) Controlled comparisons of monitored and auscultated patients

There were only a small number of deaths (20) associated with fetal distress in the study population and there were no significant differences between the monitored and auscultated groups in this respect. Much larger numbers of babies had morbid conditions associated with fetal distress and it was possible to carry out many analyses for groups which were strictly comparable in terms of factors other than whether they had been monitored or not. An example is Table IV:

Table IV
Association of morbidity with monitoring in a group of 'at risk' pregnancies

	Morbidity		
	None	Fetal Distress	Other
Monitored	51	10	33
Not Monitored	3	2	6

This table shows babies which were postmature, had passed meconium, had 'high-risk' mothers and were only delivered after long labours. These were clearly babies severely at risk and it is not surprising that most of them were monitored.

While the results are not statistically significant the monitored group does show proportionately less fetal distress. In none of our analyses of morbidity were statistically significant results obtained. For some groups the proportion of fetal distress cases was actually slightly higher in the monitored group. Babies with none of our 'at risk' factors (delivered at term, no meconium, 'low-risk' mothers, not long labour) were such a group and these are shown in Table V.

Table V
Non 'at risk' babies' morbidity related to monitoring

	None	Morbidity Fetal Distress	Other
Monitored	905	79 (5.2%)	536
Not Monitored	1255	93 (4.7%)	647

DISCUSSION

Monitoring has been assessed many times before[1-4] but no firm conclusions as to its optimum role have been reached. Pregnancy outcomes used to measure the effects of monitoring have generally included many cases which monitoring could not have influenced. Prospective studies using randomised designs have been too small[3,4]. If monitoring reduces the number of fetal distress cases by 20% a trial involving some 9,000 patients would be needed to confirm the effect. Retrospective studies have collected data at widely separated times[1] or over long periods[2]. In either case many other factors are confounded with monitoring.

This current study has solved some of these methodological problems and endeavoured to circumvent the others. Because fetal distress is uncommon (affecting less than 10% of babies) and because the effect of monitoring is not expected to be dramatic, large sample sizes are essential. Prospective studies on such a scale solely to investigate monitoring are not feasible but retrospective studies suffer from the intrinsic differences between the groups that are to be compared. Considerable effort in this study was devoted to splitting up the main monitored and not-monitored groups into directly comparable sub-groups. Our results for these show no significant benefits attributable to monitoring. The possibility however remains that the groups differ on some crucial risk factor or combination of factors for which we have not been able to control. This is an unavoidable difficulty of interpreting results of retrospective studies.

One conclusion of the study would be to dismiss the value of monitoring altogether. However it is an undeniable fact that monitoring can identify adverse reactions of the fetus to labour. We therefore recommend that instead of routine monitoring of the majority of patients (requiring one monitor for every 2-400 patients)[5] fetal cardio-tocography should be concentrated on the 'at risk' patient (requiring one monitor for every 1,500 deliveries). This enables staff to be more responsive to danger

154

signals with a consequent improvement in outcome of the 'at risk' patient and yet allow the majority to have as natural a labour as possible uncluttered by potentially stressful machines.

Acknowledgement

To Professor Browne and the Friends' of the Rotunda for their support and permission to use their data, and to the Statistics and Operations Research Laboratory, Trinity College Dublin, for their assistance.

References

1. Mueller-Meubach, E., MacDonald, H.M., Joret, D., Portman, M.A., Edelstone, D. and Caritis, S.N. (1980). Am. J. Obstet. Gynaecol. 137, 758-762

2. Neutra, R.R., Fienberg, S.E., Greenland, S. and Friedman, E.A. (1978) New Eng. J. Med., 299, 7, 324-6.

3. Haverkamp, A.D., Thompson, H.E., McFee, J.G. and Cetrulo, C. (1976). Am. J. Obstet. Gynaecol. 125, 310-320

4. Kelso, I.M., Parsons, R.J., Laurence, G.F., Arora, S.S., Edmonds, D.K. and Cooke, I.D. (1978). Am. J. Obstet. Gynaecol. 131, 526-531

5. Leading Article (1976). Br. Med. J. 2, 1466

THE LOGICAL DEVELOPMENT OF A PERINATAL
DATA BASE FOR CLINICIANS

M Maresh, P J Steer,
A M Dawson, R W Beard,

Department of Obstetrics and Gynaecology
St Mary's Hospital Medical School
London W2, England

SUMMARY

A microcomputer system has been developed which stores data for perinatal audit and produces the birth notification form and discharge summary. The system and its advantages over conventional methods are outlined. The deriation of its small, reliable and essential data base from a previous mainframe computer system is described in detail, as are the on-line validation checks on data entry.

1. INTRODUCTION

The reliable collection of obstetric and neonatal data has recently become a subject of considerable interest with the publication of the Report of the Parliamentary Select Committee on Perinatal and Neonatal Mortality (1) and of the Körner Committee set up by the Government to rationalise medical data collection (2). We have been working on the subject for the past six years latterly using a microcomputer. Our aim has been to combine the collection of data essential for perinatal audit with the production of the statutory birth notification form and maternal and neonatal discharge summaries. The philosophy underlying our system has been that it must be simple so that it can be used in busy maternity units.

2. SYSTEM DESCRIPTION

A Commodore PET microcomputer disc unit and printer which will fit on top of a desk in the labour ward office is being used at present. It has the advantage that it is a cheap system (less than £2500) and widely used.

The basis scheme is outlined in Figure 1. As soon as a mother has delivered her baby, information required for the statutory birth notification form is entered onto the microcomputer by the midwife who conducted the delivery. To produce the birth notification form 14 frames with between one and five lines, an example of which is shown in Figure 2, have to be completed. All lines (with the exception of names, addresses

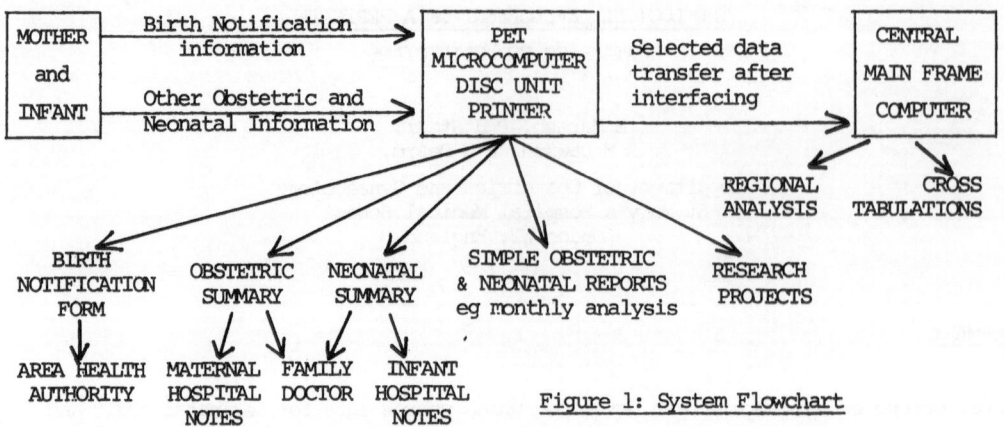

Figure 1: System Flowchart

and congenital abnormalities) have only specific answers which can be entered in the boxes and the choice is displayed beside the box. This is preferable to systems which use blank boxes for international Classification of Diseases (ICD) codes since there are bound to be errors of omission when these are filled in at a later date by coding clerks. 'On line' vetting is used (see below) and when all information has been entered, the form is printed and the data stored on five inch floppy discs. This phase has been subjected to a successful trial (3) in May 1981 and our midwives took about 10 minutes to enter the data and check the form.

Figure 2: A Frame

APGAR AT
1 MINUTE   `0 8`

APGAR AT
5 MINUTES   `1 0`

REGULAR
RESPIRATION   `0 1`
(minutes to onset)

PRESS 1 TO CORRECT ANY LINE
PRESS RETURN TO CONTINUE

The second input of data is by a trained clerical officer within 24 hours of the mother leaving hospital. This provides the data necessary for a mother and baby discharge summary and completes the information needed for perinatal audit. When the 15 frames with their validation checks have been completed the discharge summary is produced from the data entered in both inputs. The obstetrician then signs and dispatches the summary to the mother's general practitioner and the data is stored on the same disc. As a back-up the printer produces a list of all the data entered on each mother and baby in case the disc should be damaged. This phase is being subjected to clinical trial in November 1981, with a view to routine use in 1982.

The final development will be programmes to provide a regular audit of clinical practice. A monthly labour ward analysis will be produced and detailed perinatal audit will be obtained by transferring information to the Regional Computer Centre for more sophisticated cross-tabulation. Before transfer of data all means of identifying the

the mother and her baby will be removed to ensure complete confidentiality.

3. ADVANTAGES OF A MICROCOMPUTER SYSTEM

The developments in microcomputer technology imply that even detailed data collection systems can be managed by microcomputers and yet the bigger models are still relatively cheap (less than £10,000). Their compactness and mobility, and their ability to be at the site of action make them very attractive.

Mainframe computer systems like the Standard Maternity Information Service (SMIS) do not aim to produce full documentation of the pregnancy (4). This implies a duplication of data collection and wastage of medical, midwifery, clerical and secretarial time if such documentation is to be obtained. A microcomputer system whilst storing data for perinatal audit can produce immediately the birth notification form, maternal discharge summary and neonatal discharge record. With the SMIS system labour wards will still have to produce their own annual figures since results from the central computer will not be available until midway through the next year. A microcomputer can have a programme to produce a monthly labour ward analysis immediately and the annual one would be available early in the following year since all the data is stored in the individual department. Thus a microcomputer provides an incentive at the local level for collecting good data.

Mainframe systems have the problem that if errors and omissions are detected by a vetting programme it is always after the event and the hospital notes have to be found and the incorrect or missing data sought, wasting valuable clerical time. The 'on-line' vetting of a microcomputer ensures that the errors and omissions are detected as the data is entered from the notes. In addition a mainframe system employs form filling and subsequent transcribing onto the computer, giving two opportunities for errors to arise. Thus a microcomputer system should be able to provide more reliable information with a considerable financial saving and be more accessible to clinicians and administrators.

4. DERIVATION OF DATA BASE

4.1 Introduction: In busy teaching centres it is possible to collect a large amount of reliable data which can be analysed on a mainframe computer. In the past we have used such a system and it involved a considerable volume of work for the medical staff and research midwives. Only a fraction of the information collected has been used to date, which is an experience found in other units using similar schemes. This type of system may not be suitable for busy maternity units or hospitals with low staffing levels. Thus to produce a data scheme which can be used widely one must limit the amount of data collected. We have derived a small data base in the following way. Items for inclusion have been assessed to ensure that they are easy to collect, reliable and necessary, by analysing data from 2386 pregnancies on a mainframe computer file which was collected between 1976-78. The mainframe computer base needed, for singleton pregnancies, 426 numerical data items to complete the programme using 6 80 column cards One hundred and fifty eight separate variables were included, but some were in multiple choice format making over 300 possible replies.

The ease of collection of an item of data was assessed by calculating the percentages of missing values for each item after recall and checking of hospital notes. Only twelve items were found to be missing in more than 2% of cases. The reliability of an item of data was assessed by analysis of the distribution of the results. For example, analysis of the answers for blood loss at delivery showed that certain replies were always given and so these have been regarded as unreliable and have been excluded. In addition items like a past history of premature labour were considered to be difficult to document accurately. In total 25 items were thought to be unreliable and have been excluded.

Having slightly reduced the size of the data base an assessment was then made as to what data was actually needed.

4.2 Data for the birth notification form: Forty nine items were needed for the statutory birth notification form, but five could be derived by the microcomputer. With our trial of the computer-produced birth notification form (3), we were able to demonstrate high error rates for certain questions and the Area Health Authority agreed to a reduction and 13 have been omitted making only 31 items necessary. The presence or absence of fetal distress, an item of information needed for the birth notification form, is assessed by the microcomputer by fetal acidosis pH < 7.20 or abnormal cardiotocography and meconium liquor (abnormal cardiotocography or meconium on their own did not correlate well with depressed Apgar scores whilst the combination did). By including these three items individually the accuracy of the label "fetal distress" should be improved. Meconium stained liquor and abnormal cardiotocography were missing for more than 2% of cases in our mainframe computer system, but the immediate data entry facility of the microcomputer should decrease omissions.

4.3 Data for the discharge summary: Sixty three additional items were considered necessary for the summary of the mother and baby which is sent to the general practitioner. This included the postnatal haemoglobin and whether rubella vaccination was given, but omitted unreliable data such as proposed contraceptive practice.

4.4 <u>Data for perinatal audit</u>: The data considered necessary for this was derived in the following way. Tables were drawn (for example Table 1) of the types of cross tabulations wanted for an annual analysis of the perinatal service.

<u>TABLE 1</u>: Gestational Age and Mode of Delivery for Vertex Presentation

	Spont-Vertex	Straight Instru-mental	Rotat-ional Instrumental	Elective Caesarean	Intrapartum Caeseraen
≤ 28 weeks					
29 - 30					
31 - 32					
33 - 34					
35 - 36					
37 - 41					
≥ 42					

Items included were then checked to see if they conformed with the criteria for ease of collection and reliability. In addition their frequency in our population was obtained from the mainframe data file and, if less than 1%, were excluded unless they were considered to be of major importance (for example, eclampsia). The items left in the mainframe data pool which were not needed for the birth notification form or discharge summary were then critically assessed as to whether they were really of a research nature rather than being necessary for perinatal audit. Fifty items (for example Bishop score of cervix) were thus excluded. In fact only eight items were specifically required for the perinatal audit which were not needed for the forms (for example, maternal height), giving a total of 106 essential items to be divided between the two entries.

5. VERIFICATION OF DATA ENTRY

The ability of the microcomputer to have 'on-line' vetting of data entries has been used extensively to improve the reliability and completeness of the data entered. Since our system has two data inputs it is possible to enter the same data in both, and any inconsistencies between the two will be queried as soon as the second is entered. Double entry has been used for identification purposes, for mothers surname, hospital number and date of birth of infant, and for important data such as birth weight, congenital abnormalities, stillbirth and neonatal death. Gestation at delivery is crucial and in an attempt to ensure accuracy the date of the last menstrual period, the certainty of the date and the cycle regularity have been included to cross-check against the gestation. There are five more cross-checks in the first input (for example, date of entry of data must be the same or after the date of delivery) and limits are imposed on all the numerical answers so that if birth weight was entered as 350g instead of 3500g this would be queried. The second input has similar limits and a further 15 cross-checks, for example: date of birth must be later or equal to date of booking; Caesarean section must have either epidural or general anaesthesia; and if the mother is rubella immune and no vaccination is given then this is queried. There are ten cross-checks between the two inputs and these are mainly checks on duplicate entries.

This validation process coupled with the ability for people close to the event to check immediately the printed forms, should enable a microcomputer system to produce rapid, reliable data.

6. CONCLUSIONS

Many large scale data collection schemes have been described, but the data has frequently been poorly validated making the whole effort almost worthless. By logically developing a small data base and using this in conjunction with a microcomputer we believe we have produced a system which will be advantageous to the clinician and administrator at a local level and yet still allow data to go into a national system. In addition by producing all the documentation necessary for the pregnancy it is attempting to be cost effective.

Our first objective of routinely using a computerised birth notification form, which is acceptable to our Area Health Authority, has been achieved. A discharge summary has been produced and we now await the analysis of the data collected on our 1982 deliveries to test the auditing capacity of our system. Our present programme arrangement means that data for only 140 patients can be stored on each floppy disc. However, with the major developments in microcomputer technology, our system could be adapted so as to be suitable for even the busiest obstetric units in this country.

REFERENCES

(1) Social Services Committee. Perinatal and Neonatal Mortality, London HMSO. 1980.
(2) Report of the working groups A (maternity) to the steering group on health services information, London 1981.
(3) Maresh M, Beard RW, Combe D, Gillmer MDG, Smith G, Steer PJ. Computerisation of obstetric information. The St Mary's Hospital Scheme in First International Symposium on Computers in Perinatal Medicine. Ed: Chik L, Sokol RJ. Cleveland 1981, 69-72.
(4) Thomson AM, Baron SL. A standard maternity information system in Perinatal Audit & Surveillance. Ed: Chalmers I, McIlwaine G. RCOG, London 1980, p82.

DEVELOPING A REGISTER OF

RANDOMISED CONTROLLED TRIALS

IN PERINATAL MEDICINE

Miranda Mugford
Adrian Grant
Iain Chalmers

National Perinatal Epidemiology Unit
Radcliffe Infirmary, Oxford, OX2 6HE

SUMMARY

Randomised controlled trials (RCTs) have special strengths for assessing medical
practice; yet they are difficult to identify with currently available literature
search techniques. The National Perinatal Epidemiology Unit has created a register
of RCTs in perinatal medicine, the contents of which it plans to make widely available. The current card-based information retrieval system is cumbersome and we have
investigated ways of improving the efficiency and accessibility of the register by
transferring it onto a computer.

1. INTRODUCTION

Because of its experimental design, the randomised controlled trial overcomes many of
the problems of bias and interpretation associated with the collection and analysis of
observational data. In theory, therefore, it is the preferred method for assessing
the efficacy and safety of treatments and interventions in medicine. Experience has
shown how widespread adoption of inadequately appraised methods in obstetrics and
neonatal paediatrics has sometimes been misguided, and occasionally disastrous (1).
A greater knowledge and use of the "risk-minimizing" approach of RCTs might have avoided some of these mistakes. Since its formation in 1978 the National Perinatal Epidemiology Unit (NPEU) has been compiling a register of published and ongoing randomized
controlled trials in perinatal medicine. The studies included are prospective, controlled trials in which treatment allocation was either randomised or decided by strict
alternation. All the interventions took place during human pregnancy or within four
weeks of delivery.

Our aim in creating the register is to emphasize the advantage of an experimental research design and to make the results of controlled trials more easily accessible to
those working and researching in the perinatal field.

Sometimes the results of controlled trials have clear implications for practice. If,
for example, more obstetricians had based their decisions concerning the prescription

of stilboestrol in pregnancy on the results of the randomised trials mounted to assess its effects scientifically (2-4), millions of women and fetuses might have avoided the variety of adverse consequences of exposure to the drug (5-8). Many trials do not have such clear implications for practice. This is often because they are too small to identify clinically important beneficial or adverse effects of the interventions studied. The data generated by these small trials can sometimes be reanalysed in the framework of a secondary analysis from which useful information can be obtained (9,10). The Register may help in other ways: published reports of trials may guide the enquirer to the best available observational data, and those trials registered as 'in progress' may indicate when and from where experimentally derived information may be expected. Lastly, documentation by the Register of the current scope of published and ongoing trials should indicate to investigators which elements of practice remain unevaluated by clinical experiments.

2. CREATING THE REGISTER

Current indexing systems do not reliably identify published reports of clinical research by methodology. We used the following program specificiation to search the MEDLINE and MEDLARS databases of the US National Library of Medicine (In the UK, the British Library makes these databases available through BLAISE):-

> Include
>
> 1 Random allocation
> 2 All random
> 3 Clinical and all trial
> 4 Prospective or prospectively
> 5 Double and blind
> 6 Double blind method
> 7 1 or 2 or 3 or 5 or 5 and 6
> 8 7 and human
> 9 Perinatology or infant, newborn or fetus or pregnancy or puerperium, labour or labour complications or pregnancy complications.
> 10 8 and 9

For the period 1966-1976 it is only possible to search the titles of articles in major journals. The research method used is often not clear from the title and only 25% of trials were identified when we used this approach. Since 1976 it has been possible to search abstracts of articles. Comparison of the MEDLARS search of abstracts with a hand literature search of the British Journal of Obstetrics and Gynaecology between the years 1976 and 1978 revealed that the computer search had identified 90% of the trials found during the hand search. This pickup rate may improve if the term Random Allocation (which has recently become a 'minor descriptor' at the NLM) is used by indexers, and more authors (and journal editors) include a reference to research method in the summaries of research reports. There was therefore no alternative but to back-search journals systematically by hand. Forty-four major journals have been searched back to 1950 and trials have been identified in a further fifty. To date, 1800 suitable studies have been identified.

3. CLASSIFICATION OF TRIALS

Because the Medical Subject Heading (MESH) classification of the National Library of Medicine proved inadequate for our purposes, we developed a classification (11) specifically for the Register. The classification is alphanumeric: the letters A to L are used for the various stages in the reproductive cycle from conception, through pregnancy and delivery to infancy; N is used for subjects which cross the boundaries between stages; and the letters P to S are used for the behavioural, health care delivery, and sociological aspects of reproductive medicine. The numbers 1 to 4 are used respectively for physiology, associated problems, diagnostic measures, and therapeutic measures at each stage. Decimal figures are used for further breakdown. In each subsection .0 is used for general papers on the topic, and .9 for specified miscellaneous subjects. For example, a trial of stilboestrol treatment in diabetic pregnancy would be classified C4.36 (Hormone treatment in pregnancy) C2.221 (Diabetes in pregnancy).

4. OPTIONS FOR COMPUTERISING THE REGISTER

Our aim is to make the register accessible to all those interested. Because the current card-based information retrieval system is increasingly cumbersome and inefficient, we have considered whether the Register could be managed more efficiently on a computer. The chosen computer information retrieval system would need the following attributes:-

a) The capacity to store data up to four million characters (4mb), the exact size depending on the format of the records and the degree of indexing employed by the search and retrieval software.

b) The ability to add data to the file as required.

c) Program(s) capable of accessing relevant data on one or more of the following fields:- subjects (major and secondary), author, country of research, language, journal of publication, year of research and size and quality of trial.

d) Display of progress of search on monitor screen.

e) Facilities to print list of references.

f) The ability to use the system whenever required.

g) Reliability and security from erasure of data (ie facilities to duplicate discs etc).

h) Simple updating and searching facilities.

i) Economy of time and cost in labour, computer time and printing.

The major options investigated were:

1   Integration of the Register into an existing large library database

2   Use of local large-capacity computers and existing information-retreival software.

3   Use of a commercial computer bureau for storage and retrieval purposes.

4   Acquisition of a microcomputer with commercially available and tested software compatible with the machine.

The specific investigations we made were as follows:

4.1. Database at BLAISE

Because the majority of current published trials are identified by MEDLINE search of abstracts, we had discussions with the British Library about the possibility of holding our register as a separate database at BLAISE; thus making it easily available to all other users of BLAISE data. Unfortunately this is not yet feasible for technical reasons. Although we can extract items from MEDLINE and create a file to edit and update as we require, existing software does not permit us to re-index our file to conform to the MEDLINE search and retrieval programs.

4.2. Oxford University Computing Service (OUCS)

OUCS offered the use of a batch (not interactive or on-line) index and text retrieval package called FAMULUS. Any advantages of this package were outweighed by the difficulties experienced in the Oxford University Computer Service.

4.3. Commercial Bureaux

We approached three bureaux who market information retrieval services. The raw data would have to be prepared in a specified machine readable format on, for example, magnetic tape. This would involve at least six weeks' full time work by staff who can understand and interpret the existing records. The bureaux would then enter the data and set up the files in a form suitable for searching using their programs. These are inverted index files which pose problems of updating. Connection to the bureau computer is established by telephone and so the database could be used from anywhere with a terminal, modem and GPO line.

The search procedures are fast and efficient, similar in use to a commercial on-line database. Printing of retrieved references requires the additional purchase or hire of a printer to interface with the VDU, or the use of a printer terminal, although large volumes of printing can be directed to the bureau printer and then posted to the user.

We found that the costs of these systems were prohibitive, reflecting the fact that our database is very small by commercial standards.

4.4. Micro-Computer

A micro-computer with twin 8'' floppy disc drive can, in theory, hold up to ½ megabyte of information; with hard disc drive the size of storage can be expanded to 10 or 20 megabytes.

Bearing in mind the size to which we expect the register to grow, we should ideally restrict our choice to a system able to support a hard disc and compatible software to suit our needs.

Our minimum hardware requirements are for a micro-computer of sufficient power to support a disc storage system, printer and VDU. We must be able to copy data for a secure backup. If we used floppy discs alone, we would have to partition the Register; a hard disc would allow the entire Register to be accessed simultaneously.

Our choice of computer is constrained by the need for both adequate internal memory and CP/M format discs; the choice of a CP/M operating system allows a wider choice of compatible software. These requirements rule out several well known micro-computers.

Our software must permit us to enter the records into a file, define fields for search, index the file on different fields, search the indexes to identify trials satisfying specified requirements and then print the relevant records.

Since the start of our investigations easy-to-use information retrieval software written specifically for micro-computers has become available. These create indexes on key words and offer sophisticated searching techniques. Although such systems would be very convenient, we may be obliged to consider cheaper methods. Our classification system considerably reduces the need for detailed keyword indexing by the computer and we have therefore looked at standard software for word and data processing. Such software will allow us to create records and index on chosen fields; the search facilities are not so sophisticated but may be adequate for our purposes.

5. CONCLUSIONS

During our investigation into the transfer of our Register to computer it has become clear that none of the options considered offers a perfect solution. The database will ultimately be too big for a simple micro-computer with floppy disc drive and too small for a commercial mainframe service to be economic. The rapid development of micro-computer technology and software information retrieval has necessitated frequent reappraisal of this option and we now feel that the use of a micro-computer is the method most likely to satisfy our list of requirements at lowest cost.

We acknowledge with gratitude the continuing support of the World Health Organization in creating the Register of Randomised Controlled Trials in Perinatal Medicine.

6. REFERENCES

(1) Silverman WA. Retrolental Fibroplasia – a modern parable. Monographs in Neonatology. New York: Grune and Stratton Inc., 1980.

(2) Ferguson JH. The effect of stilboestrol on pregnancy compared to the effect of a placebo. Am J Obstet Gynecol 1953; 65: 592–601.

(3) Dieckmann WJ, Paris ME, Rynkiewitz LM, Pottinger RE. Does the administration of diethylstilboestrol during pregnancy have therapeutic value? Am J Obstet Gynecol

1953; 66: 1062–1068.

(4) Conference on Diabetes and Pregnancy. The use of hormones in the management of pregnancy in diabetics. Lancet 1955; ii: 833–836.

(5) Bibbo M, Haenzel WM, Wied GL, Hubby M, Herbst AL. A twenty-five year follow-up study of women exposed to diethylstilboestrol during pregnancy. N Eng J Med 1978; 298: 763–767.

(6) Beral V, Colwell L. Randomised trial of high doses of stilboestrol and ethisterone in pregnancy: long-term follow-up of mothers. Br Med J 1980; 281: 1098–1101.

(7) Herbst AL, Hubby MM, Blough RR, Azazi F. A comparison of pregnancy experience in DES exposed and DES non-exposed daughters. J Reprod Med 1980; 24: 62–69.

(8) Beral V, Colwell L. Randomised trial of high doses of stilboestrol and ethisterone therapy in pregnancy: long-term follow-up of the children. J Epidemiol Community Health 1981; 35: 161–167.

(9) Chalmers I. Randomised controlled trials of fetal monitoring 1973–1977. In: Thalhammer O, Baumgarten K, Pollak A, (eds). Perinatal Medicine. Stuttgart: George Thieme, 1979: 260–265.

(10) Baum ML, Anish DS, Chalmers TC, Sacks HS, Smith H, Fagerstrom RM. A survey of clinical trials of antibiotic prophylaxis in colon surgery: evidence against further use of no-treatment controls. N Eng J Med 1981; 305: 795–799.

(11) Enkin E, Chalmers I, Enkin MW. An index for classifying perinatal literature pilot edition. August 1980. National Perinatal Epidemiology Unit, Radcliffe Infirmary Oxford OX2 6HE.

A Comparative Study on the merits of
CAESAREAN SECTION AND VAGINAL DELIVERY
in the management of Breech Births

Alan D.H. Browne,
Department of Obstetrics/Gynaecology
Royal College of Surgeons in Ireland
Rotunda Hospital, Dublin I, Ireland.

and

Patrick Herlihy,
Department of Statistics,
Trinity College, Dublin 2.

Summary

Spectacular advances in neonatal paediatric management have resulted in great improvements in the management of low birth weight infants, accompanied by improved results in terms of survival. This has created a new situation for obstetricians managing patients who are thought to have a very small fetus at the time when the optimum mode of delivery must be selected. This situation is particularly difficult when the fetus presents by the breech. The present study offers an attempt to clarify the position for obstetricians confronted by an imminent delivery of a breech presentation in circumstances where the fetus is thought to be of very low birth weight.

Patients and Methods

Computer assisted methods have been utilised to examine data obtained from I2,995 successive births at the Rotunda Hospital. The series consists of 523 breech deliveries. 421 of these were from singleton pregnancies, and 102 were from multiple pregnancies. There were 35 perinatal deaths, and 4 late neonatal deaths. There were 484 survivors (92.5) amongst the breech births. The overall perinatal mortality rate (stillbirths + 1st week neonatal deaths expressed as a rate against all breech deliveries) was 66.9. A small number of breech presentations (15) were excluded from this study, they delivered spontaneously in the hospital but no mode of delivery was recorded. The babies born were divided into nine birth weight groups (table I) for the purpose of the study.

The mode of deliveries of babies was considered in relation to vaginal delivery and Caesarean Section. The vaginal delivery group includes all methods of vaginal delivery that were used, and the Caesarean Section group likewise includes all cases delivered by this means, whether by the lower segment technique, or the classical technique. The results to babies from singleton pregnancies and multiple pregnancies were considered separately.

Table I.

For the purpose of the study, babies were divided into nine birth weight groups as follows:-

1 =	500 - 999g		6 =	3000 - 3499g
2 =	I000 - I499g		7 =	3500 - 3999g
3 =	I500 - I999g		8 =	4000 - 4499g
4 =	2000 - 2499g		9 =	4500 +
5 =	2500 - 2999g			

Table II shows birth weight related to perinatal mortality for all babies in each birth weight group. In table III, columns 5 and 6 are corrected by the removal of lethal congenital abnormalities from all births in each birth weight group (column 5). The corrected total is shown in column 6, and the corrected perinatal mortality rate in column 7. Table IV shows the total lethal congenital abnormalities encountered in each birth weight group separately for births from singleton pregnancies and multiple pregnancies. The ICD classification of each of these lethal conditions is shown in figures (beside each case)[1]. 740 is Anencephalus and similar conditions. 741 is Spina bifida. 742 is other serious congenital abnormalities of the nervous system. 758 is Chromosomal anomalies. In summary table III indicates the extremely high perinatal mortality actual and corrected in the first four birth weight groups. In addition to 35 perinatal deaths in the nine birth weight groups, there were four later neonatal deaths thus the total mortality in the first 28 days of life was 39 out of the 523 cases, a rate of 74.6.

The percentage survival incidence in each birth weight group is shown in column 6 of table V. Column 5 of table V shows the percentage incidence of birth weight group of the whole series. It will be noted from this table that the survival rate in birth weight groups I and 2 was extremely low - as might be expected. The precentage incidence of birth weight groups I to 3 inclusive is similar, but the survival rate in birth weight group 3 is much more satisfactory that in birth weight groups I and 2, as might be expected.

The high perinatal mortality rates in the low birth weight groups I to 4 inclusive (which together form I9.2% of the whole series) prompts a detailed break-down of the perinatal mortality rate into birth weight groups. Figures for this are shown on table II from which it may be seen that in the low birth weight groups I to 4, babies from multiple pregnancies fare better than singletons.

Table II.

The perinatal mortality rate to the B.W. groups for single and
Multiple births are as follows:-

B.W. Group	PNM Rate	
	Single	Multiple
1	700	667
2	539	400
3	100	91
4	147	133
5	12	24
6	19	53
7	12	0
8	36	0
9	200	-

Table III.

B.W. group X Total births X Corrected PNM excluding lethal
congenital abnormalities.

B.W. Group	Total	Total PNM	B.W. related PNM rate	PNM excluding lethal congenital abnormalities		Corrected PNM rate
				Lethal Congenital	Corrected total	
1	13	9	692	0	9	692
2	18	9	500	1	8	444
3	21	2	95	0	2	95
4	49	7	143	2	5	102
5	124	2	16	1	1	8
6	174	4	23	2	2	11
7	89	1	11	1	0	0
8	29	1	35	1	0	0
9	5	1	200	1	0	0

Table IV.

B.W. Group X lethal Congenital Abnormalities.

B.W. Group	Lethal Congenital		Total
	Singleton	Multiple	
I	O	O	O
2	1(742)	0	1
3	0	0	0
4	2(740)	0	2
5	1(741)	0	1
6	1(741)	1(758)	2
7	1(742)	0	1
8	1(742)	0	1
9	1(740)		1
Total	8	1	9

Table V.

The number of births, in each B.W. group, for singleton and multiple births X incidence % of group X survival % in each group.

B.W. Group	Single	Multiple	Total	B.W. Group incidence%	B.W. Group Survival %
1	10	3	13	2.5	30.8
2	13	5	18	3.4	44.4
3	10	11	21	4.0	90.5
4	34	15	49	9.4	83.7
5	83	41	124	23.7	97.6
6	155	19	174	33.3	97.1
7	83	6	89	7.0	98.9
8	28	1	29	5.5	96.6
9	5	1	6	1.1	83.3
Total	421	102	523		

Further examination of the effect of the mode of delivery in singleton pregnancy births (S) shows (table VI) that in groups I to 4, the perinatal mortality rate using Caesarean Section as the mode of delivery gives much better results than the use of vaginal breech delivery. The one late neonatal death in the vaginal breech delivery series in birth weight group 5 was unrelated to the mode of delivery. Thus it could be argued that there was no advantage in either method in this birth weight group.

In birth weight group 6 the perinatal mortality rate associated with Caesarean Section was almost double that of vaginal breech delivery. The survival incidence was almost identical in the two groups. The incidence of Caesarean Section and vaginal delivery were almost identical. The individual perinatal deaths in groups 7,8 and 9 are all judged to be associated with lethal congenital abnormalities, and the mode of delivery therefore had no effect on perinatal loss.

When the incidence of Caesarean Section and vaginal delivery, are examined in conjunction with those columns which refer to perinatal mortality and survival, it would seem to reinforce the recommendation that Caesarean Section should be seriously considered as the optimum method of delivery for singleton babies in the low birth weight group categories. As a generalisation, it could be stated that in this series the use of Caesarean Section was inversely proportional to its apparent effectiveness in terms of perinatal mortality.

Table VII presents the same information about births from multiple pregnancies (M). As regards perinatal mortality it is clear that Caesarean Section gives the best results. The same can be said following examination of the survival statistics and there appears to be an argument - though much less convincing - for increasing the Caesarean Section incidence in the management of delivery of very low birth weight infants presenting by the breech from multiple pregnancies as well as births from singleton pregnancies.

Discussion

The use of Caesarean Section for the delivery of babies in groups I to 4 requires further consideration. It is a difficult matter to assess the weight of a very small baby by clinical palpation, and where possible it would be a great advantage to have an estimate of the fetal weight provided by ultrasound measurements. In addition it would be advisable to exclude - particularly in singleton births - the presence of such lethal congenital complications as open neural tube defects, (table IV).

Table VI.
Singleton Pregnancy Births (S)

B.W. Group	PNM Rate		Survival %		Mode of delivery incidence %	
	C.S.	Vag	C.S.	Vag	C.S.	Vag
1	250	1000	75	0	40	60
2	0	636	100	27	15	85
3	0	167	100	83	40	60
4	91	174	91	78	32	68
5	0	19	100	96	36	64
6	26	13	97	97	50	50
7	23	0	98	100	53	47
8	0	77	100	92	53	46
9	0	0	100	0	100	0

Table VII
Multiple Pregnancy Births (M)

B.W. Group	PNM Rate		Survival %		Mode of delivery incidence %	
	C.S.	Vag	C.S.	Vag	C.S.	Vag
1	500	1000	50	0	67	33
2	0	500	100	50	20	80
3	0	111	100	80	10	90
4	0	154	100	85	13	87
5	143	0	85	100	17	83
6	0	83	100	85	37	63
7	0	0	100	100	33	67
8	0	0	-	100	-	100
9	-	-	-	-	-	-

Clearly the extended use of Caesarean Section for the delivery of low birth weight babies presenting by the breech should only be considered when neonatal paediatric services are available to provide the necessary life support to the babies after delivery. If this condition cannot be met, it would certainly be preferable to transport the patient to a larger centre for delivery. The question as to whether the lower segment technique or the classical technique of Caesarean Section should be used for the delivery of very low birth weight babies is bound to arise more frequently in the future. Where the lower segment is imperfectly formed, there is a real risk of trauma to the mother due to extension of the incision into the vascular pedicales of the uterus. The classical type of operation - keeping the incision low - is likely to avoid such problems, but obstetricians are aware of dangers of rupture in a subsequent pregnancy or labour associated with the classical type of operation. This traditional caution is based on information now many years old, and it is probable that modern suture materials, antibiotics, and the excellent conditions provided by modern anaesthesia may invalidate it. However this is something which remains to be settled in the future. Contemporary neonatal paediatric opinion is insistant that the avoidance of trauma during the delivery of very low birth weight babies is of paramount importance to the healthy survival of the individual concerned.

Given atraumatic delivery, and the avoidance of neonatal hypoxia, there is now a growing body of evidence that in the very low birth weight babies (I500g and less) that perinatal management including neonatal intensive care, complemented by a radical reappraisal of obstetrical management, can result in good long-term prospects for such babies. These are referred to in a Lancet editorial[2]. It must be admitted that it is still to early, in many centres, to be certain of this ground, and this underlines the need for continuing follow-up studies of the very low birth weight babies born as the result of perinatal management in individual centres wherever they may be. Successful results will depend not only on perinatal management, but also on other factors such as social economic status of the parents involved.

The problem of communication of the new situation confronting obstetricians and neonatal paediatricians involved with perinatal care is something that requries constant attention. This was recognised in a paper by Ingermarsson[3], who studing data from 7I European departments showed that only a minority of obstetricians are prepared to perform a Caesarean Section for fetal reasons before the 30th gestational week; about 50% are prepared to do so at about the 33rd week. Writing as an older obstetrician, the author is well aware of the resistance felt by himself, and possibly his contemporaries, to the use of radical methods such as are outlined in this paper, because they are diametrically opposed to what had been the experience of a professional lifetime in obstetrics. This matter is referred to in a leading article from the British Medical Journal entitled 'Quality not quantity in babies'[4]. Referring to the survival of infants weighing less than I000g at birth, it notes that the survival ranges between I5 and 50% in most series and the incidence of major handicap varies from about I0% to 30%, it continues to state that whether they survive or not will make little difference to the perinatal mortality but the cost (both financial and emotional) of their survival and of supporting the inevitable number who are handicapped may be thought disproportionate.

However it must be recognised that we are in a very rapidly developing situation, and there are probably few obstetricians who would not lean towards the increasingly optimistic information that is now coming forward such as that from University College Hospital in London[5].

The main conclusion that may be drawn from the present paper is that Caesarean Section should be seriously considered by obstetricians as the optimum mode of delivery for babies that are recognised to be of very low birth weight, particularly from singleton pregnancies. Table VIII makes this point.

Table VIII

Mode of Del.	Total Died	Survived
Vag. Breech	20	26
C.S.	2	I9

REFERENCES

I. MUTCH LMM, Brown NJ, SPEIDEL BD, Dunn PM: Perinatal mortality and neonatal survival in Avon:1976-79. Br Med J I98I;i:II9.

2. Editorial. The fate of the baby under I500g at birth. Lancet I980; i:46I-64.

3. INGERMARSSON I, WESTGREN M, SVENNINGSEN NW. Long-term follow-up of preterm infants in breech presentation delivered by Caesarean Section. Lancet I978;ii:I72-75.

4. Editorial. Quality not quantity in babies. Br Med J I980;i:347-48.

5. STEWART A, TURCAN DM, RAWLINGS G, REYNOLDS EOR, Prognosis for infants weighing I000g or less at birth. Arch Dis Child I977;52:97-I04.

FORECAST MODEL FOR THE OUTCOME OF A PREGNANCY.

Seppo Hulkko Matti Kataja,

Central Hospital, Lahti,
and Central Public Health Laboratory,
Helsinki,28,
FINLAND.

SUMMARY.

A hospital material of 411 records of fetal deaths and 424 records of matched control births are studied. The data consist of findings observable before the delivery in order to make it possible to use analogous data in a forecast model.

The forecast model is achieved applying the Bayesian method to the data and assuming that the variables are independent of each other. The model is written in a simple form which yields a score ranging from 0 to 100.   Zero implies a very bad prognosis and 100 meaning no risk factors detected.   The model has the form:

$$W = \frac{121,9}{1 + 0.219*Q}$$

where Q = the product of the coefficients of the found risk factors.

The list of the risk factors begins:

Hydramnion	11.55
Diabetes (manifest or latent)	5.89
Multifetal pregnancy	5.43
Bleeding after 24 weeks.	5.20
Preceding fetal deaths	3.84
Imminent premature delivery	3.11
Diastolic blood pressure >105 or proteinuria >0.8 g/day	2.96

If the limit W<50 were used to admit a mother into more intensive control, the expected number of fetal deaths would be about 0.4% instead of 0.65% in the population left outside the control.   The control population would be about 16% of all pregnant mothers having about 50% enrichment of the presumptive loss of the child.

Purpose.

We want to find an optimal way to handle the risk factors found during the pregnancy or even before it in order to develop a means of selecting the high risk mothers for more intensive treatment.

Materials.

The material used consists originally of 424 fetal deaths in the Central Hospital of Tampere, Finland, during the years 1965-1979.   13 cases were omitted due to incomplete data or low (<600g) birth weight. In the material there are all the relevant clinical and pathological findings from the child and most of the mother during the pregnancy.

As a control material 424 normal births just before or after the study case were chosen and the same pattern of data was recorded except that of autopsy. Further, some aspects were controlled with the total number of births in the region.

Method.

A Bayesian approach was utilized to develop a model for the pregnancy outcome. The aim of the model is to find an optimum combination of characteristics used and optimal weights or coefficients for the findings. As the tool to find the best model the concept of "false positives" were used in different starting situations.

The best model.

The number of characteristics to be chosen into the model is somewhat arbitrary but in our data 13 variables led in most situations to the optimum score. The model is written into a form which allows its use also in cases where some variables remain unknown. Further to model is written so that it yields as an output a percentage ranging from 0% to 100% where the full 100% means that no risk factors are detected. The score shall not be interpreted as a probability, because it would be that only in case of 50% prior probability.

The model has the form:

$$W = \frac{121.9}{1 + 0.210*Q}$$

where Q = the product of the coefficients of the found risk factors.

The risk factors included in the model are:

Coeff	Factor or meaning.
2.46	Some detected disturbancy in pregnancy
2.46	Long lasting usage of a drug
5.20	Bleeding after the 24 week pregnancy
2.86	Diastolic Blood pressure >105 mmHg or Proteinuria> 0.8 g/day
11.55	Hydramnion
3.11	Imminent premature delivery
5.43	Multifetal pregnancy
5.89	Diabetes of the mother
2.73	Hepatosis gravidarum
3.84	Preceding fetal deaths by mother
1.83	The number of deliveries 4 or higher.
1.81	The age of the mother 33 years or more
2.42	The mother unmarried.

The factors are calculated from the observations through a simple procedure which would be for the hypertension (not included in the model) as follows:

```
              dead     control
    no        370        401                     35 * 401
    yes        35         18      coeff  =   ─────────────  = 2.107
   Total      405        419                    370 * 18
```

In this case the presence or absence of hypertension was detected in
824 of the records studies retrospectively.

The possible usage of the model.

The model may be used to calculate the combined risk of the pregnancy to follow by a fetal death.   This may be done already in the
second trimester.   No fixed limits to the score can be given because
they depend on the strategy chosen and also on the possibilities to
control the mothers or even to take them into the hospital in good time
before the delivery.   The model may be used at any contact with the
health personnel when the delivery approaches.

The data available gives some idea what would be the number of
cases to be admitted for treatment if some specific score is used as
the lowest acceptable limit.   The data collected in Tampere region
may not be representative for other countries but it should work
accurately enough in the other parts of Finland.

In Finland the perinatal mortality is about 0.65%.   If the model
would have been applied to the Tampere data in that a way that the cases
getting a score under the limit are labelled 'high' and those with the
limit or higher 'normal' the following perinatal mortalities were found
(without any intervention);

Lowest Acceptable Score	High	Normal
90	0.86%	0.27%
75	1.35%	0.34%
50	1.89%	0.39%
25	4.48%	0.48%
10	29.2%	0.56%

The result may be studied in more detail in the following table
which gives the behaviour of the model in the data used to build it.
If e.g. the number of pregnancies to be controlled shall be calculated
it can be estimated by the frequency of "false negatives".   By higher
values of the score it will take more pregnant mothers to the control
showing a high number of false negatives (in this case negative = loss
of the child).   By low limits of the score it tends to miss more cases
indicated by growing number of false positives, but the specificity of
the model rises.   It means that those few to be controlled are the
high risk cases.

The behaviour of the model in Tampere Central Hospital material in years 1965-1979

W/%	Frequency dead	Frequency contr	Cumul dead	Cumul kontr	F	False-P	Spesif	Sensit	False-N	Accuracy	Promilles
100	55	127	55	127	8.03	13.4	30.0	86.6	70.0	58.3	2.91
95	4	6	59	133	8.10	14.4	31.4	85.6	68.6	58.5	2.99
90	0	16	59	149	8.57	14.4	35.1	85.6	64.9	60.4	2.67
85	11	19	70	168	8.91	17.0	39.6	83.0	60.4	61.3	2.80
80	68	112	138	280	12.63	33.6	66.0	66.4	34.0	66.2	3.32
75	10	14	148	294	13.47	36.0	69.3	64.0	30.7	66.7	3.39
70	3	5	151	299	13.84	36.7	70.5	63.3	29.5	66.9	3.40
65	2	8	153	307	14.66	37.2	72.4	62.8	27.6	67.6	3.35
60	8	17	161	324	16.59	39.2	76.4	60.8	23.6	68.6	3.34
55	38	25	199	349	18.72	48.4	82.3	51.6	17.7	66.9	3.83
50	7	3	206	352	18.85	50.1	83.0	49.9	17.0	66.4	3.93
45	24	17	230	369	21.73	56.0	87.0	44.0	13.0	65.5	4.19
40	3	3	233	372	22.58	56.7	87.7	43.3	12.3	65.5	4.21
35	6	6	239	378	24.62	58.2	89.2	41.8	10.9	65.5	4.28
30	24	12	263	390	28.54	64.0	92.0	36.0	8.0	64.0	4.53
25	30	17	293	407	44.75	71.3	96.0	28.7	4.0	62.4	4.84
20	16	6	309	413	58.90	75.2	97.4	24.8	2.6	61.1	5.02
15	29	9	338	422	197.66	82.2	99.5	17.8	0.5	58.6	5.38
10	12	1	350	423	291.64	85.2	99.8	14.8	0.2	57.3	5.55
9	6	0	356	423	270.72	86.6	99.8	13.4	0.2	56.6	5.65
8	5	0	361	423	252.32	87.8	99.8	12.2	0.2	56.0	5.73
7	2	0	363	423	244.70	88.3	99.8	11.7	0.2	55.7	5.76
6	15	1	378	424	1000.00	92.0	100.0	8.0	0.0	54.0	5.98
5	3	0	381	424	1000.00	92.7	100.0	7.3	0.0	53.6	6.03
4	30	0	411	424	1000.00	100.0	100.0	0.0	0.0	50.0	6.50

General coefficient = 0.2192

179

Perinatal Notification System

The Establishment of a Perinatal Notification

System in Ireland

T.V.O'Dwyer,
Department of Health, Dublin 1.

In Association with:

Dr. V. Barry   Miss M.A. Kelly

Dr. J. Clinch   Mr. M. Kelly

Dr. G. Dean   Dr. D. McDonald

Dr. M. Flynn   Ms F. Spillane

Mr. D. Garvey   Mr. S. Trant

Mr. P. Grant

2. The Perinatal Notification System has the following objectives:

   (1) the rationalisation of present methods of collecting information about childbirth for vital statistics and statistical analysis and for statutory birth registration.

   (ll) the standardization of birth notifications throughout the country and the provision of relevant information to the Directors of Community Care and Medical Officer of Health.

   (2) .the provision of basic perinatal statistics for research and planning purposes.

The operation of the Perinatal Notification System is described in this paper eg, a four part form on self copying paper is completed by the hospitals, one copy is kept by the hospital and the other copies are sent to three different destinations, of these two forms are processed by computer and statistical tables are produced.

The difficulties which have been encountered in implementing the Perinatal Notification System and the progress which has been made to date will be described.

The System here described covers approx. 70% of births at present. When the system is in operation nationally it will enable the identification of the factors associated with perinatal mortality and morbidity in this country and the evaluation of their relative importance. The paper will describe what it is hoped to achieve from the availability of national, up to date perinatal statistics.

The Establishment of a Perinatal Notification System in Ireland.

3.   A description will be given in this paper of the background to the setting
up of a new Perinatal Notification System in Ireland, how the system
operates and what it is hoped to achieve from the system.

3.1 Introduction - Any evaluation of services requires information as its raw
material and the evaluation of needs in the area of care of mothers and
babies is no exception.

The importence of good information in monitoring performances of maternity
units and in identifying areas of special need cannot be overstressed. The
usefulness of vital records, which include the listing of events births and
deaths is dependent on how much detail is obtained. Their pertinence in
terms of the accuracy of the recording and the delay before the statistics
are made available to the public are critical factors. In our Irish health
services a need is recognised for a complete system of information about
perinatal events. In recent years infant mortality has been falling rapidly
in nearly all countries, in some faster than in others with an associated
fall in morbidity.

However, it must be remembered that the risk of dying in the first week of
life, is as great as the risk of dying in the following thirty years of ones
life-span. The need is growing for a system of collecting information on the
health of the baby at the time of birth which will also give information
on morbidity after birth. This information is needed to evaluate the
existing services for the care of mothers and their infants, and also to
indicate the need for new services.

The identification of maternal and infant risk groups requires the extension
of obstetrical and paediatric health care programmes. For example,
complications of delivery may appear more often in very young or older
mothers. Congenital abnormalities may be more common in infants born to
older mothers, as, for example, 'Down's Syndrome'. So in designing a health
care system the focusing of services on those in need and at risk will
produce the greatest reward.

Obstetrics is an area of medicine where the evaluation of results has been
practised by doctors for many years. It is an area where the use of
evaluation techniques is accepted and where there is agreement about the
main indicators as the Dublin clinical reports show. Minor problems may
arise sometimes about definitions. The aim of obstetrics may be defined
quite simply, as achieving an end result of a healthy, satisfied mother

and a healthy baby.

3.2 <u>Aims</u>

The aims of the Perinatal Notification System may be summarised as follows:

(1) the rationalisation of methods of collecting information about childbirth
     for vital statistics, and statistical analysis and for statutory
     birth registration.

(2) the standardisation of birth notifications throughout the country and
     the provision of relevant information to the Director of Community
     Care and Medical Officer of Health.

(3) the provision of basic perinatal statistics for research and
     planning purposes.

It is hoped that the new system will improve the completeness of statistics.
For example it has been shown in the past that both births and deaths of
premature infants have been under-registered.

At the same time the place of occurrence of births and deaths has changed
in recent years; there are now very few domiciliary births and the number
of small maternity homes has decreased steadily.

3.3 <u>Existing Methods of Collecting Information About Childbirth</u>

The following diagram shows the existing system of collecting information
about childbirth and the various forms which are used.

<u>Method of Collection Information</u>

The existing systems of collecting information and the number
of forms in use might be illustrated as follows:-

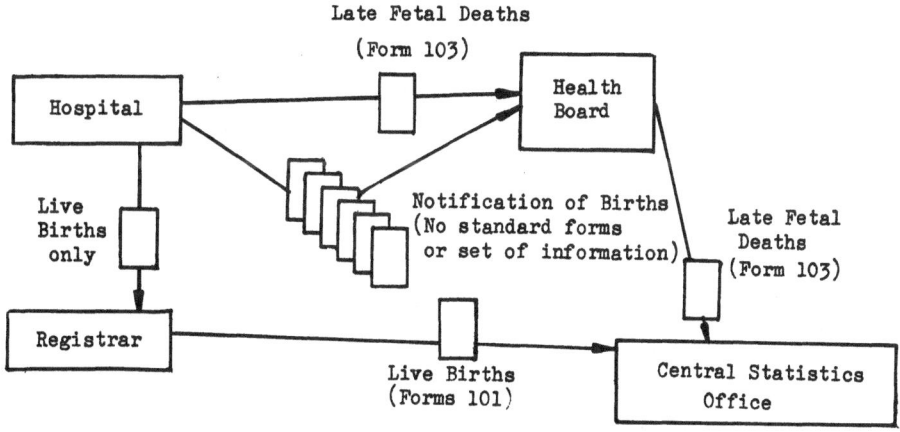

182

1) All live births are required to be registered within 42 days. The primary
   duty is on the parents of the child but in practice births are usually
   registered by the hospital staff.
2) Vital Statistics on all live births are collected via local Registrars of
   Births on a special form made available by the Central Statistics Office.
   (CSO)
3) Vital statistics on all late fetal deaths are supplied by the hospital within
   36 hours to the Director of Community Care in whose area the event occurred.
   The form used for this purpose is in two parts and the Director is required
   to retain the first part of this form and to forward the second part to the
   Director of the Central Statistics Office.
4) Lastly the hospitals are required to notify each individual birth to the
   Director of Community Care of the district within 36 hours of the birth.
   At present there is no standard form used for this notification and there
   is great variation from area to area.
   It is clear that information is collected for a number of different purposes
   in a number of different ways. It was decided to devise an integrated system
   which would meet all of these needs and also the need for national information
   on perinatal problems.

New System

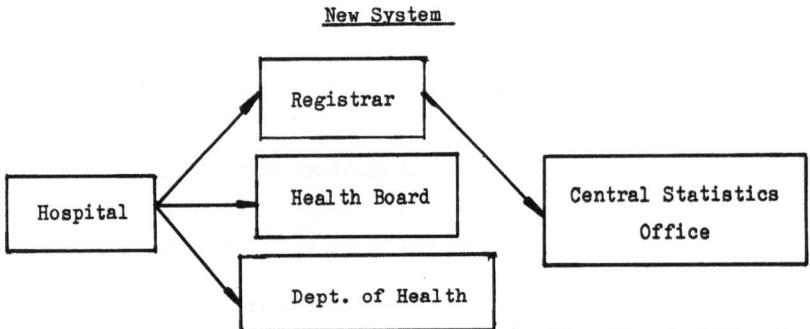

An objective of using the new four-part form is the considerable simplification
of these procedures. It also reduces the amount of paperwork and the risk
of error in copying information onto different forms.
The new form is operated as follows:
1) the top copy of the form is sent to the local Registrar of Births. All
   live births are entered in theregister and the forms are then forwarded
   to the Central Statistics Office.

2) The second copy of the form covers birth notification and is sent to the
   Director of Community Care.
3) The third copy of the form, which contains no identifying particulars,
   is sent to the Planning Unit, Department of Health for statistical
   analysis.

4) The fourth copy of the form is retained in the hospital for their own record system.

3.4 Pilot Scheme

A discussion document was drawn up and circulated to interested parties. These included the Institute of Obstetricians, Directors of Community Care, Medico-Social Research Board and Public Health Nurses. These groups were asked for their views and the information required for registration and for vital statistics was considered when the form was designed. The original form was first out on a three month basis for all births in Co. Wexford, Co Mayo and in the National Maternity Hospital Dublin. It was felt that these three areas gave a spread of experience in two Irish counties and in a large Dublin hospital. We were quickly aware that the size of the unit affected the scheme because in the smaller hospitals it was possible to organise the collection of data near the patient while this was difficult in larger hospitals. This means that in large hospitals care is required to ensure that data is available and accurate at the point of collection.

Generally, we were very satisfied with the initial pilot scheme but realised that any extension would require training of the personnel involved in the transcribing of the data. We were also aware that it would not be possible to fully dismantle the existing system until all were satisfied with the accuracy of the data collected.

Rather than abandon this scheme and start again it was proposed to extend the scheme gradually to other areas in order to obtain more experience so as to overcome any organisational difficulties and provide experience for the staff concerned in collection and transmitting information. Some revisions of the original form were required.

3.5 The Form

The form was designed to be suitable for processing by computer. At present the top copy of the form is processed in the Central Statistics Office and the third copy of the form is processed in the Public Service Computer Centre for the Department of Health. The top copy of the form contains a number of extra boxes in the left-hand column (eg, four digit county codes) which were required for the programs run by the CSO. The remaining three copies of the form are identical in layout except that the identifying particulars are blacked out on the copy of the form sent to the Department of Health. The hospitals have been given detailed instructions about the allocation of the case numbers and the general coding of the form.

The top copy of the form is now used in some areas as the unique system for registering births and it has taken over from the previous Form 101 for the collection of Vital Statistics.

The second copy of the form, the Notification of Birth is in operation alongside the existing system of birth notification as yet. The notification to the community care team has a two-fold purpose:-

(1) to notify the community care medical and nursing services which have responsibility for the subsequent care of the mother and child.

(2) to provide the basis of various health records used by the health boards.

As the information on the infant's health is useful to the Public Health Nurse when she visits the mother and infant on their return home from hospital early notification is essential. The information is also useful for completion of the Child Health Record, for immunisation purposes.

The third copy of the form is sent by the hospitals to the Planning Unit in Department of Health. The forms are sorted in the Department and the case numbers are checked to ensure that complete returns have been received from each hospital. Coding of the form is then completed. The forms are punched onto magnetic tape and sent to the Public Service Computer Centre to be validated. Rejections are corrected until the file is acceptable. When the file is complete the various reports are run. The reports are provided by hospital, health-board and survey. (These slides show the type of reports which are obtained.) They show the association between various factors (eg, background of mother) and the perinatal mortality rate.

3.6 Confidentiality

Throughout the design and development of the project we have always been concious of the problems of confidentiality and have attempted to preserve it at each stage. It is the intention that at any time data will not be made available to persons not requiring it. So the Registrar of Births and the CSO, receive the information they require and do not get medical data. The central processing point, that is the Department of Health, do not receive identification details of the patient. The only authorities getting full information are the Directors of Community Care who require it to provide for the care of the baby following hospital discharge.

3.7 Progress

The Perinatal Notification System now covers about 70% of the births occurring in the State.

One difficulty has arisen with regard to the use of the new form for birth notification. In order to comply with the wishes of the Directors of Community Care for early notification an additional form must be used as the new form cannot be completed until the end of the perinatal period (i.e. after seven days). The two main organisational difficulties which have been encountered in operating the scheme are:

(1) incorrect numbering of the forms (e.g. duplication of numbers for separate events) by the hospital staff.

(2) delays in sending forms to the Planning Unit and to the Director of Community Care.

The accuracy of the results produced has been monitored closely. The results for each hospital are circulated to the individual hospitals approx. five months after the month to which the figures refer and the hospital staffs are asked for their comments or corrections. The accuracy of the monthly tables has improved considerably since the first tables were produced in November 1980. The discrepancies which have arisen between hospital records and the Planning Unit results include:

(1) the number of perinatal deaths recorded differed. Part of the problem arises from the use of different definitions. The definition used in the scheme was for all live births and for late fetal deaths over 500 grams. Some maternity units, on the otherhand, compile their own statistics on the basis of events greater than 28 weeks gestation.

(11) the hospital record was for a greater number of events than the Planning Unit results revealed. It was found that some forms had not been forwarded to the Planning Unit.

These discrepancies indicated the type of errors which were likely to arise and it was possible to take measures to ensure that they would not recur.

As the same form is used to collect information on all obstetric events it is unlikely that late fetal deaths will be under-reported. It has been agreed that forms relating to a perinatal death will be signed by a doctor. This in effect means that we are being provided with a perinatal death certificate.

A Steering Committee was set up in March, 1981 in order to monitor the progress of the scheme and to advice on the implementation of the scheme nationally. The Steering Committee comprises a representative from the Institute of Obstetricians and Gynaecologists, the Irish Perinatal Society, Health Board, Medico-Social Research Board, a Maternity Hospital, Public Service Computer Centre, the Central Statistics Office and the Department of Health.

3.8 The Future

The system is to be extended until national coverage of births is achieved.
The system also covers domiciliary births. These now account for less than
1% of total births. Apart from improving the collection of information
for birth registration, vital statistics and birth notification the
Perinatal Notification System will provide the necessary base for a fuller
appraisal of perinatal mortality and morbidity in surving children. The
national information system will enable the identification of the factors
involved in perinatal mortality in this country and their relative importance.
Some of the major factors associated with perinatal mortality which have
been identified in international studies on the subject are:

Background factors in Mother:	Age
	Medical History
	Obstetric History
	Marital Status
	Nutritional Status
	Social Class.
Mother's practises in pregnancy:	Smoking
	Alcohol Consumption
	Drugs and Medicine
Medical care:	Antenatal Care
	Facilities for Delivery
	Method of Delivery
Factors in Infants:	Birth-Weight
	Congenital Abnormality
	Prematurity.

The association between these factors and their relative importance in
influencing perinatal mortality in Ireland must be established. It should
then be possible to take measures (e.g. an education programme for
prospective parents, improved facilities for delivery etc) to combat the
influnece of adverse factors in childbirth.

The Perinatal Notification System could also be used to set up a National
and Regional Registers of Congenital Malformations.

Lastly the Perinatal Notification System will provide information on a
continuing basis which will allow the existing services to be monitored as
well as providing pointers for the development of future services.

THE HANNOVER PERINATAL STUDY
An Example of Descriptive Epidemiology and Evaluation of Health Care

by K.-W. Hartmann and O. Rienhoff

Medical School Hannover, Institute of Medical Informatics
(Director: Prof.Dr. P.L. Reichertz)

Abstract:

Initiated by the ongoing discussion of comparatively high rates of perinatal mortality in Germany the Hannover Perinatal Study (HPS) had been implemented in about 20 voluntarily participating maternity and childrens' hospitals in the area of Hannover in January '80 (1). The HPS has been introduced into the perinatal scene for the purpose of:
- quality assurance in perinatal care,
- standardized documentation for specific scientific evaluation,
- generation of annual hospital statistics,
- comparison of epidemiological results with data from other regions,
- EDP-supported preparation of medical reports in obstetrics.

All hospitals use a specific documentation sheet to collect data-items relating to pregnancy, prenatal care, delivery, birth management and to the newborn. This form originally had been developed by the Bavarian Commission of Perinatology (2). The document becomes part of the patient record and an anonymized copy is used for data recording. When a newborn is transferred to a childrens' hospital in case of complications, the paediatricians document data of the newborn in the same way. By use of a pagination number and statistical checking of single data-items it is possible to link the perinatal and neonatal records of a newborn together. This allows for the evaluation of the complete period from pregnancy to discharge from the childrens' hospital.

A modified documentation sheet has been developed in close cooperation of the Bavarian and the Hannover study groups and will be introduced in several German studies from 1982 on.

1. History

Perinatal mortality and morbidity is considered to be a problem in Germany, comparing the relatively high rates (1979: 1.49%) with the low rates of perinatal mortality in some other European countries, especially the Scandinavian regions (e.g. Sweden 1979: 1.02%).

In 1979 some obstetricians, clinicians and practioners, paediatricians and representatives of medical organisations planned an investigation of the perinatal situation in the area of Hannover. Motivated by the Munich Perinatal Study (MPS) and a study of perinatal mortality and morbidity in Lower Saxony (1978) this group decided to install a similar study in Hannover.

From the 1. January 1980 until now all maternity hospitals and paediatric clinics of Hannover have participated in the study. In 1980 this 13 hospitals were complemented by 5 obstetric and 1 paediatric hospital in a region about 50 km around the city of Hannover. This region has been somewhat extended by 5 hospitals since January 1981. The very important fact in participating was the only voluntary decision of all hospitals. In this way the organisation, realization and execution of the study has been absolutely in the sense and the responsibility of the physicians.

2. Documentation

For data-collecting all obstetric hospitals use a specific documentation sheet, the so-called 'Perinatologischer Basis Erhebungsbogen' (perinatal basic documentation form, PBB). It is identical to the one used in Bavaria.

Starting January 1st 1982 a new documentation sheet will be introduced in Bavaria, Hannover and some other states. The selection of parameters included could mainly be based on Bavarian experiences while the layout of the sheet and organisational changes within the formular flow were introduced from Hannover (Fig. 1). The documentation sheet is a NCR-Paper consisting of three sheets.

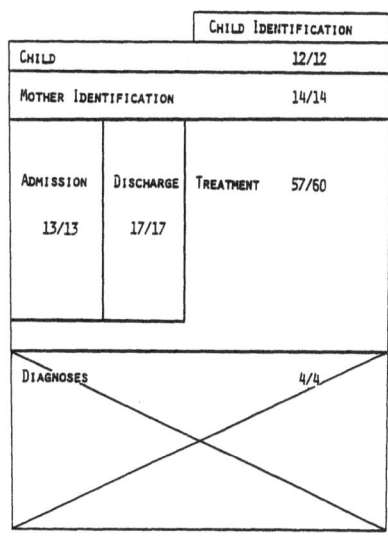

```
CLINIC IDENTIFICATION  4/4
                        PATIENT IDENTIFICATION
MOTHER, PRENATAL  12/12

PREGNANCY         27/35

DELIVERY          40/52

CHILD             27/39

MOTHER, POSTNATAL  8/8
```

```
                    CHILD IDENTIFICATION
CHILD                       12/12
MOTHER IDENTIFICATION       14/14

ADMISSION  DISCHARGE  TREATMENT  57/60
  13/13      17/17

DIAGNOSES                        4/4
```

Fig. 1: Perinatal Basic
     Documentation Form (PBB),
     structure of data groups
     and number of parameters
     per group, second value
     including catalog entries.

Fig. 2: Newborn Discharge Record
     (NEB), structure of data
     groups and number of pa-
     rameters per group, se-
     cond value including ca-
     talog entries.

In case of transferring a newborn, because of malformations, disfunc-
tions, premature birth etc., to a childrens' hospital the third sheet,
another copy of all gathered data, is sent with the newborn. So the
paeditrician gets a first overview information of delivery and the
newborn.

The aspect of information passing is a new detail developed in the HPS
and not used in Bavaria. Another new essential in the HPS is the
development of a complete newborn documentation in the childrens' hospital (Fig. 2).

Whenever a newborn reaches the hospital within the first seven days
of life this documentation takes place. Using a documentation sheet
which is formed analogously to the PBB the paediatrician can document
the whole period of the newborn in care. This documentation sheet is

called 'Neugeborenen Entlassungs Bogen' (newborn discharge record, NEB) and consists of three NCR-sheets as the PBB does. Data groups in this form are:

- physiological data from birth of the newborn
- personal data of the mother
- status of admission
- events of hospital stay
- status of discharge

which use only the first half of the page. The second part has in difference to the PBB a specific function. This part is preformed as a condensed report to the practioner by discharge of the newborn. Therefore this part consists of freetext-lines for diagnoses, operations, timings for ongoing care, medication and food recommendations.

The NEB is handled similar to the PBB, first sheet acts as a standardized neonatal documentation for the patient record, second sheet is sent to the documentation staff for data recording and the third sheet is used for information to the practioner as described above.

3. Data Recording

All anonymized copies of the documentation sheets are sent to the documentation staff residing in the 'Kassenaerztliche Vereinigung Niedersachsen' (KVN) in Hannover. The functions of communication, organisation, documentation are centralized there. The incoming documentation sheets are first checked by a midwife with special documentation knowledge. Most of errors, missings, uncertainties are detected and corrected by telephon contacting of the hospitals. In other cases the sheets are rejected and sent back for correction to the hospitals.

After passing this 'control station' the data of the sheets are recorded with a multi-user disquet-system by data-typists. All disquet-data are joined together, formatted and checked by formal errors with EDP-support. Then the constructed data records are processed by a complex program system. Hardcopies of missing documentations of all hospitals are produced and can be used for checking completeness.

More important is the checking of various logical relations within the data and listing out the detected errors or inconsistencies. In a next step the data of each hospital are grouped to generate a hospital statistic. This statistic shows the absolut and in some cases the relative frequency of all parameters from the documentation sheet. At last a summary statistic with data of all hospitals is produced. These steps happen simultaneously for the PBB- and the NEB-data. But there is difference in the programs and the statistics. Data of the PBB are processed by a program-system developed in the MPS and transferred to the HPS. Processing of NEB-data is done by programs developed by the Institute of Medical Informatics. The hospital and summary statistics from NEB-data are presented in a condensed form of only one page, containing basic values of vitality status, treatment and morbidity.

Every three months all gathered data are processed and error lists and statistics are sent to hospitals to give a short-time feedback of the clinical situation. For specific scientific analyses of data SPSS (Statistical Package for the Social Sciences) can be used in a wide range. But it is also planned to implement a SIR database (Scientific Information Retrieval) to give a short-time response to questions of the obstetricians or paediatricians by taking the interactive options of the system.

4. Intentions

In generating clinical statistics the obstetrician or paediatrician gets a feedback of his management in hospital. He can discuss the results with his colleagues and thereby get new interpretations of his own actions in perinatal care. The comparison of clinical and summary statistics gives the possibility to determine the state of his management to all others. If this approach of critical reviewing is extended by using detailed analysis of the data it is possible to get better knowledge of underlying structures and relations in birth and neonatal management. These results then can be used for continuing medical education in perinatal conferences.

New aspects in morbidity will be derived from statistics of another dataset, the linkage of the perinatal record (PBB) and the neonatal record (NEB). The linkage is attempted by a formal fact, the pagination number. It is a printed serialization number on all PBB. If a newborn is transferred to a childrens' hospital and documentation is started there, the pagination number from the PBB sent with the newborn is written to the NEB, acting as a pointer to the matching perinatal record.

Programs for linkage automatic are developed in the Institute for Medical Informatics. The linkage of records is done as described above. If no pointer is present in a neonatal record other routines are started which build a so called 'indikator' for matching PBB. The 'indikator' is derived by comparisons of specific data-items in NEB and PBB and gives a measure for matching.

The longtime data recording of perinatal data in the Hannover area also opens the way to countrywide comparison of results. First national comparison can be done with the Bavarian region. For identical methods are used in both regions best conditions of comparability are given. Also international comparison is possible with data from southern Finland where the same documentation sheet is used as in Bavaria. In Germany also Hesse, North-Rhine-Westphalia, Bremen and other states are planning or starting documentation of perinatal data.

5. Conclusion

The first two years of the Hannover Perinatal Study have given first impressions of the perinatal scene in this region. Annual and quarterly statistics have proved to be useable and practical instruments of reflecting outcome of perinatal and neonatal management. By this a basic approach to quality assurance in perinatology is done. Continuing evaluation and transformation of results by medical education can be a starting point for improved perinatal care and accordingly decreasing mortality and morbidity.

Literature:

(1) Rienhoff O, Hartmann KW. Perinatologische Arbeitsgemeinschaft in der Kassenaertzlichen Vereinigung Niedersachsen. Programm-Satzung-Gliederung, Kassenaerztliche Vereinigung Niedersachsen, Hannover, Feb. 1980.

(2) Selbmann HK et al. Muenchner Perinatal-Studie 1975-1977. Koeln-Loevenich, Deutscher Aerzte-Verlag GmbH, 1980.

(3) Weitzel H, Hartmann KW. Zur Epidemiologie der Fruehgeburt. Reihe Wissenschaftliche Information, Milupa AG (in print).

(4) Rienhoff O, Selbmann HK, Hartmann KW. Zur epidemiologischen Nutzung flaechendeckender Qualitaetskontrollen in der Perinatologie. Berlin, Springer Verlag, (in print).

(5) Hartmann KW, Weitzel H, Rienhoff O. Zeitliche Muster in der Inanspruchnahme der Schwangerschaftsvorsorge. (unpublished).

Acknowledgement:

This Study is supported by the Kassenaerztliche Vereinigung Niedersachsen.

HIP PROSTHESIS DESIGN

Ph. CINQUIN[x], B. CHALMOND[x], D. BERARD[x], L. DUSSERRE[x], P. TROUILLOUD[xx],
P. GRAMMONT[xx], D. BINNERT[xxx], J.P. MABILLE[xxx], C. CARASSO[xxxx].

x Département d'Informatique Médicale
xx Service d'Orthopédie
xxx Service de Radiologie

Centre Hospitalier Régional de DIJON, 2 Bd Maréchal de Lattre
de Tassigny, 21034 DIJON CEDEX.

xxxx Université de Saint Etienne.

ABSTRACT

A method of automatic hip prosthesis design is presented.

The shape of the tail of the prosthesis is optimized with respect to the anatomical surface of the medullary canal of the femur.

Four conventional hip roetgengrams are performed ; each of them is processed by an edge detector which defines the edge of the projection of the medullary canal.

The available information about the unknown surface of the canal is made of four sheafs of straight lines originating in the X-ray focus and leaning on the edges : all those straight lines are tangent to the unknown surface.

Once mathematically translated, this information is the input to a surface "recognizer" using parametric surface spline functions that were devised for that purpose.

The resulting surface will then be used for the definition of the optimal shape of the tail of the prosthesis, and the final step will be tooling of the prosthesis by a numerically controlled millingcutter.

The major medical interests of this work lie in the reduction of the risks of loosening of the prosthesis and in the improvement of the mechanical properties of the whole.

INTRODUCTION

The aim of this paper is to present a sequence of processes leading to hip prosthesis exactly fitting the anatomy of any individual.

Hip prosthesis are composed of a sphere (the femoral head) screwed on a tail. The tail is hammered and cemented into the medullary canal of the femur. (fig. 1 and 2)

There are about ten tails available, and the surgeon chooses the one whose front projection best suits the shape of the medullary canal of the femur as it appears on an antero-posterior hip roetgenogram.

Therefore, with conventional methods, the tail roughly fits the canal and the resulting gaps between prosthesis and bone are filled with cement.

Orthopaedist surgeons think that the fitting of the tail on the actual anatomy of the individual would greatly reduce the risks of loosening of the prosthesis and would improve the mechanical characteristics of the whole. Indeed, it would be possible to reduce the amount of necessary cement, whose elasticity is zero.

The achievement of this anatomical fitting raises three problems :

1) We have to define the actual shape of the canal.
2) From this actual shape, we have to define the desirable shape of the prosthesis (which must match several constraints such as convexity constraints for the sake of tooling, constraints inherent in the way the prosthesis is hammered into the duct, and so on).
3) This desirable shape must be numerically defined, and will be the input to a numerically controlled milling-cutter.

As soon as the roetgenograms are performed, the sequence of processes is fully automatic.

This paper mostly deals with the first of those three points. The canal is defined by numerical processing of four hip roetgengrams. We first present the radiological procedure and the information each roetgenogram of the canal enables us to derive about its shape. Each roetgenogram is processed to extract the edges of the duct and we describe the algorithms we use. Then, the actual mathematical reconstruction of the inner surface of the canal is performed through the use of surface spline functions that were modified to suit our problem.

I - RADIOLOGICAL PROCEDURE

1.1 - Computed tomography versus conventional radiology

The Total Body Computed Tomography provides an obvious solution to our problem : indeed, the shape of the medullary canal of the femur can be precisely defined by serveral spaced slides of the femur.

But some of the requirements of the surgeons were that the process should not be too expensive and might be used for all hip prostheses. Therefore, we could not consider the possibility of using Computed Tomography and had to do with conventional radiological technics.

1.2 - Mathematical setting of the problem

So, we want to define the shape of the medullary canal of the femur with four hip roetgenogrames. We shall successively study what we can derive from one, then from four roetgenograms.

A two-dimensional equivalent of the problem will enlighten it. Then we shall state the constraints defining the unknown surface of the canal.

1.2/1 - Information derived from one roetgenogram

On a hip roetgenogram, the medullary canal is outlined by two curves Γ_1 and Γ_2 (fig. 1 and 4).

The laws of radiology state that the unknown surface S of the canal is tangent to the straight lines D and D' in P and P' respectively.

More precisely, it is clear that S is tangent to the plane defined by $\vec{OM}$ and $\vec{d}$, as defined on fig. 4.

And this is true for any M belonging to Γ_1 or Γ_2.

1.2/2 - Information brought up by four roetgenograms

The positions of the sources and of the films of the performed roetgen-grams are indicated in fig. 5. All the sources are in the same plan.

Thus the available information is made of four sheafs of straight lines tangent to the unknown surface S.

1.2/3 - Bi-dimensional equivalent of the problem

A 3.D display of the available information about S is not easy to carry out.

But let $(M_i)_{i=1,2,...,8}$ be the intersection points between the curves $(\Gamma_i)_{i=1,2,...,8}$ and the plan of the sources.

Then the curve $\mathcal{C}$ represented in dotted-lines in fig. 6 is the intersection of the unknown surface S with the plan of the sources.

In fact, $\mathcal{C}$ is the solution of the bidimensional following problem : find a plane curve tangent to the straight lines $(O_i M_i)_{i=1,2,...,8}$

It is clear that the usual interpolation methods cannot solve this problem : indeed, we have no mesh on which an unknown function would be imposed definite values.

That is why we have to parametrize the problem.

1.2/4 - Constraints defining surface S

The 2.D display of fig. 6 should easily be 3 - Dimensionally completed in the reader's mind. Thus, it is clear that the actual problem also calls for parametrization.

This means that we are looking for a function $x : T \subset R^2 \to R^3$, such as the corresponding parametric surface be tangent to the four sheafs previously defined.

An auxiliary condition is that the surface be closed.

We have found out that an acceptable choice for T was the rectangular region R : $t = (t_1, t_2) \in R \Leftrightarrow \begin{cases} 1 \leqslant t_1 \leqslant 9 \\ z_{min} \leqslant t_2 \leqslant z_{max} \end{cases}$

Remarks :

      - z_{min} and z_{max} are the lower and upper bounds of the z coordinates of curves Γ_i (the z axis is the axis of the femur).

      - the region $8 \leqslant t \leqslant 9$ is neccessary for the closing of the surface.

The tangency between S and the four sheafs of straight lines reduces to a linear system of equations involving the values of x and of its partial derivatives of order one.

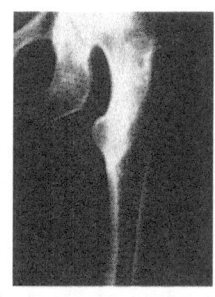

fig. 1

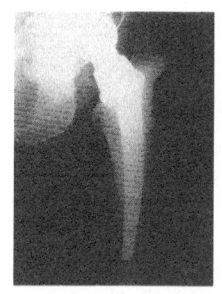

fig. 2

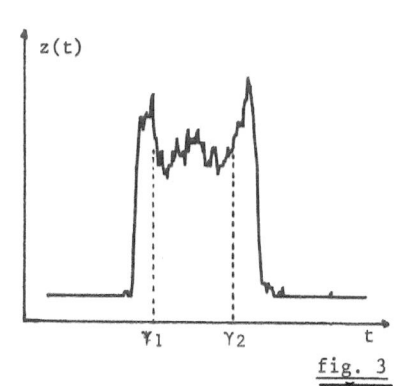

fig. 3

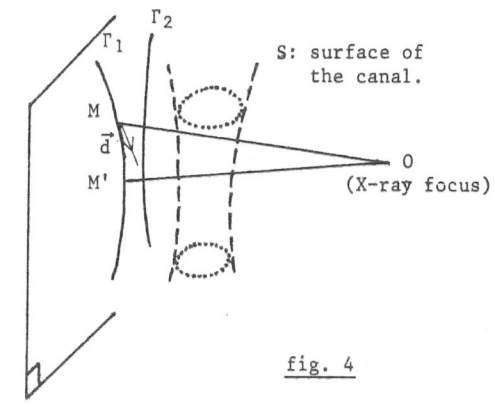

Γ_2

Γ_1

M

$\vec{d}$

M'

S: surface of the canal.

O
(X-ray focus)

fig. 4

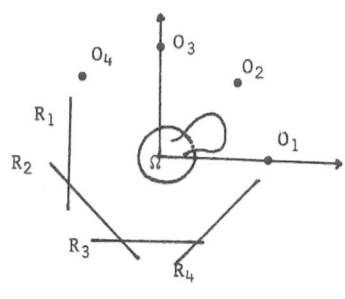

O_4 O_3 O_2

R_1

R_2 O_1

Ω

R_3

R_4

Upper sight   fig. 5

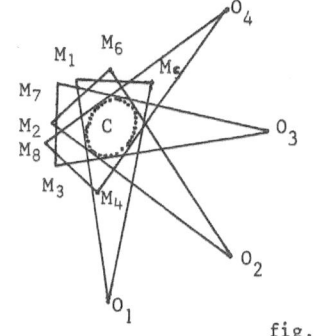

M_1 M_6 O_4

M_7 M_5

M_2 C O_3

M_8

M_3 M_4 O_2

O_1

fig. 6

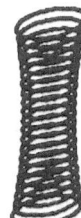

Reconstructed phantom
$r = z^2/12 + 0.25$

fig. 7

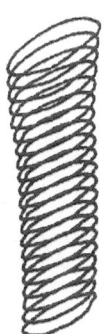

Reconstruction of an actual medullary canal.

fig. 8

II - PATTERN RECOGNITION OF THE MEDULLARY CANAL

2.1 - Introduction

A roetgengram of a femur is characterized by the two edges of the bone and by the two edges of the medullary canal. The latter may be very blurred, as we can see on figure 1. The image is digitized into 512 x 512 picture elements with 64 gray levels.

The edge detections are made row after row. It means that for each row of the digitized image, we determine the two points which belong to the edges of the medullary canal. When the 512 rows have been scanned, the edges are enhanced by a non linear smoother.

2.2 - The procedure

A row is considered as a digital signal $\{z(t), t = 1 \ldots 512\}$, where $z(t)$ is the brightness level of the tth digitization of the current row. An example of a such row is given in figure 3. The signal is assumed gaussian and generated by the model $z(t) = \delta(t) + u(t)$, where $\delta(t)$ is the expected value of $z(t)$, and $u(t)$ is gaussian $N(0, \sigma^2)$. The non-stationarity of the signal is caused mainly by changes in $\delta(t)$. In general, these variations are smooth, except for the abrupt change of the edge of the bone, and maybe for the edges of the canal.

First, a sequential detection of the two edges of the femur is processed. Each line is scaned through a moving window of size n, in which the "cumulative sum of the deviations" is calculated :

$$CS = \underset{k<r<n}{\text{Max}} \left| \sum_{j=k+1}^{r} (z(j) - \bar{z}(j-1)) \right| / \hat{\sigma} \sqrt{n-k} \ ,$$

where $\bar{z}(j-1)$ is the mean of the first $(j-1)$ brightness levels of the window and k is a starting parameter. An edge is detected as soon as CS becomes greater than a theorical value. The ticklish point of this method is the estimation, or the choice, of the "parameter of variations" σ.

Secondly, as we have an a-priori knowledge of the position of the edges of the canal with regard to the edges of the femur, a bayesian estimation of those positions can be developped. For that purpose, the bayesian estimation of a square signal in an autoregressive noise is used (3).

III - ACTUAL RECONSTRUCTION OF THE SHAPE OF THE CANAL

Conventional interpolation methods provide an estimate of an unknown function $f : R^2 \rightarrow R$, when the values of f or of some of its derivatives are known for the mesh points of a grid in R^2.

Among these interpolation methods, spline functions are very interesting for their minimization properties that ensure good smoothness.

Bi-dimensional spline functions can roughly be divided into functions defined by tensorial product of one-dimensional splines and surface spline functions, as introduced by DUCHON. (6)

We have applied those two kinds of methods to our problem, which is the interpolation of a function $x : R^2 \rightarrow R^3$, defined by the values of linear combinations of x and of its first partial derivatives.

Therefore, we defined parametric bicubic spline functions and parametric surface splines functions. (5)

A parametric bicubic spline functions is a function $x : R^2 \rightarrow R^3$, whose components are bicubic functions. The constraints defining the surface of the canal (see section 1.2/4), associated with the continuity conditions on the derivatives deriving from the definition of a bicubic spline function, provide a linear system of equations that fully defines the parametric bicubic spline functions. In this system, the unknowns are the values of x and of its partial derivatives of order two in the points of the grid.

Likewise, the results of DUCHON for surface spline functions were generalized to the case of parametrice surface spline functions and presented in (2).

IV - CONCLUSION

These methods were experimented for the reconstruction of a phantom surface and an actual medullary canal. These results were promising : indeed, the inaccuracy of the method lies within acceptable bounds. (See fig. 7 and 8).

This study has been carried out with a micro-computer Hewlett Packard 9845 B driving a Grinnel GMR 274 image processing-display device.

We are now going to brood over the problem of the definition of the desirable shape for the tail. The last step, which should raise no technical difficulty will be the numerical control of the milling-cutter that will tool the prosthesis.

References

(1) AHLBERG, NILSON and WALSH : The theory of splines and their applications.
Academic Press, NEW YORK 1967.

(2) CARASSO and CINQUIN : Optimal reconstruction of surfaces using parametric spline functions.
Colloque d'optimisation, théorie et algorithmes, 16 - 20 Mars 1981 à CONFOLANT.

(3) CHALMOND B. : Rupture de modèles pour des processus autorégressifs,
Thèse, ORSAY, n° 2711, Octobre 1979.

(4) CINQUIN P. , TROUILLOUD P., GRAMMONT P., AUTISSIER J.M., CHALMOND B. :
Morphologie osseuse, intérêt de l'Informatique associée à la radiologie.
Congrès d'anatomie, FLORENCE, Mai 1981.

(5) CINQUIN P., "Splines unidimensionnelles sous tension et bidimensionnelles paramétrées. Deux applications médicales".
Thèse, SAINT ETIENNE, 28 Octobre 1981.

(6) DUCHON J. : Interpolation des fonctions de deux variables par des fonctions splines du type plaque mince.
R.A.I.R.O. Analyse Numérique vol. 10 n°12, 1976, pages 5 à 12.

(7) LAURENT P.J. : Approximation et Optimisation.
Hermann - PARIS - 1972.

AUTOMATED ECG ANALYSIS IN SCREENING FOR CORONARY HEART DISEASE .*

Jörg Michaelis, Pia Beyermann, Ewald Glück, Peter Hain, Rainer
Lippold, Eberhard Scheidt, Wilhelm Schindler

Institut für Medizinische Statistik und Dokumentation der Universität
Langenbeckstr.1, 6500 Mainz, F.R.G.

1. SUMMARY.

In 1980 a cohort study was set up in order to evaluate the performance of existing ECG-computer programs in a screening situation
and to develop specific algorithms for early detection and prognosis of coronary heart disease. The study is based on regular occupational health examinations of about 8000 individuals.
In the present paper the visual interpretation of 2850 ECGs is compared with the automated analysis by the programs of BONNER and PIPBERGER.
The latter program showed a greater specificity and appeared therefore to be somewhat better suited for the screening purpose. We feel,
however, that new criteria are needed for this task.

2. PROBLEM.

At present available computer programs for automated ECG and VCG
analysis are exclusively designed to detect existing diseases, their
sensitivity and specificity are mainly adjusted to a clinical decision situation. The ease of automatically processing large numbers
of ECGs suggests the application for screening purposes. Although
this specific application area has been frequently emphasized
in discussions and is already established in preventive medical programs - see e.g. Okajima (1) - the practical value of automated
ECG - screening has not been systematically analysed so far.
Therefore we started in 1980 a cohort study in order to evaluate
and to compare some of the existing programs in a screening situation as well as to develop specific algorithms for early detection
and prognosis of coronary heart disease. For this purpose we will
combine the commonly known risk factors and ECG measurements with
specific respect to short and long term variability of these measurements. It is expected that these variabilities will differ be-

* Supported by the Bundesminister für Forschung und Technologie,
  Projekt HKP 303

tween persons who stay healthy and those developing coronary heart
disease.

3. MATERIAL AND METHODS.
3.1 Study design.

Our study is based on regular occupational health examinations of
about 8000 individuals. One subgroup consists out of aviation personnel which is highly preselected towards healthy persons. A
second subcohort is formed by employees of a pharmaceutical company
in leading positions. The third group is recruited from members
of the Mainz University who have to undergo regular health examinations and are of age above 30 or show high occasional blood
pressure measurements or other risk factors. ECGs and clinical data
are recorded for each individual once a year, some of the aviation
personnel have two examinations per year.
Data acquisition of resting ECG and VCG and post-exercise ECG is
performed by a MARQUETTE (MAC DR) recording system - with preprocessing (quality control, a/d-conversion, data compression and
storage on a digital cassette) by a microcomputer. In addition
clinical laboratory measurements (glucose, cholesterol, LDL/HDL,
etc.) are obtained, further a standardized report on smoking habits,
physical activity, drug intake, present and past diseases.A modified ROSE questionnaire is also used in individuals complaining
about related symptoms.
ECG interpretation is performed by medical doctors in their conventional fashion. The comparison of visual and automated analysis
is performed by an independend person and is restricted to a set
of basic diagnostic entities. For each ECG it is marked whether
there is complete agreement,partial agreement or disagreement between the visual and automated interpretations. All cases with dis-
crepances are reviewed in a second round by the first human interpreter together with two other members from our group and it is
tried to characterize the underlying cause of disagreement as due
to measurement errors, different criteria or additional clinical information available to the medical doctor during interpretation of
the ECG.

3.2 Data processing

Details of the data flow within our cohort study have already been

published elsewhere (2). Automated ECG- and VCG-analysis is performed by the computer programs AVA 3.6, BONNER I and II (for serial
comparisons), SICARD and MARQUETTE. In addition an automated MINNE-
SOTA-coding is performed by the program developed by TUINSTRA and
coworkers (3).

The measurements and diagnostic classification results generated by
these programs are stored sequentially on magnetic tapes.
In order to assure a proper record linkage we developed a specific
data storage and retrieval system for the study. Figure 1 illustrates the record linkage of the data steming from different sources:
Each study participant receives a unique identification number which
contains a control digit. This number is entered together with
other identifying information (dates of birth and ECG recording,
recording location etc.) into the data acquisition carts and the
protocol sheets with clinical data and results of visual interpretation. In addition sequential numbers are automatically generated for each preprocessed ECG and VCG record and the clinical data
in order to avoid errors in the record linkage and to detect inconsistencies. The program for the record linkage does look for such
errors and generates a protocol which serves as a basis for interactive correction. During the process of interactive correction a
corresponding file is generated which serves for automated corrections if certain errors had occured in multiple records.
"Data base level I" refers to an index sequential storage system

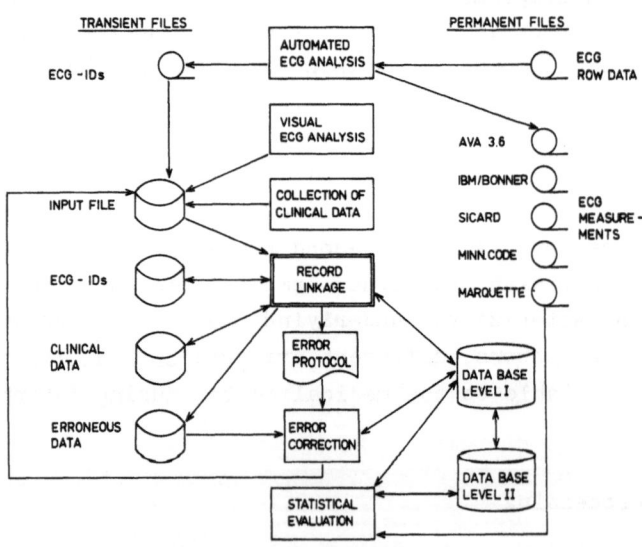

Figure 1: Record linkage and data storage

which we developed for a primary storage of the clinical data
and the information about the status of automated ECG-/VCG-
processing of the individual records, further the location of
the measurements on the sequential tapes. This data base is mainly used for the record linkage, error corrections, regular
updates and generating lists indicating which participants have
to be called for follow-up examinations.
"Data base level II" refers to the commercially available data
base system ADABAS which contains the basic clinical informations
from the study participants and supports the flexible definition
and composition of subcohorts for the statistical evaluation.

4. RESULTS

Recruitment of study participants started succesively for the different recording sites, the latest in April 1981. Until November
1981 about 5500 participants could be included with about
17000 single ECG and VCG recordings.
The recording carts proved to be well suited for the use within
field studies, most of the technicians took advantage of the
quality control features so that in general we obtained a much
better signal quality than formerly within clinical studies using
other equipment. Loss of ECG raw data due to malfunction of the
digital recording occurred only in about 1‰ of all recordings.
In the present paper we compare within one subcohort the visual
interpretation of 2850 ECGs and VCGs by one cardiologist with those
obtained by the BONNER/IBM programs, the VA program and the
automated Minnesota-coding.
From 2850 ECGs analysed by the BONNER/IBM I program 2378 (83%) were
classified as normal both by visual and automated analysis. There was
partial or complete agreement on 49 cases of LVH, however 40 cases were
classified as definite hypertrophies by the cardiologist only.
The results obtained by version II of the BONNER/IBM program showed
only minor changes. Within our study this program will mainly serve
for the evaluation of serial changes observed in the follow-up of the
participants.
The results of the automated Minnesota-coding cannot be reported in
detail within this paper. Only 53 % of 2850 ECGs were coded "0"; out of
this 99 % had been classified as normal by the visual interpretation.
With respect to the visual interpretation also the codes indicating
coronary heart disease and hypertrophies showed a low specificity. As

we are planning to evaluate the Minnesota Code with respect to its prognostic value we have to wait for the results from the follow-up observations.

Comparisons of automated ECG and VCG interpretations was at present restricted to 1732 cases analysed by the BONNER/IBM I- and VA-programs. Some of the results are shown in table 1.

Compared to the visual interpretation the specificity of the VA-program was greater than that of the IBM-program: 86,2 % of all VCGs were classified as normal both by visual and automated analysis compared to 79,8 % of the ECGs. The sensitivity of recognising LVH and RVH is somewhat higher for the VA-program than for the IBM program: 49 vs. 31 LVH-cases and 25 vs. 13 RVH-cases. There were, however, also a lot more false positive hypertrophies produced by the VA-program , especially LVH. The false negatives with respect to the visual interpretation (called "disagreement / visual only" in table 1) were to about the same amount classified as "possible" and "definite" hypertrophies by the cardiologist. Myocardial infarcts were detected equivalently by both programs. 6 respectively 4 of the infarcts not detected by the VA- or the IBM-program were classified as "definite" by the cardiologist. Table 1 shows that the threshold for "bradycardia" used within both programs is higher than that used by the cardiologist, especially within the IBM-program. Only very few of the observed discrepancies were due to appearant measurement errors.

5. DISCUSSION

Evaluation of conventional or automated ECG - interpretation is optimally performed if the true diagnostic classifications are obtained by ECG-independent clinical or pathological data. Within our study it is not feasible to perform extensive cardiological examinations in order to obtain correct ECG-independent diagnostic classifications. Therefore, in a first step, we could only compare the results of automated and visual ECG - interpretations. During the course of our study it will be possible to obtain exact relevant clinical data from the participants developing cardiac diseases. Therefore the results we obtained so far have to be regarded as preliminary.

We may, however, conclude from our present analysis that neither the automated ECG analysis nor the ECG interpretation by a cardiologist in his usual clinical fashion is suited for the special purpose of mass screening because both produce an amount of pathological or questionable diagnostic statements which appears not to be adequate for a scree-

DIAGNOSTIC CATEGORY	AGREEMENT				DISAGREEMENT			
	COMPLETE		PARTIAL		VISUAL ONLY		PROGRAM ONLY	
	AVA 3.6	IBM I	AVA 3.6	IBM I	AVA 3.6	IBM I	AVA 3.6	IBM I
NORMAL	728	768	765	615	10	110	199	80
L V H	34	28	15	3	57	76	81	56
R V H	23	13	2	–	92	104	87	10
M. INFARCT	13	16	3	1	18	17	31	7
ST-T CHANGES	8	34	2	3	80	69	48	33
EXTRASYSTOLES	9	18	–	–	11	6	3	26
BRADYCARDIA	13	29	–	–	4	2	231	446
TACHYCARDIA	4	4	–	–	2	2	11	7
L A H	12	14	–	–	5	3	30	5
R B B	–	2	–	–	4	2	–	3
L B B	1	2	–	–	1	–	–	–

Table 1   Comparison of visual and automated analysis of 1732 ECGs and VCGs

ning examination of clinically healthy persons.

We therefore would conclude that it is necessary to develop specific diagnostic algorithms which are better suited for the screening situation. We hope that we will be able to develop such criteria from our prospective study.

In the present situation the program AVA 3.6 showed a higher specificity than the BONNER/IBM program version I. The sensitivity of both programs with respect to diagnoses of major importance within a cardiovascular screening appeared to be equivalent with a small superiority of the VA - program in recognising ventricular hypertophies.

6.REFERENCES

1. Okajima, M. A series of questionnaire studies on usage of computerized ECG interpretation systems in Japan. Current facts and comparison between '79 and '81 surveys. IEEE Computers in Cardiology 1981, in press
2. Michaelis, J., Hain, P., Lippold, R., Scheidt, E., Schindler, W., Value of automated ECG-analysis for screening purposes. IEEE Computers in Cardiology 1981 ,in press
3. Tuinstra, C.L., Bonjar, F.H.: Validation of a Minnesota code program. p.353 - 355 in van Bemmel, J.H., Willems, J.L. (eds.) Trends in computer processed electrocardiograms. Amsterdam - New York - Oxford, 1977
4. Pipberger, H.V.: Comparative evaluation of ECG computer programs. IEEE Computers in Cardiology, p. 85 - 87, Long Beach, 1976.
5. Macfarlane, P.W., Melville, D.I., Horton, R.M., Bailey, J.J.: Comparative evaluation of the IBM (12-lead) and Royal Infirmary (orthogonal three-lead) ECG computer programs. Circulation 63, 354 - 359, 1981
6. Tuinstra, C.L., Rautaharju, P.M., Prineas, R.J., Duisterhout, J.S., Comparison of the operational value of six systems to asses the Minnesota Code. p. 487 - 492 in de Padua, F., Macfarlane, P.W.. (eds.) New frontiers of electrocardiology, Research Studies Press, Chichester, 1981

Information-theoretic analysis of human epileptic seizure EEGs

N.J.I. Mars

Section Medical Data Processing
University of Leiden
2333 AL Leiden
The Netherlands

Summary

This paper discusses the analysis of human EEGs, recorded during epileptic seizures, to determine the area in the brain -the so-called epileptogenic focus- responsible for the synchrony seen during seizures.

Because the pathways of propagation of epileptic activity in the brain are highly non-linear, conventional methods of measuring the time delays between derivations (like crosscorrelation) can not be used. Instead, a new analysis method -based on information theory- has been developed, the AAMI-function (Average Amount of Mutual Information).

Like the crosscorrelation, the AAMI-function provides a measure of the predictability of one signal, given another. By computing the AAMI for a range of lag-values -in analogy to the crosscorrelation function- time delays between signals can be determined.

To estimate AAMI, an algorithm has been developed which comprises an iterative probability density function estimation procedure. Simulations have been performed to determine the quality of our estimator. The technique has been applied to EEGs of artificially provoked seizures in dogs and of spontaneous human seizures.

The method appears also suitable for investigation of other non-linear phenomena in the brain.

1.0 Introduction

The study of EEGs, recorded during epileptic seizures in humans, is difficult because the pathways of propagation of epileptic activity in the brain are highly non-linear.

Conventional techniques for measuring time delays between derivations, based on the cross correlation function, require the assumption of linear channels of propagation.

In this paper we describe a new method for the analysis of non-linear no-memory systems, using the concept of Average Amount of Mutual Information (AAMI). A measure for Mutual Information was introduced in Shannon's landmark paper [1] and extended and generalized by Gel'fand and Yaglom [2]. AAMI can be used to characterize the relation between input and output signals of non-linear systems.

Although the main goal in the development of our method has been the construction of a tool for the estimation of time delay in non-linear systems, we feel that our approach is of more general use. Recently, reports on the application of a comparable technique to studies in psychiatry have appeared [3].

2.0 Theory

Using the mathematical theory of communication of Shannon, Gel'fand and Yaglom extended and generalized Shannon's measure of mutual information [2]. Their measure provides the amount of information about a random vector contained in another such vector.

This measure of mutual information can be defined for stochastic variables with realizations which only assume a finite number of discrete values and for stochastic variables in which the realizations assume continuous values. We will show the definition of Average Amount of Mutual Information (AAMI) only for the discrete case.

We consider two stochastic variables X and Y. We assume that the realizations assume values from the finite sets $\{x_i\}$, i=1,N and $\{y_j\}$, j=1,M, respectively. The elements x_i and y_j have a probability of occurence given by $p_X(x_i)$ and $p_Y(y_j)$ in which:

$$p_X(x_i) = \text{Prob}(X = x_i) \tag{1}$$

$$p_Y(y_j) = \text{Prob}(Y = y_j) \tag{2}$$

$$p_X(x_i) \geqslant 0 \quad i=1,2,\ldots M \tag{3}$$

$$p_Y(y_j) \geqslant 0 \quad j=1,2,\ldots N \tag{4}$$

$$\sum_i p_X(x_i) = 1 \tag{5}$$

$$\sum_j p_Y(y_j) = 1 \tag{6}$$

The joint probability of occurence is given by $p_{XY}(x_i,y_j)$ with:

$$p_{XY}(x_i,y_j) = \text{Prob}(X = x_i, Y = y_j) \tag{7}$$

$$p_{XY}(x_i, y_j) \geqslant 0 \quad i=1,2,\ldots M \tag{8}$$

$$j=1,2,\ldots N$$

$$\sum_i \sum_j p_{XY}(x_i, y_j) = 1 \tag{9}$$

For this discrete case the AAMI is defined as:

$$\text{AAMI}(X,Y) = \sum_i \sum_j p_{XY}(x_i,y_j) \log \frac{p_{XY}(x_i,y_j)}{p_X(x_i) \cdot p_Y(y_j)} \tag{10a}$$

In the continuous case, we find analogously

$$AAMI(X,Y) = \int_{-\infty}^{\infty}\int_{-\infty}^{\infty} f_{XY}(x,y) \log \frac{f_{XY}(x,y)}{f_X(x).f_Y(y)} \, dx \, dy \qquad (10b)$$

(When $p_{XY}(x_i,y_j) = 0$, the corresponding term in the summation is taken to be zero.)

The unit is bits, nats or hartleys, if the base of the logarithm is respectively 2, e (2.71828...) or 10.

AAMI is equal to zero if the variables are independent and greater than zero if the variables are interdependent.

Estimation of AAMI requires knowledge of the joint and marginal densities. Because these densities are normally not known a priori, they have to be estimated. We will first discuss methods for estimating these densities.

3.0 Estimation of probability density functions

3.1 Choice of method

The problem of estimating a probability density function from a number of samples has been discussed extensively in the literature. Wegman [4,5] and Fryer [6] have given reviews of this literature. Following Wegman, we distinguish four methods for density estimation: orthogonal series, kernels (or windows), histograms and maximum likelihood estimators.

Of the four methods, the kernel estimator appears to be the most suitable one for our application. This estimator has been studied by Parzen [7].

The kernel estimator in general is given by:

$$f_N(y_1,y_2,...y_M) = \frac{1}{N} \sum_{n=1}^{N} \prod_{m=1}^{M} \frac{1}{h_m(N)h} \, K(\frac{y_m-x_{mn}}{h_m(N)}) \qquad (11)$$

Here M is the number of dimensions of the density, N the number of M-dimensional samples, $h_m(N)$ the kernel width for N samples, y_m the variable in the m'th dimension, x_{mn} the n'th sample value in the m'th dimension and K(.) the kernel function.

Parzen [7] has derived conditions for K(.) which assure asymptotic unbiasedness, asymptotic consistency and uniform consistency. These properties can be achieved with a wide class of kernel functions.

Epanechnikov [8] has used this freedom in the choice of K(.) to derive the non-negative kernel form and kernel width which give the minimum relative global approximation error over all densities, in case the true probability density function has a Taylor expansion in all its arguments everywhere under the restriction that $h_m(N) = h(N)$, i.e., that the kernel width is independent of m.

The optimal kernel function derived by Epanechnikov is given by:

$$K_{opt}(y) = \frac{3}{4\sqrt{5}}(1 - \frac{y^2}{\sqrt{5}}) \qquad \text{if } -\sqrt{5} < y < +\sqrt{5} \qquad (12)$$

$$= 0 \text{ elsewhere}$$

Note that the optimal kernel function has a simple quadratic form and is independent of the true probability density and of the sample size. The function has finite support which makes the computation easier.

Within this class of optimal kernel functions, the optimal kernel width which minimizes the relative global approximation error of the density to be estimated is given by [8]:

$$h_{opt}(N) \approx \left[\frac{ML^M}{ND} \right]^{1/(M+4)} \qquad (13)$$

in which:

$$L = \int_{-\infty}^{\infty} K^2_{opt}(y) \, dy = \int_{-\sqrt{5}}^{\sqrt{5}} \left[\frac{3}{4\sqrt{5}}(1- \frac{y^2}{\sqrt{5}}) \right]^2 \, dy = \frac{3}{5\sqrt{5}} \qquad (14)$$

and:

$$D = \int_{-\infty}^{\infty} \cdots \int_{-\infty}^{\infty} \sum_{m=1}^{M} \left[\frac{\partial^2}{\partial x_m} f(x_1,x_2,\ldots,x_M) \right]^2 \, dx_1 dx_2 \ldots dx_M \qquad (15)$$

The kernel width which is optimal for the estimation of the density is thus a function of the number of samples and of the density itself.

We have used the Epanechnikov kernel estimator in an iterative way, in which an estimated kernel width is used to provide an estimate of the probability density function (using (11)), which in turn is used to provide an improved estimate of the optimal kernel width, etc. We have been unable to prove the convergence of this iterative procedure. In our experiments with estimation of densities based on samples from known probability density functions, we have not experienced any problems in this respect.

3.2 Computation of AAMI.

The algorithm described above is used to compute the density values on a rectangular grid within a range of -3σ to $+3\sigma$. To compute the AAMI value according to (10b), the integrand of (10b) is integrated, using Simpson's rule [9, p. 231]. The use of the range -3σ to $+3\sigma$ for the estimation of the probability density function implies that the densities are assumed to be zero outside that range.

We tried two different methods for the the computation of (10b). In the first method the marginal densities $f_x(x)$ and $f_y(y)$ were obtained by numerical integration of $f_{xy}(x,y)$. In the second approach the marginal densities were estimated independently, using the one-dimensional equivalent of (11). Extensive simulations showed that the second method always gave superior results (i.e., closer to the theoretically expected values). In the applications to be described the second method has been used.

To assess the feasibility of the computational procedure described and the practical usefulness of AAMI, we performed experiments with three known systems: a linear system, a rectifying system and a squaring system. The input signal for all three systems was recursively low-pass filtered Gaussian noise. The effects of number of samples, correlation between samples, and signal- to-noise ratio have been studied. Very high correlations between samples (> .95) cause our estimator of the probability density functions to degenerate. However, this problem can be lessened by adding known amounts of white noise to the signals. Sequences of 256 to 1024 samples appeared to be usable for the purpose of estimating reliable AAMI-values.

4.0 Application of AAMI to time delay estimation

To estimate time delays in non-linear systems we computed the value of AAMI between the input and output signal for a range of lag-values, in analogy to the crosscorrelation function. The lag-value where the AAMI reaches a maximum is an estimate of the time delay of the system studied. (By using this procedure one circumvents the problem of assigning meaning to the AAMI, as only AAMI values from the same system are mutually compared.)

Simulations have been performed using the same three systems described above for a wide range of signal-to-noise ratio, number of samples and correlation between samples. These simulations showed that for linear systems the AAMI-function is almost as good an estimator of time delay as the cross correlation function. For non-linear systems the cross correlation function is useless (in the two non-linear systems described, the cross correlation between input and output signals is zero); the performance of the AAMI-function is only marginally less than for linear systems.

5.0 Application to biological systems

Our motivation for the development of this time delay estimator comes from a medical problem: the localization of an epileptogenic focus in the brain of patients suffering from epileptic seizures. Localization of this focus is be done by computing time delays between EEG-signals recorded during epileptic seizures with electrodes implanted in the brain.

To validate our approach, we analysed seizures recorded with implanted electrodes from dogs with artificially induced epileptogenic foci. The results showed that the (known) focus localization could be found by our method with a sufficient degree of reliability.

Having stood this first test, we applied the method to recordings obtained from patients which have undergone surgical treatment for intractable epilepsy and in whom the localization of the focus is more or less known (post-operatively).

We are currently assessing the outcome of these experiments as a prerequisite to the clinical use of our method for focus localization. More detailed results from this research will be reported elsewhere [10].

References

[1] C.E. Shannon and W. Weaver 1949
The Mathematical Theory of Communication
University of Illinois Press, Chicago, Ill.

[2] Gel'fand, I.M. and Yaglom, A.M. 1959.
Calculation of the amount of information about a random function contained in another such function.
American Mathematical Society Translations Vol. 12, pp. 199- 246.

[3] Inouye, T., Yagasaki, A., Takahashi, H. and Shinosaki, K. 1981.
The dominant direction of interhemispheric EEG changes in the linguistic process.
Electroencephalography and Clinical Neurophysiology Vol. 51, pp. 265- 275.

[4] Wegman, E.J. 1972.
Nonparametric probability density estimation: I. A summary of available methods.
Technometrics Vol. 14, No. 3, pp. 533- 546.

[5] Wegman, E.J. 1972.
Nonparametric probability density estimation: II. A comparison of density estimation methods.
Journal of Statistical Computation and Simulation Vol. 1, pp. 225- 245.

[6] Fryer, M.J. 1977.
A review of some non-parametric methods of density estimation.
Journal of the Institute of Mathematics and its Applications Vol. 20, pp. 335- 354.

[7] Parzen, E.   1962.
On estimation of a probability density function and mode.
Annals of Mathematical Statistics Vol.   35, pp.   1065- 1076.

[8] Epanechnikov, V.A.   1969.
Non-parametric estimation of a multivariate probability density.
Theory of Probability and its Applications Vol.   14, pp.   153- 158.

[9] A.H.   Stroud 1971
Approximate calculation of multiple integrals
Prentice-Hall, Englewood Cliffs, N.J.

[10] N.J.I.   Mars and G.W.   van Arragon 1981
Submitted for publication in Electroencephalography and Clinical
Neurophysiology.

CLOSED LOOP EP-PROCESSING*)

Helfrid MARESCH
Gert PFURTSCHELLER
Institute of Biomedical Engineering, Technical University Graz
Inffeldgasse 18, A-8010 Graz

Abstract

Closed loop EP-processing means a choice of the stimulus onset according to the the ongoing EEG activity analyzed on line. Out of many other possibilities we choose the phase of the EEG as the determining parameter for stimulation. The difference between random phase and alternating phase stimulation is pointed out, also a study of the influence of the stimulation phase on the amplitude and phase of the EEG after the alpha blocking phenomenon is performed. The differences between random stimulation and closed loop stimulation are expressed also as signal to noise ratio and give so an objective judgement about the method.

Method

For closed loop EP processing a special system was designed, consisting of a PDP 11/23 computer and an acoustic and visual stimulation unit (Amplaid, SLE), both controlled by the computer (fig. 1). For data acquisition two amplifiers with a frequency range from 0.01 Hz to 10 kHz are available. The amplifier output is sampled by an 8 channel differential input A/D-converter with direct memory access and a maximum throughput rate of 100 kHz.

The control of the stimulators if performed by a parallel I/O board with 16 bits for each of two ports, connected to the amplaid mk5 (as501, as502) stimulators. All acoustic parameters (frequency, burst plateau time, raise-decay time, stimulus level, repetition rate) are controlled by the computer. The visual stimulator (flash) is triggered by the computer.

The computer programs make an online analysis of the EEG data possible, as well as a storage of the raw data on the magnetic disk for later offline processing. Data acquisition is performed into a circular buffer in the background at choosable sampling rates. The usage of a circular buffer technique enables us to regard also events which occur before the trigger point, as well as to monitor the EEG continuously. After a trigger event which can be chosen to be set by the computer or by another device, a predefined rest of the buffer is filled and the whole buffer area to be analyzed is written to another RAM area within a few milliseconds. First investigations by this system were performed to study the influence of the EEG

---

*) supported by the "Fonds zur Förderung der wissenschaftlichen Forschung in Österreich", proj.no.4279

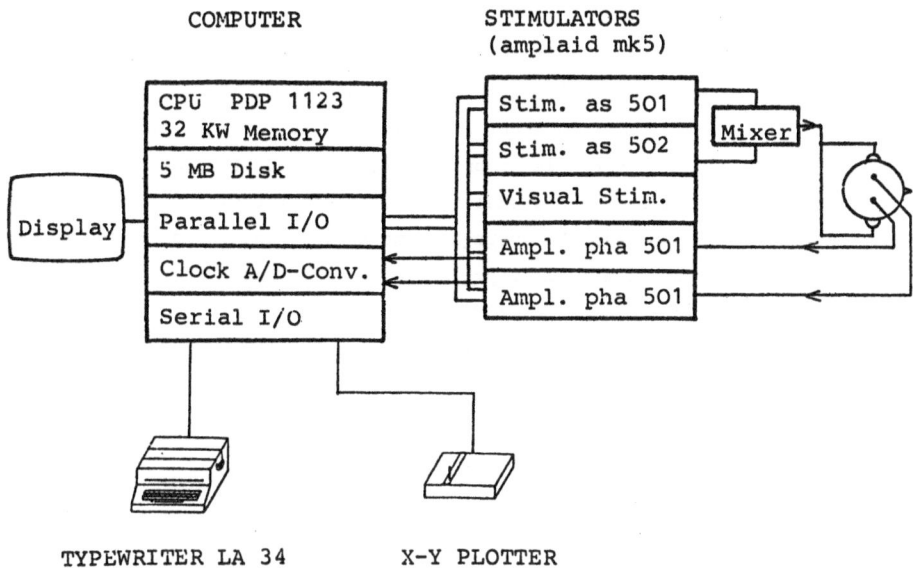

COMPUTER   STIMULATORS
                           (amplaid mk5)

CPU   PDP 1123 | Stim. as 501
32 KW Memory | Stim. as 502   Mixer
5 MB Disk | Visual Stim.
Display | Parallel I/O | Ampl. pha 501
Clock A/D-Conv. | Ampl. pha 501
Serial I/O

TYPEWRITER LA 34   X-Y PLOTTER

Fig.1: Blockdiagramm of the computer- stimulator system

dependent of the time of visual stimulation in relation to the alpha phase. The subject was sitting in a quiet, not darkened room with eyes closed, having the flash
light at a short distance (appr. 20 cm) in front of his eyes. The analyzed EEG epoch
was 2 seconds, 0.5 sec before and 1.5 sec after the stimulus. The sampling rate was
128/sec. The stimulation point was choosen in relation to a maximum or minimum of the
EEG: 1,2,..,6 sampling points after a maximum or a minimum, that means the following
time delays after the maximum and the equivalent phase angles at an average alpha
frequency of 9.7 Hz, yielding an average sycle time of 104 msec (see also fig. 2):
delay msec   8   16   23   31   39   47   60   68   75   83   91   99
phase angle 28   55   80 107 135 163 208 235 260 287 315 343   (degrees)

To get a fair comparision of the phase locked stimuli with those at random stimulation, the following stimulation sequence was performed:
1. random
2. after maximum
3. random
4. after minimum
This sequence was repeated 50 times. For the investigation of the phase influence to
the EP and the following EEG the random stimuli were omitted. The time distance between two flashes was randomized in the range between 3.0 and 3.5 sec.

The electrodes were posed on Pz and Oz (positive:Pz), with ground on mastoid. This
bipolar derivation was already used at normative VEP studies(1,2). As the negativity
of Oz means usual an upward deflection in the drawing of the averaged time series,

216

we speek in the following of a maximum in respect to Pz. The amplifier had a time constant of 0.3 sec and an upper cutoff frequency of 20 Hz (6 dB point). For the comparison of reverse phase stimulation with random phase stimulation Pz-A2 derivation (positive: Pz) was used. A study about unipolar and bipolar derivations in respect to the signal to noise ratio is in preparation. The evaluation of the EEG trials included the estimation of the signal to noise-ratio for 0.25 sec epochs and the calculation of the variance of the averaged time series. The signal to noise-ratio was computed according to a formula presented in (3) .

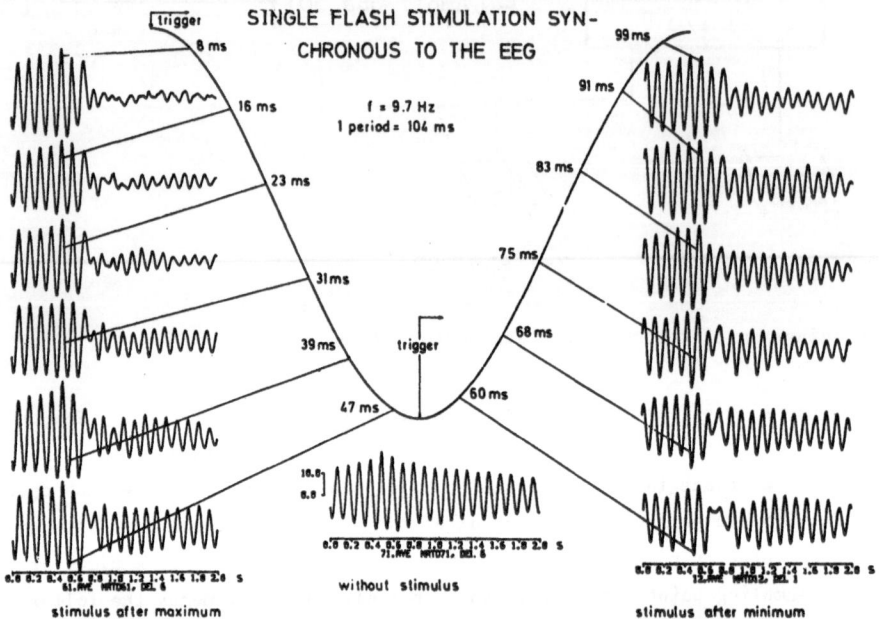

Fig.2: Points of stimulation at certain phase angles of the alpha rhythm. The averages of 50 single trials each, recorded synchronous to maxima and minima, are also drawn.

Results

In 6 experiments the optimum phase for reverse stimulation could be determined. As from the analysis of the EEG after the evoked potential could be seen, the fastest recovering of the alpha, aliasing the late components of the VEP most,occurs at phase angles between 135-180 and 315-360 degrees, so that a stimulation phase outside this regions should be preferred. As to be seen in Table 1, the amplitude of the VEP is not so much influenced as the signal to noise ratio. The averages are displayed in Fig. 2. The influence of the stimulation phase to the latency of the 3 main components of the VEP was very small. The latencies were the same within 1 sampling point (7.8 msec).

max: N100 at 87 msec, min: P150 at 149 msec, max: N200 at 204 msec.

The according averages are drawn in fig. 3.

Three further experiments were performed to compare random phase with reverse phase
stimulation. For these experiments a delay of 8 ms after maximum and minimum (28 and
208 deg.) was selected. The results, again regarding the periods 0-0.25 and
0.25-0.50 sec after the stimulus, are to be seen in Table 2. (Fig. 4).

Table 1: SNR and amplitudes of the VEP for different phase-pairs at reverse
phase stimulation.

angle (degrees)	SNR (Ps/Pn)		amplitude
	0.00-0.25	0.25-0.50	
28 - 208	39.7	9.06	27.2
55 - 235	32.8	15.0	27.5
80 - 260	43.0	11.6	28.5
107- 287	24.1	12.1	25.0
135- 315	26.6	15.7	23.0
163- 343	26.5	13.6	28.3

Table 2:VEP-SNR and amplitude comparision: random and alternating phase stimulation

	random			alternating phase		
	SNR		amplitude	SNR		amplitude (uV)
	0-0.25	0.25-0.5		0-0.25		0.25-0.5
exp.1	20.1	25.0	39.0	35.3	36.2	49.0
exp.2	18.4	4.6	39.2	47.7	15.6	45.8
exp.3	38.9	7.1	41.6	48.0	28.2	42.2

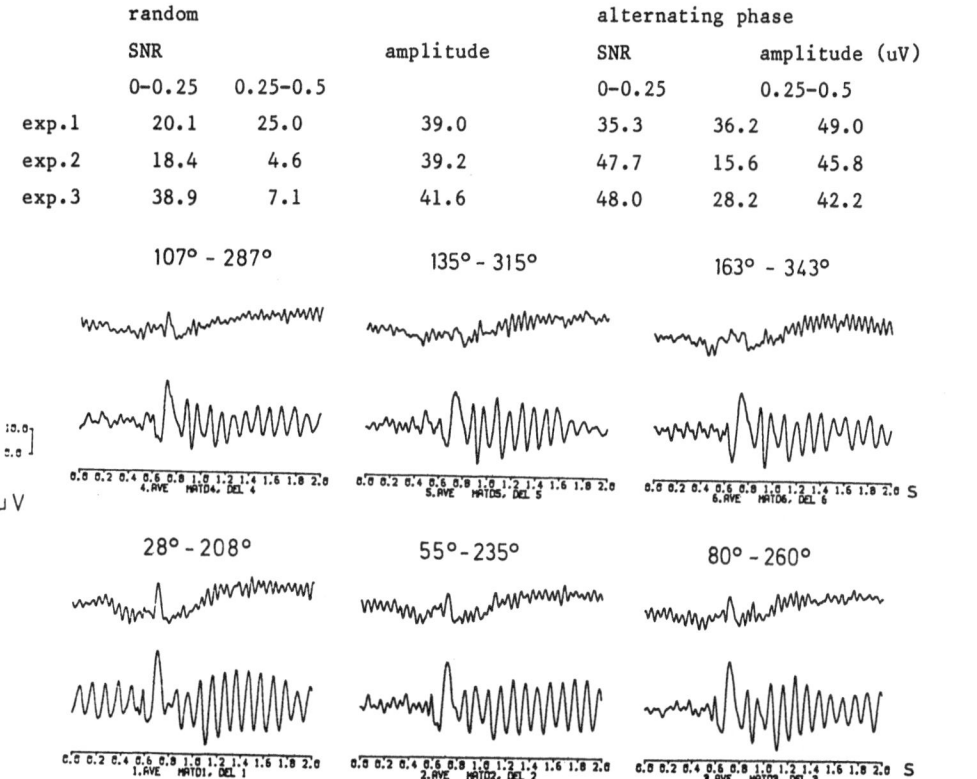

Fig.3: Averages of 100 time series each, recorded at opposite phase angles acording
to table 1. (reverse phase stimulation)

The number of averages in these experiments was 100. In all three cases the reverse phase stimulation yields better SNR-values as well as higher VEP-amplitudes. The attention was not only directed to the VEP but also to the time after it, up to 1200 msec after the stimulus. As a typical time point where especially the greatest changes of the amplitude of the averaged time series and the greatest changes of the variance could be observed, the period of 0.5 sec to 0.75 sec after the stimulus was regarded. Table 3 gives an impression of the dependence of the SNR, the amplitude and the variance from the alpha phase at stimulation time.

Table 3: Amplitudes of the average, SNR and variance at different stimulation phase angles

phase	delay	ampl.of uV	average %	var. %	SNR	%
28	8	5	19	68	1.15	5
55	16	7	27	60	2.73	11
80	23	11	42	68	5.48	22
107	31	12	46	77	5.48	11
135	39	18	69	84	7.00	29
163	47	22	85	96	9.69	40
208	60	23	88	103	21.5	88
235	68	21	81	98	15.7	64
260	75	19	73	95	19.5	80
287	83	17	65	86	16.0	65
315	91	16	62	95	6.40	26
343	99	13	50	84	6.20	25

The %-values are referred to the values measured at no stimulation:

SNR = 24.5

Amp. = 26.0

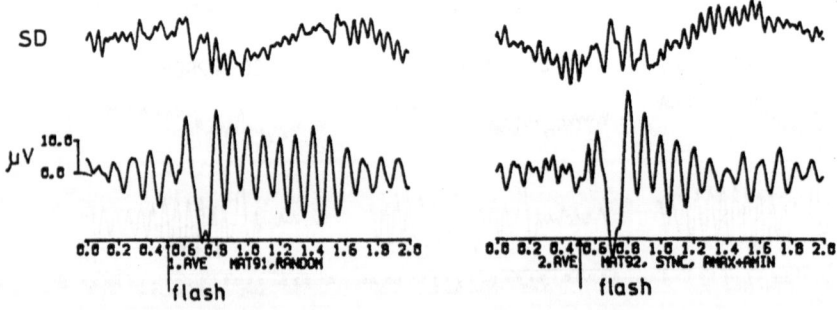

Fig.4: Comparision of random phase with reverse phase stimulation.
left: random phase   right: reverse phase
The number of averages is 100

Finally the latencies of the alpha rhythm after the stimulus were regarded. Fig.5 shows the latency changes referred to the undisturbed latencies measured without stimulation. As to be seen in fig.6, the amplitude of the alpha rhythm is reduced shortly after the stimulus. After 350 - 500 msec it recovers, dependent from the phase in which the stimulus was set. The alpha rhythm is blocking more at stimulation times shortly after the maximum. Also the alpha recovering occurs faster at after minimum stimulations, as to be seen in table 3. At 1 sec after stimulation alpha rhythm is completely at the amplitude level observed before stimulation, but

latency of maxima (ms) without stimulation

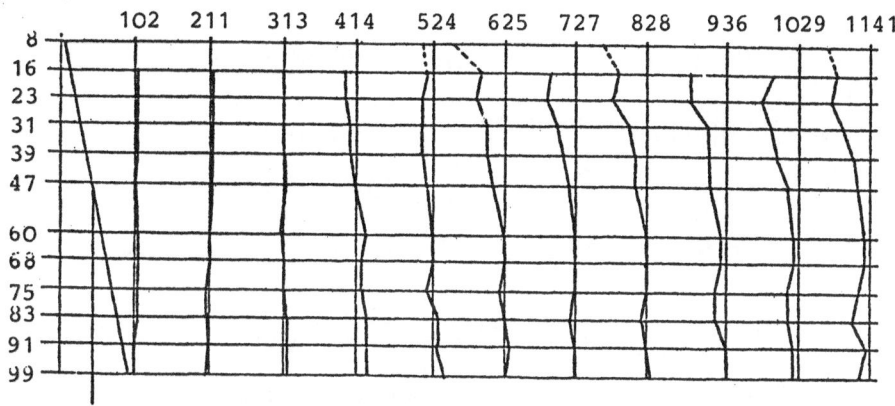

stimulation time

Fig.5: Latencies of the undisturbed EEG, recorded synchronous to an alpha maximum (vertical lines) and latencies of averaged EEG trials, influenced by a single flash. The time of stimulation is drawn at the left side.

the average amplitude is reduced due to the randomization of the phase at stimulation times -5 to 30 msec after maximum. The latencies are shifted to earlier times, when the flash occured in the declining slope (maximum to minimum) of the EEG. At the stimulation point 8 msec after the maximum the phase of the following EEG was completely randomized and could hardly be measured up to 1500 msec later. At later stimulation phases in the falling slope a complete phase reversion by pi (180 deg.) appr. 1 sec after the stimulus could be observed.

Discussion:
Compared with random phase stimulation, the inverse phase stimulation could be shown to be more efficient in respect to the signal to noise ratio at VEPs. This fact could also be found at auditory evoked potentials in an earlier study.(4)

An influenc of the stimulation phase to the phase of the recovering alpha rhythm after blocking could also be seen. Stimulations into a positiv slope of the alpha rhythm (increasing negativity at Oz) seem not to alter the phase in respect to the phase before the stimulus.

At a stimulation into the negativ slope a phase shift is induced, also a distortion of the stability of the phase from trial to trial could be observed.

The latencies of the VEP components however were not influenced at all, as well as the amplitude did only reduce at the 135 - 315 degr, stimulation. An assumption, that the alpha activity should be the same as the phase of the expected VEP, could not be found. In contrary, if the stimulation (at 8 - 16 msec after maximum) lets a coincidence of the 90 msec VEP component expect, the alpha provocation is delayed and the phase is independent from the prestimulus phase.

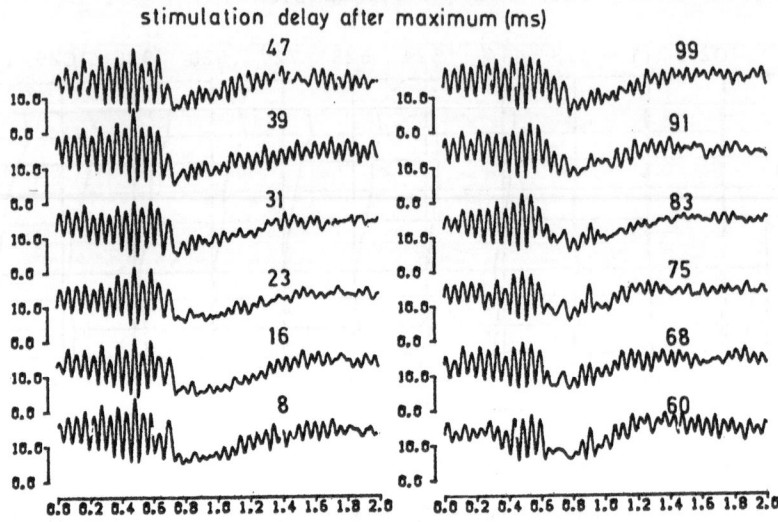

Fig.6: Square root of the variance of the averages drawn in fig.2, giving an impression of the time course of the amplitude at single EEG recordings. The numbers indicate the time lag between the synchronization maximum and the stimulation.

References:
(1) Ciganek, L.: Variability of the human visual evoked potential: normative data. Electroenceph.clin.Neurophys.,1969, 27:35-42
(2) Jasper, H.: The ten-twenty electrode system of the International Federation. Electroenceph.clin.Neurophys.,1958, 10:371-375
(3) Maresch, H., Pfurtscheller, G. and Schuy, S.: Objectivation of single and averaged evoked potentials by means of statistical methods. Proceedings of the second mediterranean conference on medical and biological engineering, Marseille,1980, 71-73
(4) Maresch, H., Pfurtscheller, G., and Schuy, S.: Evoked potentials at EEG-controlled acoustial stimulation. Proceedings of the 6-th annual meeting of the Austrian Society of Biomedical Engineering, Graz, 1981:115-118

THERMO-BLOOD-FLOWMETRY, MICROPROCESSOR PROCESSED THERMOGRAMS

Iwao Fujimasa, Kou Imachi, *Hitoshi Miyake, **Masahiro Iwatani,
Kazuhiko Atsumi

Institute of Medical Electronics, Faculty of Medicine,
University of Tokyo, 7-3-1, Hongo, Bunkyo-ku, Tokyo, Japan

*Health Care Center, Technology and Science University of Nagaoka

**1st Surgical Department, Tokyo University Hospital

(SUMMARY)

Infrared thermograms indicate skin bloodflow distribution
pattern under relatively warm environment (physiologically neutral
thermal environment). The paper shows a new conversion method from
thermograms to skin blood flow rate using a stand alone microcomputer. Under neutral thermal condition, the skin blood flow can be
calculated from a formula which includes five parameters; local skin
temperature, local deep body temperature, body temperature, environment temperature and dimension of the object. The system consisted of
a microcomputer (PC-8001) with an I/O interface (PC-8011) and a
mini-floppy disk drive (PC-8031) and a digital memory infrared
thermography camera (Infraeye 150). A themogram image of Infraeye 150
includes more than 100 k words (1 word is 10 bits.) and the signals
are send to the I/O port with 100 kHz. As the PC8001 has only 64k
bytes memory and I/O speed is less than 10kHz, the data reduction was
requested. Firstly, one dimension thermoprofile was converted blood
flow profile. Secondly, the thermal image was reduced to 40x20 input
image and converted blood flow image. The software was written in
assemblar and N-BASIC and the image was displayed on a color CRT and
a graphic printer. Skin blood flow rate distribution display can
contribute quantitative diagnosis for peripheral vascular disorders.
The prototype system was tested and evaluated 88 clinical cases in
Tokyo University Hospital.

1. Introduction

Infrared thermography has been developed as a remote sensing
technology for surface thermal pattern measurement. The diagnosing
technique of clinical thermography has been based on pattern recognition of thermograms and not based on thermal physiological
analysis. Abnormal hot or cold region indicate the existence of
local thermal abnormality under the skin and abnormal vascular
pattern indicate inflammatory or malignant tumor under the skin. But
the climatic environment of thermography in clinic is generally mild
and warm temperature condition. The condition are called physiologically neutral thermal condition and skin temperature is kept
constant. The temperature mainly depends upon blood flow rate in the
skin. Objects of the work are to find an algorithm to calculate skin
blood flow rate from skin surface temperature and some complementary
physiological parameters and to develop a thermo-blood-flowmetry
method using a micro computer system.

2. Theory and Formula

Skin blood flow rate is affected mainly by environmental thermal condition and heart production in the body. Surface skin temperature is decided the balance between heat loss and heat production. Supply of heat to the skin depend on heat transportation by blood flow, on conduction from deep tissue, and on the metabolic production in the skin. On the other hand, the skin loses the heat to environment by radiation, by evaporation and by convection. In relatively warm room temperature, skin temperature maintaines stable value. The balanced condition is called 'thermally neutral condition or skin blood flow controlling condition' and the skin temperature can be expressed in a function of skin blood flow rate.

The function was described in the formula (1):

$$Vs = \frac{Kr(Ts-Tw)+Kf \cdot D^{0.25}(Ts-Ta)^{1.25}+Ev-Kc\left(\frac{Tc-Ts}{d}\right)-Mo \cdot 2^{\frac{Ts-Tm}{10}} \cdot d}{\alpha \rho c(Tb-Ts) \cdot d} \qquad (1)$$

where,

```
Kr,Kf,Kc = constant
Tb = blood temperature
Tc = core temperature
Ts = skin temperature
Tw = wall temperarture
Ta = ambient temperature
Ev = heat by evapolation
α  = counter current rate
ρc = density x specific heat of blood
D  = diameter of body or extremity
Mo = basal metabolic rate
Tm = basal metabolic temperature
ts = skin thickness
```

The blood temperature (Tb) was substitute body temperature, the core temperature was measured by a deep body termometer 'Coretemp' and skin temperature was measured by an infrared thermography 'Infraeye 150'.

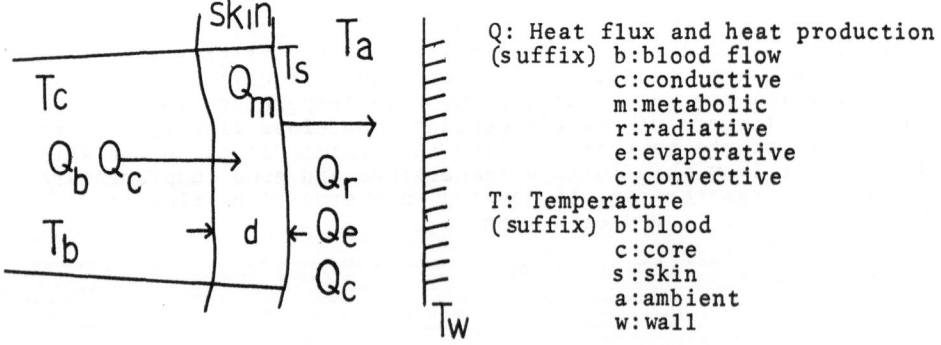

Q: Heat flux and heat production
(suffix) b:blood flow
c:conductive
m:metabolic
r:radiative
e:evaporative
c:convective
T: Temperature
(suffix) b:blood
c:core
s:skin
a:ambient
w:wall

Figure 1. Thermal model of skin and its neighbourhood

3. System Configuration

The thermo-blood-flowmetry system was composed of an infrared thermography instrument, 6 channel deep body thermometers, a 32k microcomputer, a 32k interface unit and two minifloppy disk drives. A thermal pattern was memorized in the infrared thermography 'Infraeye' memory with 10 bit digital images. The picture is composed of 224 scan line x 448 elements, and then the total elements exceed 100kw. As frequency response speed of computer input from the thermogram is required 100kHz, the image processing of the thermogram using microcomputer inheres request to data reduction. Fortunately, the precis of skin tissue blood flow rate shows relatively coarse, because the spacial resolution of deep body temperature is larger than 1 cm^2. We tried to reduce 40 x 20 elements from a thermogram. (Fig.2)

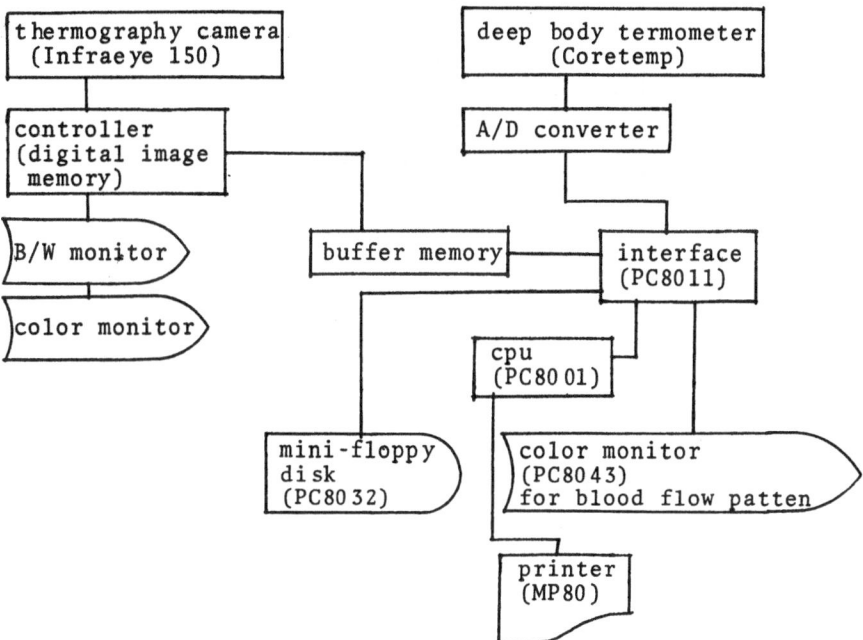

Figure 2. System configuration of skin blood flowmetry system

The software was written in assemblar and N-BASIC. In future, the system shall be expand and can convert all information of thermal images into blood flow data.

4. Clinical Evaluation

Firstly, the system was evaluated by an experiment animal and normal persons. The culculated blood flow rate was validated with a tissue blood flow metry method of H2 gas clearance method and past research data of plethysmography and radio-active xenon clearance method from documentations. Secondly, blood flow rate of lower extremities of patients with peripheral circulatory disturbance was measured.

The skin blood flow rate calculated by this method was 9.7 to 15.0 ml/ 100 g/ min on thigh, 10 to 14.5 ml/ 100 g/ min on leg and 11.0 to 13.3 ml/ 10 0g/ min on foot.

The culculated results were displayed on a color monitor and a graphic protter as shown in Fig.3a and 3b.

These results coincided well with previous studies. Therefore this noninvasisive method to evaluate the skin blood flow rate is practically useful.

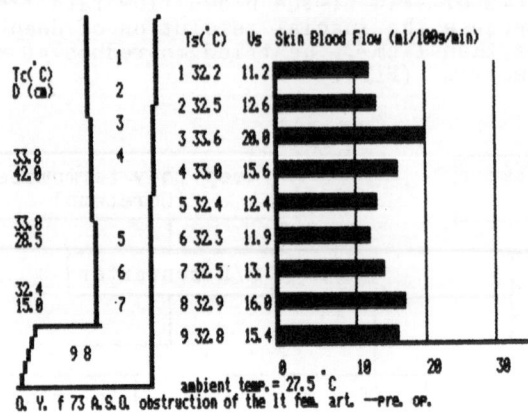

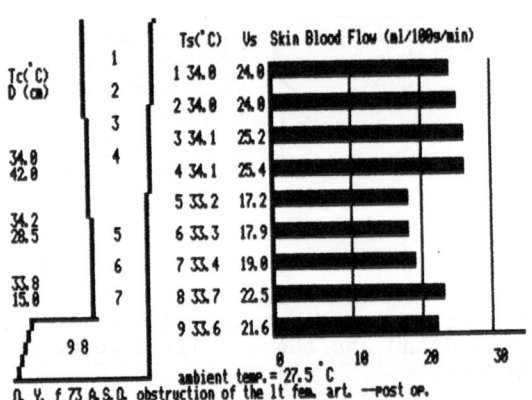

Figure 3. Typical thermo-blood-flowmetry displays
Two figures show estimated blood flow rate on a left lower extremity. Upper (a) shows pre-sympatectomy data and lower (b) shows post-sympathectomy data.

The system has been introduced into differential diagnosis of peripheral circulatory diseases of lower extremities. 88 cases of sclerotic arterial obstruction or obstructive thrombo-angitis were taken thermograms and deep body temperature and analysed by the method.

5. Discussion

The patterns of thermogram can tell us thermal abnormality of the surface of skin noninvasively. Blood flow rate in the skin tissue is the most predominant factor to decide the skin temperature. Then, the ability to display blood flow pattern of skin inhares in a thermogram. For varidation of the results obtained from the system, relationship between skin temperature and skin blood flow rate was drawn in figure 4. As from a textbook of physiology, the relation between the blood flow rate and the temperature of skin was projected as exponential curve.

As a practical application, evaluation of blood flow regeneration after lumbar sympathectomy was tried in 13 cases. The surface temperature and blood flow rate of feet were significantly increased in those cases.

The 40 x 20 graphic image display method has been developed and evaluated in normal object. Today, sensitivity analysis of each parameters of the model revealed that the effect of deep body tempeature to blood flow of the skin was neglectfully small at neutral temperature condition. Then the formula (1) will become simple and thermograms will be easily converted to blood flow pattern.

As a conclusion, thermo-blood-flowmetry method is a powerful aid of diagnosis of peripheral vascular disease and give us a quantitative data processing methodology for analysing thermograms. data processing methodology for analysing thermograms.

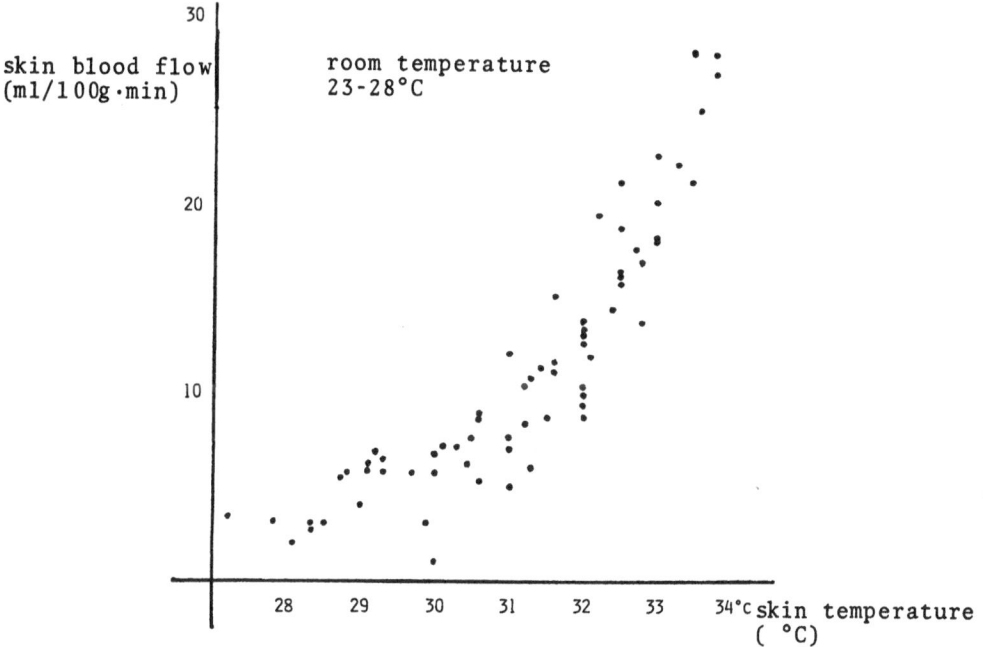

Figure 4. Relationship between skin temperature and skin blood flowrate

5. References

1) Iwatani,M., et al.; Evaluation of the skin blood flow rate by
   heat flow analysis. Bio-Medical Thermography 1(1), 70-72, (1981)
2) Fujimasa,I., et al.; Algolithm of thermogram analysis under
   thermal stress. Bio-Medical Thermography 1(1), 54-56, (1981)

Request for reprints: Dr. I. Fujimasa, Institute of Medical
Electronics, Faculty of Medicine, University of Tokyo, 7-3-1, Hongo
Bunkyo-ku, Tokyo, 113, Japan

EEG ANALYSIS METHODS IN EXPERIMENTAL NEUROPHYSIOLOGICAL RESEARCH

P.Rappelsberger[+], H.Pockberger[+], H.Petsche[+], R.Vollmer[++]
[+]Neurophysiological Institute, University of Vienna
[+]Brain Research Institute, Academy of Sciences
[++]Ludwig Boltzmann Institute of Clinical Neurobiology
Währingerstraße 17
A-1090 Wien
Austria

SUMMARY

This paper deals with the application of spectral analytical methods to field potentials (EEG) recorded simultaneously with arrays of
electrodes from the cortical surface or from intracortically. An essential point is the appropriate presentation of the results, in which 4
parameters have to be taken into consideration: the amplitudes of the
spectral values, the different frequency components, the time dependence of the spectra and the local variations of the spectra due to
the different recording sites. The figures show some examples where
alternatively one or two of these parameters are kept constant to
study the mutual dependence of the other parameters.

INTRODUCTION

The aim of our study is to find links between the anatomy of the
cortex and the electrical signals (field potentials, EEG) which are
generated within the cortex (Rappelsberger et al, 1981). The purpose
of this research is to get a better understanding of the basic mechanisms of EEG generation, e.g. evoked potentials which become more and
more important in clinical diagnosis (Pockberger et al, 1981). A further important research program is the study of the basic mechanisms
of epileptic seizures, their synchronization and the effect of anti-
convulsive drugs (Petsche et al, 1979; Rappelsberger et al, 1979).

METHODS

The studies are performed in animals where it is possible to record
either directly from the cortical surface with sets of electrodes or
from intracortically with semi-microelectrodes produced in thin-film
technology (Prohaska et al, 1979). In every case, recordings are made

with up to 16 electrodes simultaneously. This raises the problem to manage the great amount of data. A first data selection is obtained by storing the data on analogue tape and by converting them off-line. The sampled date are stored on disc or on computer tape.

For the application of spectral analytical methods a program package was developed which performs the different calculation procedures and which manages the different kinds of presentations of the results on a storage disply. The calculations include: power spectra, coherence- and phase spectra, partial coherence- and phase spectra, multiple spectra etc. (Jenkins and Watts, 1968).

EXAMPLES AND PRESENTATION OF THE RESULTS

Figure 1 shows examples of raw data. For the visual inspection of the EEG signals the amplitude scale, the time scale, the number of traces and finally the individual channel numbers according to the denotions of the electrodes can be varied appropriately.

The possibility of a correct interpretation of the results with respect to the individual question of interest depends heavily on an

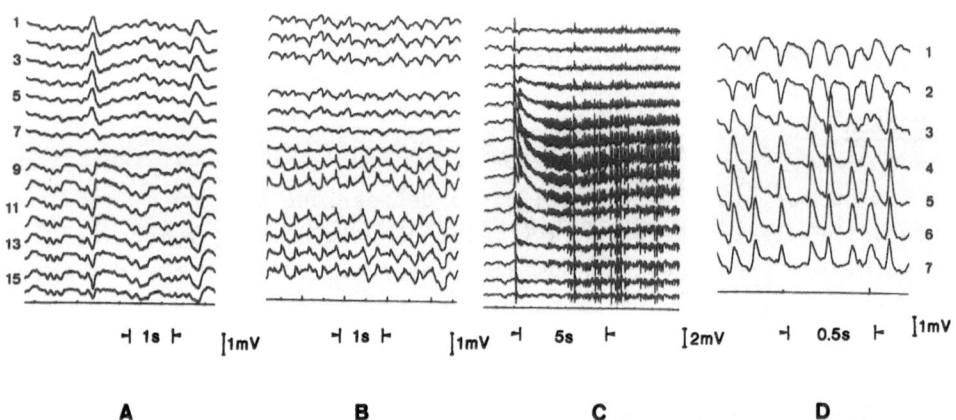

Fig.1: Intracortical EEG examples recorded simultaneously with multi-electrodes from the rabbit's cortex. In all examples the uppermost trace is from close to the cortical surface. The numbers to the left and to the right denote the electrode contacts which are either 10 x 10 μm^2, 150 μm apart for 16-fold electrodes, or 50 x 50 μm^2, 300 μm apart for 8-fold electrodes.
A: Spontaneous activity.
B: Photic driving. In this example traces 4,11 and 16 are omitted.
C: Seizure activity on a compressed time scale to study the course of the seizure.
D: Seizure activity recorded with the 7 uppermost contacts of an 8-fold electrode. The enlarged time scale enables the study of single seizure potentials.

appropriate presentation. In our case, up to 4 parameters have to be taken into consideration. These parameters can either be kept constant or are treated as variables.

The first parameter is the amplitude of the spectral estimates. In the examples of this paper the amplitudes are variables and either functions of frequency (Fig.2) or time (Fig.3) or space (Fig.4).

The second parameter is the frequency. In figure 3 the frequency scale is from 0 to 40 Hz whereas the plots in figures 2 and 4 are obtained for a constant frequency of 7 Hz and 1 Hz, respectively.

The third parameter is time. Figure 2 shows the time dependence of the 7 Hz frequency component in different spectra. In the plots of figures 3 and 4 time was kept constant, i.e. the spectral values of both figures were obtained for a constant time interval of 42 s.

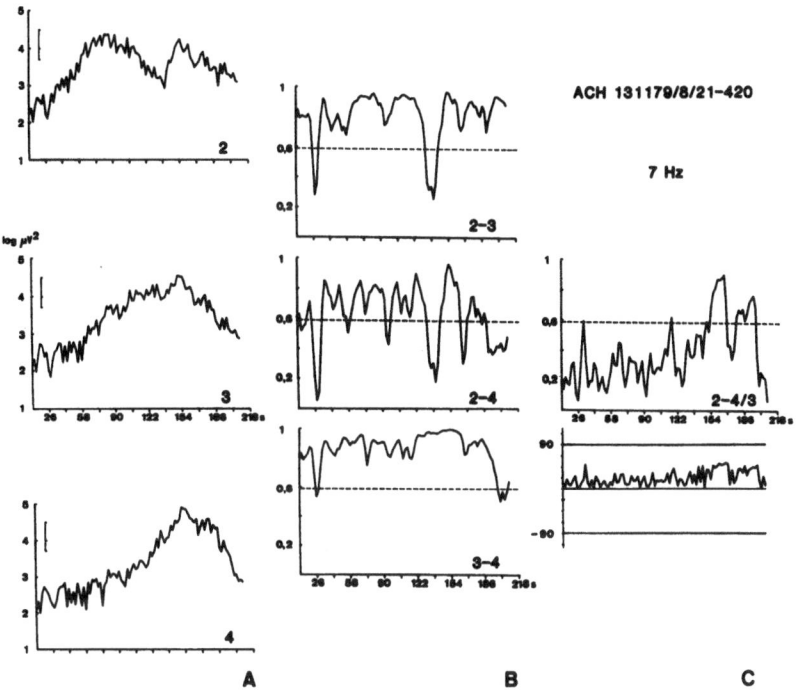

Fig.2: Time dependence of spectral values in the 7 Hz band. The numbers 2,3 and 4 denote electrodes placed at different sites of the cortical surface. Each graph is the result of the computation of 100 short time spectra of successive 2 s EEG sections.
A: Time dependence of power in the 7 Hz band for three different recording sites. Power is plotted on a logarithmic scale. The bars denote the 95 % confidence intervals.
B: Time dependence of the squared coherence values. The dashed lines indicate the upper 95 % confidence limit of zero coherence.
C: Time dependence of the squared partial coherence between signal 2 and 4 with exclusion of the influence of signal 3. In the lower part the corresponding phase plot is shown.

The fourth parameter which has to be taken into consideration in our presentations is the space coordinate according to the different positions of the electrodes on the cortical surface or the different intracortical locations of the electrode contacts. The plots of figure 2 show the analysis of seizure activity recorded with 3 electrodes (No 2, 3 and 4) located on the cortical surface.

Figure 3 shows a three-dimensional plot of power spectra in dependence of a space coordinate (1...16) according to simultaneously recorded EEG signals from the different cortical layers at distances of 150 μm. Additionally, in figure 4 the space dependence of different spectra in the 1 Hz frequency band are shown. In these plots the amplitudes i. e. power, squared coherence (K^2) and phase (φ) are functions of the spatial coordinate.

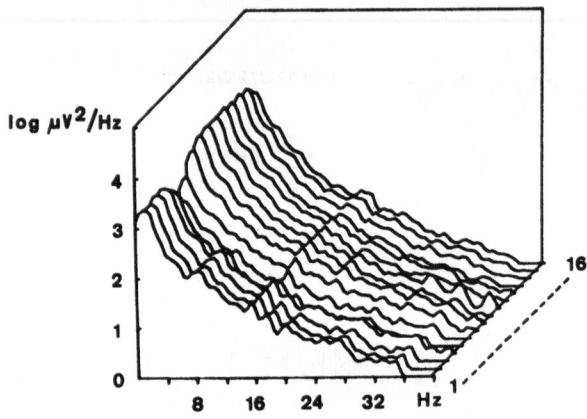

Fig.3: Power spectra of a 42 s EEG sample in a three-dimensional plot. The numbers 1 to 16 denote the electrode contacts and represent the spatial coordinate. The frequency scale is on the abszissa. Power is plotted on a logarithmic scale.

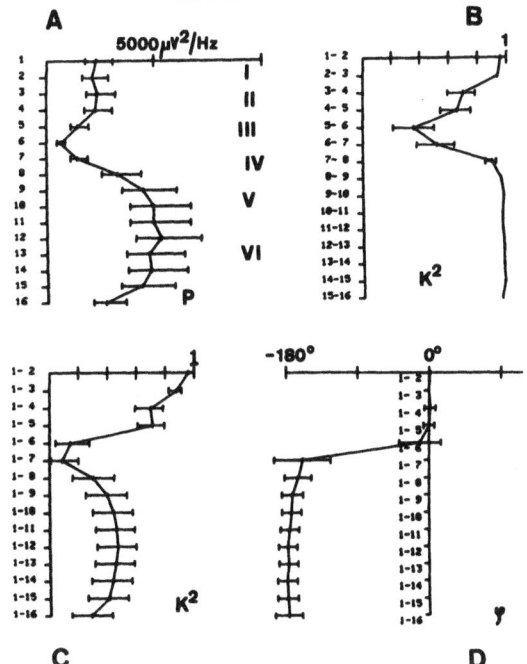

Fig.4:
A: Power distribution (P) in the 1 Hz frequency band within the cortex according to Fig.3. Power is plotted on a linear scale. The bars denote the 95 % confidence intervals. The roman numbers denote the cortical layers and the numbers 1 to 16 are the electrode contacts at distances of 150 μm.
B: Squared coherence values ($\overline{K^2}$) in the 1 Hz band between adjacent electrode contact signals.
C: Squared coherence values ($\overline{K^2}$) between the field potentials at contact 1 and all other contact signals plotted with increasing distance.
D: Phase plot (φ) according to C.

REFERENCES

Jenkins G.M., Watts D.G.: Spectral analysis and its application. Holden-Day, San Francisco, 1968.

Petsche H., Rappelsberger P., Lapins R., Vollmer R.: Rhythmicity in seizure patterns: topographical aspects. In: E.J.Speckmann and H. Caspers (Eds.): Origin of Cerebral Field Potentials. G. Thieme, Stuttgart, 60-79, 1979.

Pockberger H., Petsche H., Rappelsberger P.: Die Wirkung von Clonazepam auf das visuell evozierte Potential des Kaninchens. EEG-EMG 12: 14-20, 1981.

Prohaska O., Pacha F., Pfundner P., Petsche H.: A 16-fold semi-microelectrode for intracortical recordings of field potentials. Electroenceph. clin. Neurophysiol. 47: 629-631, 1979.

Rappelsberger P., Petsche H., Vollmer R., Lapins R.: Rhythmicity in seizure patterns: intracortical aspects. In: E.J.Speckmann and H. Caspers (Eds.): Origin of Cerebral Field Potentials. G.Thieme, Stuttgart, 80-97, 1979.

Rappelsberger P., Pockberger H., Petsche H.: The contribution of the cortical layers to the generation of the EEG: field potential and current source density analyses in the rabbit's visual cortex. Electroenceph. clin. Neurophysiol. 1981, in press.

COUNT RATE DISTORTIONS INTRODUCED IN GAMMA CAMERA DATA

BY A NUCLEAR MEDICAL IMAGE ANALYSIS SYSTEM

A. Brennan, J. F. Malone
Trinity College, Dublin
College of Technology, Kevin St., Dublin
and Saint James's Hospital, Dublin.

SUMMARY

A well established Nuclear Medicine Imaging Computer has been found to
interfere with the data presented to it by a gamma camera at high count-
rates.   The form of the interference found was highly unexpected, previously unreported, and occurred at count-rates that overlapped the clinically relevant range.   Explanations for this behaviour were derived
by examining the response of the system to a controlled range of count-
rate data.   From these observations the main features limiting the performance of the system were deduced.   These included data acquisition
into a remote memory of limited size (rather than core) and relatively
slow software operation for moving data from the remote memory to core
and processing it there.   The performance of the system has been greatly
improved by increasing the speed of the software operations and increasing the size of the remote memory.

1. INTRODUCTION

The combination of a gamma camera and dedicated image processing minicomputer is now standard equipment in many nuclear medicine departments.
These systems have found extensive application particularly in cardiology
(1).   Some cardiac studies require that compact boluses of high activity
be imaged.   It has been found that these activities are such that in
some cases gamma cameras are incapable of responding correctly to the
count-rates involved.   This has given rise to a wide range of studies
on count-rate losses in gamma cameras and a systematic literature in this
field now exists (2), (3), (4).   One study exists in which the influence
of the computer on count-rate response of the overall imaging system has
been demonstrated and corrections have been proposed (5).

We have examined in detail the influence of a modern highly complex
commercially available Image Processing System (MDS - A^2 System) on known
input count-rates.   The results demonstrate that the system significantly
distorts the count-rates in an unexpected fashion.   The output count-rate
from the computer was found to be dependent on (a) the input count-rate,

(b) the matrix size into which the image is acquired, (c) the duration of each frame in the image, (d) the size of the source, (e) aspects of the hardware configuration of the system, (f) aspects of the system software. From a study of these phenomena we have been able to deduce the critical features of the system that contribute to the count-rate response and determine a configuration which is unlikely to give misleading results in the clinically relevant range.

2. MATERIALS AND METHODS

The imaging system used is a Medical Data Systems A^2 Two Terminal System. It essentially consists of a Nova 3 Minicomputer with 48K 16 bit words of core, and three disc drives, 2 X 2.5 Megabyte and 1 X 80 Megabyte. Each terminal has 64K 16 bit words of remote memory associated with it. Images from the gamma camera are initially acquired into this memory, and subsequently transferred to disc via the core memory. Images are acquired into the system in a array of pixels. The field of view may be divided into 32 X 32, 64 X 64, 128 X 128 or 256 X 256 pixels. For simplicity all of the work described in this study has been limited to the 64 X 64 array which is the one commonly used for acquisition of dynamic studies in Nuclear Medicines.

Each pixel in the array in remote memory consists of a memory location 8 bits deep. Thus it is capable of storing up to 255 counts at each location, and each array occupies 2K 16 bit words. If one pixel in an image overruns 255 counts the system automatically advances to another 64 X 64 array and subsequently adds the contents of the two arrays to provide a complete image. To avoid confusion in terminology we have designated a complete image as a "frame" and from the above it is clear that a frame may consist of the sum of a number of arrays which will be referred to as "subframes". After processing in the core, images are stored on disc in arrays 8 bits deep referred to as byte mode or 16 bits deep referred to as work mode. The system is interfaced to an I.G.E. Maxicamera II which was used to feed data at various rates to the computer. Two sets of source configurations were used, one was the BSI phantom used with the collimator in position (4). The other was a point source situated 5 cm from the crystal with the collimator removed. The latter allowed the main features of the system be characterised with sources of relatively low activity.

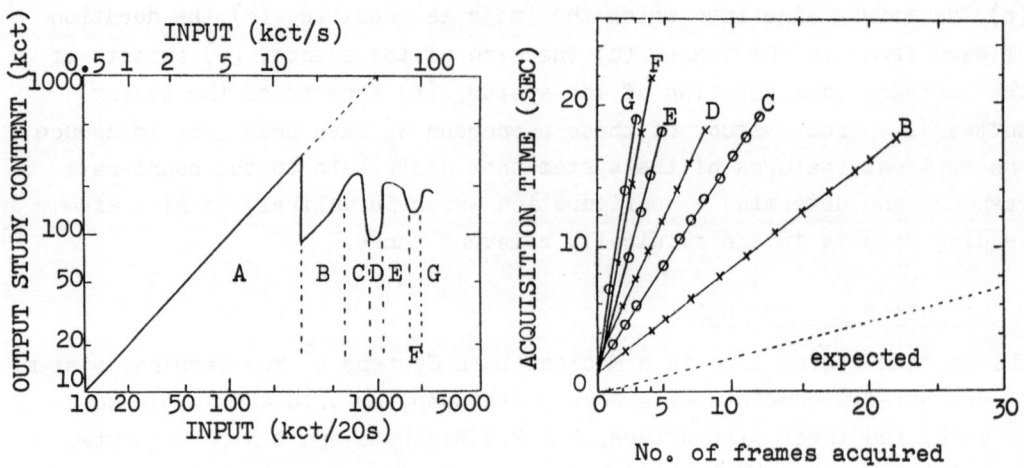

Figure 1. Output count as a function of the input count. The broken line gives the expected output count.

Figure 2. The time taken to acquire a number of frames versus the number of frames. The broken line gives the expected time in all cases.

3. RESULTS

3.1 Response of System to Wide Range of Count Rates

The gamma camera was exposed to sources of gradually increasing activity under standardized conditions. The computer was programmed to acquire 20 seconds of data into eighty 64 X 64 byte arrays, each of 0.25 seconds duration in dynamic sequence. The total number of counts in the frames acquired by the computer was summed and compared with the counts recorded in 20 seconds by the gamma camera scaler. The results are presented in figure 1. The output counts from the computer increases linearly with activity up to an input count-rate of 15K c.p.s. This corresponds to an activity of 370MBq (10mCi) in the BSI phantom and is in the clinically relevant range (1), (4). At greater input count-rates the output count from the computer decreases rather than increases. Further increases lead to a step like increase and decrease in the computer output. This pattern was qualitatively reproducible but its quantitative features are dependent on the factors listed in the introduction. Furthermore, the pattern is highly unusual, has not previously been described in a nuclear medicine system and could give rise to misleading results. To facilitate discussion, the regions on the curve are identified by the labels A - G as indicated.

With a view to determining the reasons for the failure of the computer
to respond to increasing count-rates the contents of the studies that
had been acquired were analysed in detail.   Each study has features
that were reproducibly related to the region A - G in which it was acquired.   These features are listed in Table 1 as can be seen, (a) each
region on the curve corresponds to characteristic number of sub-frames,
(b) studies acquired outside of region A did not have data in the full
compliment of 80 frames, (c) the acquisition process did not terminate
in 20 seconds exactly once the count-rate exceeded that for region A.

3.2 Time taken for acquisition of less than 80 frames

It was decided to determine the time required for the system to acquire
a number of frames less than or equal to the maximum number that could
be acquired in each region.   The results are presented in Figure 2 for
the regions B - G.   The time taken to acquire a number of frames is
plotted against the number of frames.   The figure demonstrates the following features (a) there is a strong linear relationship between the
number of frames acquired and the total time taken to acquire them (p
0.98 in all cases), (b) frames with a larger number of subframes take
longer to acquire than those with a smaller number of subframes, (c)
all the curves intercept the time axis at about 1.7 seconds indicating
that this is the minimum time required to acquire even one 0.25 seconds
frame.   These observations were confirmed for other acquisition modes
where in all cases the qualitative features were consistent although
the quantitative features can be different.

Region	Subframes per frame	K word per frame	Frames with data	Acquisition Period
A	1	2	80	0 min.20s.
B	2	4	22	0 min.18s.
C	3	6	14	18 min.20s.
D	4	8	8	0 min.18s.
E	5,6,7	10,12,14	8,7,6	22 min.10s.
F	8	16	4	0 min.18s.
G	9	18	5	23 min 0s.

Table 1: Main features of acquired studies for
regions A -G.

Region	R(s)	t(s)
B	1.6	0.7
C	1.9	0.7
D	1.8	0.7
	1.7	0.7
E	1.4	0.7
	1.3	0.7
F	1.3	0.7
G	1.1	0.8
Mean	1.6 ± 0.3	0.7 ± 0.02

Table II: Value of R
and t for regions
B - G.

4. HYPOTHESIS

The above consistent observations on the performance of the computer system lead to the development of a hypothesis with regard to its features that limited acquisition. The hypothesis contains two components (a) that acquisition will fail when conditions leave the balance between data entering and leaving remote memory such that more than 64K words are required to store the portion of the study still in remote memory, and (b) that the time T required for acquisition of a study is

$$T = R + SFAt$$

The terms have the following meanings: $\underline{R}$ is a "dead time" of the system that occurs before it initiates removal of subframes from the remote memory. $\underline{SFA}$ is the total number of subframe additions that must be performed in core to construct full frames. This in fact is given by $SFA = N (sf - 1)$ where N is the total number of frames and sf is the number of subframes per frame. $\underline{t}$ is the time required to clear a subframe from remote memory to core and perform the addition in core.

The results of Figure 2 are completely consistent with this hypothesis and analysis of these results gives the series of values for R and t listed in Table 2. The values are remarkably consistent given that there are errors in the measurement of acquisition time which had to be estimated using a stop watch. The mean value of $\underline{R}$ is 1.6 seconds and the mean value of $\underline{t}$ is 0.7 seconds. Both these are relatively long compared with the frame rates used in some dynamic studies in nuclear medicine.

5. CONCLUSIONS AND REMEDIES

The results and hypothesis presented above refer to Version 80-B(V80-B) of the software produced by the manufacturers of the system. They demonstrate that a modern nuclear medicine system can significantly interfere with acquisition of data from a gamma camera in the clinically relevant range. The principal features of the system that contribute to this are (a) acquisition into a remote memory rather than core, (b) the size of the remote memory, (c) acquisition into the remote memory in byte mode only, (d) the time required to initiate the process of removing data from remote memory (R), (e) the time required to effect the addition of subframes (t). Additionally, the size of the source viewed was found to be very important. Many approaches could be taken to resolving these problems. The manufacturers have concentrated on improving (d) and (e) in a revised version of software (V80-C). Times which closely approximate to $\underline{R}$ and $\underline{t}$ for V80-C software have been greatly reduced. Other improvements have also been made. Additionally, we have elected to modify (b) by increasing the size of remote memory from 64K to 256K thereby increasing the size of study that can be accommodated before the effects described become apparent. With these improvements it is necessary to go considerably beyond the clinical range before count-rate distortions become evident.

REFERENCES

(1) Bachrach SL, Green MV and Borer JS. Instrumentation and Data Processing in Cardiovascular Nuclear Medicine: Evaluation of Ventricular Function. Seminars in Nucl. Med. 1979; 9: 257 - 274.

(2) Sorenson JA. Methods of Correcting Anger Camera Deadtime Losses. J Nucl Med. 1976; 17: 137-141.

(3) Adams H, Hine GJ and Zimmerman CD. Deadtime Measurements in Scintillation Cameras under Scatter Conditions simulating Quantitative Nuclear Cardiography. J Nucl Med. 1978; 19: 538-544.

(4) HPA. The Theory, Specification and Testing of Anger Type Gamma Cameras. 1980.

(5) Cranley K, Millar R and Bell TK. Correction for Deadtime Losses in a Gamma Camera/Data Analysis System. Eur J Nucl Med. 1980; 5: 377-382.

A COMPUTERISED SYSTEM FOR ELECTROCOCHLEOGRAPHIC (ECOG)

MEASUREMENT

Wellner U , Biesalski H.K. , Harth O.

Institute of Physiology

Johannes Gutenberg University of Mainz

D 6500 MAINZ , West - Germany

To study the influence of vitamin A on hearing we choose to examine ECoGs induced by an audible stimulus.The basis of this project is a suitable experimental equipment for inducing and recording inner ear electrical responses in guinea pigs.
The problem to be studied asks for a high number of animals and measurements within one animal;furthermore the ECoGs of each animal have to be examined over a long period of time.This calls for a simple and automated measurement and evaluation procedure.
In contrats to most ECoG experiments we do not study the influence of special oto - toxic agents (noise,drugs etc) but examine the variation of ECoG signals as caused by different metabolic states of vitamin A.Consequntly only slight variations in the electrophysiological signals are expected.This demands for an exact and highly reliable measurement apparatus.To fullfill these requirements we choose to design a highly computorised equipment.

The experimental setup designed by us yields the following advantages :
1. It offers all the features of a commercial system as a subset of its
   features.
2. The following tasks are software defined and therefore easily alterable:
   a. Audible stimulus generation
   b. Signal aquisition and - conditioning (e.g. sampling rate,digital filtering)
   c. Averaging
   d. Patternrecognition
   e. Patternevaluation
   f. Filing of signals and results
3. Audible stimulus generation and signal aquisition are both under supervision
   of the main computer.This allows for the establishment of a feed back loop
   in order to optimize an experimental run.
4. Less discrete devices than in commercial system.
5. Easy handling;the operator is guarded by messages from the programm.
6. Quality checking can be encorporated as a standard programm task thus
   inhibiting experiments which would yield erranous data.
7. A data base for results can be encorporated.

A   HARDWARE

Picture 1 shows the main components of the electronic equipment.The main computer is a PRIME P 300 with 112 k bytes of memory,two disk drives,two mag tapes and a digital i/o system,ten asynchronous by directional serial interfaces (with control lines) and an analogue-digital conversion system.
At the experimental site the second computer system is installed . this system is composed of two single-board computers based on the Z 80 processor.The system is compatible to INTELs multibus.It is equipped with several V.24 interfaces and an ADC and DAC-system.The microcomputer is connected to the prime computer via a V.24 communication link operating at 9600 baud.
The mentioned loud speaker ,the animal,the intracochlear electrodes and the pre - amplifier are contained in a special isolated chamber.

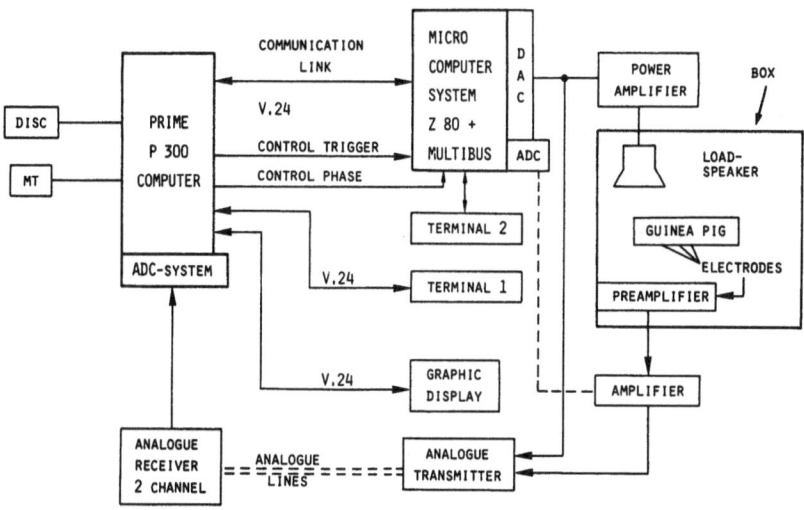

Picture 1 : Main components of the electronic equipment

B   SOFTWARE DESIGN

The software is grouped into three divisions :
1. Communication software for the connection of the microcomputer to the
   PRIME computer.
2. Special software - organized in three levels - to be run on the PRIME
   computer.
   2.1 First level software
       a. Data aquisition
       b. Stimulus generation
   2.2 Second level software
       This software performs the following tasks:
       - Non real time signal conditioning
       - Averaging
       - Patternrecognition
       - Patternevaluation
       - Filing of results of a single experiment
       - Display of results on the graphical display
These programms are organized as subroutines which are called by third level software.
   2.3 Third level software
       This software resembles the experimental design. The flow of an experiment
       is governed by the sequence of calls of second level software,of messages
       to the operator and responses of the operator.
       At this level the modularity of the programm system allows for an easy
       redesign of the experimental procedure.

240

A general frame for the experiment we have to conduct is described by the following sequence of tasks :
1. Calibration and quality check of transmission line.
2. Loading the appropriate microcomputer programm and setting its static parameters.
3. Single ECoG experiment
   - recording the responses to a number of stimuli
   - averaging of responses
   - patterrecognition
   - patternevaluation
   - display of averaged signal
4. Filing the results.

C   CONCLUSIONS

The proposed experimental setup has proved to be very usefull in standard experiments for screening purposes.It is furthermore higly flexible so that it can be used in research projects which directly involve signal analysis itself.
For standard experiments the PRIME P 300 computer can be ommitted by letting the microcomputer system perform the signal aquisition and - evaluation.
Thus our system can be used for the development of a microcomputer based ECoG system for clinical purposes.

TOWARD A MONITORING OF THE ANESTHESIA LEVEL ON THE BASIS OF THE EEG.

S. Cerutti°, G. Avanzini[+], A. Cefalà°, S. Franceschetti[+]

(°) Politechnic, Institute of Electrical Engineering, P.za Leonardo da Vinci,32 - 20133 Milano

(+) Neurological Institute "C.Besta", Via Celoria 11, 20133 Milan, Italy

1. INTRODUCTION

The EEG signal provides relevant information about the functional status of CNS. Its usefulness in monitoring the anesthesia level has been repeatedly demonstrated (1) (2) (3) since 1937. More recently automatic analysis techniques (4) (5) have been successfully introduced, providing a quantitative evaluation of the main EEG parameters during anesthesia, but they have not become routinary in most of the cli nical applications.
The present paper illustrates the first results of a research aiming at quantifying the effect of the anesthetic level on the EEG signal, using spectral techniques to enhance the information and to display it in such a way as to provide an immediate and easy tool for the anesthetist.
To avoid direct effect of surgery on CNS,patients undergoing operation on peripheral nervous system were selected.

2. MATERIALS AND METHODS

Ten patients, aged from 35 to 50, hospitalized for herniated lumbar intervertebral disk at Istituto Neurologico "C. Besta" underwent EEG recording session during surgery. The basic EEG was normal in all of the patients. Anesthesia was induced by I.V. Penthobarbital (2 to 3 mg/kg) and maintained by Halothane and Nitrous Oxide (N_2O). For each patient ECG and blood pressure were continuously monitored during surgery. Occasionally blood gas analysis was performed. Operatory sessions lasted between 60 and 90 minutes. EEG samples (10 minutes each) have been recorded in relation to the most significant epochs of anesthesia :

1 - Basal EEG (patient awake with closed eyes)
2 - I.V. Penthobarbital infusion
3 - Alothane + N_2O administration (first 10 minutes)
4 - Alothane + N_2O (steady state prior to surgery)
5 - Dorsal root manipulation
6 - Alothane and N_2O discontinuation
7 - Awakening.

EEG signal was recorded from bilateral temporo-parietal leads by means of silver-silver chloride needle electrodes. Bipolar derivations were employed. For a detailed description of the acquisition and processing system see fig. 1.

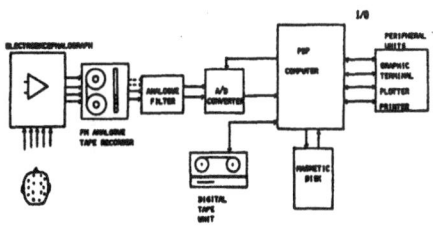

Fig. 1 - Block diagram of the acquisition and Processing system

Off-line analysis has been performed at Institute of Electrical Engineering, Politechnic of Milan.

Basic procedures of EEG Automatic Analysis include spectral analysis and power computation. Signal is reconstructed on a video terminal and inspected to eliminate unwanted or noisy records. Power Spectrum is computed on a block of 1024 samples, corresponding to 5.12 sec., by means of the Fast Fourier Transform. For each block of
data the program computes: 512 harmonics (0-100 Hz) and associated power; power associated to delta (0-4 Hz), theta (4-8 Hz), alpha (8-12 Hz), beta (12-25 Hz) frequency bands.

Fig. 2A shows a plotted reconstruction of a 5.12 sec basal record of a sampled EEG
signal and (fig. 2B) its associated power spectrum with the computed power for each
frequency band (absolute and percentage values). Average power computed on 10 single
spectra is plotted in fig. 3 for each band.

3. EXPERIMENTAL RESULTS AND CONCLUSIONS

Data representation plotted for all 10 patients to describe EEG power change by
varying anesthesia levels, show a regular pattern which well charaterizes anesthetic
action and surgical steps. A typical example is shown in fig. 3. Following infusion
of Penthobarbital EEG shows a quick change defined by slow and high amplitude waves
which abruptly increase total power, whereas fast frequencies almost disappear. During surgery,by maintaining constant N_2O and Alothane,power associated to delta
waves remains high, theta is slightly increased,alpha and beta remain low. Pattern
is reversed as anesthesia ends.

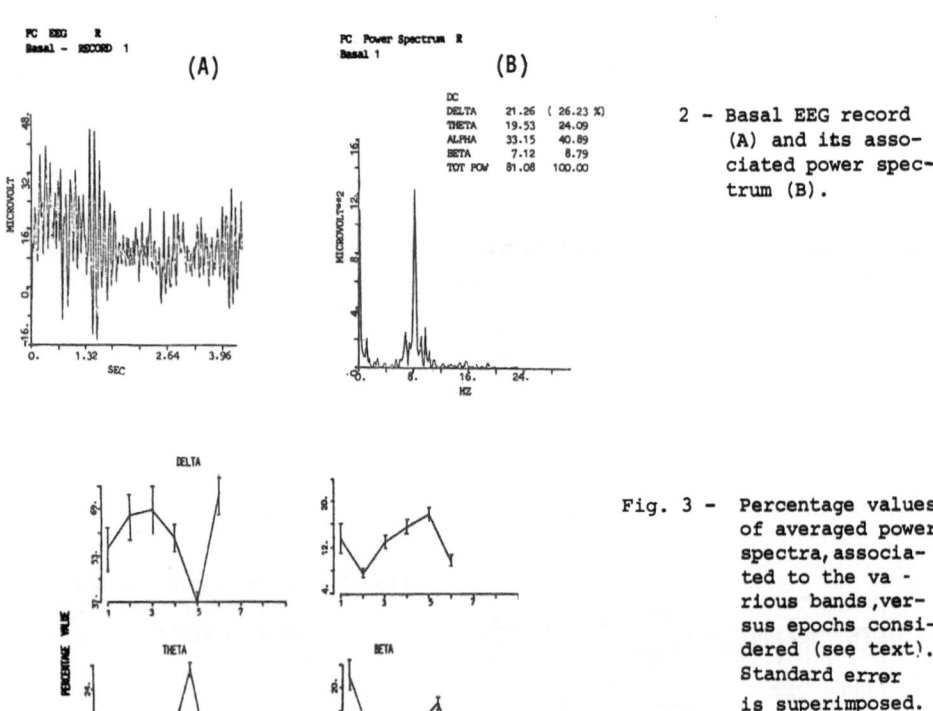

2 - Basal EEG record
   (A) and its asso-
   ciated power spec-
   trum (B).

Fig. 3 - Percentage values
   of averaged power
   spectra, associa-
   ted to the va -
   rious bands, ver-
   sus epochs consi-
   dered (see text).
   Standard error
   is superimposed.

This constant pattern was found to be sensitive to variations in the concentration of single drugs (i.e. +.2,.3% Halothane) or to the different drugs involved in anesthesia (i.e. Penthobarbital, see epoch 2 in fig. 3). Under an external sensorial input such as manipulation of dorsal root, EEG spectral power distribution suddenly changes showing a relevant decrease of delta power and a reciprocal increase of the other components, with particular regard to theta frequencies (epoch 5 in fig.3). These changes are typical of the arousal reaction evoked by sensory stimulation. It has to be noted that in our patients the dorsal root stimulation (very powerful in the awake state) fails to elicit any vegetative reaction to pain (i.e. changes in the blood pressure and heart rate). It may be concluded that the EEG monitoring Provides in this case parameters much more sensitive than those usually employed.

REFERENCES

(1) Gibbs F.A., Gibbs E.L., Lennox W.G., "Effect on the EEG of certain drugs which influence nervous activity", Arch. Intern. Med., Vol. 60, 1937: 154-166.

(2) Klein F.F., Davis A.D., "The use of the Time Domain Analyzed EEG in conjunction with cardiovascular Parameters for monitoring anesthetic levels",IEEE Trans. Biomed. Eng. vol. BME-28, No.1, 1981: 36-40.

(3) Valenta H.L. Jr., "Detection of electroencephalographic response following changes in the anesthetic dose", ISA, ISBN 87664-405-1, 1978:47-54.

(4) Butler L.A., "A Real-time software system on the PDP-11 for two-channel EEG spectral analysis during surgery", Computer Programs Biomed., 6, 1976: 1-10

(5) Mc Ewen J.A., Anderson G.B., Low M.D. and Jenkins L.C., "Monitoring the level of anesthesia by automatic analysis of spontaneous EEG activity", IEEE Trans. Biomed. Eng. Vol. BME-22, July 1975:845-856.

The present paper was partially supported by a Grant from the Italian Research Council (CNR).

AN EEG MACHINE WITH AN INTEGRAL MICROPROCESSOR.

Dr.H.R.A. Townsend,
The National Hospital,
Queen Square,
London.

Electroencephalography (EEG) is concerned with recording and interpreting the small potential fluctuations which appear on the surface of
the scalp, and are related to the functioning of the brain.

The EEG machine consists of a bank (usually 8 or 16) of sensitive
amplifiers, and a similar number of pen recorders.

The pen recorders produce a set of graphical records representing
fluctuations of voltage with time.   The voltage applied to the pen
recorder input deflects the trace up or down, while the paper on which
the pens write is drawn along at a constant speed (usually 1.5 or
3 cm/Sec) to provide a common time axis for the graphs.

Certain phenomena can only be seen if the signals are processed
before display, and many of the larger centres today use mini- or
micro-computers which either process magnetic tape records of EEG
activity, or in some cases are directly connected to the EEG machine.
The output from such processing is displayed on an oscilloscope and
permanent records are produced by a graph plotter.   The computer
itself usually has magnetic discs for program and data storage and is
controlled by a keyboard and visual display unit.   All these peripheral
devices are convenient but expensive;   much more expensive than the
microprocessor itself, which only costs a few pounds.

Other laboratories have "special purpose" computer based devices
adapted with amplifiers for recording EEG signals, but otherwise small
general purpose computers in all but name, and correspondingly priced.
These devices need a special laboratory and specially trained staff.
Additionally these special purpose "Evoked response computers" suffer
from the difficulty of relating their outputs to the "conventional"
Electroencephalogram.

By building a microprocessor as an integral part of the machine
deriving its input from the EEG amplifiers and using the EEG recorders
to display the results of its computations considerable savings can
be achieved both in equipment costs and in the time of the skilled
personnel who make the recordings.   This approach is almost mandatory
if, as now seems practically and clinically desirable, multiple
channels have to be analysed simultaneously and the results are to be

available in "real-time" (i.e. immediately).

An apparatus will be demonstrated which makes use of a Motorola 6802 microprocessor to analyse each 4 channels of EEG activity. When the pens are not required to display the results of processing (which is most of the time) the potentials are simply copied from the outputs of the EEG amplifiers to the inputs of the pen recorders, sampling the potentials 1000 times a second. The effect is that it is impossible to tell that a microprocessor is interposed and the machine behaves exactly as a conventional EEG. (This is a valuable feature as it provides a constant check on the correct functioning of the processor and its associated Analog to Digital and Digital to Analog convertors).

A good deal of thought has gone into the design of the control interface, which has been reduced to the absolute essentials; viz. two press-buttons, an on/off switch, and a sixteen position rotary switch.

a) A press-button RESET/CLEAR starts the processor obeying the program and at the same time clears the internal memory.
b) The on/off switch is used to select a suitable portion, or portions, of the recording for analysis.
c) A further push-button INTERRUPT/DISPLAY switches off the EEG monitoring feature described above and uses the EEG pens to display a graph of the information held in the microporcessor memory.
d) The rotary 16-position switch controls the amplitude (or gain) of the function displayed by operating (c) above.

Programs are available to allow the EEG apparatus to record responses evoked by most of the stimuli commonly used for routine clinical testing, for example:

a) Far-afield potentials evoked by a click stimulus, during the first 10 millisec.
b) Far-afield potentials evoked by a stimulus to a peripheral nerve and recorded over the nerve roots and spinal column, as well as the early components of the cortical evoked potential occurring at about 20 millisec.
c) The potentials recorded over the occipital region in response to a pattern-reversal visual stimulus, which are a useful physical sign in the diagnosis of Disseminated (Multiple) Sclerosis.
d) Event-related slow potentials such as the Contingent Negative Variation and "Bereitschaftspotential".

Provision is made for four built-in programs, any one of which can be selected at the touch of a button.

COMPUTATION OF THE PRESSURE DERIVATIVE AND RELAXATION

INDICES USING DIGITAL SIGNAL TECHNIQUES

G. Martín, J. Cosín, A. Ramirez and J.V. Gimeno
Centro Investigación. C.S. La Fe.
Valencia (Spain)

The present study was designed in order to know the sources of errors in the determination of the most used relaxation indices, obtained from the left ventricular pressure (LVP) wave: Maximum negative dP/dt (max neg dP/dt) (10) and the relaxation rate, T (11). The experimental models (awake and anaesthetized dogs) and the processing methods (based on a 12 bits A/D converter and 700 Hz of sampling rate) are described in other papers (5,6,7,8).

Max neg dP/dt: The Figure 1 shows a simultaneous display of original and resynthesized curves (LVP and dP/dt) from a tip-manometer recording. The resynthesized curves were obtained, using the corresponding sums of Fourier series and the dP/dt curves differentiating these series (6,7). The max neg dP/dt augmented uniformly as the number of harmonics was increased showing an important dependency of the higher frequencies. Moreover (Fig 2), P at max neg dP/dt varied slowly, to the effect that max neg dP/dt tends to appear inmediately after the cessation of the aortic flow when the number of harmonics increases (8). The behaviour of dP/dt was in agreement with the studies of other authors (4,9).

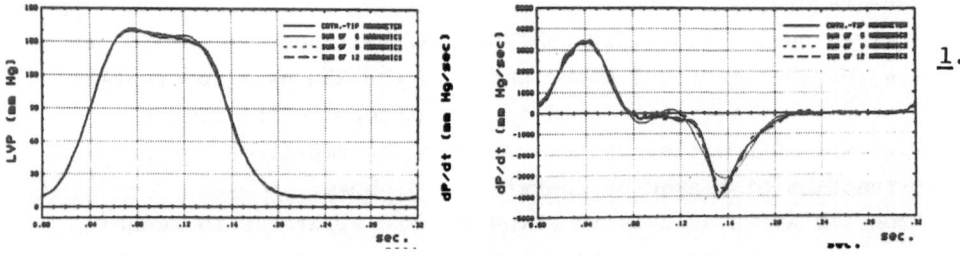

1.

The Figure 3 shows an example of the results obtained using different algorithms as piececurse approximation for dP/dt function (linear interpolation, three and five point aproximation and five and seven parabolic data fit). As a standard noise-free data model we employed the reconstructed derivative from 20 harmonics of LVP. The derivative waveform obtained were compared to the model derivative on the basis of root-mean-squared error (Similar results as published by Marble et al (4)) and specially comparing the max neg dP/dt values. The most appro-

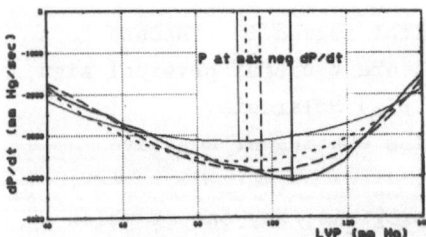

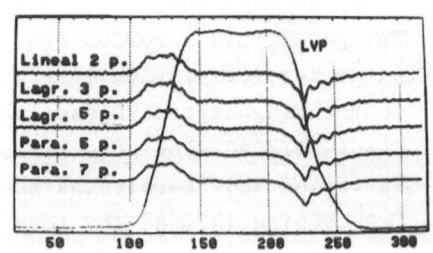

Fig 2. Same function that Fig 1.   Fig 3.

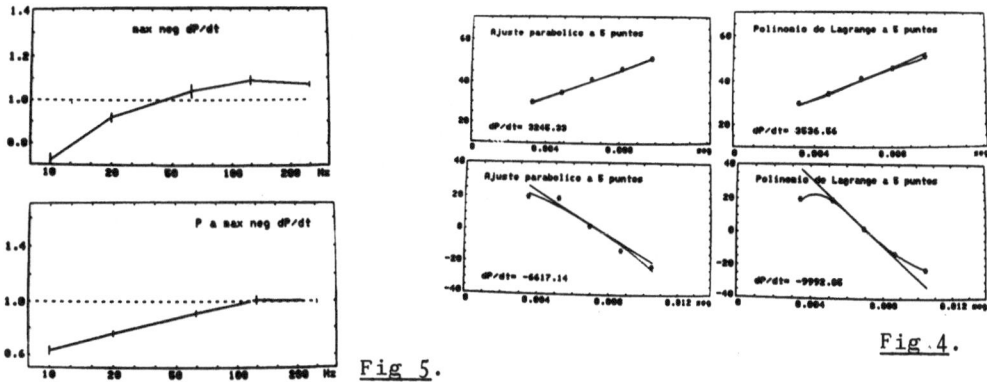

Fig 5.

Fig.4.

piate algorithms were both based on 5 points. However in same particular examples (See Fig 4), the Lagrange algorithm produced important
overestimulation of dP/dt maxima.

The Figure 5 shows the effects on max neg dP/dt and P at max
neg dP/dt varying the analog differentiator cutoff frequency (7). They
are expressed as the ratio between the analogical value and the corres
ponding model derivative. The results were compatible with those published by Barry et al (1) studying the same problem on max pos dP/dt.

Relaxation rate T: For using T index (11) is necessary to examine how
precisely the LVP fall during isovolumic relaxation follows an exponen
tial function.

When we fit exponential with independent term (P=A+B exp
(k.t)) using Chebysev polynomial (2,3) (Fig 6) we obtained that the fi
tting was better, than when we use only a function of the type $P=P_0$
$exp((-1/T).t)$. In all studied beats, the values of A were negatives,
ranging from -20.8 to -3.5 mm Hg and consequently the value of expo-

nent k, were much more greater
than the exponent (-1/T). These
findings, were in agreement with
the fact that the ln P vs. t
plot deviate from linearity in
the sense that always the line
curve down (Fig 6), indicating a
negative errors in all curves.

The values of T calcu-
lated from the logarithm of LVP
were significantly smaller than
those calculated in the same
beat from the linear regression
of dP/dt against P. In the 20
dogs studied, the values of T
were respectively: 23.68±2.32
(range:14.8-29.3) and 34.06±6.93
(range:21.8-44.8)(p<0.01). Both
plots (Fig 7)(6,7) showed an ana
logous pattern, the LVP fall fas
ter than an exponential would
predict during the latter por-

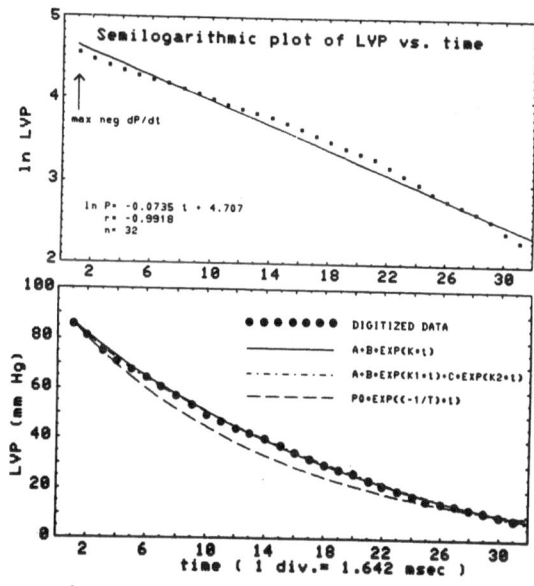

Fig 6. Exponential fitting to LVP fall

248

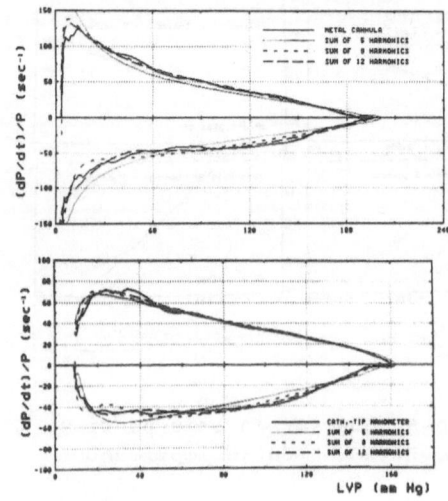

tion of isovolumic relaxation.

We conclude:
(1) There exist some evidences on the possible effects of the events at or near the time of aortic valve closure on the max neg dP/dt values
(2) The LVP fall is not strictly monoexponential.

Fig 7. P-dP/dt representation of two waves.

REFERENCES
(1) Barry WH, Marlon AM, Adams M and Harrison DC. Effects of varying differentiator frequency response on recorded peak dP/dt. Cardiovasc Res. 1975; 9:433-39.
(2) Malachowski GC. Exponential fitting using the Chebyshev transformation. BIOENG 80. Biological Engineering. pp 400-03. University College London.
(3) Malachowski GC. Regression Methods in Biology. The Physiological Laboratory. (to be published). Cambridge.
(4) Marble AE, McIntyre M, Hastings-James R and Hor ChW. A comparison of digital algorithms used in computing the derivative of left ventricular pressure. IEEE Trans. BME-26. pp 524-29. 1981.
(5) Martín G, Gimeno JV, Ramirez A and Cosín J. A digitized analysis of isovolumic pressure fall. Computers in Cardiology. IEEE Computer Society. pp 359-62. 1979.
(6) Martín G, Gimeno JV, Ramirez A, Cosín J and Báguena J. Effects of high-frequency harmonics on cardiac relaxation indices. Am J Physiol. 1981; 240:H669-75.
(7) Martín G, Gimeno JV, Ramirez A, cosín J and Báguena J. Determination of cardiac pressure derivative maxima. Proc International Conference on Digital Signal Processing. pp 212-19. Florence. 1981.
(8) Martín G, Ramirez A, Cosín J and Gimeno JV. Resynthesis from harmonics of left ventricular pressure and its derivatives: A study on cardiac relaxation. Computers in Cardiology. IEEE Computer Society (in press). Florence. 1981.
(9) Spitz AL, Alderman EL and Harrison DC. Digital filtering and interpolation of intracardiac pressure data. Computer in Cardiology. IEEE Computer Society. pp 365-67. St Louis. 1976.
(10) Weisfeldt ML, Scully HE, Frederiksen J, Rubenstein JJ, Pohost GM, Beierholm E, Bello AG and Daggett WM. Hemodynamic determinants of maximum negative dP/dt and periods of diastole. Am J Physiol. 1974; 227:613-21.
(11) Weiss JL, Frederiksen JW and Weisfeldt ML. Hemodynamic determinants of the time course of fall in canine left ventricular pressure. J Clin Invest. 1976; 58:751-60.

COMPUTATIONAL REQUIREMENTS FOR DIGITAL FLUOROSCOPY - SPECIFICATION OF EXISTING
SYSTEMS AND THEIR RELATIONSHIP WITH NUCLEAR MEDICINE IMAGE PROCESSORS.

[o+]K.P. Maher; [o+]J.F. Malone; [*]G.D. Hurley; [*]D.P. McInerney.

* Dept. of Radiology, Meath/Adelaide Hospitals, Dublin 8, Ireland.

o Dept. of Physics, Dublin Institute of Technology, Kevin St., Dublin 8, Ireland.

+ Federated Dublin Voluntary Hospitals, James's St., Dublin 8, Ireland.

1. INTRODUCTION

Digital techniques are presently being applied to conventional radiology, particularly
fluoroscopy, following their successful application to Nuclear Medicine and Computerised
Tomography. The most common approach has been to digitise an image obtained from an
image intensifier-TV chain and to perform the required processing on this data (1,2).
In 1981 a large number of clinical papers have been published on this subject, but
little attention has been paid to the computational aspects. This paper discusses the
approaches that have been taken, compares them where relevant, with Nuclear Medicine
and describes an approach that may be taken using relatively inexpensive microcomputer
systems.

Digital Fluoroscopy offers the following advantages over conventional fluoroscopy:
a) increased patient safety due to the development of less invasive procedures (3);
b) decreased examination costs due to (i) reduction in the need for patient preparation
or postcare in hospital and (ii) recording of images on media less expensive than film
(4); c) increased diagnostic capabilities of present systems due to the capabilities of
modern image processing - specifically, the high resolution and low noise features of
digital intravenous fluoroscopy systems are expected to provide more accurate results
compared to Nuclear Medicine first pass angiography (5).

2. SPECIFICATION OF DIGITAL FLUOROSCOPIC IMAGES

Matrix size and data rate requirements in Nuclear Medicine image processing have been
adequately satisfied using minicomputers. The large amount of software developed for
this modality would benefit Digital Fluoroscopy if such computers could be modified to
process video images. However, the minicomputer storage and manipulation of nuclear
images is a slow process in comparison to the requirements of Digital Fluoroscopy. This
is due to a) the higher spatial resolution of video images; b) the higher data rates
involved; c) the contribution of fluoroscopic apparatus to image noise.

Since a CCIR video image contains roughly 580 lines of visual information, a 512 x 512
pixel array may store such an immage without much loss of spatial resolution. This
resolution is rarely encountered in routine medical imge processing since useful nuclear
images are frequently obtained from 64 x 64 arrays (Table 1). Further, video data rates

are quite high since the brightness of each pixel must be digitised. This seems to be adequately catered for by 8 bits (6). Thus, to store a video frame, a 2 Mbit memory would be required, which would be filled every 40 ms, giving a data rate of roughly 50 Mbit/s. Data rates in nuclear imaging are much lower - of the order of 10 kbit/s. Because of the quantum and electrical noise sources associated with fluoroscopic imaging some image averaging must be performed to improve SNR. Since a number of video frames are required for such algorithms, a minicomputer approach would require a very large memory.

IMAGE	NUCLEAR	FLUOROSCOPIC
Matrix Size	64 x 64	512 x 512
Bit Rate	10^4/s	10^7/s
Bits/Frame	5×10^5	2×10^6
Frame Time	1s - 3min	0.04s

Table 1 : Comparison of Nuclear and Fluoroscopic Digital Images.

3. TYPES OF IMAGE PROCESSING REQUIRED AND DESCRIPTION OF PRESENT SYSTEMS

The exact type of processing required depends on the application, but from the above, it is evident that it would be desirable for a processor to perform a) frame averaging for noise reduction; b) image subtraction for use in angiography; c) logarithmic amplification of contrast levels; d) contrast and edge enhancement; e) videodensitometry; f) fast transfer to bulk storage.
Three types of processor have been developed to date, which incorporate some of these processes. These developments have been stimulated by encouraging results of research in the USA and West Germany. One approach has centered around building hard-wired digital algorithms for the real-time processing of video images (6,7). Another approach has concentrated on the high speed processing of stored data (2,3). These systems are minicomputer based and are much slower and more expensive than the real-time systems, but they offer greater flexibility in the definition of the processing algorithms. A third (5) is a combination of both the real-time and minicomputer systems.

4. A SIMPLIFIED APPROACH

Due to the expense of implementing any of the above approaches, we have concentrated on the evaluation of the feasability of low-cost systems, so that the potential of commercial systems, which are just appearing on the market, may be appreciated. As an input device, both a 256 x 256 x 8 Charge-Injection-Device and a 1" Vidicon TV camera have been used for viewing x-rays placed on a viewing box. Further, an analogue Video Tape Recorder has been employed for image post-processing.

251

The images obtained using these devices have been digitised using both a 6 bit slow-scan converter and an 8 bit real-time Analogue-to-Digital converter and used for storing images in a commercially-available microcomputer and a Nuclear Medicine image processor, respectively. Areas of investigation have so far been confined to angiographic images and the results and conclusions of these investigations will be presented.

5. REFERENCES

1. Nudelman S, Capp MP, Fisher HD, Frost MM, Roehrig H. Photoelectronic imaging for diagnostic radiology and the digital computer. Proc SPIE. 1978; 164:138-146.

2. Hohne KH, Bohm M, Erbe W, Niedre GC, Pfeiffer G, Sonne B. Computer angiography A new tool for x-ray functional diagnostics. Med Progr Technol. 1978; 6:23-28.

3. Christenson PC, Ovitt TW, Fisher HD, Frost MM, Nudelman S, Roehrig H. Intravenous cervicocerebrovascular angiography. Amer J. Roentgenology, 1980; 135: 1145-1152.

4. Roehrig H, Nudelman S, Fisher HD, Frost M, Capp MP. Photoelectronic imaging for radiology. IEEE Trans Nucl Sci. 1981; NS-28:190-204.

5. Nalcioglu O, Roeck WW, Pearce JG, Gillan GD, Milne ENC. Quantative fluoroscopy. IEEE Trans Nucl Sci. 1981; NS-28: 219-223.

6. Kruger RA, Mistretta CA, Riederer SJ. Physical and technical considerations of computerised fluoroscopic difference imaging. IEEE Trans Nucl Sci. 1981; NS-28: 205-212.

7. Gould RG, Lipton MJ, Mengers P, Dahlberg R. A digital subtraction fluoroscopic system with tandem video processing units. Proc SPIE. 1981; 273-21.

CLASSIFICATION PROCEDURES IN CONNECTION WITH BIOLOGICAL SIGNALS: COMPUTERIZED RECOGNITION OF PERSONS BY EEG SPECTRAL PATTERNS

H.H. Stassen, R. Günter, G. Bomben
Psychiatric University Clinic Zurich
Research Department
8029 Zurich, Switzerland

The intra-individual stability of EEG and its characteristic variability are well-known phenomena of EEG analysis and the object of several studies (1), (2), (3), (4), (5). The aim of our investigations was to formalize the stability concept and to decompose the original EEG signal in a static part (representing the organic components) and a dynamic part (representing the reactive components).

Modified techniques of communication theory were applied to Fourier-transformed EEG time series (6), (7) leading to the definition of EEG spectral patterns (5). The most difficult problem concerning the analysis of these quantities was the development of an appropriate similarity-measure that considers not only the power distributions but also the corresponding variabilities. A set-theoretical measure was found to be an adequate solution (5).

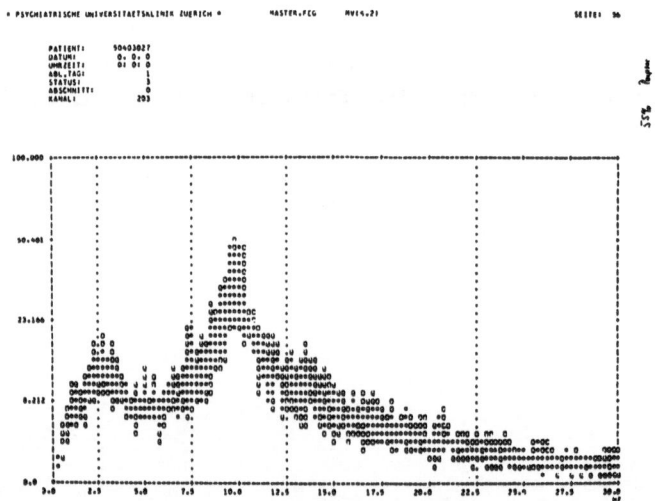

Figure 1: EEG spectral pattern for 1 channel estimated from 4x20 seconds EEG time series

Results

The results of our investigations show that the intra-individual similarity of
"static" EEG spectral patterns ("within subjects") is significantly greater than the
inter-individual similarity ("between subjects"). Consequently a subject can be
recognized by his EEG spectral pattern with a confidence probability of about 90 %.
In other words, if the coputer system once becomes acquainted with the pattern of
a specific person, additional measurements allow a computerized recognition of that
person with an unreliability of only 10 % under similar experimental conditions.
This is based on 6560 spectra from 82 persons (5). The estimates of the "static" EEG
spectral patterns were tested by means of repeated measurements in connection with
multivariate statistical procedures such as nonmetric multidimensional scaling,
cluster analysis and decision functions. Preliminary results of our present investigation (a specially controlled longitudinal study comprising 50 persons: 2 measurements in an interval of 14 days, a 3rd measurement after 1 year ist planned) verify
the above conclusions impressively. The analysis of the inter-individual similarity
coefficients leads to distinct natural groupings according to the fine graduations
of mutual differences. This discriminating effect of "static" EEG spectral patterns
also holds for different experimental situations, suggesting an organic or genetic
predisposition of each subject.

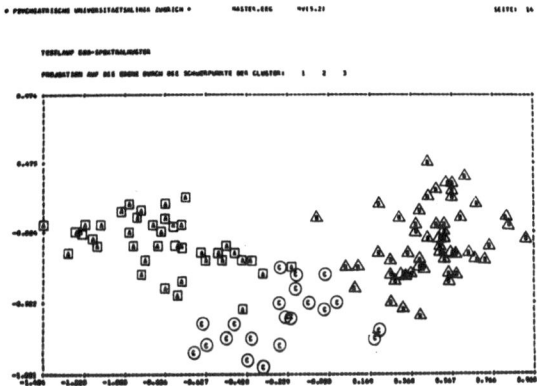

Figure 2: Projection of the elements of 3 "natural" groupings onto the plane defined
by the corresponding cluster centers

As a direct consequence, it seems to be very promising for "dynamic" EEG experiments,
to eliminate the "static" part as a non-interesting background information. This

approach to pattern recognition has been applied with great success in the field of digital image processing and led to a better resolution in most cases.

Remarks

EEG's were provided by Dr. M. Koukkou-Lehmann, digitized online and stored on magnetic tape. Mr. W. Manske performed the coding of data and artefacts. The program system and the databank are installed on an IBM 3033/MVS.

References

(1) Berkhout, J and Walter, DO. Temporal stability and individual differences in the human EEG: an analysis of variance of spectral values. IEEE Trans. biomed. Engng, 1968, BME 15: 165-168
(2) Kennard, MA and Schwartzman, AE. A longitudinal study of electroencephalographic frequency patterns in mental hospital patients and normal controls. Electroenceph. clin. Neurophysiol., 1957, 9: 263-274
(3) Matousek, M, Arvidsson, A and Friberg, S. Serial quantitative electroencephalography. Electroenceph. clin. Neurophysiol., 1979, 47: 614-622
(4) Van Dis, H, Corner, M, Dapper, R, Hanewald, G and Kok, H. Individual differences in the human electroencephalogram during quiet wakefulness. Electroenceph. clin. Neurophysiol., 1979, 47: 87-94
(5) Stassen, HH. Computerized Recognition of Persons by EEG Spectral Patterns. Electroenceph. clin. Neurophysiol., 1980, 49: 190-194
(6) Brown, TJ. Program for the Analysis of Time series. NASA TM·X-2988, 1974
(7) Batchelor, BG. Pattern Recognition. Plenum Press, New York, 1978: 418-424

AN INTERPRETER FOR MATRIX GRAPHICS

H.P. Meinzer

Institute of Documentation, Information and Statistics,

German Cancer Research Center,

Heidelberg, FRG.

SUMMARY

The language PIC is an interpretative command language which can be applied to digitized matrix images. The routines collected in the language PIC are all quite general. Therefore there is no restriction as to where the images actually originate. It is also suited for the education of beginners in the field of pattern recognition. If some problem-dependant specialized programs are included, sophisticated application programs can be constructed.

INTRODUCTION

Up to now no integrated software is available to deal with the problems in the field of matrix images. At the most there is a pool of FORTRAN callable subroutines.

In a research and development environment this approach to computer graphics is a very costly one as it is very man power-dependent. Experience shows that it is more promising to develop an easy-to-use interaktive package which can be applied by the researcher himself.

THE LANGUAGE PIC

This language consists of seven groups of commands.
- dataset management functions
- simple image manipulations
- gradient operators
- smoothing algorithms
- fourier manipulations
- display functions
- auxiliary functions

A few commands of every group will be described in more detail. For reading a command it must be explained that all expressions in brackets can be dropped. The sign '|' is the logical OR function.

The dataset management functions are:

STORE NAME

ERASE NAME

All images are stored online on disc. The user addresses a picture only via its name and must not deal with the actual size. Most of the following operations are performed on the image stored in the workspace. Some simple image manipulations are

    WINDOW IX, IY, IDELTAX, IDELTAY
    SCALE N(/M)
    SELECT N-M (SET IVALUE)

With these commands both the size and the grayvalues of an image can be influenced. There are seven gradient operators available in PIC, e.g.

    SOBEL
    ROBERTS

For smoothing we have three commands.

    MEDIAN N
    SMOOTH
    FLAT

MEDIAN is a simple median filter, FLAT is a non-linear operation on the grayvalues. There are four FOURIER operations available:

    POWER
    AUTOCORR
    CORR
    FOURIER (REV)

POWER and AUTOCORR evaluate the power spectrum and the autocorrelation of a given image. CORR correlates two pictures. FOURIER evaluates the real and imaginary parts of a given picture. FOURIER REV reverses this process. Operations on the resulting FOURIER pictures like high pass or low pass filters are also available.

For the display of images there are a number of commands:

    PRINT (REV) (ON WHITE PAPER)
    PLOT HISTO
    PLOT TOPO
    PLOT CONTOUR

PRINT permits a low quality print on a standard alphanumeric printer. All PLOT functions need a graphic terminal TEKTRONIX 4014 for the display of the output. Finally there are a few auxiliary functions.

Though PIC already includes a number of generally useful commands, there will always be something missing. PIC can be connected to other programs in two ways. One is that PIC can include specially written algorithms via some kind of general DUMMY commands, or PIC itself can be included into other FORTRAN programs. Technically both alternatives are very different.

THE IMPLEMENTATION

PIC runs on an IBM 3032 with the operating system TSS (time sharing system). It needs at least one graphic output device like a TEKTRONIX 4014 storage tube (3).

The software is written in FORTRAN. The analysis of the input strings (commands) is done by a parser which was generated by the parser and lexical analyser generating system PAULA (1,2,5) which was developed in our institution (4). Some of the image processing software was copied from literature or contributed by others (6).

APPLICATION

PIC was developed at the German Cancer Research Center (DKFZ), Heidelberg. Therefore, all our applications are in the medical-biological field. We applied PIC to one- and two-dimensional electrophoresis gels. These gels are produced by thousands in all groups working on DNA and RNA mapping and sequencing. In a further project we tried to analyse the different stages of tumor growth in the colon of rats.

ACKNOWLEDGEMENTS

Quite a few people contributed ideas and programs to PIC. I want to thank J. Dengler, U. Engelmann, M. Jaksch and G. Zinser for the software they made available, and Dr. Komitowski who delivered images. Special thanks go to Prof. G. Zajicek who helped a lot in many aspects.

REFERENCES

1. AHO, A.V., ULLMANN, J.D.: The Theory of Parsing, Translation and Compiling. Vol. 1 and 2. (Englewood Cliffs, N.J.: Prentice Hall 1972).

2. BECKER, N., OSTERBURG, G., SCHADEWALDT, K.: PAULA - Generator für LL (1)-Parser und lexikalische Analyseprogramme. DKFZ, Heidelberg, Technical Report No. 10, 1977.

3. HAHNE, H.: TEKTRONIX: TCS und AG-II. DKFZ, Heidelberg, Technical Report No. 8, 1976.

4. MEINZER, H.P.: Command Languages in Application Programming. In Lindberg, D.A.B., Kaihara, S. (Eds.): MEDINFO 80, pp. 719-722. (Amsterdam, New York, Oxford. North-Holland Publ. Co. 1980).

5. WIRTH, N.: Compilerbau. (Stuttgart: Teubner 1977).

6. ROSENFELD, A., KAK, A.C.: Digital Picture Processing. (New York: Academic Press 1976).

COMPUTERIZED ANALYSIS OF SOMATOSENSORIAL EVOKED POTENTIAL.

E. Amori*, A.Andraghetti*, A.Benini*, G.Lommi**, S.Lotta**.
Department of Medical Physics Parma*/ Department of Rehabilitation
Villanova**.

Methods and Materials:

The examination was performed by stimulating the median nerve near
the wrist controlaterally at the lesioned hemisphere.   The lead was
obtained by placing the electrodes on the scalp at 7cm from the medium
point between nasio-inion;   the reference electrode was placed on the
forehead.   The analysis of the waveform was performed by means of a
DISA 1500 Digital EMG System.

The computer analysis was performed with an on-line implementation
made available by using a Hewlett Packard multiprogrammar and a P 6060
Olivetti minicomputer with 48K memory.   An analog tape recorder was
also connected with the system (Figure 2).   In this way we obtained a
real-time and a deferred analysis.   The compatibility of the devices
employed guaranteed a correct information flow, utilising an appropriate input-output program following the IEEE 488 standard specifications.

The numerical data referred at a distance(between the wrist and
7th cervical)of 65cm were obtained from a program which calculated all
the significant maximum and minimum   relative latencies, zero-
crossing latencies and the first three components upslopes and down-
slopes.   The presence of quasi-isoelectric responses have induced us
to take into consideration also the areas, related to the zero-line.
Between the two minimums if above the zero-line or the maximum and minimum
if under it.

Description of the problem:

The study of the components of somestethic evoked potential(SEP)
is an effective clinical test to deduce important information relative
to the transmission of an electric stimulus either through the peri-
pherical nervous trunk or through the spinal medulla (1).   Pathology
related to the posterior columns of the spinal medulla produces, in
fact, significant modifications on the latencies, amplitudes of the
normal components of SEP (2,3,4,5).   The multiplicity of locations
serving as sources of the various components of SEP is presumably the reason
for the extreme difficulty in determining their participation with
utmost exactitude.   Due to the ability   to evaluate the state of
continuity of the posterior cords, many authors (6,7,8) have investig-

ated to see if the modifications occurred after incomplete or complete
traumatic lesions.   This is in order to find some prognostic indices
especially where non-conforming SEP was present.

This study describes an attempt to find an appropriate set of
parameters to evaluate the modifications of SEP waveforms in subjects
with cerebral vascular focal lesions both before and after   rehabilitation.   The set of parameters was chosen from a control group of 60
subjects on the basis of clinical normality (Figure 1).

Results and Discussion.

The pre and post treatment data collected were compared with the
results provided by a clinical test also performed before and after
therapy.   The clinical test made on 50 subjects with pathological
findings consisted in the evaluation of the aphasia, aphrassia, movement and sensitivity scores.   On analysing the electrophysiological
results 12 of the 22 patients with an initial isoelectric SEP had
modified the response by the end of the treatment.   In 7 cases the
complete set of components partially reduced in their early amplitudes
and new tardy components appeared in 5 cases.   A very interesting
comparison was made between the clinical and electrophysiological test.
The 12 patients who showed modification from the initial isoelectric
condition had an improvement also in the clinical test.   In particular
the appearance of tardy components and formation of early components
manifested respectively a good recovery of movement, aphasia, and
improvements in sensitivity.   Patients with modified but complete SEP
showed no important modifications.   More complex appeared to be the
comparison of cases in which more components were involved.   However
the possibility of having a constant and immediate verification of the
validity of a rehabilitative therapy via a frequent SEP control analysis
seems to us very promising especially in those patients who show an
electrophysiological improvement at the same rate with a clinical
improvement.

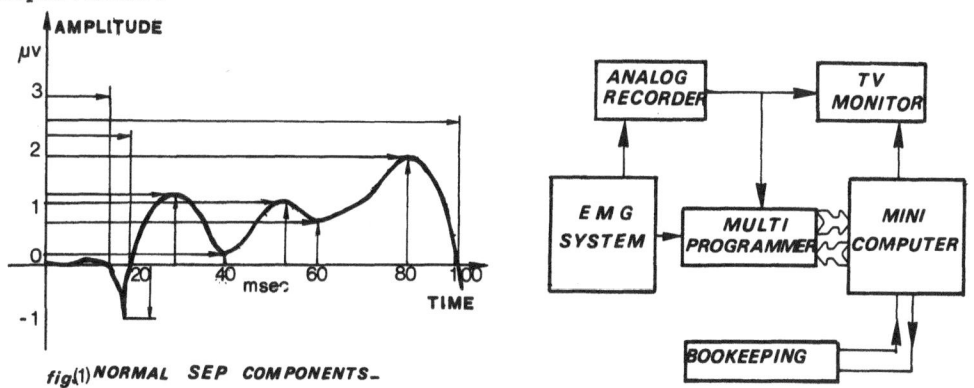

fig.(1) NORMAL SEP COMPONENTS.

260   fig.(2) SCHEMATIC BLOCK OF THE SYSTEM.

REFERENCES.

1) Desmedt J.E. Prog.Clin.Neurophysiol. Ed.J.E.Desmedt, Basel 1980.
2) Halliday A.M. and Wakefield G.S. J.Neurol. Neurosurg. Psychiat., 26, 211-219, 1963.
3) Oester Y.T., Azlis A.W. and Ridriquez A.A. Arch.Phys.Med.Rehabil. 51, 21-27, 1972.
4) Cracco R.Q. International Journal of Neurology, 3, 233-246, 1975.
5) Cadilhac J., Georgesco M., Benezech J., Duday H., Dapres G. Electroencephalography and Clinical Neurophysiology, 43, 160-167, 1977.
6) Kaplan P.E., Rosen J.S.. Paraplegia, 19, 118-122, 1981.
7) Rossini P.M., Greco F., David P., Pisano L., De Palma L.,Tonali P. Giornale Italiano di Ortopedia e Tramuatologia. Vol.5, 379-390, 1979.
8) Engler G.L., Spielholz N.I., Bernhard W.N., Danziger F., Martin H. Wolff T. Journal of Bone and Joint Surgery, 160 A, 528-532, 1978.

TEXT PROCESSING SYSTEMS FOR THE DOCTOR'S OFFICE

by

J.R. Möhr[+], G. Peter[*], H. Krayl[*], H. Runge[#], S. Marquardt[•],

[+]Institut für Medizinische Dokumentation, Statistik und Datenverarbeitung der
Universität Heidelberg
Im Neuenheimer Feld 325, D-6900 Heidelberg, FRG

ABSTRACT:

A series of investigations was conducted in order to assess the need for
automated text processing among physicians in the FRG. These included a
survey of existing text processing systems, qualitative and quantitative
analysis of individual practices, statistical analysis of volume of
correspondence of all (approximately 3000) physicians in private practice
in the region of Nordwürttemberg, and computer simulation of office
organization in general and specialized practice.

The results show that text processing can result in economic gains and
improvement of office organization in approximately 10 % of physicians'
practices. One equally important motive for applying text processing is
analysis of office structure and function. This means that primitive text
processing techniques do not suffice. An outline for the functions of a
text processing suitable for physicians' offices is given.

1. INTRODUCTION

There is a definite trend towards support of practicing physicians through small in
house computer systems (1). In countries where reimbursement procedures are based
on a fee service system, there exists a preoccupation with administrative functions
in order to support this system. The support of medical functions is desirable. The
processing of medical reports has a key role as a link between the adminstrative
functions:

- billing
- scheduling
- surveillance

and medical functions in the proper sense:

- generation of reports
- patient in information system
- categorial analysis of medical characteristics
  of office functions.

There exists considerable experience on the principles of medical text processing

[*]Fachbereich Medizinische Informatik, Fachhochschule Heilbronn,
[•]Arzt für Radiologie, Neckarstr. 136, D-7000 Stuttgart,
[#]Städt. Kliniken, Heilbronn

(2,3,4,5). Most of it was gained in the hospital environment (4,5,6,7,8,9). Also the employment of these principles by practicing physicians has been suggested for more than a decade and tested to some extent (2,4,10). However available systems did gain only limited acceptance. This may have two reasons:

- the available systems are not adequate
- there is actually no need for text processing among physicians.

Both aspects were examined in a series of investigations in 1980, the results of which shall briefly be summarized in the following. Since the results indicate a need for text processing systems, the principal features of such a system will also be outlined.

2. ADEQUACY OF AVAILABLE TEXT PROCESSING SYSTEMS.

In 1980, a comprehensive survey of commercially available text processing systems was compiled and made available to interested physicians (11). It includes some 80 products of close to 50 vendors.

The results show that despite a great variety of systems ranging from electronic typewriters with storage capacity and textediting capabilities to micro and mini computer based systems with more complex computing capabilities, there are hardly any systems that support the spectrum of functions which is desirable for text processing in physician's offices. The systems offered need improvement in order to be acceptable on a broad scale by physicians. This is particularly necessary at a time when computers for application in doctors offices are increasingly available, since the investment for a computer supporting mainly administrative functions and that for an adequate text processing system tends to be in the same range (fifty to hundredandfifty thousand DM). It is therefore essential to know, whether text processing is a useful adjunct to doctors office computers if provided in an adequate manner. This question was approached by investigating individual offices, by analyzing the volume of correspondence of all physicians in a region of the F.R.G., and by using the results of such investigations in computer simulation of offices.

3. INVESTIGATIONS OF INDIVIDUAL OFFICES

One of us (S.M.) is practicing as radiologist in the central area of a large industrial city of South West Germany. In this radiologic practice, textprocessing using text fragments stored on magnetic tape cassettes and an electronic typewriter is employed routinely for over ten years.

In another practice which is almost exclusively spezialized on diagnostic gastro-enterology, a thourough investigation was carried out concerning applicability of text processing (12). In this practice, approximately 250 to 300 patients are treated per month in 2 to 3 sessions. For practically all of them, a letter is prepared informing the referring physicians of the obtained findings. This investigation showed the following:

- As found elsewhere (2,3,13) standardized text predominates, the reports
  being made up to a large extent of very few phrases or words and
  a great number of different expressions used rather rarely.
- The time needed for preparation of a report is in the range of twenty minutes (physician's and secretarial time accumulated).
- Using automated text processing, the time spent for preparation of
  an individual report could be decreased to perhaps five minutes.
- The production cost for reports decreases in such a way that even a
  medium scale computer system costing approximately 100 thousand DM
  would be cost effective if more than 200 patients were treated per
  month.
- Although the economic gains are the primary consequence of time savings, these effects were not the primary motive for the physician.
  The physician was primarily interested in the analysis of the office
  operation and medical performance.

A similar experience was made in a large group practice with inpatient facilities
specialized on the treatment of cardiovascular diseases (14).

The analysis of office structure and function may be particularly relevant in a
country with high density of physicians and a resultant tendency towards subspe-
zialization. If this type of demand would exist universally, it should represent a
strong incentive for improving commercially available text processing systems for
the use in physicians' practices.

4. STATISTICAL ANALYSIS OF VOLUME OF CORRESPONDENCE OF PHYSICIANS IN THE REGION OF NORTH-WÜRTTEMBERG

The fee for service system adopted in the F.R.G. has the advantage of making some
aspects of office operation fairly transparent. Preparation of reports and letters
is a reembursable service in most types of practice. An analysis of the data of the
KV (Kassenärztliche Vereinigung) North Württemberg *, a region in South Western
Germany, was therefore undertaken in order to assess the distribution of the
requirement for text processing in this region (15).

Table I shows the distribution of reimbursed letters among specialists and general
practitioners. The majority of physicians produce very few reimburseable letters.
While there are practically no general practitioners producing more than 100
letters per quarter or 35 letters per month, there is a definite group of specialists (660) producing from 35 to 400 letters per month.

The data is broken up for selected specialists in Table II. It shows that there are
certain specialists like urologists, ENT specialists, surgeons and orthopedists who

* We are endebted to Prof. Dr. Häussler, president of the KV North Württemberg, and
  Mr. Herles, executive officer, for permission and Mr. Wrona for assistance in
  obtaining anonymous data.

Table I

Volume of Correspondence of
Internists and Specialists

Data based on an analysis of reimbursed services in the 4th quarter (Oct.-Dec.) 1979 of
physicians in the region of North Württemberg

Volume of Correspondence in No. of Letters per Month	No. of Doctors				Total	
	Specialists		General Practitioners			
	abs.	%	abs.	%	abs.	%
0	162	10	563	43	725	26
0- 1	129	8	350	27	479	16
2- 5	148	9	178	14	326	11
6- 10	155	10	124	9	279	10
11- 17	125	8	53	4	178	6
18- 25	137	9	25	2	162	5
26- 35	98	6	14	1	112	4
36- 50	156	10	5	0	161	5
51- 70	111	7	2	0	113	4
71-100	122	8			122	4
101-135	84	5	1	0	85	3
136-180	88	5			88	3
181-235	48	3			48	1
236-300	23	1			23	1
301-365	18	1			18	1
366-435	8	0			8	0
436-500						
501-650						
> 651	2	0			2	0
	1614	100	1315	100	2929	100

Table II

Volume of Correspondence of Selected Specialists
(analysis of same data as in table 1)

Volume of Correspondence in No. of Letters per Month	No. of Doctors											
	PED		INT		SURG		ENT		UROL		ORTH	
	abs.	%	abs.	%	abs.	%	abs.	%	abs.	%	abs.	%
0	41	23	45	10	1	1	0	0	0	0	3	3
0- 1	51	29	40	9	2	2	1	1	1	2		
2- 5	30	17	74	17	2	2	2	2				
6- 10	31	17	60	13	8	9	2	2	1	2	1	1
11- 17	11	6	54	12	4	5	6	6				
18- 25	3	2	42	9	7	8	9	9	3	5	4	4
26- 35	4	2	29	7	6	6	5	5	1	2	1	1
36- 50	4	2	42	9	14	16	8	8	4	7	7	7
51- 70	3	2	21	5	14	16	10	10	3	6	6	6
71-100			18	4	12	14	16	15	10	19	11	12
101-135			9	2	9	10	11	11	7	13	8	9
136-180			4	1	3	3	16	15	11	20	23	24
181-235			3	1	4	5	11	11	9	17	10	11
236-300			4	1			3	3	2	4	10	11
301-365			1	0			4	4	2	4	5	5
366-435							2	2			1	1
436-500												
501-650												
> 651											1	1
	178	100	446	100	86	100	104	100	54	100	91	100

PED - pediatricts, INT - internists, SURG - surgeons, ENT - ear nose and throat, UROL - urologists
ORH - orthopedists

start at a volume of correspondece where general practitioners and even internists level off. Assuming that similar time characteristics apply for the preparation of letters in these practices as in the investigated individual ones, considerable gains should be expected in approximately 200 to 300 practices out of the total of close to 3000 included in the investigation.

The actual relevance of text processing may even be greater than reflected in these figures since the preparation of reports is sometimes included in the basic service. Examples are all radiologic examinations. Therefore radiologists do not show up in these figures. Using a different technique of analysis (15) we showed that twenty out of the fifty radiologists included in this investigation prepare between 15 and 40 letters per day (1) and may be able to save between 1 1/4 and 6 1/2 hours per day if they save between 5 and 10 minutes per report for various types of reports.

5. COMPUTER SIMULATION OF OFFICE OPERATION

Although the evidence obtained so far indicates the possibility of considerable time savings per prepared letter, there remains the question, whether the time gained can be used effectively for other duties or is absorbed in office routine. For investigating this, computer models were built, using GPSS as simulation language:

1 Model of general practice/common type of practice for internal medicine (16).

2 Specialized highly structured practice with different separated functional entities such as diagnostic radiology, endoscopy, different types of examinations (17).

The first model was used to simulate different organizational settings varying in type of access control (drop in access versus scheduling), types and quantity of staff (varying number of aides/secretaries employed) amount of correspondence (letters prepared for varying fraction of patients) and organizational backup (conventional organization versus computer supported organization). The different characteristics were represented in the model by varying distributions of activities and varying associated time characteristics. These characteristics were based on a number of available quantitative analyses (12,18,19).

The volume and type of correspondence in this model is characterized by a marked predominance of short notes the preparation of which require less than a minute, and the rare occurence of letters requiring more than five minutes of preparation. It was assumed that these time characteristics can hardly be altered by automated support. The simulation experiments with the first model showed that office function can be smoothed by introducing scheduled access, but that the volume of correspondence can not be increased without additional staff.

The second model was closely oriented at the simulation of the diagnostically oriented gastroenterologic practice mentioned above. In this case computer support was mainly supposed to affect documentation and preparation of reports. Assuming a documentation procedure that allows for automated generation of reports, the simulation results indicate that all letters may be prepared by the office persounell and are available immediately at the time of the last visit of the patient while in the current system 70% of the correspondence is prepared by external secretarial services and becomes available only a week after completion of investigations. Still the extent of occupation of the practice personnell decreases while that of the physician remains essentially unchanged.

6. GENERAL PRINCIPLES FOR A TEXT PROCESSING SYSTEM

Text processing and report generation are functions with multiple relations to other functions in office practice. If based on an integrated medical documentation system, a variety of reports (letter to referring physicians, reports on special investigations etc.) may be generated as well as lists of services rendered. This forms the basis of administrative functions like billing and accounting as well as the core of a patient information system. Both functions serve to evaluate medical operations within the office as well as global office operation. Medical reports concern usually a wide variety of individual characteristics of different patients and are produced in small quantities. Layout, correction, features, formating etc. are of minor importance than in the industrial environment. The desirable characteristics for a text processing system to be used in the medical environment are therefore:

- support of an integrating database
- incoupeling of the processes of data acquisition/
  documentation and of report generation
- adequate features for control and correction of reports
- support of inquiry functions concerning documented entities (e.g.
  patients, specimens from patients)
- support of statistical analysis accross documented entities.

The principal functions are

- data acquisition
- textsynthesis
- text processing and printing.

While text processing and printing are available on a variety of commercial systems for business applications, the synthesis of text from text blocks is less common and usually not based on an integrated documentation and information system. Also data acquisition in the business environment is usually supported by dialogue at fixed work places and directly linked to the preparation of a report whereas in the doctor's office environment considerably greater flexibility is desirable.

In particular the support of offline data acquisition is needed.

General construction principles for medical reporting systems are therefore

- efficient handling
- correctness
- adaptivity.

Efficient handling refers to data acquisition, data correction, specification of reports and initiation of printout. Offline data acquisition may be realized alternatively to or as preparation for input via terminal. In any case, dialogue has to be realized in such a way as to give the user simultaneous control of the available alternatives of text and of the resulting documentation. If data is input to an integrated data base, efficient input procedures may conflict with efficient handling of corrections. Concerning report generation it is essential that a procedure for generating a given type of report be specified once and for good with possible modifications or additions in individual cases and that the printing of the results be controllable independently of the input manipulation and documentation. In order to support the functions which are more remotely connected with report generation - such as data analysis and evaluation - efficient procedures for generating tables and statistics have also to be provided.

Plausibility checks are also an essential part of a reporting system in order to achieve correctness of documented data and generated reports. These concern types of data, values of variables, relations between values of different variables etc.

Adaptivity refers to differing requirements of different users as well as to varying and evolving needs of a given user. Therefore an application independent basic concept has to be realized which can be adapted efficiently to different and changing applications. The following characteristics should therefore be definable for a particular environment

- type, format and contents of offline acquisition media
- structure of CRT frames
- logic of user guidance
- type and value of input fields
- plausibility checks, error promptings
- type and contents of reports
- number, type and characteristics of output devices.

Realization of these demands has to resolve a conflict between the complexity that a comprehensive implementation of all requirements entails and the lack of support of essential functions that might result from a more restricted solution. Our concept for implementation shall subsequently be outlined.

7. GLOBAL CONCEPT FOR REALIZATION

Our global concept is based on interactive dialogue for data acquisition, with optional offline procedures for preparation of data input. The dialogue is frame oriented. Input frames may be defined interactively through dialogue. Frames are referred to as chapters ("Kapitel") which consists of lines ("Zeilen"). Each line consists of fixed texts and input fields. Input fields have to be specified in the following manner:

- optional or mandatory input
- data field length
- data field type
- name (as reference for output synthesis)

The following types are permitted:

1 alphanumeric codes (specification of acceptable codes optional)

2 text strings, optionally including codes

3 numeric, including specification of thresholds which may or may not be exceeded

4 calendar date

5 time.

Data access may be achieved hierarchially proceeding from specification of application area ("Formularname") to data field or directly using a unique field identification.

This information is somewhat complemented for realization of the branching logic of the dialogue and the execution of plausibility checks. The language elements used for realization of text synthesis are derived from the elements of structured programming. The following types are realized:

Print ("Drucke")   Initiates text output

Assign ("Setze")   Assigns a value to a variable

For ("Für")   Permits repetition of a statement or sequence of statements. The number of statements and/or repetition is controlled through an accumulator or depends on a condition. This allows to search all available values connected to a given application as well as inclusion of values meeting specified conditions.

If ("Wenn")   This type of statement specifies a condition for a statement of a sequence of statements. AND ("UND") and OR ("ODER") are allowed to specify logic relations between operands. Field contents, variables, constants or expressions are allowed for operands.

The possibilities of subroutine techniques are also made available. The synthesis of a text paragraph may be specified and included in a different program by subroutine call. Every output specification may be called by a unique identifier. The user may specify identical names for several applications or programms. The system generates unique identifiers. A release management is considered for later implementation. It will control different versions of a given application (input specification, plausibility checks, output specification).

Data acquisition is made independent of generation of an actual report. The user identifies a given application and inputs the relevant data. Several data sets for a given object are stored under unique identification in the data base. A report is generated by calling a given output routine for an object represented in the data base. All available data for an object may be included in this report. The generated report may be examined, modified and printed.

This concept is realized on the basis of standard MUMPS on PDP 11/40 hardware (20,21) and will later be converted for use on Z80 based microcomputers using CP/M.

8. INTERMEDIARY REALIZATION

Parallel to the development of the system outlined above, a solution based on the only suitable commercially available system for business application, which was identified during our survey, is being tested.[*] This system provides for realization of user dialogue in a "dialogue module" and of text synthesis through an "evaluation module".

In order to define the dialogue, frames are generated which are identified by a unique name, and delimited by a special character. So is every input field for which specifications are given above.

Data acquisition results in the production of an abreviated expression consisting of variable names and their values. These may be accessed by specifying the generating frame for control and correction. The abbreviated expressions are also the basis for report generation by calling an evaluation module.

The synthetized text may be formatted and corrected prior to printout. The printout may include additional constants or variables such as the address of the recipient. Implementation of the system is completed, as far as outlined above. The system has been realized in COBOL on medium scale DDC computer systems, using IDAS as data base system. The textbox in use in the radiologic practice with different equipment for more than ten years have to a large extent been converted into this system with an effort of approximately three hundred hours.

The currently employed software has to be complemented by evaluation modules in order to exploit fully the possibilities opened up by compact storage of patient information. Also the development of administrative modules for more comprehensive support of the practicing physician is at present taken into consideration.

Routine application of this system is scheduled to start in Nov. 1981. The results of the routine test of this version will be accounted for in the implementation of the system outlined above.

---

[*] INTEXT marketed by STRÄSSLE for use on DDC Systems.

REFERENCES:

1. Rienhoff, O.; Abrams, M.E. (ed.): The computer in the Doctor's Office
   (North Holland: Amsterdam, 1980)
2. Giere, W.; Baumann, H.; Schmidt, H.A.E.: Der programmierte Arztbrief, ein
   Weg zur klinischen Volldokumentation
   IBM Nachrichten 193 505-511 (1969)
3. Giere, W.: Einführung der Datenverarbeitung in der ärztlichen Praxis-Dokumen-
   tation und Informationsverbesserung in der Praxis der niedergelassenen Arztes
   mittel EDV-Service. (DIPAS)
   DVM Bericht 3, Gesellschaft f. Strahlen- und Umweltforschung, 8042 Neuherberg
   (1975)
4. Pocklington, P.R.: The necessity for and requirements of, and Basic Design of
   a General Data Interpretation and Evaluation System,
   In: Anderson, J.; Forsythe, J.M.: Medinfo 74
   (Amsterdam: North Holland, 1974) 411-418
5. Thurmayr, R.: Über ein neues Verfahren der Dokumentation digitaler Daten und
   der automatischen Berichterstattung in der Klinik
   Habilitationsschrift (München GSF Bericht MD 85, 1974)
6. Thurmayr, R.; Schnabel, M.; Schulze, R.: 15 Jahre Erfahrungen mit Dokumenta-
   tionssystemen für medizinische Basisdaten. In: Reichertz, P.L.; Schwarz, B.
   (ed.): Informationssysteme in der medizinischen Versorgung - Ökologie der
   Systeme (F.K. Schattauer, Stuttgart,1978)
7. Thurmayr, R.; Schnabel, M.; Thurmayr, G.R.; Laux, S.; Schöffel, J.; Sieber, I.:
   Präsentation von Basis- und medizinischen Berichtsdaten. In: Möhr, J.R.,
   Köhler, C.O. (ed.): Datenpräsentation
   (Springer, Berlin, Heidelberg, New York, 1979) 164-176
8. Elsässer, K.H.; Hepperle, G.; Hoenicke, E.; Offenhäuser, K.H.: Datenpräsentation und Verlaufsdarstellung im Arztbrief und am Bildschirm. In: Möhr,J.R.,
   Köhler, C.O. (ed): Datenpräsentation
   (Springer, Berlin, Heidelberg, New York, 1979) 177-185
9. Pocklingtion, P.R.: A critical survey of 30 months OMR form processing within
   the Medical System Hannover. In: Reichertz, P.L. (ed): Informationssysteme in
   der Medizinischen Versorgung (Schattauer: Stuttgart, 1977) 619-625
10. Giere, W.: EDP use in free practice: motivation of physicians and paramedical
    staff after two years of routine difficulties
    Journees d'Informatique Medicale, Toulouse, 1975
11. Haas, P.; Schattmeier, F.; Möhr, J.R.; Peter, G.: Textverarbeitung - eine
    Geräteübersicht für Ärzte (Rationelle Praxis, Albstadtweg 11, Stuttgart 1981)
12. Möhr, J.R.; Boese, J. (Hrsg.): Berichte aus dem Praktikum Systemanalyse im
    Gesundheitswesen: Textverarbeitung in der Arztpraxis
    Intl. Report, Univ. Heidelberg, 1980
13. Möhr, J.R.: Einsatzmöglichkeiten und Bedeutung der Textverarbeitung in der
    Medizin. (Rationelle Praxis, Albstadtweg 11, Stuttgart 1981)
14. Stelzer, H.: Computerunterstützung für eine Praxisklinik - Systemanalyse
    Thesis, Univ. Heidelberg, 1980
15. Schlienz, R.: Quantitative Analyse des Textverarbeitungs- und Dokumentations-
    volumen in Arztpraxen Nordwürttembergs im 4. Quartal 1979.
    Seminararbeit, Fachhochschule Heilbronn 1981
16. Lange, M.: Entwicklung eines Simulationsmodells zur Untersuchung der Ablauf-
    organisation allgemeinmedizinischer Praxen. Thesis, Univ. Heidelberg, 1980
17. Eiermann, H.: Computermodell einer Azrtpraxis zur Untersuchung des Einflußes
    von Textautomation. Thesis, Univ. Heidelberg, in preparation
18. Möhr, J.R.; Haehn, K.D. (Hrsg.): Verdenstudie, Strukturanalyse allgemeinmedi-
    zinischer Praxen. (Dtsch. Ärzteverlag, Köln, 1977)
19. Reichertz, P.L. et al.: Praxiscomputer im Routinetest / Eine Begleitstudie zu
    einem Feldversuch (Dtsch. Ärzteverlag, Köln, 1980)
20. Klumpp, I.: Entwurf und Realisierung eines Textgenerierungs- und Verarbei-
    tungssystems, Thesis, Univ. Heidelberg, 1981
21. Boschert, W.: Entwurf und Realisierung eines Maskengenerators zur Erstellung
    von Erfassungsdialogen. Thesis, Univ. Heidelberg, 1981

271

RESEARCH INTO DECISION - MAKING STRATEGIES USED IN GENERAL PRACTICE

J. Ridderikhoff

Department of Family Medicine, Erasmus University
Rotterdam, 3000 Dr Rotterdam, The Netherlands.

SUMMARY

Do recognisable strategies exist according to which a family physician reaches a decision? Or are there as many strategies as there are dictors? I think the latter may be true, but these strategies can be clustered into two main directions: inductive and deductive. The characteristics of the former exist mainly in the early generation of hypotheses and the attachment of the estimation of chances to the argumentatation-steps.

The latter can be described as a process of sequential logical steps with prior probabilities attached to a limited number of hypotheses. A research protocol, according to which about 50 family physicians will be interviewed, is described.

RESEARCH INTO DECISION - MAKING STRATEGIES USED IN GENERAL PRACTICE

Introduction

Research into decision-making strategies used in general practice is aimed to learn more about the procedure family physicians follow in order to arrive at a decision concerning their patients. The result of this process is not just the name of a disease but a judgment about the present state of a patient, based on observed symptoms, which leads to choices for treatment.

I conjecture three strategies according to which a physician can gather and digest information. On the one hand we can recognize an inductive method, which can be divided in two submethods: pattern-recognition and inductiveheuristic. On the other hand there is the systematic-deductive form, a deterministic approach to medical problem solving.

In the search for these strategiesaat least three elements play major roles:
- the character of the medical problem;
- the time available for the problem-solving process;
- the testing of hypotheses.

Because of the broad area of patient complaints in general practice I focus at medical-somatic diseases. The prevalence rate for these diseases helps us to sort the desired different characters of the medical problems. Time is a major factor for everly family physician. "The essence of the doctor's art actually is to make decisions, a tremendous number every day, often on the basis of insufficient evidence, under the pressure of time (..) and to make them with (at least outwardly) the appearance of a claim, dedicated and warmly human personality." (Biörck, 1977).

The testing of hypotheses is one of the cruces in diagnostic procedures. How can a doctor test a hazy hypothesis without knowing the precise results?

Points to be investigated

I discern four points to be investigated:
1) Do recognisable strategies exist according to which a family physician reaches a decision?
2) If so, can these strategies be formalized?
3) Do they depend on influences from the physician's background and surrounding?
4) Do they essentially differ from the strategies taught at the Universities?

The model

In essence the diagnostic process is a separating one: separating one disease from another in order to arrive at a diagnosis = a judgment about the present state of a patient.

The family doctor deals with a broad, often immense area of symptoms, diseases and related health disturbances. This is contrast to the clinician whose scope reaches only to medical science itself and a special field within this science.

So the question is do family physicians use a specially assigned strategy in their everyday work?

Two preliminary remarks on this subject.

- in general, experienced family physicians identify clusters of symptoms and/or diseases (Categories). This notion has also been briefly mentioned in literature (Derouesné: see Salamon et al, 1976). "Categories are sets of diseases and sets of symptoms which are not mutually exclusive and whose subsets suggest multidirectionality, that is more than one disease". (Jaquez & Norusis, 1976). Sorting out illnesses according to their symptoms depends upon the ability to recognize the symptoms, but this assumes that the diseases and the symptoms in fact appear - in sufficient frequency - in the patient population. In other words, this means that the prior probabilities depends upon how the symptoms appear, their frequency of appearance, how serious they are when they appear and their appearance in the context of the variables (e.g. age and sex).

- "People tend te make their choices based more on likeliness than using the logic of prior probabilities" (Tversky & Kahnemann, 1974).
"Experts are very good at generating new data from early hypothesis formation" (Balla, 1980).
"The initial steps in the diagnostic process are entirely human (without instruments)

273

and aimed at a striking reduction in uncertainty" (Bolinger & Ahlers, 1975).

Out of these thoughts came the notion for the three strategies and the criteria for recognizing them. The deductive strategy is based on an analysis of sequential steps of explanation and verification, with the probabilities attached to the conclusion (diagnosis). In the inductive strategy probablilties (in terms of likeliness) are attached to the argumentation-steps. Diagnosis here is a maximization of chances or a minimization of the uncertainty (of the doctor). "Eine solche probabilistische Kennzeichnung des Argumentationsschrittes bedeutet dass kein deduktiver (syllogistischer) sondern ein Induktiever Wahrscheinlichkeitsschluss vorliegt. Die einen solchen induktieven Schritt kennzeichnende Probabilitas ist keine statistische Wahrscheinlichkeit, sondern eine induktieve Wahrscheinlichkeit." (Sadegh-Zadeh, 1977).
Pattern - recognition is not only the first step but also the shortest version of inductive stategy, a kind of basic theme.
Inductive-heuristic strategy is the iterative process of this basic theme. This gives the following scheme:

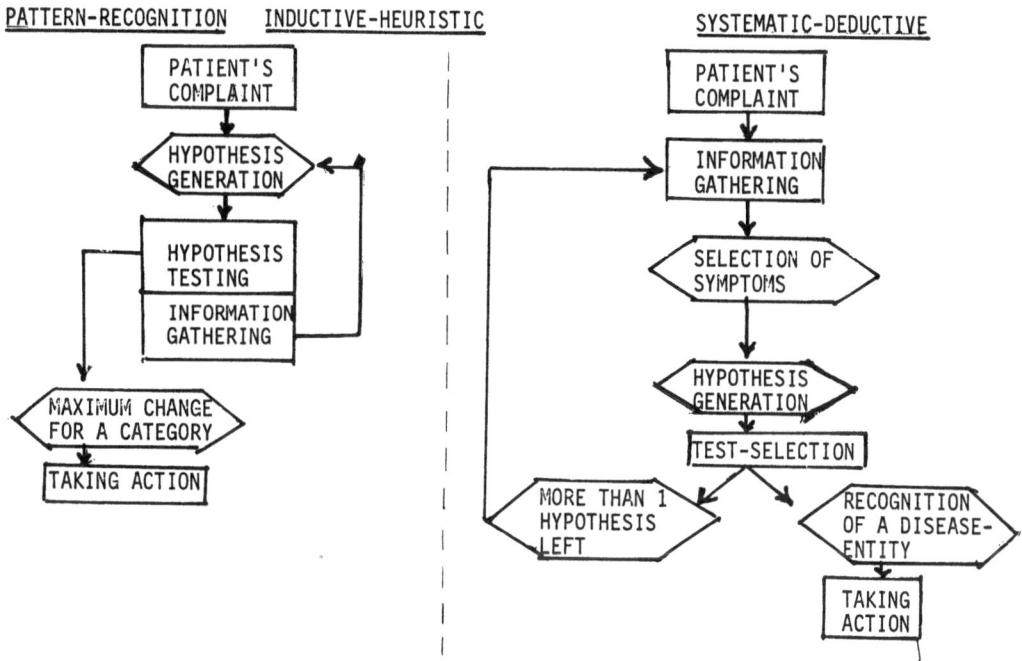

PATTERN-RECOGNITION   INDUCTIVE-HEURISTIC   SYSTEMATIC-DEDUCTIVE

To test this scheme I had to develop four instruments:
- a model for a paper patient;
- a questionnaire;
- Calculus of probabilities scale;
- Uncertainty scale.

Instruments

1) Paper patient. In order to standardize the input in the decision-making process the paper patient represents the real patient. Realizing the disadvantages of paper patients we try to minimize these effects.

Starting from the Portable Patient Problem Pack (P 4) of Tramblyn & Barrows (1978), I developed the following model:

- a situation card with a statement about the patient's presenting problem and situation. This informatation is handed over to the doctor;
- a design of all possible symptoms split into 8 classes:
  - general social information
  - general medical information
  - current existing diseases
  - history
  - examinations
  - tests
  - referral & consultation
  - treatment

Symptoms are indicated by their aspects (e.g. symptom Pain is set out by the aspects location, intensity, irradiation etc).

The paper patient will be developed from actual patients. To get some idea about the prevalence rate in general practice I make use of two studies in Rotterdam or neighbourhood (Monitoring project, Lamberts, 1980 and EPOZ, Valkenburg, 1978).

2. Questionnaire. The family physician's characteristics can be split into several sectors, as shown in the scheme.

CHARACTERISTICS OF THE GENERAL PRACTITIONER

Training and experience		
PRACTICE	Organisation - general form - daily pressure	Technical Sector - practice equipment - use of laboratories - use of x ray departments
Professional sector: - special medical interests - continuing education		

Data pertaining to these charactristics will be gathered by means of a questionnaire.

3. Calculus of probabilities scale. This instrument consists of an open scale into which the testee draws his bars of estimation. The distances between the bars can be measured. This scale is related to the hypotheses.

4. Uncertainty scale. This scale is principalty the same as the former one, but related to the testing-units.

Criteria

To recognize the strategies I shall make use of 19 criteria grouped as follows:
- character of the problem: the frequency of occurrence of a certain disease in the practice of a family physician;
- time: simulating the time-limits in the doctor's everyday work;
- information-units: every bit of information to a related question of the physician;
- testing-units: bits of information related to a certain hypothesis. Only in the context there is a difference between information- and testing-units;
- estimation of chances. This criterion will give information about the way doctors use probabilities in their decision-making process. Essential for this criterion is the quantification (measurement) of the probabilities;
- uncertainty reduction. Family physicians try to minimize the obligatory companion of their decision-making process: uncertainty. This criterion gives further information about the family physician's digestion of large amounts of information under time pressure;
- hypotheses: although one can presume a difference between hypotheses in the deductive and the inductive strategy, hypotheses are principally all the same: premises of the doctor;
- sequency of steps: see model on page 2.

Implementation

"Most doctors (..) do not practice in the fashion in which they have been trained. The pressures of time, patients and competition leads the doctor to adopt a variety of short-cuts and other useful strategies which may be detract from the quality he renders, but which allow him to function more effectively within the context and settings within the works." (Mechanic, 1978). What I am looking for is the claim of the general practitioner that he has a specific strategy. Alas, he was unable to define this strategy, so this research can only be an explorative one. In that case can choose out of two methodologies each divided into two methods:
1) Observation.
   a. Looking for elements that can be observed in doctor - patient encounter and try to find common denominators. As far as I know only a limited experiment has been carried out in Utrecht, Netherlands. They found far over 2500 elements almost without common denaminators.
   b. Looking for special elements in doctor - patient management e.g. choosing drugs (Lilja, 1976), use of diagnostic x - rays (Childs & Hunter, 1972), number and kind of questions (Smith & McWhinney, 1975).
   These studies leave strategies and contents out of consideration. Perhaps the lack of specificity of primary care has fostered studies to define its content and methodologies, while the subspecialties are by their nature defined by relatively

clear knowledge boundaries and/or technical skills.

2. Theoretical Model

    a. designing (a) theoretical model(s) to optimize the diagnostic process, with or without a doctor, by means of statistical and/or computer aids. Innumerable schemes and programmes have been originated, despite little practical success in their application to routine patient care. The explanation of this lack of succes is complex and includes, according to Taylor (1976):

    - lack of understanding of the decision - making process itself, and

    - the need for a theoretical framework within which such systems can be developed.

To this end I think one has to design one's model as closely as possible to the real practice situation in the appropriate area of the healt care system so that from the beginning the proposed system will fit as closely as possible to the needs of the existing system and to the physicians who will use it.

    b. designing (a) theoretical model(s) to examine the decision - making strategy(gies) of the family physician by structured observation (e.g. Elstein). There will no specific appreciation of the physician, because the aim of this investigation is to try to find his routes to his decision, i.e. his specific thinking process. Some procedure criteria I found in the excellent study of Elstein (1978), but, especially for the inductive strategy I had to design some new criteria.

To minimalize the bias I had to be sure that most of the (continuous) variables were uniform in each situation. Therefore I had to make use of paper patients, because real patients or actors simulating real patients are too changeable in the long run. Also the feed back to the process must be given by the testee. The only unrestricted variable is time. This not only fits to the real practice situation but also because there "were no studies indentified in which "real" time was examined in relation to decision - making" (Barr & Norem, 1978). I consider the criteria as continuous due to lack of precedented research to rely on. As one of the results of this research Prof.Dr. Abrahams (mathematician/statistician of the Economic Faculty of Erasmus University Rotterdam) will try to dichotomize the criteria by means of multivariate analysis.

I hope some 50 family physicians and 8 - 10 internists form the Rotterdam area will co-operate with the experiment. If possible, they will be stratefied according to:

- age and sex
- spread over the research area
- a patient population between 2000 - 3000 persons
- university of study

As I have to depend on the voluntary co-operation of the family physicians we can probably not adhere strictly to the above - mentioned stratification. The produce with the physician (and the clinician) will be as follows:

- the doctor is given the situation card
- he now choosen his own strategy asking for information, generating hypotheses (noting on a form) etc.
- answers to his questions are given by the paper patient (transmitted by an independent

interviewer)

- he notes down changes in estimation of chances and uncertainty
- the testee chooses his own closure of the process by making a proposition for treatment (e.g. writing a prescription, referring to a clinician)
- each doctor has to work through 4 paper patients
- total available for these 4 patients is 80 minutes.

The whole procedure is videotaped and time - labelled in the testee's surgery. After a week, to give the operator time to work out the acquired data, the tape is re-examined together with te testee. I shall ask him/her to think aloud together with the presented process, thus testing some of the criteria (e.g. testing units, their relation to certain hypotheses).

The questionnaire is handed over to the physician asking him to mail the forms within a week. Clustering the data and statistical analysis will follow. If everything works out smoothly research starts mid 1982.

References:

1. Balla, J.I.: Logical thinking and the diagnostic process, Meth. Inf. Med., 1980, 19, 88-95
2. Barr, D.M. & Norem, D.G.: Factors in influencing clinical decision making by physicians, Report Community Health Research, Rockford School of medicine, 1978
3. Betaque, N.E. & Gorry, G.A.: Automating judgmental decision making for a serious medical problem, Management Science, 1971, 17, 421-434
4. Bolinger, R.E. & Ahlers, P.: The science of "pattern recognition". J.A.M.A., 1975, 233, 1289-1291
5. Childs, A.W. & Hunter, E.D.: Non - medical factors influencing use of diagnostic x - rays by physicians, Medical Care, 1972, 10, 323-335
6. de Dombal, F.T., Horrocks, J.C., Walmsley, G., Wilson, P.D.: Computer - aided diagnosis and decision - making in the acute abdomen., J. Royal Coll. Phycns., London, 1975, 9, 211-218
7. Jacquez, J.A. & Norusis, M.J.: The importance of symptom non - independence, in: Decision making and Medical Care, F.T. de Dombal & F. Grémy, N. Holl. Pub.Cy., 1976, Amsterdam, 227-239
8. Lamberts, H.: Psychosocial problems and the disease model: two major determinants for health care delivery. Personal Information
9. Lilja, J.: How physicians chosse their drugs, Soc. Science and Med., 1976, 10, 363-365
10. Mechanic, D.: Medical Sociology, Free Press, New York, 1978
11. Muller-Sloos, A.J. & Ridderikhoff, J.: Research into decision - making strategies used in General Practice. Preceedings International Conference in Health Care, Montreal, 1980
12. Sadegh-Zadeh, K.: Subjektive Wahrscheinlichkeit und Diagnose, Meth. Inf. Med., 1974, 13, 97-102
13. Salamon, R., Derouesné, C., Samsom, M., Bernadet, M., Grémy, F.: Decision-making aids used to determine the content of medical teaching in: Decision-making and Medical Care, F.T. de Bombal & F. Grémy eds., N.Holl. Pub. Cy., 1976, Amsterdam , 379-393
14. Smith, D.H. & Mcwhinney, I.R.: Comparison of the diagnostic methods of family physicians and internists, J. Med. Ed., 1975, 50, 264-270.
15. Tamblyn, R. & Barrows, H.: Teaching guide for the P 4 system, Problem based learning systems, Monograph 5 4/78

16. Tamblyn, R. & Barrows, H.: Evaluation Trail of the P 4 system, Problem based learning systems, Monograph 4 4/78. Mc Master University, Faculty of Health Sciences
17. Taylor, T.R.: Clinical Decision Analysis, Meth. Inf. Med., 1976, 15, 216-224
18. Tversky, A. & Kahnemann, D.: Judgment under Uncertainty, Science, 1974, 185, 1124-1131
19. Valkenburg, H.A.: Epidemiologisch Preventief Onderzoek, Zoetermeer, 4e voortgangsverslag, 1978, Erasmus Universiteit Rotterdam, Medical Faculty, Institute of Epidemiology

REFLECTIONS ON AN INTERACTIVE COMPUTERISED HISTORY-TAKING SYSTEM IN A GENERAL
MEDICAL PRACTICE

G.A.W. Dove
General Practitioner, North End Medical Centre
211 North End Road, London W14 9NP, England
Honorary Lecturer, Charing Cross Hospital, London

P.M. Norris
Senior Clinical Psychologist

Summary

An interactive micro computer-based questionnaire has been devised, using simple,
friendly language to interview patients in a general practice. The social history
obtained from the programme was made available to the doctor before his subsequent
consultation with the patient. The paper explores the nature of the patient
experience with the computer and the implications for future medical practice.

An interactive computer programme was designed for patients in a West London surgery.
The questions all concerned the social history of the patients, and medical questions
were excluded. The questions were deliberately designed to create a friendly,
informal atmosphere, and one question followed on from another to maintain continuity.
The questions were presented to the patient on a video screen, and the patient had a
choice of three answers to each question - 'Yes', 'No' and 'Don't Know'. This
limitation inevitably reduced the amount of information that could be obtained but
the patients were free to take as long as they liked to answer questions in order to
encourage fantasy and conjecture about the questions asked.

Previous studies have been undertaken that showed that the patients enjoyed interacting with a computer [1] [2] and that they found it easier to talk to their doctor
following the computer interview [3] The patients' were of all ages and both sexes.
Some were new to the practice. They were selected by the doctors because they felt
that the social history taken by the computer would help them in their understanding
of the patient's problem. Part of the procedure has been to collect ideas from the
patients themselves. The value of this exercise was to highlight those areas that
the patient was most interested in, both to help the doctor in his subsequent interview and at the same time to broaden the basis of the programme.

Doctors' surgeries, especially in central London, are not places that are ideally
suited for reflection, or indeed for thorough medical interviewing and examination.
There are constant pressures; patients seeking immediate attention, limited
resources, and an emphasis on action rather than introspection [4]. Observation of
interactions in a crowded surgery points to the considerable difference between the
patient's attitudes to the doctor and to other members of the team. If a doctor is
late for surgery or keeps the patient waiting for an unduly long period, it is seldom
he who experiences the patient's wrath and frustration. A patient who appears

polite and submissive to the doctor may be the same patient who has upset the receptionist with his anger and rudeness. To collect research information, to attempt a quantitative or qualitative evaluation of what is actually happening in such a situation is a difficult and challenging analytical problem. These variables make it important for research in a practice to collect the patients' reactions not only from the doctor but from other sources, since they may present a placatory and over positive reaction to a doctor who is evidently keen and involved in the research. Twenty-five of the patients in this study were given questionnaires to be filled in and handed to the receptionist.

In the original published work the patients' expressions were enthusiastic and suggested that the patient felt the doctor's interest throughout the interview.[5] Not all our patients were so strongly positive. Reasons for this may vary. One of the striking differences was the environment in which the computer interview took place. Whilst in the original study the patients were alone with the computer to reflect and ponder their replies in a peaceful atmosphere, in this study they had to undertake the interview in a crowded waiting room. However, the overall results suggest that the majority of patients enjoyed completing the progamme, and many of them expressed strongly positive reactions. "It made me think about myself", "It eased the tension and helped me talk", "It's like talking to a person" - statements like these recurred. Of the twenty-five patients who completed the questionnaire the majority expressed positive reactions, said they felt it had helped them to think about their problems and felt that it had positively enabled them to talk to their doctor more openly and freely after the interview.

It is the facilitating nature of the programme that we are particularly interested in. That the programme is introduced by the doctor and the patient completes it with the knowledge that he will be seeing the doctor afterwards means that the computer interview acts as an adjunct to the relationship between the patient and doctor. Not only does it provide the patient with space and stimulation to think about himself, but it also gives him the message that the doctor is interested in all aspects of his life. One might compare the computer experience with the child's first toy, his transitional object as coined by Winnicott; for just as the child cannot make use of the benefit from an experience of a transitional object without a good enough mother, so the facilitating and creative process involved in the patient's use of the computer interview needs a good enough doctor to work with the experience. Not to recognise this is a dangerous overestimation of the powers of the computer.

The following clinical examples illustrate some of these points.

Example 1

A twenty-one year old girl came to the practice complaining of migraine, which had been investigated with no physical cause having been found. She was a girl who found it hard to talk to the doctor about her life, and the computer interview evidently left her feeling stirred up and upset. She scornfully told the psychologist she thought the questions were silly and irrelevant, and particularly objected to being asked questions about her relationship with her father and about her feelings about her body. However, to the doctor her reaction was different. She was compliant and submissive, saying she had enjoyed the experience. Exploration of her answers led to the uncovering of a great deal of family disturbance, and she broke into a tirade about her "hateful" stepmother. Here we see that the computer interview had stirred up a lot of feeling in this girl what was now open to exploration, but it demanded skilful handling to make the experience helpful and increase her understanding of herself, rather than make it a frightening experience to be scorned and rejected. Was the difference between the reactions to the psychologist and to the doctor due to the psychologist being a woman and a further indication of the girl's difficulties in relation to other women and to herself as a woman? Questions of this kind led us to wondering how far this girl's emotional struggles underlay her problem with migraine.

Example 2

A fourteen year old girl was brought to the surgery by her mother, complaining of periods of giddiness. Physical investigation revealed no apparent cause, and the mother appeared to be extremely anxious about her daughter's condition, which had resulted in her daughter missing time at school. The girl complained of an attack of giddiness at the start of the computer interview, and she was surprised to find that it diminished as the interview wore on. Her answers expressed uncertainty about her relationship with her parents, and after the interview she was concerned to know if it was a "lie detector", and more anxiously she asked "does Mummy know the answers". It was then a short step to discussing with her her anxieties about her mother's intrusiveness and her difficulties in keeping her thoughts secret from her mother. Although the doctor was aware of these aspects of the mother/daughter relationship previously, the computer interview was a step in enabling the girl to think about the problem and openly express it.

Example 3

The last example is of a twenty year old schizophrenic man, who we shall call John, who had been coming to the practice for some years, and whose family was well known to the doctor. The boy had had a breakdown seven months before, and had suffered from auditory hallucinations ever since despite the medication given. The relationship with the doctor had been an important aspect of John leaving home and setting up a life in a hostel following his breakdown. John was very struck by his interview with the computer and said that it had shown him himself; "It showed me who I am". Following this he had several supportive sessions with the psychologist and visited the doctor. However, he stopped coming after talking in great depth about his feelings of not having any sexual drive, and feeling empty and "not a person". Shortly after John returned to work his father died, but said to John before he died that the computer had done John good. A while later John was hospitalised for two weeks and then returned to resume his sessions at the practice.

The computer interview was a tool through which it was possible to build up a relationship with John that incorporated the sense of help and understanding. The computer as a medical tool in no way reduces the doctor's contribution to patient care. If anything it increases the importance of the doctor's role in the aspect of medicine that cannot be automated, involving interpersonal skills. The success of the computer interview in helping the patient to think more deeply about himself and communicate his thoughts to the doctor, depends on the skill of the doctor, while at the same time the computer allows the doctor to utilise his experience and learning more objectively.

Society is faced with a dilemma in its attitude to computer technology. Computers can be used as tools to facilitate man's development, aiding the exploration of new avenues of growth, or they can be seen as competitors for men's roles, threatening jobs and taking over all important functions. The latter is the path of great danger, for in it lies the assumption, expressed by John, that the machine is more powerful and effective than the men who created it. Psychologists have a heavy responsibility in determining the effects of increasingly sophisticated computer research. This study is specifically aimed at looking at the computer as a facilitating tool, enriching the potential understanding between a doctor and his patient and gathering important data to further exploration of the aetiology of disease.

References

(1) Evans C.R., Evans R.J., Marjot D.G., Matthews A.E.B., Somerville S., Whitfield S. (1977).   Some experiments in interviewing immigrant patients in their own language, using automated presentation of questionnaires.   Medinfo. Shires/Walt Editors. I.F.I.P. North Holland Publishing Company 225-227.

(2) Lucas R.W. (1977).   A study of patients' attitudes to computer interrogation. Int.J.Man-Machine Studies. 9.69-86.

(3) Dove G.A.W. et al (1977).   The Therapeutic effect of taking a patient's history by computer.   Journal of the Royal College of General Practitioners 1977.   27, 181, 477-481.

(4) Balint E. and Norrell J.S. (1973).   Six Minutes for the Patient.   London: Tavistock Publications.

(5) Dove G.A.W., Gordon M, Lucas R., De Wardener Prof. H., (1979).   History Taking By Computer: A "Psychotropic" Effect.   Published in Medical Informatics Berlin 1979. Proceedings 253-260.

CAPOS - COMPUTER - AIDED - PHYSICIANS - OFFICE - SYSTEM.

W.J.Klaring,
Computer Centre of the Veterinary University of Vienna.

Modern science has confused people's understanding about their environment in many fields, which is in direct contrast to what scientific knowledge wants to achieve. Partly the causes of this uncertainty lie, I am sure, in the so far defective structures of the various information flows - the single person knows less and less of the whole and thus loses confidence.

The methods of modern electronic data processing have proved an indispensible aid both when we gather profound medical knowledge in research and when we apply and spread this knowledge in our daily medical practice.

A relatively well defined field in this wide spectrum is the surgery of the doctor. Especially to deal with administrative business rationally and to attempt the application of promising medical discoveries in the service of his patients present obstacles hard to overcome in the running of a surgery because the human performance has a time limit.

In our days it is possible to manage the numerous tasks of a surgery rationally with the help of computerised organisation systems that are carefully planned and optimally adapted to the individual demands, and in the way to save time and money.

PHILOSOPHY AND STRATEGIES.

A suitable Computer Aided Practice Organisation System will be worked out after the respective careful analysis of the present and the desired conditions in the various medical organisation unit (surgeries of a general practitioner or a specialist, group practice, clinic laboratory etc.) has been made. For this purpose a complete micro-computer system will be handed over to the doctor "key ready", i.e. it is at his disposal in working order as soon as it has been installed and started, corresponding to his requirements together with all the necessary organisation details, program systems, training and know-how.

A strictly modular structure of such a system is desirable. The parts should be a great number of modules that are completely compatible with each other and can be installed in as many combinations as possible. In this way it is possible in every single case after deciding the dimension of the hardware to adapt the desired organisation concept to the

285

current needs of the medical organisation unit. Such a computerised
system serves the doctor subjectively, locally and directly.

POSSIBLE USES OF COMPUTER IN MEDICAL PRACTICE.
Following the worldwide experiences in the use of computers in medical
practice such systems have now been adapted to the conditions prevailing in Austria. Such an organisation concept can after due analysis
be realised in every single case by installing a complete microcomputer
system which contains the optimised program modules and can be set up
in the surgery. The immediate data collection concerning different
tasks in electronic storage permits through computer programs the
electronic availability and processibility of all these data at any
time.

Primarily important administrative business as well as important
medical activities can be performed more rationally. Private bills
and health insurance claims and other accounts can be carried out with
program modules according to the individual wishes and needs of the
doctor.

The appointment book should be an integral part of the system.
It facilitates coordination and planning of work in the surgery and
his communication surroundings. A text-editing system makes essential
rationalising in certain routine work possible, e.g. the writing of
diagnoses, case histories, letters, bills, automatic demands of payment
etc.

The center of this organisation concept is the medical information
system. In it must be stored all information and data of the patients
from the medical and adminstrative viewpoint which are important for a
doctor subject to the Austrian law concerning data protection.

This is the base of the immediate medical uses of a computer-
aided organisation system for the medical doctor. In this way case
histories, diagnoses, therapies, medicaments etc. of all his patients
are available at any given time.

It enables him by means of statistical or biomathematical modules
to process topical information, e.g. about the successes of his own
therapies, the calculation of forecasts from defined symptoms, correlations, differences or analyses of certain problems but especially to
gain evidence on the efficiency of his surgery.

Direct measurement-reading, computer-aided ECG analyses, control
of laboratory equipment can be integrated into such a system. Prices
based on current hard- and software rates for a complete key-ready
computer-aided organisation system will range from AS 150.000 to about
AS 900.000. In addition a computer-aided organisation system in the

surgery gives access to international medical data banks through
present-day rapid technological development.

In the near future personal services will be easy to realise with
the help of such systems, e.g. the handling of financial transactions
or the calling to topical information services like daily papers etc.

The question I put at the beginning must already be answered with
an unequivocal "yes" for Austria. Similar to developments in the
economic fields where computer-aided methods have been of great use to
mankind, a sensibly dimensioned and adapted computer system will help
the general practitioner to save time and money after initial financial
expenditure which can already be justified, and therefore give him
scope for his original medical activity to the benefit of his patients.
At the same time he need not be without the knowledge of topical medical and technological discoveries.

SUMMARY.

The concept of a computer-aided physician office organisation
system comprises a complete key-ready package to be used in all types
and sizes of physicians's offices to support the doctor in his work.
Philosophy, strategies, possible uses of computers in the physician's
office are presented with regard to rationalising administration,
evidence of efficiency, medical information processing as well as
better use of the doctor's time in his surgery, group practice, clinic
or laboratory. Aspects of application and prices of such a micro-
computer-system in the administrative and medical fields are discussed.

LITERATURE.
Klaring,W.J.: "Mikrocomputer-Systeme in medizinischer Forschung und
Praxis", Wien, tierarztl. Mschr. 5, 1980.

PATIENT COMPLIANCE IN HYPERTENSION CARE: THE CRITICAL ROLE OF THE COMPUTER

Patrice DEGOULET (1), Hong An VU (1), Gilles CHATELLIER (1), Claude DEVRIES (2) Pierre-François PLOUIN (3), Jean-Claude HIREL (2), Pierre CORVOL(3), Joël MENARD (3)

(1) Service d'Informatique Médicale, Hôpital Pitié, 91 bd de l'Hôpital, 75634 Paris Cédex 13.
(2) Centre Inter-Universitaire de Traitement de l'Information (CITI2), Paris.
(3) Hôpital Saint-Joseph and Hôpital Broussais, Paris.

The role of the computer in improving patient compliance with the medical treatment of arterial hypertension is analyzed in the light of the experience obtained with the computerized ARTEMIS system in a Hypertension Clinic in Paris. The efforts required include organizational, educational and therapeutic measures, as well as perseverance in identifying the factors associated with poor compliance. Appointment automation, development of a personalized computer record and the education of patients are ways of improving their awareness of the disease and their knowledge of its medical environment. An epidemiological search for factors enabling prediction of poor compliance, and the adaptation of surveillance and treatment to patient behaviour are also necessary. Among the factors associated with poor compliance, socio-environmental elements seem as important as the severity of the hypertensive disease.

1. THE IMPORTANCE OF COMPLIANCE

In day to day practice, the benefits derived from the medical treatment of permanent arterial hypertension are often considerably less than expected (1). There are several possible reasons for this lack of success : 1- insufficient screening of hypertensive patients (2), 2- insufficient or delayed access to care of certain social categories (3), 3- insufficient or inadequate treatment and, 4- low compliance with medical or dietary prescriptions (4). Although screening, access to care, adequate treatment and a good compliance with medical prescriptions are necessary to reduce the incidence of cardiovascular complications, compliance is certainly the critical requirement. Any efforts to improve the screening of hypertensive disease and care distribution are useless if compliance is poor (5). When this is so, benefits for the individuals are nil, but expenses for the community are maximal.

The Veterans Administration Trial of 1970, showing a reduced incidence of cardiovascular events in treated compared with untreated groups (6,7), gave the decisive impulse to a worldwide campaign against arterial hypertension. However 50 % of the patients initially fitting the inclusion criteria were later excluded from the trial after a preliminary period of follow-up because they were not attending their consultation or were not taking the entire course of prescribed treatment. More than half the patients followed by Caldwell and Finnerty in the early seventies were lost to follow-up after one year of treatment (8,9). When, during the same period the benefits of the medical treatment of hypertension were demonstrated, the major importance of the patient's compliance with medical recommendations became obvious. (1)

The reasons for poor compliance with hypertension treatment are numerous (table I). Hypertension is a silent disease, necessitating long-life treatment which is sometimes poorly tolerated or difficult to follow and always costly (1). Improving compliance requires the combined efforts of both the therapeutic receiver and provider as shown in table II. The aim of this paper is to show the possible or already effective place of the computer in relation to all potential measures to improve compliance. Most of the suggestions made result from the experience acquired in the Saint-Joseph Hospital Hypertension Clinic between 1975 and 1981 through the daily use of the computerized ARTEMIS system (10,11).

TABLE I : Main reasons for poor compliance in hypertension.

- Hypertension is an asymptomatic disease. Treatment may be difficult to justify to the patients concerned

- Treatment is of life-long duration

- Treatment includes drugs and dietary recommendations which are easier to prescribe than to follow (body weight reduction, stopping cigarette smoking, etc.)

- Unpleasant side-effects of anti-hypertensive drugs are common

- Adequate treatment requires considerable participation by the patient, as well as time and perseverance

- Cost of treatment may be high and not completely covered by public and/or private insurances

2. ROLE OF THE COMPUTER IN IMPROVING COMPLIANCE

2.1. The computer and patient management

2.1.1. Appointment automation

Creation of a pleasant functional environment (1), efficient organization of appointments and reduction of waiting (12) are known to facilitate compliance. At least for the two last measures, the computer may be particularly helpful. The ARTEMIS system registers all appointments in computer files (10). Personalized reminder letters are sent to the patient and to his general practitioner six months or two months before the next appointment and in long term cases, once a year. A different letter of reminder is sent to patients who fail to keep their appointments. If they do not answer a final letter of recall is sent which includes a short questionnaire on the reasons for non-attendance at the Clinic. Specific recall letters are also sent when dates of appointments are changed to suit either the patient or the physician.

2.1.2. Planning of clinical examinations

The investigation of a newly referred hypertensive patient includes confirmation of the diagnosis, evaluation of the severity of hypertension and a search for an endocrine or a renal cause (13). The planning of these investigations will probably remain the complete responsibility of the physician for a long time. However, direct help from the computer can now be expected for the indication and optimization of the schedule of the initial investigations (14) and for retrospective evaluation of their efficiency (15).

TABLE II : The scope of efforts for improving compliance in hypertension : the role of the computer.

PROCEDURES	COMPUTER FUNCTIONS
PATIENT MANAGEMENT	
.Creation of a pleasant functional environment (1)	
.Efficient organization of appointments and reduction of waiting time (9)	.Appointment automation (10) * Computerized recall letters (10) *
.Minimal adapted investigations (13)	.Computer generated work-up
PATIENT EDUCATION	
.about the disease (14)	.Computer-assisted teaching (21)
.about his or her disease (17,20)	.Personalized computer record (10) *
MEDICAL STAFF TRAINING	
.about the disease (22)	.Computer-assisted teaching (21)
.about his or her results	.Personalized care quality control (10,11,23) *
THERAPEUTIC EFFORT	
.Minimization of treatment, avoidance of side-effects, minimization of costs (1)	.Systematic search for contraindications or previous intolerance (10)* .Computerized optimization of prescriptions (24)
EPIDEMIOLOGICAL RESEARCH	
.Comparative epidemiology (1)	
.Search for high-risk patients (1)	.Standardized and computerized medical records (10,11) *
.Randomized trials (16)	

* = Functions carried out by the computerized ARTEMIS system

2.2. Patient education

With or without computers patients can be educated about hypertension. In a randomized trial among Canadian industrial workers, 95% of the 80 patients who were given such education acquired a good knowledge of hypertension, compared to only 20% in the non educated group ; however this effort failed to improve compliance which was desperately low in both groups (16). More specific education of patients about their own hypertension may be more rewarding as regards compliance. Factors which may have a positive effect include exact awareness of the severity of their disease (17, 18) and direct participation in treatment procedures (e.g. patients' measurement of their own blood pressure and participation in adapting pill-taking to their daily routine). In the ARTEMIS system, each patient is given a duplicate of his computerized record (10). At each clinical examination a summary of this record is produced including a table of blood pressure, body weight values, cigarette consumption, main laboratory follow-up tests (cholesterol, glucose, uric acid, etc...), so that the patient is kept permanently aware of his health status. Direct involvement of the patient in computer-assisted teaching programs is a feasible approach (21) but further cost-benefit analyses are necessary before they can come into general use.

2.3. Medical staff training and personalized care quality assesment

Training physicians to obtain compliance in hypertension was found to be effective both in reducing the drop-out rate and facilitating blood pressure control (22). The result for the 62 physicians involved in such a trial argue clearly in favour of including specific education on compliance problems in the curriculum of medical studies, with or without a computer.

Another approach, used in the ARTEMIS system since 1979 is to provide each physician with regular feed-back information on his own results (e.g. the drop-out rate or the percentage of patients whose hypertension is well controlled). Such personalized care quality assessment greatly stimulated physicians in detecting deviation or fatigability when managing chronic conditions in large numbers of patients (10,23).

2.4. Therapeutic efforts to reduce non-compliance

Optimization of treatment has three components: 1- The search for the minimum treatment (i.e. lowest number of drugs and doses), 2- The search for better tolerance (i.e. no contraindications or side effects) and 3- The search for the best cost-benefit ratio (i.e. the best result for the lowest price). The ARTEMIS records include a standardized questionnaire on drug contraindications and previous drug intolerance (10). In addition the patient is specifically questioned on compliance with drug prescriptions and observed side effects during each visit to the Clinic. All this information is summarized on a special print-out which is a useful guide to the physician for further prescriptions or recommendations. Direct computer optimization of drug prescriptions, as attempted by Coe and coworkers (24), is probably the next step, but will obviously require cautious evaluation.

2.5. Epidemiological research

2.5.1. Comparative epidemiology

Indications about the compliance level in a population of patients may be obtained by measuring the regularity with which appointments are kept, by interviewing patients, measuring plasma or urinary drug levels or by appreciating the secondary effects of drugs (1). The simplest indication, i.e. the attendance of consultations, is often sufficient in practice to appreciate the degree of non-compliance and allow comparative epidemiology, as shown in table III. Between January 1976 and December 1978, 1830 patients with systolic blood pressure >= 160 mmHg and/or diastolic blood pressure >= 95 mmHg were referred to the out-patients' Clinic of the Saint-Joseph Hospital. Of these, 484 were referred back to their general practitioner or cardiovascular consultant because they had only been sent for therapeutical advice, for geographical or personal reasons, or because their blood pressure fell during the visits that followed their initial consultation. The other 1346 patients were cared for by the clinic and followed up with the ARTEMIS system. After a one year follow-up, 11 (0.8%) were dead and 209 (15.5 %) were lost to follow-up, a drop-out rate comparable to the rates observed in countries with either similar or different health care environments (25-29).

TABLE III : Drop-out rate in different health care systems.

LOCATING OF STUDY	NUMBER OF PATIENTS	HEALTH CARE SYSTEM	DURATION OF STUDY (months)	DROPOUTS (%)
Hamilton (25)	224	Practitioners	12	12.0
New-York (26)	206	Specialists	12	50.5
Göteborg (27)	646	Clinic	12	6.0
U.S.A. (28)	5314	Clinics	12	18.1
Australia (29)	3427	Clinics	36	20.4
Paris, ARTEMIS system	1346	Clinic	12	15.5

2.5.2. Factors predictive of poor compliance

Certain factors in non-compliance are patient-dependent, (e.g. behavioral, clinical and biological factors), others depend on the medical environment (waiting time, duration of visits or physician characteristics) and others again, on the interaction between patients and their medical environment (conception of this environment or awareness of the disease). A list of as many as 200 parameters able to influence compliance was compiled by Sackett and Haynes (30,31). Although so long a list, obtained under non-homogeneous health care delivery conditions, is unlikely to fit any particular medical environment, it may be used as a guide-line in epidemiological studies on compliance, each medical staff being responsible for identifying the major factors corresponding to its environment.

This attitude was adopted towards the information collected in the ARTEMIS system between 1976 and 1978. The computerized records for the 209 non-compliant patients mentioned in the preceding paragraph were analyzed and their characteristics compared to those of the 1126 patients still under surveillance after one year (Table IV). The patients who dropped out were more often males, were younger and had lower blood pressure levels, were more frequently overweight excess at entry, had higher cigarette consumption and more often belonged to lower social categories than the compliant patients. Patients directly referred from screening on their work-site had a higher drop-out rate (29.0%) than those referred by a general practitioner or specialist (13.1%) (p<0.001). Inside the Hypertension Clinic, the drop-out rate was lower (14.1%) among the patients followed up by the Clinic's four permanent physicians than among those treated by the non-resident physicians (24.4%). In all cases, the use of a computerized and standardized medical record facilitates the search for the factors predictive of poor compliance and the evaluation of their relative importance. In the particular

TABLE IV : Factors predictive of low compliance with appointments. ARTEMIS system, Saint-Joseph Hospital (1976-1978).

CHARACTERISTICS	PATIENTS FOLLOWED	DROPOUTS	p
No of patients	1126	209	
Male sex (%)	55.1	65.1	<0.01
Age (years)	51.4±12.5	47.4±13.5	<0.001
Referred by work-site physicians (%)	13.9	30.4	<0.001
Manual workers, employees, service personnel (%)	48.7	59.1	<0.05
Systolic blood pressure at first visit (mmHg)	178.0±23.1	171.1±20.8	<0.001
Previous antihypertensive treatment (%)	66.2	45.5	<0.001
Cigarette consumption at first visit (cig/day)	3.6±8.3	6.1±11.9	<0.01
Weight index (Kg/m2)	25.2±4.0	26.5±4.6	<0.001

Hypertension Clinic studied, socio-behavioral parameters (e.g. patients' socio-professional categories, body weight or cigarette consumption) as well as the severity of their hypertensive disease were closely related to compliance with appointments. A systematic search for these parameters, as conducted in a standardized record, may be of a great value in predicting good or poor compliance for a newly referred patient, and may constitute the first step in the appreciation of each patient's Health Belief Model (18).

3. A COMPREHENSIVE APPROACH TO THE PROBLEM OF COMPLIANCE

We have reviewed here the potential or already effective role of the computer when dealing with the problem of compliance in a large population, mainly by drawing on our experience acquired with the ARTEMIS system. Other heath care systems may require different or at least adapted strategies for improving compliance. In addition, the importance of the part played by the computer should not be over-emphasized. Computerized functions have to be integrated with non computerized functions in an overall approach, as shown in table II. In this approach, the physician must never forget the permanent impact of his first contact with patient on the results of future treatment.

4. CONCLUSION

Compliance, which is the concordance between the physician's wishes and the reality of medical practice, is of major concern when dealing with a chronic condition like hypertension . Improving compliance requires thorough knowledge of its mechanisms , the ability to measure it regularly and reliably , and the development of a whole set of organizational, educational and therapeutical procedures. To obtain a 100% compliance may seem like the quest of the Graal, in which physicians and health personnel consume all their energy; but the computer could help to bring them salvation by relieving them of part of their burden.

5. REFERENCES

1. Ménard J, Plouin PF, Degoulet P, Ducrocq MB, Tugayé A, Corvol P. L'observance, clé du traitement antihypertenseur. Médecine Cardiovasculaire. 1980;1:43-48.
2. Miall WE, Chinn S. Screening for hypertension: some epidemiologial observations. Br Med J. 1974; 3:595-600.
3. Degoulet P, Devriès C, Wolf JP, Plouin PF, Ménard J. L' accès aux soins de l' hypertendu: influence des catégories socio-professionnelles. Nouv Presse Med. 1980; 9:15-19.
4. Sackett DL. Patients and therapies: getting the two together. N Engl J Med. 1978; 296:278-279.
5. Stason WB, Weinstein MC. Allocation of resources to manage hypertension. N Engl J Med. 1977; 296:732-739.
6. Veterans Administration Cooperative Study Group on Antihypertensive Agents. Effects of treatment on morbidity in hypertension: results in patients with diastolic blood pressure averaging 115 through 129 mmHg. JAMA. 1967; 202:1028-1034.
7. Veterans Administration Cooperative Study Group on Antihypertensive Agents. Effects of treatment on morbidity in hypertension: II results in patients with diastolic blood pressure averaging 90 through 114 mmHg. JAMA. 1970; 213:1143-1152.
8. Caldwell JR, Cobb S, Dowling MD, De Jongh D. The drop-out problem in antihypertensive treatment. J Chron Dis. 1970; 22:579-592.
9. Finnerty FA, Mattie EC, Finnerty FA. Hypertension in the Inner City: I analysis of Clinic dropouts. Circulation. 1973; 47:73-75.
10. Degoulet P, Ménard J, Berger C, Plouin PF, Devriès C, Hirel JC. Hypertension management: the computer as a participant. Am J Med. 1980; 68:559-567.
11. Degoulet P, Ménard J, Devriès C, Berger C, Hirel JC. Computerized evaluation of medical activities in Hypertension care. In: Lindberg DAB and Kaihara S. Medinfo 80. Amsterdam: North-Holland, 1980; 607-610.
12. Fletcher SW, Appel FA, Bourgeois MA. Management of hypertension: effect of improving patient compliance for follow-up care. JAMA. 1975; 233:242-244.
13. Report of a WHO expert committee: Arterial Hypertension. Technical Report Series No 628. Geneva: World Health Organization, 1978.
14. Gascuel O. Un programme d' aide à la décision médicale structurant automatiquement ses connaissances. in Rapport du congrès Intelligence artificielle et Reconnaissance des Formes, Nancy 1981. (in press).
15. Fineberg HV, Hiatt HH. Evaluation of medical practices : the case for technology assessment. N Engl J Med. 1979; 301:1086-1091.
16. Sackett DL, Haynes RB, Gibson ES, Hackett BC, Taylor DN, Roberts RS, Johnson AL. Randomized clinical trials of strategies for improving medication compliance in hypertension. Lancet. 1975; 1:1205-1207.
17. Nelson EC, Stason WB, Neutra RR, Solomon HS, McArdle PJ. Impact of patient perceptions on compliance with treatment for hypertension. Medical Care. 1978; 16:893-906.
18. Taylor DW. A test of the Health Belief Model in hypertension. In: Haynes RB, Taylor DW, Sackett DL. Compliance in health care. Baltimore and London: The John Hopkins University Press, 1979; 103-109.

19. Haynes RB, Sackett DL, Gibson ES, Taylor DW, Hackett BC, Roberts RS, Johnson AL. Improvment of medication compliance in uncontrolled hypertension. Lancet. 1976; 1:1265-1268.

20. Schulman BA. Active patients orientation and outcomes in hypertensive treatment: application of a socio-organizational perspective. Medical Care. 1979; 17:267-280.

21. Houziaux MO, Bartholomé M, Bartsch P, Bovy P, De La Broissine M, Lefèvre P. SIAM-DOCEO: anamnèse et enseignement médical assistés par ordinateur. In: Lecture Notes in Medical Informatics. Berlin: Springer-Verlag, 1981; 11:959-962.

22. Inui TS, Yourtee EL, Williamson JW. Improved outcomes in hypertension after physician tutorials. Ann Int Med. 1976; 84:646-651.

23. Degoulet P, Chatellier G, Devriès C, Plouin PF, Hirel JC, Ménard J. Etude de la variabilité intra et intermédecins dans l' utilisation d' un dossier standardisé de surveillance des malades hypertendus. In: Lecture Notes in Medical Informatics. Berlin: Springer-Verlag, 1981; 11:471-477.

24. Coe FL, Norton E, Oparil S et al. Treatment of hypertension by computer and physician,a prospective controlled study. J Chron Dis. 1977; 30:81-92.

25. Rudnick KV, Sackett DL, Hirst S, Holmes C. Hypertension in family practice. Can Med Ass. 1977; 117:492-497.

26. Engelland AL, Alderman MH, Powell HB. Blood pressure control in private practice: a case report. Am J Public Health. 1979; 69:25-29.

27. Andersson O, Berglund G, Hansson L, Sannerstedt R, Silvertsson R, Wikstrand J, Wilhemsen l. Organization and efficacy of an outpatient hypertension Clinic. Acta Med Scand. 1978; 203:391-398.

28. Hypertension Detection and Follow-up Program Cooperative Group. Patient participation in an hypertension control program. JAMA. 1978; 239:1507-1514.

29. The Australian Therapeutic Trial in Mild Hypertension. Report by the management committee. Lancet. 1980; 1:1261-1267.

30. Sackett DL and Haynes RB. Compliance with regimen. Baltimore and London: The John Hopkins University Press, 1976.

31. Haynes RB, Taylor DW, Sackett DL. Compliance in health care. Baltimore and London: The John Hopkins University Press, 1979.

The MISSION System:
Application of New Technology to Improvement of Physician-System Interfaces In Ambulatory Care Information Systems.

Arthur Clayton Curtis
Indian Health Service, Office of Research and Development
P.O. Box 11340
Tucson, Arizona 85716/USA

This paper describes current efforts to establish an experimental facility for research into innovative, highly interactive interfaces between health care providers and computer-based medical databases. Oriented toward ambulatory care settings, the MISSION system (Medical Information System Supporting Interactive Online Networking) is intended as a demonstration of the potential for increasing the efficiency and effectiveness of medical care by improving physician access to, and consequently utilization of, computer-supported health information systems.

Introduction

In spite of the obvious need for assistance in managing burgeoning amounts of patient-oriented clinical data, physician utilization of computer-based information systems has remained rather low-key. Not surprisingly, resistance to the use of automated systems in the routine delivery of health care by other than ancillary personnel has centered on the provider-system interface: the degree to which any innovation interferes with the physician's accustomed mode of patient care determines how well it will be accepted. Although in the short run physicians can apparently be induced to try almost anything, it is clear that long-term success rests on the ability of information systems to adapt to the provider rather than the other way around. The general scarcity of directly physician-interactive information systems is evidence that insufficient attention has been paid to both the human factors inherent in such interaction and the importance of a flexible interface which is acceptable to providers of care -- notably, but not exclusively, physicians. Fortunately, increasing ease of access to newer technology supports an optimistic view of the potential for realization of an acceptable means of user-system communication, and thus the eventual success of direct provider interaction.

Background

The Indian Health Service (IHS), a part of the U. S. Public Health Service, has been responsible since 1955 for the health of some 700,000 American Indians and Alaskan Natives. A computer-based Patient Care Information System (PCIS) implemented by the IHS Office of Research and Development has been in concurrent development and operation in selected locations since 1969. An encounter form - oriented batch system with limited capability for on-line retrieval of health summaries, the system is based on a comprehensive data collection system which in the areas of implementation captures information on every encounter with the health care system by a patient population of approximately 340,000. The constantly-growing off-line database currently totals approximately 630 million characters. Provider support is primarily through batch reports and periodic generation of health summaries in microfiche form.

The PCIS has been a valuable tool in applied health care systems research, as well as certain aspects of program and patient management. However, even in limited operation it has been faced with user requirements to which its ability to respond has been severely limited by its underlying technology as well as by resource constraints. The inability of average users to effectively integrate the system into their day-to-day activities eventually led to the decision to develop a truly interactive system which would complement the PCIS and improve its usefulness in the direct delivery of health care.

Design Goals

(1) The system must satisfy major needs unmet by the PCIS, including: (a) Interactive access to patient managment data (especially in the area of chronic disease): to provide better care by encouraging standardization of management on recognized principles and by maximizing communication between multiple providers, (b) Clinical database maintenance: to increase user satisfaction with, and trust in, data provided by the system, (c) Clinical database queries: to increase utilization of the data stored by the system, with an expected secondary benefit of improvement in the quality of data supplied to the system.

(2) The system must achieve high provider acceptance. Thus, beyond the implicit requirement of functional utility an attempt is being made to construct a comfortable interface which is: (a) highly interactive and responsive, (b) easily learned, (c) forgiving of user mistakes, (d) polite in its interactions, (e) supportive of users with varying levels of sophistication, (f) adaptive to individual user preferences, (g) readily changed by the user as user requirements change. High priority is being given to investigation of the usefulness of non-keyboard input devices and flexibility of display modalities.

(3) Other ingredients are necessary for operational success: (a) relatively low cost, (b) highly local control of installation and operation, (c) non-redundant acquisition and entry of data, (d) modularity of function, installation, and operation, (e) capability for interfacing with existing systems.

Application Structure

The primary goal of the project is to develop a system which will satisfactorily implement the previously summarized applications at a facility level, although it should be kept in mind that these local systems may one day serve as nodes in a larger IHS-wide network. The basic model of the operating environment is that of a small clinic, generally in a relatively rural location, without provision for special air conditioning, raised flooring, power supply, etc. The clinic may or may not include pharmacy, lab, or radiology functions, and the system must be able to accomodate the presence or absence of those functions, with appropriate adjustments in cost. System cost must not exceed that of typically available lab instruments -- in the $50,000 range or lower for a fully-configured system. Staff will usually include one to four physicians, two to four nurses, and additional personnel from medical records, lab, and pharmacy as a function of the size of the facility. Specialized computer support will generally not be available.

Information flow can be diagrammed roughly as follows:

```
MEDICAL RECORDS
     !
     +
     TRIAGE ----!-----+ NURSING --------!
         +     !                        !---+ PROVIDER ----!
         !     !-----+ LAB ------------!                   !
         !     !                        !                   !
         !     !----------------------!                    !
         !                                                  !
         !----------- PHARMACY +---------------------------!
         !                                                  !
         !--------------------------------------------------!
```

This structure depends on a multi-level storage hierarchy which distributes the data base to a limited extent while still allowing for: (1) local short-term data storage and manipulation by users, thus maximizing its usefulness and emphasizing local quality control, and (2) host-level long-term storage and processing for large scale analysis and aggregation for higher-level processing.

System Architecture

Hardware and software organization were shaped by three concepts:

1. An appreciation of the value of an adequate means of experimenting with various design architectures, state-of-the-art hardware and software technology, and varying operational settings prior to serious commitment to development and implementation of a system of significant size or complexity. This motivated building a development system capable of dynamic change rather than to issuing a competitive procurement for a completely specified product.

2. A belief that adequate understanding of the principles involved in effective provider-system interaction is so crucial to the eventual success of a truly interactive medical data system that every effort must be made from the outset to support a realistic, flexible, research and testing environment. The importance of the opportunity to experiment with hardware and software approaches to the human-machine interface, although frequently underestimated by line management, cannot be overemphasized.

3. A commitment to sufficiently powerful technology from the start. It was felt that major compromises with this philosophy could be made only at the risk of creating a design which could prove to be inflexible, incapable of growth, and performance-wise unacceptable to its intended users.

Based on these considerations, the decision was made to configure a small, highly local system specifically suited for and dedicated to the proposed applications. A microprocessor-based, distributed, multiprocessor structure was felt to best meet the strong requirements for reliability, simplicity, ease of operation at local sites, responsiveness, and support for a non-traditional user interface. Excellent commercial versions of this architecture are currently available "off the shelf" (e.g., the Datapoint ARC, Zilog Z-NET, Three Rivers' PERQ, and Xerox STAR systems). Although these systems already embody crucial decisions on interface design, each of which could preempt certain research approaches, it would nonetheless have been eminently desireable to build around any of these products. However, only a locally developed system could be expected to meet current funding constraints. This is unfortunate, since it will certainly be impossible to duplicate many of the features of the more powerful systems. Oddly enough, few commercially available systems support much in the way of non-keyboard input-output. This, together with cost considerations, ironically limited equipment selection to the "hobby" level. Since the IHS has no in-house capability for building and supporting hardware, selection was further limited to packaged systems with vendor support. Due to availability of color graphics, devices such as the graphics tablet, and recently- announced local network support, the APPLE II was finally selected as the basic microprocessor element.

The original local network design was based on multiple symmetric small systems sharing access to mass storage (disk) and using common regions on the disk to implement inter-processor communications. The archetype for this was the Winchester-based CORVUS with the CONSTELLATION intelligent multiplexor and MIRROR videotape backup system. However, NESTAR recently introduced CLUSTER ONE, an "Ethernet"-like local network product, and CORVUS has recently announced OMNINET -- one of these will be used if economics allow.

Communication between the local network and the host will be via telecommunications implemented on one of the small processors, and will take place on a transaction-oriented basis through a shell which hides the exact format required by the host from the local system. An effort will be made to minimize traffic levels due to limitations on transmission speed imposed by affordable equipment.

Initial considerations included the use of intelligent terminals for implementing many of the complex portions of the user interface, thus unburdening the application system of high-overhead tasks and making possible system-independent interface enhancement through the use of specialized hardware. Some of this was sacrificed when the decision was made to adopt a more distributed microprocessor-based organization. However, a "shell" approach to software design has provided some degree of application isolation from interface hardware specifics while still making it possible to experiment with multiple approaches to philosophies of communication. Devices to be evaluated in this respect include: speech synthesis and recognition equipment, graphics displays, selection devices (touch-sensitive screens, light pens, graphics tablet, "mouse").

It should be noted that the relatively recent availability of multi-processor micro-based systems may significantly alter system configuration plans as the system evolves.

Although not as visible as the hardware, the software component of the user interface is equally significant. Choice of an implementation language represented an extremely important decision, since the applications software is being developed from scratch and is expected to be highly volatile. Therefore, several criteria entered into its selection: (a) high programmer productivity, (b) wide availability (especially on small processors), (c) high efficiency, (d) good mass storage utilization, (e) powerful string manipulation capability, (f) flexibility of program structure In order to maximize these considerations, the decision was made early on to write the system in a high-level language. MUMPS was finally selected for its balanced tree-structured file system, pattern-matching and string-manipulating facilities, and availability in both multi-user form on larger systems as well as single-user versions on microcomputers running the CP/M operating system.

RESEARCH TOPICS

The scarcity of reasonable models imposed an unanticipated requirement for significant basic research as a critical component of the development process. This is targeted at issues such as:

- better understanding of patterns of information usage,
- effects of information presentation formats on intelligibility and comprehension of content,
- analysis of conditions conducive to maximal information transfer rate between user and system,
- effects of user-tailorable interfaces (for characteristics such as dialog structure) on user satisfaction and efficiency,
- dissemination of new technology beyond original development sites with minimum requirements for on-going technical support which might stifle further research and development,
- system evolution, essential to the satisfaction of varying local needs, with maintenance of the degree of commonality essential to permit sharing of data and system enhancements.

Summary

This paper has outlined current efforts to establish a sophisticated experimental facility for research into innovative interfaces between health care providers and computerized medical databases. Although the primary goal is to demonstrate the potential for increasing the efficiency and effectiveness of ambulatory medical care through the use of computer-based information systems, the development of the projected system offers an excellent opportunity for investigation of ways to improve the interfaces to, and consequently utilization of, computer-based medical information systems in general. The information thus gained may have widespread application in attempts to satisfy the the information-handling needs of providers of ambulatory care.

THE AUTOMATIC TREATMENT OF THE INFORMATION IN THE MEDICAL RECORDS AT THE LEVEL OF THE GENERAL PRACTITIONER

Sergio Cerutti

Institute of Electrical Engineering, Politechnic, P.za Leonardo da Vinci, 32 - 20133 MILANO - Italy

1. INTRODUCTION

The noticeable evolution of the techniques of microelectronics has caused low-cost and small-size computers to have access to a very wide class of users. That has been true in the medical field also for the general practitioner (GP) who may find in the personal computer a very precious instrument of work (1). Recently in Italy a new law has been issued which institutes a National Health Service with particular tasks to the GP who is in charge of being the first interface between the patient and the distributed health government structures. The present work is supported by a Special Project of the Italian Research Council aiming at the definition, the analysis and the implementation of an operation system for the collection and the distribution of the information at the various levels of health operators and, hence, even at the GP's. The first results of this research are briefly illustrated.

2. FUNCTIONS REQUIRED TO THE GP'S PERSONAL COMPUTER

Prior to any attempt of automatizing the functions of the GP operation system, it is important to stress the main functions which today are required to such doctors both by law and by the fulfillment of a high level professional standard: in Table 1 such functions are listed at this regard.

- Patient Records
- Patient-Control Programs
- Clinical Protocols
- Various programs for Clerical Jobs
- Programs to get local statistical and epidemiological Indicators
- Training and professional Updating Programs

Tab. 1 - Functional requirements of a General Practitioner's operation system.

- PATIENT RECORDS. That is required both for administrative (updating of the list of conventioned patients) and for clinical purposes (creation of patient files with possibility of information storing and retrieving: history data, laboratory examinations, previous diagnoses etc.). Part of the record is conceived in a fixed-text and part in a "quasi-free" text approaches (2).
- PATIENT-CONTROL PROGRAMS. This is for patient subsets gathered by age, sex, dege-

nerative or chronic pathologies (diabetes, hypertension, cardiopathy, etc.). There is chance to get trend analysis, diagnosis check, therapy control for a more suitable action on the patient.

- CLINICAL PROTOCOLS. For particular screening or aimed investigations (infections or seasonal diseases, preventive intervenctions etc.) to be agreed with other physicians and the Health National Service.
- VARIOUS PROGRAMS FOR CLERICAL JOBS. For the routinary tasks of GP's (filling in of the prescriptions, of the certificates, of all the tasks required by law and/or dependent from the professional activity). It is estimated that about 30% of the physician's time is dedicated to them.
- PROGRAMS TO GET LOCAL STATISTICAL AND EPIDEMIOLOGICAL INDICATORS. These data from GP's must converge to a higher level concentrator for the relevant routines (Health Local Unit, District or similar).
- TRAINING AND PROFESSIONAL UPDATING PROGRAMS. E.g. the opportunity of using a personal computer for training and professional updating by means of interactive programs (new drugs, new therapies, computer-aided diagnosis, differential diagnosis, drug side-effects and so on).

3. THE PERSONAL COMPUTER AND THE TECHNOLOGICAL DEVELOPMENTS.

The basic project for the GP personal computer is constituted by :
i) 8 bit CPU + 32 K (or 48 Kbytes) as a core memory (RAM) + a keyboard. They are generally assembled in single enclosure
ii) the peripherals are: back-up memory (2x8" floppy disk units with 1Mbyte or 2M byte on-line) a printer and a CRT video display.
    A rough average cost of the hardware plus the basic software is estimated about 8000 $ for a single ready-to-use commercial equipment. In the future we think to develop a prototype which, with great quantities, could be sold for less than 5000 $ with the design criteria illustrated above.
Some recent reviews in the field of personal computing applications (3) (4) have considerably stressed the dramatic improvements that the technological developments will put at disposal of the potential user in the future. For the GP that could imply :
- An interconnection between doctors and distributed databases via telephone cable (the so-called "telemedicine"). That allows to read medical,statistical and clinical data, to make diagnosis in real time at distance by evaluating patient's biological signals (ECG, EEG, pressures) and to get an easier and closer connection with the other decentralized health structures.
- The development of optical disks (with the possibility to store on a single disk 2.10^{10} bit, i.e. 100.000 pages of printed text) will allow to store and retrieve

directly signal patterns, laboratory data, X-rays, drawings, figures, photos,etc.
- The voice communication between physician and computer will greatly simplify many input/output operations, expecially from the side of users who are certainly untrai ned and unexpert, as medical doctors are.

4. CONCLUSION

The first results have been shown towards the design of a special purpose personal computer for GP's. Taking into account the development of microelectronics it is possible today to think of a 5000 $ equipment or less. Furthermore, it is important to point out that not only price criteria are fundamental for the penetration into the market of such a model but the use easiness, the flexibility and the smooth integrability of the system at the doctor's office as well.
As a conclusion it is important to stress the point that medical personal computing can not do miracles, of course, but is able to change many aspects of physician's work. This change will surely be in positive if physicians are well trained in using such a new machine and new methodologies,even starting from university studies.

REFERENCES

(1) Reinhoff O., Abrams M.E. eds., "The Computer in the Doctor's Office", North Holland Publ. Co., 1980.
(2) Cerutti S., Timò Pieri C., "A Method for the Quantification of the Decision-Making Process in a Computer-Oriented Medical Record", Int. Jour. Bio-Med. Comp. 1981, vol. 12: 29-57.
(3) Nilles J.M., "Personal Computers in the future: an Overview", IEEE Trans. SMC-10, 1980 n. 8: 474-476.
(4) Hayes J.P. "Technology Changes in Personal Computers", IEEE Trans. SMC-10,1980. 476-480, n. 8.

ACKNOWLEGMENTS

The present paper has been partially supported by a Grant of the Italian Research Council (CNR), Special Project on Informatics.

GENERAL PRACTITIONERS INFORMATION SYSTEM;
an automated informationsystem for the
practice and research in the Netherlands.

Jacob de Moel
Netherlands Institute of General Practitioners
Postbox 2570
Utrecht
Netherlands

A GP information system has been employed at the Netherlands Institute of General Practitioners since March 1981. The information system is intended to serve
two major objectives, namely to support the provision of information within general practices and further to provide an instrument to facilitate health service and epidemiological research.
A fully decentralized network system is being developed, characterized by a
stand alone computer system within the practice, which, for reasons of research
is connected with the institute by means of dial-up lines. In this system the
accessibility of information would be realized for all parties concerned with
full protection of the patient's privacy. The GP remains manager, owner and operator of his database, so that big institutionalized information banks are superfluous.

History

The Netherlands Institute of General Practitioners exists since 1970. The Institute is charged with introducing new developments and carrying out scientific
research into the general practice. In the Netherlands is little knowledge about
the demands for and supply of assistance in the general practice. This is partly
caused by a system of remuneration within the sick-funds which does not require
the GP to report back to the system. In the first place the GP has a control monitoring role in the total health care system in the Netherlands : before patients
may consult a specialist they must be referred by a GP; and specialists, in their
turn, report their findings in respect of the patient back to the GP. Secondary,
the GP has his own medical role. Most GP's keep files on their patients. For
some time, researchers and policy-making agencies have been concerned in making
these files accessible for investigation. The project described here is an attempt to do precisely that.

General Practice

Most GP's have their own practices. Recently however there has been an increased tendency for GP's to work cooperatively and various forms of cooperation have been introduced. With the introduction of cooperative forms and the growing complexity of medicine we find an increase of communication problems and information needs.

After an extensive inventory the following information system related functions within the practice have been distinguished:
- medical assistance
- general administrative and miscellaneous supportive activities within the practice
- provision and processing of information
- financial administration
- practice management
- dispensary (in rural practices).

The patients file is pivotal among these functions. In order to achieve access for the benefit of research as well as for the general practice, the project is based on integrated automatised data processing which includes the patient's file. The systematization of the data processing system has to be subdivided in such a way that individual differences of opinion between GP's are preserved. The various methods to be found in the medical literature distinguishes information according to either content, SOAP (subjective, objective, assessment, plan) or to presentation and/ or level of abstraction P.O.R. (problem oriented record). There are objections to both systems. SOAP is a method of contact-registration, without the possibility to record the central aim of a series of contacts. POR distinguishes problems which are not uniformly defined and it relegates the complaints to the status of an after thought rather than making them the object of the investigation. An automated registrationsystem should be more dynamic than the existing paper based systems. In automated surroundings a more dimensional classification of the elements to be registered should provide remarkable advantages for doctors as well as researchers.

Scientific Research

The automatization of patient-records provides an entry point for processing for research purposes. If the contents of the information system are allowed to follow established data definition and classification systems they would become processable. The processing benefits the GP as well as the researchers.

Discussion of the results of the processing with the GP's would motivate them to collect a greater part of the registration information in accordance with the norms for confidentiality and completeness established by the researcher (social process). They should be supported by modern means : touch-sensitive screens and network communicative facilities (technical process).

In this setting, we shall test the extent to which patients files are suitable for research (empirical process). The researchers require accessible raw data and flexible conditions. This is in part the reason for the development of a network system.

Network system/ carrying the project out

Each practice would receive a mini-computer which would process the raw data completely independently as wel as storing it. These computers would be linked via auto dialing telephone lines to a central computer. The central computer will be used for system development and research purposes.

Data processing for the research would be devided into three phases:

1. preprocessing of raw data; in the practice
2. principal statistical processing: centrally
3. post processing of raw data in the practice.

Raw data will not come form the practice and the patients privacy is fully protected without removing access.

The network system proposed in this project has a variety of potential applications; for example : as an independent GP system, in a regional medical information system, in a national system and in a combination of these.

THE COMPUTERISED NURSING RECORD - AN EFFECTIVE MEANS OF COMMUNICATION

Paula Procter SRN
Computer Liaison Nursing Officer

Jean G. Jarvis SRN HV
Divisional Nursing Officer

Alison E. Head BSc FRSA
Senior Systems Analyst
Royal Devon & Exeter Hospital (Wonford), Exeter, UK.

The paper describes the development of the Exeter Computer System designed to help nurses to maintain the Nursing Records of individual patients. Apart from enumerating the benefits and identifying the system as a powerful research tool, it shows the system to be beneficial in the implementation of the Nursing Process.

INTRODUCTION

'In the nursing sphere in the United Kingdom, much discussion and experimentation is taking place with a view to defining the use, content and design of the Nursing Record. According to the Central Health Services Council Report, chaired by Tunbridge,[1] the purpose of the nursing documentation "is to provide a running record of the nursing care given to the patient during his stay in hospital, together with the observations on his progress and response to treatment".'

These were the opening words of a paper given in Berlin at the first MEDCOMP conference in 1977[2]. In view of the current emphasis on effective communication, and bearing in mind the General Nursing Council commitment to the principles of the Nursing Process, these words are even more appropriate today, in any hospital where learners are trained. The Royal Devon & Exeter Hospital (Wonford), is such a District General Hospital, with 420 beds treating some 13,000 inpatients annually, 60% of whom are emergencies.

HISTORY

The approach adopted by Exeter in the 1970s was to use an on-line interactive computer system to maintain an Integrated Patient Record, containing Administrative, Nursing and GP information. Access is controlled by strict use of individual passwords with individually set access rights. The design of the Nursing System was influenced by many considerations the following being perhaps the most important.

   i)   Nurses exist primarily to nurse patients.

  ii)   Maintaining a Nursing Record is an essential part of nurses communication with one another about a patient but it is no more than a means to an end.

 iii)   The increasing number of part time and bank nurses highlight the need for improved communication methods.

  iv)   The computer system should be designed in a self-teaching manner, not relying on nurses to remember codes, but allowing short cuts if their familiarity with the system enables them to use these.

   v)   The system should enable nurses to view and amend details of patients' records

in one transaction. The resultant Care Plans should be able to be printed immediately either for individual patients or for a whole ward or group of patients.

vi) Each Care Plan should be patient orientated expressing his individual needs.

vii) It should be possible to produce lists eg Diet, Transport.

viii) It should be possible to calculate workload by patient and ward directly from
Care Plan information.

ix) Transfer of all Nursing Information should be possible between beds and wards.

x) The originator of any piece of information should be the person adding it to
the patient's record. Her unique identity and initials should automatically
accompany any amendments made by her to a record.

xi) A nurse signing onto the system at the ward based VDU should have access
directly to that ward's information, but those with appropriate authority
could view other wards' information.

xii) Both emergency and pre-registered patients should be allowed on the system.

SYSTEM OUTLINE

In order to achieve these aims the following Nursing Systems were designed for a network of one VDU for each ward and one hard copy printer between two wards on the same
floor level:

i) Admission, Transfer into a ward and Change Admission details.

ii) Change record of position of patients' beds within a ward.

iii) Set up and amend Patients' Care Plans.

iv) Print Care Plans, Name Lists, etc in several different ways.

v) Report that care has been given according to the care prescribed by the Care
Plan.

vi) Transfer and Discharge with automatic printing of a Discharge summary.

The systems were implemented in 4 wards from 1976 onwards and Working Parties guided
their development at all stages.

Other systems available in read only mode include:

i) Surname search on Master Patient Index to find a patient's Hospital Number and
view his Hospital Patient Administration Summary.

ii) Direct access to Patient Administration Summary if Hospital Number is known.

iii) Urgent and Unexpected Pathology Results.

iv) Nursing Procedures as defined by Procedure Working Party (120 such procedures).

v) GP list with associated Community Nurses names and telephone numbers.

vi) Pharmacy Information Service (600 drugs accessible by 1600 different names).

vii) What's On - showing local events, Nursing Diary Dates, Post Graduate Medical
Centre functions etc.

DEVELOPMENT

In 1979 the Exeter Reporting system became operational and the Nursing Management
then committed themselves to the system. A Nursing Officer responsible for liaising
between the wards and the Computer Project was appointed to organise training and

implementation of the system on the remainder of the fourteen Wonford words.
Additional design considerations agreed by 1979 were:

i) Information from Reporting should enable
    a) an evaluation of the care given and the resultant outcome.
    b) the production of a record of learners specific experience.

ii) Bedstates should be produced automatically.

iii) Nursing Officer night/day report should be produced automatically.

iv) Care Profiles specific to individual wards should be introduced, formalising
    the most frequent use of the 'short cut' facilities.

v) It should be possible to mark an order at any time during the day, for
    termination at midnight.

In parallel with the system development during the last 3 years, the Nursing Process
has been presented and discussed both by Working Parties and informally throughout
the district. This year Exeter became one of 12 participating centres in the WHO
medium term research programme on the Nursing Process. In 4 Wonford wards and 4 wards
at a hospital where the computer is not in use, pilot schemes have been in progress
since Spring 1981 to compare the different techniques employed in this total patient
care approach. In this time it has become clear that the computer system has great
potential for use in the process of defining, reporting on and evaluating care.

CURRENT STATE

It is not possible here to give a description of all the applications listed in the
system outline. This paper concentrates on the area of Orders and Reports and the
day to day maintenance of the patient record.

A standard phraseology for most Nursing Orders is in use in the nursing system and is
constantly under review by a working group of all grades of staff. The Phrases are
grouped together under titles such as Mouth and Eye Hygiene, Urine Tests (Ward) and
Urine Tests (Lab), Recordings, Assessment on Admission, etc each group being referred
to as a Page. When selected by its number, Phrases of this Page are displayed on the
screen for selection of those required to form any number of orders or statements. By
using Phrase 99 on any Page and following it by free text, eg 99 $\sqrt{\text{text}}$ it is possible
to make any statement which is required but not found among the preset Phrases. The
computer analysis of the use of free text is a major input to the Phrase Review Working
Party.

Care Profiles, tailored to suit the individual requirements laid down by each ward
sister, are made up of orders chosen from Pages, or actual Pages themselves which are
displayed for items to be selected, eg from Assessment Pages 77-79. The orders may be
accepted directly or rejected. Care Profiles can contain orders which require a data
entry and these are displayed for the nurse to complete or reject as appropriate.

The list of numbers and titles of all Pages and of each Ward's own Care Profiles is
attached at the side of the VDU for easy reference.

EXAMPLE OF A FICTITIOUS CASE

The best way to demonstrate the use of the system is to take a fictitious patient,
Bill Jones, say, who is a 39 year old single schoolmaster who is known to be diabetic
and on insulin. He has been on a strenuous walking holiday in Austria staying in moun-
tain refuges and did not remove his socks for several days. He is now being admitted
as an emergency with extensive ulceration of the right foot which is heavily infected
and has small black areas. He is rather thin and wears contact lenses to correct his
shortsightedness. He is for theatre for de-sloughing and toileting. The nurse takes
note of the patient's history on admission using a prompt sheet and expressing her
assessment in her own words. At the VDU she then sets up the initial nursing care
plan to enable her knowledge to be communicated to all the other staff who require it.
The nurse gains access to the system by typing in her own password. This is not displayed on the screen, but is passed direct to the system which checks its validity and
retrieves her user access code, initials and unique identity from the User Detail File.
The ward's layout screen is transmitted to the VDU together with the choice of nursing
systems. She selects Orders for the patient by typing O and number 15, underlined in
figure 1.

```
)                                    AVON                    NURSING SYSTEMS
   SINGLE ROOMS  -----------------------------------------------------------
                 ----------------------   14 AUDREY FARMER    30 ALYS B CHANDLER
    11 ANDREA OSTLER                       5 ALFRED MILLINER  28 ALBERT BAKER
  BAY G                                   ----------------------------------
   29 ALEXIA HAWKER                                           18 ANN AMELIA COOPER
                 ----------------------   3 ANNABEL C GROCER  17 AMANDA M POTTER
  BAY H          ----------------------------------------------------------
    15 BILL J JONES                       10 ALAN L COLLIER   4 ANTHONY COOK
     2 ARTHUR JOHN SAWYER                 19 ARAN G CARPENTER
  BAY J          ----------------------------------------------------------
    22 ALISON JANE SKINNER                13 ANNIE S FORRESTER 16 ALICE MARY PRINTER
     9 AGATHA T TAYLOR                    25 AUGUSTA BUTLER   20 ANTONIA L MILLER
  BAY K          ----------------------------------------------------------
     8 ALGERNON FOWLER                    24 ANTONY D BUTCHER  6 ADRIAN GARDNER
     7 ALDRED JAMES SMITH                 27 ALLEN E SHEPHERD 23 ALBAN A LAWYER
  DAY/EXTRA BEDS ----------------------------------------------------------
                 ----------------------   ----------------------  ----------------------
                 ----------------------   ----------------------  ----------------------
```

Indicate by O,R,A,D or P the order in which Orders,Reports,Admission,Discharge
or Position in Ward is required:-(O   )
If Orders or Reports is required then type the numbers of the patients in the
order required:-(15

)
If printing is required,indicate here( )

                              Figure 1

Bill Jones has nothing yet set up on his Care Plan, so the choice of this ward's Care
Profiles is displayed. These include "80 - Assessment on Admission" and "81 -
Emergency Admission" etc.
Having just taken note of the patient's condition on admission the nurse first wishes
to communicate the salient items and the care she deems appropriate to cope with the
individual requirements of the patient. She has noted that he is diabetic and will
need Urine Tests (Page 20) and Blood Tests (Page 22). He is very thin and will need

```
                    10.11.81------Today-
                    ((  )WEARS CONTACT LENS(ES), BOTH,NOT TO WEAR LENSES WHILE DROWSY,REPLACE AS SOON
                    (       AS SAFE.
Profile—(  ( )MOBILITY,INFECTED FOOT ULCER:CONTROL INFECTION.
   80    (  ( )THIN,RELIEVE PRESSURE.
         (  ( )DIABETIC.
         ((  )APPLY SHEEPSKIN BOOT(S), LEFT.
Page 4 —{(  )NURSE PATIENT ON SHEEPSKIN.
         ((  )KEEP RIGHT HEEL OFF BED.
Page 20—(  )TEST URINE FOR SUGAR & KETONE BODIES, EVERY SPECIMEN.
Page 22—(  )BLOOD GLUCOSE ESTIMATIONS (B.M.STIX).
                                                    ——Profile 81 selected next

         Type C, D or T before an order to be CHANGED, DELETED or TERMINATED
         List other page numbers:-(81 ←                                         )
         Next patient( )Continue preset path( )Report for this patient( )WRONG PATIENT( )
```

Figure 2

additional pressure area care, so the Page containing Phrases specific to Relief of
Pressure (4) is also selected. The Assessment on Admission Profile, 80, follows these
Pages and the result of this use of the system is to be seen in the top part of
figure 2 where we have noted beside each order the Page or Profile from which it was
selected. On this screen the nurse then selects Profile 81, Emergency Admission.
Figure 3 then shows all the orders automatically offered as a result of this Profile.

```
)MR   WILLIAM JAMES JONES            M  39YEARS    WHO  333333
10.11.81------Today-
  ( )WEARS CONTACT LENS(ES), BOTH,NOT TO WEAR LENSES WHILE DROWSY,REPLACE AS SOON
      AS SAFE.
  ( )MOBILITY,INFECTED FOOT ULCER:CONTROL INFECTION.
  ( )THIN,RELIEVE PRESSURE.
  ( )DIABETIC.
  ( )APPLY SHEEPSKIN BOOT(S), LEFT.
  ( )NURSE PATIENT ON SHEEPSKIN.                                        **
Mark deletions,terminations: accept orders,from Today, Tomorrow  or Date  WRONG
BED BATH.----------------------------------------- (/)    ( )  ( .11.81) ( )
MOUTHWASH,AS REQUIRED.----------------------------- (/)    ( )  ( .11.81) ( )
CHANGE POSITION OF PATIENT 2-HOURLY.--------------- (/)    ( )  ( .11.81) ( )
BED REST.------------------------------------------ (/)    ( )  ( .11.81) ( )
INTRAVENOUS FLUIDS AS PRESCRIPTION SHEET.---------- (/)    ( )  ( .11.81) ( )
RECORD TEMPERATURE,PULSE,BLOOD PRESSURE
    6xDAILY.---------------------------------------- (/)    ( )  ( .11.81) ( )
RECORD WEIGHT WEEKLY ON MON.----------------------- (/)    ( )  ( .11.81) ( )
ROUTINE URINE TEST.-------------------------------- (/)    ( )  ( .11.81) ( )
MIDSTREAM SPECIMEN OF URINE.----------------------- ( )    ( )  ( .11.81) (/)
PASS NASO-GASTRIC TUBE.---------------------------- ( )    ( )  ( .11.81) (/)
NOTHING BY MOUTH,TILL SEEN BY DR.------------------ (/)    ( )  ( .11.81) ( )
CHECK CONSENT FORM.-------------------------------- (/)    ( )  ( .11.81) ( )
PREMEDICATION.------------------------------------- (/)    ( )  ( .11.81) ( )
INFORM RELATIVES OF PROCEDURE.--------------------- (/)    ( )  ( .11.81) ( )
```

Figure 3

The orders required have been accepted by marking in the 'Today' column whereas unwanted ones must be marked in the 'WRONG' column. One order SHAVE /named part/ will
have been displayed on an intermediate screen as a data entry would be required and
in this case it was rejected at that stage. The end result is a specifically set up
Care Plan tailored to correspond to the needs of Bill Jones, see figure 4.

BILL JONES   333333 WHO ------------1557-HOURS-10.11.81---Tuesday
----

          Special Needs & Precautions
WEARS CONTACT LENS(ES), BOTH,NOT TO WEAR LENSES WHILE
 DROWSY,REPLACE AS SOON AS SAFE.
MOBILITY,INFECTED FOOT ULCER:CONTROL INFECTION.
THIN,RELIEVE PRESSURE.
DIABETIC.

          Basic Care
BED BATH.   (AEH)
MOUTHWASH,AS REQUIRED.   (AEH)
CHANGE POSITION OF PATIENT 2-HOURLY.   (chart)
APPLY SHEEPSKIN BOOT(S), LEFT.   (AEH)
NURSE PATIENT ON SHEEPSKIN.   (AEH)
KEEP RIGHT HEEL OFF BED.   (AEH)

          Mobility
BED REST.   (AEH)

          Diet & Fluids
INTRAVENOUS FLUIDS AS PRESCRIPTION SHEET.   (TTT)

          Observations & Recordings
RECORD TEMPERATURE,PULSE,BLOOD PRESSURE 6xDAILY.   (TTT,TTT,AEH,AEH,
                                                      18,22)
RECORD WEIGHT WEEKLY ON MON.   (--)

          Tests & Investigations
ROUTINE URINE TEST.   (TTT)
TEST URINE FOR SUGAR & KETONE BODIES, EVERY SPECIMEN. (TTT)
BLOOD GLUCOSE ESTIMATIONS (B.M.STIX).   (AEH)

          Technical Care
NOTHING BY MOUTH,TILL SEEN BY DR.
CHECK CONSENT FORM.   (AEH)
PREMEDICATION.   (chart)
INFORM RELATIVES OF PROCEDURE.   (AEH)

Figure 4

As the various requirements for our patient are met the nurse reports those carried out
by signing-on as usual with her individual password and marking on the VDU by the side
of the order carried out. The Reporting System supplies her initials, see Care Plan,
figure 4, and her unique identity is retained for legal purposes on the daily record.
This record is eventually microfiched for long term storage. The order remains there
the following day so that the care and a report are prompted each day, and recorded
each day until the nurse consciously removes the order from the Care Plan. Post oper-
atively, when the patient is fully conscious, the note about his lenses may be amended,
but the fact of their use is easily retained, thus, a problem and its action are
amended without cluttering the record or losing any information as the original phrase
will be retained both on microfiche and in the Discharge Summary.
As he progresses Bill will require instructions concerning his diet from the point of
view of his diabetes and a noted loss of weight. He is to be weighed twice weekly and

needs to see a dietician to organise some diet suitable to build up weight, while still controlling his diabetes. The daily care is constantly being reviewed, for example, "Full weight bearing, wearing special shoe" now replacing "Non weight bearing". In each case the phrase is amended simply, efficiently, and legibly and the old record is always retained. Figure 5 shows the VDU display at this stage. The amended statements are underlined.

```
)MR   WILLIAM JAMES JONES                M  39YEARS    WHO  333333
20.11.81------Today-
     WEARS CONTACT LENS(ES), BOTH.
     MOBILITY:RIGHT FOOT:KEEP INFECTION FREE:MOBILISE.
     THIN,LOSING WEIGHT.
     DIABETIC:CONTROL.
     BATH WITH HELP.
     APPLY SHEEPSKIN BOOT(S), LEFT.
     NURSE PATIENT ON SHEEPSKIN.
     KEEP RIGHT HEEL OFF BED.
*    WALK, FULL WEIGHT BEARING,WEARING SPECIAL SHOE, RIGHT LEG.
     DIET:DIABETIC 180-GRAMS CARBOHYDRATE.
     RECORD TEMPERATURE,PULSE 2xDAILY.
     RECORD WEIGHT 2xWEEKLY ON MON & THUR.
     TEST URINE FOR SUGAR & KETONE BODIES, BEFORE MEALS.
     BLOOD GLUCOSE ESTIMATIONS (B.M.STIX).
     CLEAN WOUND WITH EUSOL, HALF STRENGTH.
     APPLY DRESSING AS PRESCRIPTION SHEET.



  )**) If Update is correct, make choice below & SEND to RECORD this UPDATE )**)
  Continue  preset path( )         Nursing Reports for this patient( )
  More Orders for this patient( )  Nothing further( )      WRONG UPD/TES/PATIENT( )
```

Figure 5

BENEFITS AND CONCLUSIONS

A quantitative evaluation of the effects of computerisation on the Nursing Record has been carried out and a paper presented on the subject at this conference.[3] At the time the study was carried out in Exeter (1978) the concept of Care Profiles had not been introduced nor was initialled reporting taking place. This would influence the only adverse conclusion "that the Nursing record took longer to maintain". In addition we now cannot ignore the fact of the cyclic "process" in Nursing and all the essential extra documentation which this leads to in manually maintained records. Thus the conclusions of Kumpel and Davis would, even in 1978 point to significant improvement in the record. However, the system in Exeter gives not only an improved orders record but also a clear record of care actually carried out and a summary of all care given to each individual patient, available on the printer at any time on request and automatically provided on discharge. In addition the system has shown great potential for use in the process of defining, reporting on and evaluating care.

Admission, Transfer and Discharge not only append information to the Hospital Administration system giving current patient whereabouts, accessible on VDU by patient name or number, but also enable bedstates to be produced automatically for Hospital Administration, Ward and Management purposes.

The patient's Nursing records provide further management information, not the least being daily workload figures for all patients and all wards. These, plotted monthly, show some obvious areas needing investigation eg Weekend ward use. The Profiles set minimum standards agreed by ward and management. Study of their use and of the individual Care Plans can give useful information leading to predicted workload patterns, the scheduling of waiting list admissions to smooth out workload levels, and afford a basis for accurate costing of individual cases. We consider that gaps in communication are hazardous to patients. It is observed by nurses in Exeter that the system leads to an improved record of care and to more effective communication.

ACKNOWLEDGEMENTS

The authors would like to acknowledge the work of the Computer Liaison Nurse, Mrs. C. Brenton and the Ward Sisters and staff of the Royal Devon & Exeter Hospital (Wonford).

REFERENCES

(1) Central Health Services Council (1956). The Standardisation of Hospital Medical Records (Tunbridge Report) HMSO, London.
(2) HEAD A.E. Maintaining the Nursing Record with the Aid of a Computer. MEDCOMP 77, Berlin. ISBN 0 903796 16X, ONLINE Conferences Ltd, 1977, Uxbridge, UK. pp469-483.
(3) KUMPEL Z. DAVIS A. Quantitative Evaluation of the effects of Computerisation on the Nursing Record. MIE 82, Dublin, Conference Proceedings to be published by Springer-Verlag - Lecture notes in Medical Informatics.

NURSE ALLOCATION WITH COMPUTER ASSISTANCE -

EXTENSION TO A MANPOWER PLANNER

George Maguire, Jean Roberts
Lancaster District Health Authority
Lancaster
United Kingdom

SUMMARY

The School of Nursing in the Lancaster District is relatively small with three
hundred nurses in training at any time. The task of scheduling School/Block, Leave
and Specialty training periods falls to the Nurse Allocations Officer. The manual
calculation of course interactions is very time consuming. The time required for
testing possible alternative schemes and modifications becomes prohibitive. A computer program was designed to allow the input and definition of data on training
courses of differing durations and with different numbers of trainees per intake.
The overlaying of these course structures produced the potential local on each location per week. Extensions to the program provide management information on available resources.

1. INTRODUCTION

The Lancaster District School has one hundred and seventy eight students and one
hundred and twelve pupil nurses in training at any time. The learners have a dual
role both to undertake relevant training to result in qualification and to offer
'pairs of hands' on the wards. About thirty per cent of the nursing manpower is
provided by learners and the proportion of bedside care provided by them is significantly greater.

At any time it is necessary for both service and school managers to know the potential workload in their department. This indication should be made available as early
as possible. The Allocations Officer has the task of tuning the training schemes
within the General Nursing Council (GNC) training requirements (1) to provide an
even flow of nurses to the wards. The skill lies in minimizing the peaks and
troughs and wide divergences of skills offered to the wards. A computer program is
an aid, releasing the Allocations Officer to integrate ad hoc courses and modified
schemes effectively.

2. THE LOCAL SITUATION

Contrary to the requirements of a large Nursing School, Lancaster has to specifically allocate to ward level not specialties because of the limited locations available for teaching. The complex mathematical wastage factors build into models such as at the London Hospital (2) cannot be applied to a school where the wasting of one learner imposes a seven per cent wastage immediately. The allocations officer can instinctively predict in which year (and intake) wastage is most likely to occur but no finite quantification can be applied.

WEEK NO.	157	158	159	160	161	162	163	164	165
LOCATION									
School	14		28	28		14			28
Surg.1	2	4	4	4	4	4	4	5	5
Night	1	1	1	1	1	1	1		
Surg.2	3	5	5	5	5	5	5	6	6
Night	1	1	1	1	1	1	1		
Surg.4	3	5	5	5	5	5	5	6	6
Night	1	1	1	1	1	1	1		
Surg.5	2	4	4	4	3	3	3	4	4
Night	1				1	1	1		
Chest	5	4	4	1	5	5	5	6	5
Night	3	2	2	1	1	1	1		1
Med.3	6	4	5	1	6	6	5	6	6
Night	3	3	2	1	1	1	2	1	1
Med.6	8	5	6	2	6	6	5	7	7
Night	3	3	2	1	2	2	3	1	1
Geriatric	13	13	13	12	12	12	13	13	13
District	1	1	1	2	2	2	1	1	1
Paediatrics	5	5	5	5	5	5	5		
SCBU	4	4	4	4	4	4	4		
Child	5	5	5	5	5	5	5		
Theatre	7	7	7	7	7	7		7	7
Casualty	7	7	7	7	7	7		7	7
CCU			2	2	2	2	2	2	2
ICU			2	2	2	2	2	2	2
Ortho.	6	6	6	6	6	6	6	7	6
Night	1	1	1	1	1	1	1		1
Gynae	6	6	6	6	6	5	7	7	6
Night	1	1	1	1	1	2			1
Opthal.			2	2	2	2	2	2	2
ENT			2	2	2	2	2	2	2
Derm.			3	3	3	3	3	3	3
Cubicles			2	2	2	2	2	2	2
G/U			1	1	1	1	1	1	1
Pool					14	14	14		
Leave	42	42		14	14		28	42	14

FIGURE 1: SECTION OF A PROPOSED TRAINING SCHEME SHOWING THE PROJECTED LOAD ON EACH WARD LOCATION USED FOR TRAINING.

This tool starts off as a projected forecast of the potential load brought about by the implementation of particular schemes (Figure 1). Once a scheme is operational it should not be altered for the learners on that course. The service managers need an up to date monitor of the actual personnel available to them.

3. THE SERVICE REQUIREMENT

The actual manpower must be identifiable by night/day duty. The general aim in the Lancaster District is to deploy the limited known resources as efficiently as possible.

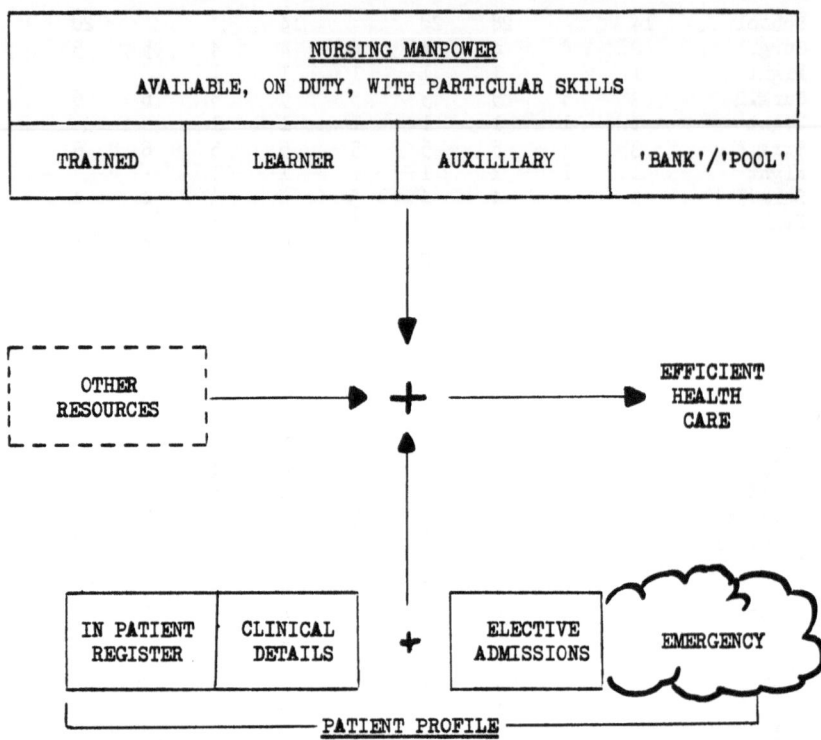

FIGURE 2: SOME FACTORS INVOLVED IN PROVIDING EFFICIENT HEALTH CARE

4. COMPUTER PROGRAM

The computer program is written in the high level language Coral-66 (3) operational on the Ferranti Argus 700 equipment located in the Lancaster Health District. Currently the program is run by Computer Services personnel under instructions from the Allocations Officer about proposed training schemes. The policy of the District (4) is to make systems operable without requiring trained computer operations staff. This Nursing project is designed to be runnable by the user department. It will be transferred when a visual display unit is installed in the School of Nursing.

5. DEVELOPMENT

It will become increasingly necessary to have accurate information on nursing manpower available as we move towards the calculation of nursing care required by each
ward (Figure 2). Our In-patient register will be used to create a requirement based
on clinical patient state. For example, if a ward has on a particular day a high
proportion of immediately post-operative patients the absence of the one nurse may
require more immediate cover than on a ward with mainly pre-operative patients and
the workforce may be transferred temporarily on this account.

The creation of the Nursing Manpower Planner is a phased procedure. Firstly the
projected training load is modified by actual attendances, transfers to other locations, sickness and absences. When nurses terminate training this needs to be
input to the schedule as this will cause an ongoing shortfall in the remaining
specialties which the nurse would have moved into subsequently.

To give Nurse managers a tool to more effectively assess the 'pairs of hands' on a
ward we must map the trained nurses on duty onto the actual nurses in training
available to the District to cover shortfalls for whatever cause. No attempt is
made at this stage to consider the quality or grade of the staff available. Assessment of this overall availability then allows more effective use of the "Nurse Bank"
or "Pool of Trained Nurses" available to the District to cover shortfalls for whatever cause. Frustration of the service centres round getting the nurse at the point
of delivery of care at the right time. There can, of course, be too much reliance
upon learners as service pairs of hands.

6. CONCLUSIONS

One benefit that has been found from using computer assistance in assessing potential nurse training plans is that alternatives can be calculated and considered
quickly. Once a scheme is approved it can be made available to service managers/
nurse tutors and the learner nurses in a short period of time. The Allocations
Officer is then able to devote more time to integrating ad hoc courses efficiently.

The extension of the computer produced projection to a manpower planner gives early
warnings of shortfalls and overloads to service managers allowing them to react in a
more timely (and hopefully successful) way to the situation. In Lancaster, areas of
shortfall have been identified and information passed onto service managers. Modification of Leave arrangements, duty rotas and the use of Bank Nurses avoided

potential crisis situations on the wards.

The principles of good training, better patient care and better resource management will all benefit from the controlled use of computer assistance.

REFERENCES

1. Directory of Schools of Nursing "GNC Requirements" HMSO (1980) 4th Edition p.4

2. A computer-aided interactive procedure to improve nurse training programmes.
   A.R. Shah Med. Inform. (1979) Vol.4 No.4 209-218

3. CORAL-66 LANGUAGE SPECIFICATION (Ferranti Computer Systems Ltd).

4. Computer Applications Working Group - Policy Statement concerning the Application of Computers in the Lancaster Health District (Internal Document KB/BB/34) March 1981.

UTILIZING AN ON-LINE COMPUTER SYSTEM FOR PATIENT
CLASSIFICATION AND STAFF DETERMINATION

Anne N. Gebhardt
Director Special Projects, Nursing
Brigham and Women's Hospital
75 Francis St., Boston, MA   02115

SUMMARY

This paper describes an on-line patient classification program operated from each nursing care unit. The patients are evaluated according to CRT screen menus of care needs by the care unit nurses. The program then weights each patient and assigns a care level. Daily summaries of these weights and their attendant staffing levels are available to administrators for guidance and justification in assigning personnel, establishing costs of care, and future planning. The logic and input/output of this program are a joint development between nursing and computer personnel.

INTRODUCTION

The need to determine, evaluate, and document patient care needs and nursing interventions in relation to the amount and cost of nursing care provided per patient has been a concern of nursing administrators, hospital administrators, trustees, and/or private and public agencies that have responsibility for the financial well-being of an institution and cost containment of health care. No longer can a nursing director justify the need for increased budgetary allowance by such categorical statements as "our patients are sicker" or "patient care is more complex." Hospital administrators or those who hold the purse strings need documentation, facts, and figures to validate such requests. As health care has become a big business, its components must conduct their affairs in a businesslike fashion. JCAH regulations, Cost Containment, Cost Effectiveness, Fee for Service, Case Mix Payment Systems, and DRGs (Diagnostic Related Grouping for Reimbursement) are terms which are here with us now and will surely become significantly more important in the near future.[1,2]

How can a nursing director justify staffing requests or requirements? What kind of data is needed? How is it accumulated, stored, rearranged, retrieved, and interpreted in light of other data? What data is available if one of the proposed reimbursement programs becomes a reality and nursing care requirements for specific patient groupings must be predicted? One source of valuable data can be obtained through a good patient classification system.[3,4,5,6] In this age of computer technology used by a wide variety of businesses and industries, it behooves nursing to develop computerized applications which will enhance the business aspect of a nursing department.[7,8]

BACKGROUND

The merger of three hospitals to form the Brigham and Women's Hospital and the subsequent move of these three divisions into one large new 638-bed facility provided the impetus for the Nursing Department to review its Patient Classification Systems. Although each of the hospitals has had a classification system that served them reasonably well in their former settings, no one of these would suffice for all in the new agency. This paper does not intend to deal with the methodology of establishing a patient categorization system, but rather with the implementation of the resulting assessment tool in an on-line computer system to facilitate use of the tool for patient classification, nurse staffing prediction, patient acuity levels, trends, and storage of data for future retrieval.

However, for background information purposes, a Patient Classification Committee was established by the Nursing Department with representation from in-house clinical divisions representing Critical Care, Medical-Surgical, Obstetrics/Gynecology, and Rheumatology and Orthopedic nursing. This committee, with input from all levels of nursing staff, determined the need for five categories ranging from minimal care to critical care with a prototype definition for each. Then a list of 24 patient care indicators, which would be common to all patient needs, was developed and each indicator was assigned a weight. In order to accommodate the differences in patient needs in each of the specialties for any one indicator, each specialty developed its own weighting system (Obstetrics/Gynecology is not completed at this time). Next, parameters were established to classify patients as Class I, II, III, IV, or V according to the sum of the indicators, again by specialty. Nurse staffing requirements or Full Time Equivalents (FTEs) can be based on these five classifications.

The use of any classification tool in the past has been cumbersome and time consuming. Nursing staff on the patient care units usually place patient categorization low on the priority list when patient care activity levels are high. The person most qualified to use the classification tool is the nurse at the patient bedside. She/he is most cognizant of the patient needs and this knowledge should be utilized in determining patient classifications. All too often the nurse sees such work as a chore, busy work, or something "the office" requires that has little relevance to her or him in the daily performance of nursing care. In many situations, the finished product may not truly reflect the patient care needs because of either underestimation or overestimation. Furthermore, tally sheets are usually forwarded to a nursing office where secretarial or supervisory staff total, compute, record, and interpret the data -- a tedious and routine task. All this, of course, leads to haphazard classification, inadequate or untimely data for staffing determinations, and incomplete or unreliable statistics.

No matter how sophisticated a classification system is, or how objective the assessment tool is, the success of the program is dependent on the individuals responsible for the completion of the tool. Therefore, any measure to simplify this process will enhance the probability of complete and reliable results. The staff should understand the program and be given periodic feedback on the results of their efforts.

METHOD

The Brigham and Women's Hospital is fortunate to have an on-line computer system with a CRT (cathode-ray tube) on each nursing unit. This is being utilized by the nursing staff for such programs as nursing care plans, laboratory orders and results, etc. Therefore, it is logical that such a system available to the nurse who is actually giving the patient care should be utilized on the patient care unit as the entry point for the classification program. While the assessment tool is on trial in a manual application, the computer program design is in process and minor changes can be made if necessary.

The computer system is an on-line system with remote communications from the nursing units. Response time is about one-second delay. Each station has a CRT, keyboard, selector pen (light pen), and printer. The nursing staff has been instructed in the use of this equipment and a variety of programs. The nurse can complete an individual patient classification assessment tool via CRT very rapidly (within 5 to 15 seconds). Typically, the nurse will be responsible for assessing 15 patients.

The nurse enters the Patient Order Entry screen and light pens "Care Level." See Figure 1.

INPATIENT MASTER FILE
```
    ROOM = 14A112    NAME = DOE, JANE                       MRN = 000-000-0
ADMITTED = 06/01/81 @ 10.30  EST LOS = 000  ACT LOS = 001   BIRTH = 12/15/1913
 SERVICE = ORT    ADMITTING DIAG = RHEUMATOID ARTHRITIS     SEX = FEMALE
                  WORKING DIAG =
 ATT DOC = 00000-0                        SPEC = ORT              AGE =
 REF DOC = 00000-0
    COND =      ACCOM =    CARE LEVEL =                     RELIG =
 ADDRESS =                                                  BLOOD =
  STREET =                                      DISCHARGED ON = / /
    CITY =                    STATE =       ZIP = 00000
ALLERGIES=
    TEAM =      RES PHY =                          H.O. =
ROOM TEL = 0000  PRIMARY NURSE =

PROBLEM LIST      DOCTORS ORDRS      CARE PLAN          VITAL SIGNS
                  CHANGE             CARE LEVEL                    GO BACK

 PFK = 1-UPDATE    2-ADD    3-NEXT    4-PREVIOUS    9-DELETE
                                                         LAST-UPD=
```

FIGURE 1

This displays the Patient Categorization screen. See Figure 2.

PATIENT CATEGORIZATION -   SELECT APPROPRIATE INDICATORS FOR THIS PATIENT

```
? ADM/TRANS/DISCH.                    ? EMOTIONAL NEEDS - COMPLEX
> PHYSICAL ACTIVITY/ADL - PARTIAL     ? EMOTIONAL NEEDS - CRISIS
? PHYSICAL ACTIVITY/ADL - COMPLETE    ? RESPIRATORY NEEDS - I
> ELIMINATION NEEDS - PARTIAL         ? RESPIRATORY NEEDS - II
? ELIMINATION NEEDS - COMPLETE        > DRESSINGS - SIMPLE
> NUTRITIONAL NEEDS - I               ? DRESSINGS - COMPLEX
? NUTRITIONAL NEEDS - II              ? ISOLATION - SIMPLE
> FLUID & ELECTROLYTES - I            ? ISOLATION - COMPLEX
? FLUID & ELECTROLYTES - II           > SPECIAL INTEGUMENTARY NEEDS
? FLUID & ELECTROLYTES - III          > ASSESSMENT, OBSERVATION - I
? SPECIAL MEDICATIONS                 ? ASSESSMENT, OBSERVATION - II
> LEARNING NEEDS - I
? LEARNING NEEDS - II
                        COMPLETED BY:

         READY       LAST UPDATED ON 00/00/00 AT 00/00/00 BY:

 PFK =   1-UPDATE    2-ADD    3-NEXT    4-PREVIOUS    9-DELETE
 RECORD HAS BEEN UPDATED.                             LAST-UPD= 07/16/81
```

FIGURE 2

     As the nurse selects an appropriate indicator with the light pen, the question
mark changes to a pointer and the indicator is highlighted. If the nurse selects
the wrong indicator, the error can be quickly corrected by light penning the indicator again and the pointer will return to the question mark. When the list has
been completed, the nurse signs (types in) her name and light pens "READY" to fina-
lize the process. The computer will respond with the update time, date, and name
of nurse.

What is not seen by the nurse during this process is the weighting program. Figure 3 shows the weights for the indicators for a Rheumatology/Orthopedic patient. The weight of the indicators selected has been underlined in this illustration. These weights will be totalled and the computer will classify the patient according to the specific parameters into Class I, II, III, IV, or V. This will not be displayed.

```
PATIENT CATEGORIZATION  -   SELECT APPROPRIATE INDICATORS FOR THIS PATIENT

5  ADM/TRANS/DISCH.                    5  EMOTIONAL NEEDS - COMPLEX
3  PHYSICAL ACTIVITY/ADL - PARTIAL     7  EMOTIONAL NEEDS - CRISIS
6  PHYSICAL ACTIVITY/ADL - COMPLETE    1  RESPIRATORY NEEDS - I
3  ELIMINATION NEEDS - PARTIAL         4  RESPIRATORY NEEDS - II
4  ELIMINATION NEEDS - COMPLETE        1  DRESSINGS - SIMPLE
2  NUTRITIONAL NEEDS - I               6  DRESSINGS - COMPLEX
6  NUTRITIONAL NEEDS - II              2  ISOLATION - SIMPLE
3  FLUID & ELECTROLYTES - I            6  ISOLATION - COMPLEX
5  FLUID & ELECTROLYTES - II           5  SPECIAL INTEGUMENTARY NEEDS
6  FLUID & ELECTROLYTES - III          3  ASSESSMENT, OBSERVATION - I
5  SPECIAL MEDICATIONS                 5  ASSESSMENT, OBSERVATION - II
3  LEARNING NEEDS - I
6  LEARNING NEEDS - II
                         COMPLETED BY:

          READY      LAST UPDATED ON 00/00/00 AT 00/00/00 BY:

PFK=   1-UPDATE   2-ADD   3-NEXT   4-PREVIOUS   9-DELETE
                                                 LAST-UPD= 07/16/81
                         FIGURE 3
```

The Nursing Department must determine the frequency of classification of patients -- whether it should be completed by a specified time each day or prior to each shift change. The computer will then compute the total number of patients in each class, and according to predetermined formula, indicate the number of staff required for each care level for three shifts. See Figure 4.

```
07/16/81             ** NURSING STATION MASTER **              14.09.30

           NURSING STATION:  14A                STATUS: A
              DESCRIPTION:   FLOOR 14  POD A
                     UNIT:   1  LOCATION: P
               FIRST ROOM:   14AV01  AUTHORIZED BEDS: 018

              FTE STAFF REQUIRED PER CARE LEVEL

     CARE LEVEL: 1    STAFF REQUIRED/SHIFT - 1: 00.200  2: 00.090  3: 00.080
     CARE LEVEL: 2    STAFF REQUIRED/SHIFT - 1: 00.300  2: 00.250  3: 00.160
     CARE LEVEL: 3    STAFF REQUIRED/SHIFT - 1: 00.450  2: 00.400  3: 00.325
     CARE LEVEL: 4    STAFF REQUIRED/SHIFT - 1: 00.750  2: 00.750  3: 00.650
     CARE LEVEL: 5    STAFF REQUIRED/SHIFT - 1: 01.000  2: 01.000  3: 01.000

PFK=   1-UPDATE   2-ADD   3-NEXT   4-PREVIOUS   9-DELETE
                                                 LAST-UPD=
                         FIGURE 4
```

This information can be obtained for each nursing unit or other summary combination. If the classification is to be completed by a specific time each day, the computer will indicate whether or not all patient classification menus have been completed. Future plans are that it will inform the user which ones need updating.

To take this program a step further, the data for each clinical nursing division will be displayed in summary form and may be used in the Staffing Office as a guide for daily allocation of staff.

CRITIQUE

What are some of the problems that might be encountered? How is feedback provided to the staff nurse? Staff allocation might be one direct effect. Earlier it was stated that the patient's class (I, II, III, IV, V) would not be displayed. This is intentional on the part of the designers of the Classification System in an attempt to maintain objectivity in the program. For instance, if the nurse thought that a higher classification might result in more nurse staff for the unit, manipulation of the tool might occur. On the other hand, if class levels are consistently low and staff predictions not adequate, the Head Nurse might reorient the staff to the use of the assessment menu or reevaluate the weight program. These types of problems can occur in a manual system also.

Often due to unavailability of a bed on the specialty unit of choice for a patient, the patient is located on a unit whose care has a different focus than that required for this patient. Therefore, the program design must include provision for weighting the patient according to his care specialty rather than his location within the hospital. For example, an orthopedic patient on a medical unit would be automatically weighted with orthopedic values.

Weekly, monthly, quarterly, or yearly summaries of data can be easily retrieved. The data may indicate overstaffing for particular mixes of patients. Other information which can be entered into the program might include how many staff are actually provided, how many are float or supplementary staff.

In summary, classification of patients using an on-line system can be accomplished with ease with the added benefit of a data base for a variety of programs. The most important point here is that the Nursing Director must interact with the computer development staff to indicate what information is desired, what is relevant to the day-to-day operation of the department, and what is necessary documentation for budget justification or other statistical programs.

BIBLIOGRAPHY

(1) Bentley JD, Ph.D., Butler PW, MHSA. "Describing and paying hospitals - developments in patient case mix." Association of American Medical Colleges May 1980.

(2) Fetter RB, et al. "Case mix definition by diagnosis-related groups." Supplement to Medical Care February 1980; 18.2.

(3) Chagnon M, et al. A patient classification system by level of nursing care requirements. Nursing Research 1978; 27(2): 107.

(4) Giovannetti P. Understanding patient classification systems. J. Nursing Administration 1979; 9(2): 4-9.

(5) Reinert P, Grant D. A classification system to meet today's needs. J. Nursing Administration 1981; 11(1): 21-30.

(6) Barham V, Schneider WR. Matrix: a unique patient classification system. J. Nursing Administration 1980; 10(12): 25-31.

(7) Somers JB. Information systems: the process of development. J. Nursing Administration 1979; 9(1): 53-58.

(8) Duraiswamy N, et al. Using computer simulation to predict ICU staffing needs. J. Nursing Administration 1981; 11(2): 39-44.

REGIONAL STUDY OF COMMUNITY NURSING POLICY

T. Bates,   Senior Operational Research Scientist

S.A. Dobra, Operational Research Scientist,
             North East Thames Regional Health Authority,
             The John Ellicott Centre,
             Cavell Street,
             The London Hospital,
             Whitechapel, London,
             England.

L. Harding, Regional Nurse (Personnel and Training),
             North East Thames Regional Health Authority,
             40, Eastbourne Terrace,
             Paddington, London,
             England.

SUMMARY

At the invitation of the Nursing Division of the North East Thames Regional Health
Authority, a study of community nursing has been undertaken.   The objectives of the
study were to assess how resources are used, to suggest how resources could be more
effectively deployed, to determine indicators of need and to suggest appropriate
staffing levels throughout the Region.   Implementation of the findings has been
achieved in two of the districts surveyed;   further implementation is expected in
subsequent health districts.

1   INTRODUCTION

1.1 Background to Study

In order to plan future allocation of resources to community nursing services, the
Regional Nursing Division requested the Operational Research Section to conduct a broad
study of community nursing in the Region.   In this paper the research findings with
respect to general practitioner attachment for home nurses will be discussed.   At
present, the North East Thames Regional Health Authority supports the introduction of
general practitioner attachment schemes.   With general practitioner attachment each
nurse is allocated to a specific general practitioner's patients, in comparison with
the traditional method of allocating nurses to geographical zones.   With attachment
schemes, communication between the nurse and the GP is likely to be improved.   There
have been many early studies and enquiries conducted into the formation of GP attachment schemes, for example the Harvard-Davis Report (1), R. Ann Abel of the Department
of Health's Social Science Research Unit (2), most early papers reported favourably
towards GP attachment.

It should, however, be recognised that these early studies were conducted on attachment schemes, where there was commitment from all members of the team. More recently there has been a growing view that GP attachment schemes do not function as well as was previously thought. A recent study by J. Hughes and J.A. Roberts of The London School of Hygiene and Tropical Medicine, into nurse managers' views of community nursing services (3), outlined the many problems faced at present in community nursing. In general, nurse managers of non GP attached nurses reported far fewer problems than nurse managers of attached nurses. There were few districts where 'satisfactory' attachment had been achieved. Most problems reported can be classified into logistic and resource problems.

1.2 Other Quantitative Studies

There have been few published quantitative studies of community nursing directed at assessing the resource implications of the range of operational policies that could be implemented by the district management. However there is a noteworthy paper on this subject by A. Fernendez, G. Gregory, A. Hindle and A.C. Lee (4). The authors developed a mathematical model of community nursing in Westmorland. The model was used to evaluate alternative attachment schemes for the district, in terms of additional mileage and staffing costs.

1.3 Present DHSS Norms

The present planning of the service is based on meeting target DHSS per capita norms (5) without taking specific regard of opportunity costs or actual costs. The DHSS circular 13/72 recommends as a minimum norm of one home nurse per 4,000 persons resident in a district. For districts with 'extensive attachment schemes or with a high proportion of old and/or disabled people in the population' it recommends a ratio of one home nurse per 2,500 persons.

2   DATA COLLECTION

2.1 Sample

At present there is little routinely collected statistical data for community nursing which is of use to regional planners. The problem is largely due to the time needed to be spent by nurses on data collection, time which some nurses argue would be better spent in patient care. In carrying out this study, detailed surveys of the nurses' work were conducted in four districts within the Region, one in Essex, one in Outer London and two in Inner London. At present over 400 community nurses have taken part in the study, covering more than 10,000 patient visits.

2.2 Database

Each nurse filled in a coded computer entry diary sheet for each day of the survey. From this, a detailed database of community nursing, including home nursing and health visiting has been created. This has allowed detailed analysis of the work carried out and has provided parameters for mathematical modelling.

3 ANALYSIS OF DATA

3.1 General Results

The analysis of the data has shown both differences and similarities in home nursing between the districts. The data showed that on average clerical and administrative duties occupied each nurse for about one fifth of the working day. Time spent travelling occupied over one fifth of the working day, leaving less than three fifths of the day for treating patients. In a typical day the nurse will treat between six to nine patients. There is considerable variation in where 'visits' take place; in one district the nurse makes 80 percent of the visits at the patient's home, while in another district over 95 percent of the visits took place in the patient's home, the remaining visits take place at health centres, clinics and surgeries.

3.2 The Need for a Mathematical Model

At present the method of allocating community nursing resources does not include details of a districts age/sex profile, social needs, present provision of primary and secondary care facilities, and the type of nursing deployment. The research programme aimed to include all appropriate parameters into a mathematical model which would allow alternative options of deployment of resources to be assessed.

3.3 The Model

A computer based mathematical model has been developed. The model computes the whole time equivalent staffing level required and the total mileage covered in order to meet a given level of demand within a district. The model takes into account the following factors:-

a)   The percentage of visits to be carried out at health centres, clinics and surgeries.

b)   The density of visiting within the district.

c)   The mode of transport of the nurse and travel speed.

d)   The level of general practitioner attachment.

e)   The level of administrative and clerical duties undertaken by a nurse.

f)   The percentage of 'ineffective visits'.

In essence the model dynamically balances the nurses time available in half day sessions of visiting between:-

1)   Travelling

2)   Making home visits

3)   Working in a health centre, clinic or surgery.

4)   Administrative and clerical duties.

3.4 'Travelling Salesman Problem'

An element of the model involves the solution of a 'travelling salesman problem'. The incorporation of the 'travelling salesman problem' into the model, introduces an important non-linearity, which expresses the fact that as the number of visits to be made in a tour in a fixed area increases, the average distance between visits decreases. If one takes a unit square, choosing points at random where visits are to take place and also a random base point, then taking an optimum route between visits, figures 1 and 2 shows the relationship between the total visits made against the average total distance travelled and the average distance between visits.

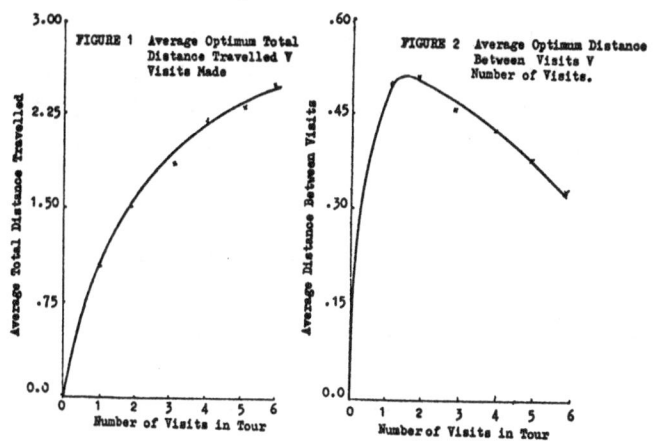

3.5   Description of Model

The model combines factors a) to f), expressed in terms of analytical functions, together with an empirical solution of the 'travelling salesman problem' discussed, to form a single expression of the total time a nurse spends in an average session of nursing work, this is the summation of factors 1) to 4).   The model numerically solves this expression by the Newton-Raphson method, in order to compute the number of 'visits' that can be made by a nurse in a half day session of visiting.   The model then derives the total staffing requirement of a district, and an estimate of the total distance travelled by the nurses, based upon the parameters of the model.

3.6   Implementation of Model

The model has been implemented, in 500 FORTRAN Program Statements and operates in an interactive mode.

4   RESULTS

4.1   General Results

The model explains the variation in the data collected between the districts.   The survey data, showed that for the Essex District, which did not have GP attachment schemes, the average time spent travelling was 25 percent of the nurses' working day. For the Outer London District, which operated an attachment scheme, home nurses spent 21 percent of the day travelling.   The visiting density per square mile for the Outer London District was five times greater than for the Essex District.   This is largely due to the higher population density of London compared with Essex.

The average travel speed was 6 miles per hour in the Outer London District, in comparison to 15 miles per hour recorded in Essex.   In both districts, approximately 95 percent of the 'visits' take place in the patient's home. The combination of these conflicting factors, leads to both districts having their home nurses spending the same proportion of the day travelling. But with the Outer London District operating an attachment scheme and the Essex District deploying its nurses geographically.

4.2   Staffing

The survey data for the Inner London Districts showed an even slower travel speed. By car nurses travelled at an average of 4 miles per hour, and by all modes of transport at an average of 3 miles per hour. The combination of travel speed and density of visiting leads to the Essex District requiring an additional 15 percent of resources so as to provide the same standard of care as that of a typical London District, with the same level of visiting and with geographical deployment of its nurses. If full GP attachment is introduced into a London District, the model predicts that an additional 7 to 14 percent increase in establishment, would be required so as to provide the same level of visiting as a non attached district. For the Essex District, an additional 30 to 80 percent increase in staff is required, in order to provide the same level of visiting, than if the district deployed its nurses geographically.

4.3   Cost Implications for an Essex District

The model predicted that GP attachment for the Essex District would lead to an additional mileage cost of between £125,000 to £375,000 per annum at 1979 prices, for each district, which would make the total cost for a district including staffing costs at between £270,000 to £740,000 per annum at 1979 costs. The amount of increase depends on the level of GP provision.

4.4   Cost Implications for a London District

For London Districts the cost implications for attachment schemes are less severe. If up to 40 percent of the patient visits are treated in the GP's surgery, this has the effect of balancing the savings in the nurses' time for central treatment, with the increase in staff required to support an attachment scheme. There are however additional mileage costs of between £25,000 to £50,000 per annum. In terms of opportunity costs this represents 4 to 8 whole time equivalent staff, who could be deployed geographically at the same total cost.

4.5   Other Options

From these figures it can be seen why full GP attachment is rarely achieved. In order to overcome these fundamental problems of attachment schemes, districts often geographically zone patients to attached nurses or limit attachment to selected practises in an effort to reduce travelling. As a consequence these schemes lack the advantages of either full GP attachment or geographical deployment of nurses.

5   CONCLUSION

5.1   General

With attachment schemes the information flow between the GP and the nurse is said to be greater, which in turn leads to better patient care. Balanced against this is the opportunity cost measured in terms of lost patient care, brought about by increased travelling. It is not possible to quantify the benefit of GP attachment, although it is possible to quantify the cost.

5.2 Staffing Levels

The mathematical model described, with the age/sex profile of a district as an estimator of demand, has been used to derive home nursing staffing levels across the Region. The model has variations in home nursing staffing levels across the Region, taking into account population densities, traffic conditions and morbidity. These results have yet to be discussed with nurse managers. The districts location and method of deployment of staff, has a significant affect on the resources required, in order to provide a given level of care, measured in terms of visits. Without further detailed research into social factors that may affect demand for service, the age/sex indicator of demand combined with the use of the mathematical model developed, adequately describes the present situation within the Region.

5.3 Summary of the Main Findings of the Regional Study

The study of GP attachment for home nurses described in this paper, is one part of a broader study into community nursing. Research findings on both attachment for home nurses and health visitors have been produced, the method of referral and the patient's present contact with secondary care has been analysed. Further information of these studies are available in Management Services Reports, A Study of Community Nursing in Colchester District (7), Home Nursing in City and Hackney (8), Home Nursing in Tower Hamlets (9), A Study of Home Nursing Services in Haringey District (10), Health Visiting in Haringey Health District Survey Results (11) and Home Nursing Services in North East Thames Regional Health Authority (12). Further reports are in preparation. In general the GP initiates approximately 50 percent of the home nurses visits, irrespective of attachment arrangements. For health visitors, the GP initiates less than 5 percent of the visits. The data showed that in general home nurses spend less than 5 percent of the day with early discharged patients and also less than 5 percent of the day with waiting list patients. The survey data recorded the type of treatment that was carried out, where the visit took place and the grade of nurse who carried out the treatment. The data showed that a substantial proportion of the visits, up to 40 percent of all patients seen, could have been treated centrally, if there was provision for this type of service. In one of the survey districts 20 percent of all visits take place in health centres, the data showed that this figure could be almost doubled. It also showed that between 30 to 50 percent of visits could be carried out by nursing auxiliaries. At present the ratio of qualified to un-qualified staff does not reflect the nursing procedures undertaken. This result is in agreement with L. Hockey's Study (6) of the work carried out by SRN and SENs, which showed that many qualified staff considered that parts of their work could be carried out by less qualified staff.

5.4 Acceptance and Implementation

The findings of the study have been accepted in the two initial study districts, and some policy changes have been introduced with respect to attachment, grades of nurse employed and central treatment of patients; further implementation is expected in subsequent districts.

REFERENCES

1   Central Health Services Council.   The Organisation of Group Practise:
    A Report of a Sub-Committee of the Standing Medical Advisory Committee.
    (Chairman: Harvard Davis R.) London, HMSO, 1971.

2   Department of Health and Social Security, Social Science Research Unit.
    Nursing Attachments to General Practise: Staff Implications of Schemes
    for Attachment of Local Authority Staff (Health Visitors and Home Nurses)
    to General Practise, Abel R.A., DHSS Social Science Research Unit Study
    Number 1, London, HMSO, 1969.

3   Hughes J., Roberts J.A., Nurses Managers' Views of Community Nursing
    Services. Department of Community Health, London School of Hygiene and
    Tropical Medicine. London. April 1981.

4   Fernandez A., Gregory G., Hindle A., Lee A.C.   A Model of Community
    Nursing in a Rural County.   Operational Research Quarterly, 25, 231,
    Birmingham, 1974.

5   DHSS Circular 13/72. London.

6   Hockey L., Use or Abuse? A Study of the State Enrolled Nurse in the Local
    Authority Nursing Services.   Queens' Institute of District Nursing.
    London. 1972.

7   Bates T., A Study of Community Nursing Services in Colchester District
    Survey Results.   Management Services Report 1112.   North East Thames
    Regional Health Authority. London. 1981.

8   Bates T., Home Nursing in City and Hackney.   Management Services Report 1110.
    North East Thames Regional Health Authority. London. 1981.

9   Bates T., Home Nursing in Tower Hamlets.   Management Services Report 1111.
    North East Thames Regional Health Authority. London. 1981.

10 Bates T., A Study of Home Nursing Services in Haringey District.
    Management Services Report 1074.   North East Thames Regional Health
    Authority. London. 1981.

11 Bates T., Health Visiting in Haringey Health District Survey Results.
    Management Services Report 1090.   North East Thames Regional Health
    Authority. London. 1981.

12 Bates T., Home Nursing Services in North East Thames Regional Health
    Authority.   Management Services Report 1091.   North East Thames
    Regional Health Authority. London. 1981.

QUANTITATIVE EVALUATION OF THE EFFECTS OF COMPUTERISATION
ON THE NURSING RECORD

Zdenek Kumpel PhD
Exeter Community Health Services Computer Project,
Royal Devon & Exeter Hospital (Wonford),
Barrack Road, Exeter, Devon.
UK

Allen Davis,
West Midlands Regional Health Authority,
Norton Court, Queen Elizabeth Medical Centre,
Edgbaston, Birmingham.
UK

Two projects, one in Exeter and the other in Birmingham, have computerised the nursing orders section of the nursing record. Evaluation was carried out at both sites and covered both the situation before and after the introduction of the computer. Although the computer systems have been developed independently the evaluation has enabled the authors to draw conclusions about the effect of computerisation on the nursing record in general. The main effects of computerisation are:

(a) The nursing record gives a more complete and more accurate picture of the patient's needs.
(b) Clinical condition of patients is assessed more readily and quickly.
(c) The use of non-approved abbreviations has virtually been eradicated.
(d) Computer based nursing orders take slightly longer to maintain. This is outweighed by their better quality as well as by a decrease in time spent on reporting.
(e) A system similar to that in Exeter would require capital expenditure of some £10,000 per ward and over £2,900 per ward per annum to run.

1. INTRODUCTION

The nursing record is defined in this document as a permanent cumulative record of nursing care received by a patient during the inpatient episode together with observations on progress and response to treatment (other than charts). It provides the main source of information for the nursing staff for monitoring the care and treatment of patients and communicating about it, and usually consists of a nursing orders section and a nursing reports section.

Two computerised nursing record systems have been evaluated on the basis of values for performance criteria (1) that have been measured in most cases before and after the introduction of the computer. These systems are in operation at Royal Devon and Exeter Hospital (Wonford) at Exeter and Queen Elizabeth Hospital in Birmingham. The main purpose of this paper is to show that in spite of some differences in systems design there are common conclusions to be drawn about the effects of computerisation.

2. MANUAL SYSTEM

At Exeter the manual system of nursing records was based on the Kardex. It contained 30 card holders, each of which corresponded to a particular bed in the ward. Each holder contained a record for one patient only and that record consisted of at least a nursing orders card, which held patient identification information and a synopsis of the nursing care (past and present) required for that patient, and a nursing reports card which held, in addition to patient identification information, details of the patient's condition, behaviour, response to treatment etc. Frequently, continuation cards of each type were necessary.

Until 1972 a similar manual system of nursing records was in operation at Birmingham. The proliferation of other nursing documentation there, which was mainly caused by the fact that the patient-orientated orders section of the Kardex did not give the ward sister a good picture of the total ward workload, led to the separation of the nursing record into two documents. The nursing orders section of the Kardex was abolished and replaced by a nursing care list. This was a daily form (one for each ward), onto which patients' names and their nursing orders for the day were written. Each row on the form corresponded to a patient and the orders were grouped into several columns corresponding to hygiene, mobility, technical care and so on. Nursing reports section of the Kardex remained unchanged.

3. COMPUTER SYSTEM

The basic philosophies of the Birmingham and Exeter computer nursing records systems are similar (2, 3). As currently implemented only the nursing orders are operational; nursing reports and observations are still maintained manually. A structured list of a variety of phrases that constitute nursing orders is kept on a computer file. Nursing staff use ward VDUs to access this file (using tree branching techniques) in order to maintain the record of nursing orders for patients on wards. As well as the current nursing orders the computer also maintains a record of all deleted orders, thus making available the cumulative record of nursing orders for each patient. A system of passwords means that only authorised users have access to information and also makes any entry traceable back to its originator. Within this common framework the two systems show some differences.

The Exeter system makes use of a ward VDU and a ward printer terminal (the latter is shared between two wards). There is no ward printer terminal in Birmingham. Thus the Exeter system offers a greater variety of printing facilities. Although both Birmingham and Exeter systems structure the list of nursing orders by body systems, type of care, care packages, etc, the Birmingham system provides for each ward an individually tailored list of those basic and technical orders that occur most frequently on that ward. On both computer systems nursing orders are available in two modes: on the VDU and in hard copy. The Exeter hard copy is in the same form as the nursing orders on the VDU, ie patient orientated. The hard copy at Birmingham is the ward orientated nursing care list while the VDU records are patient orientated. Another useful feature of the Birmingham system is the automatic cancellation of some types of orders after a specific time.

4. RESULTS OF PERFORMANCE CRITERIA MEASUREMENTS

Out of the many recommended performance criteria (4) that were measured for nursing records this paper reports on only those that are felt by the authors to be the most relevant when determining the potential impact of computerisation on the nursing record.

4.1 Completeness and accuracy of nursing records

This performance criterion is defined as the extent to which patients' needs are covered by orders in the nursing record at any given time. It has been expected that under a computer system, a better presentation of potential orders on the ward VDU may lead to an increase of orders actually present in the nursing record. It is also argued that the automatic retention in the record of any orders that are not cancelled (Exeter), or those orders that are not subject to automatic cancellation (Birmingham), will lead to a more complete record. On the debit side it may also be argued that this facility will result in an increase in the number of superfluous orders and/or different orders.

The method adopted to measure this criterion was a peer audit using a predetermined checklist. A random selection of patient records was made on every ward included in the audit. The nurse in charge was then asked, against the checklist, to specify the nursing needs of these patients at that time. Having noted the needs a check was made against the nursing record (by a qualified nurse together with the nurse in charge) as to the presence or absence of corresponding orders. The orders were categorised into accurate, missing, different and superfluous.

An accurate order is a written order which, in the opinion of the nurse-auditor, corresponded exactly to a specific patient need. If a written order did not correspond exactly to the patient need (for instance, if "light diet" was entered where the patient need was "normal diet"), the order was categorised as different. If no written order was entered against a given need the order was classified as missing. Finally, if an order appeared in the nursing record but no patient need corresponding to that order had been stated, it was treated as superfluous.

Table I: Completeness and accuracy of nursing records (%)

	Manual		Computer	
	Birmingham	Exeter	Birmingham	Exeter
Accurate	36	32	64	52
Different	10	10	15	13
Missing	54	58	21	35
Superfluous	0	2	2	3

Table I shows, for instance, that 36% of patient needs were accurately reflected as nursing orders in the manually kept nursing orders at Birmingham. The corresponding figure for Exeter is 32%. After the introduction of computerised nursing records these figures rose to 64% and 52% for Birmingham and Exeter respectively.

The most remarkable feature of the above Table I is the high level of agreement between the Birmingham and Exeter results. In the cases of superfluous orders and different orders neither the differences between sites nor the differences between systems are statistically significant. However, the introduction of computer systems at their respective sites has resulted in a statistically significant increase in the proportion of accurate orders, ie orders that are present in the nursing record and correspond to the patient's needs; and in the correspondingly statistically significant decrease in the proportion of missing orders. As the proportion of different orders has not changed significantly, the increase in the proportion of accurate orders is due to the decrease in the proportion of missing orders, ie mainly to the fact that under both computer systems the outstanding orders are carried forward automatically which was not the case with manually kept nursing records.

A general conclusion can therefore be drawn from the above figures, viz that computerisation of nursing records in a way similar to that of Birmingham or Exeter can be expected to reduce the number of missing nursing orders by half, resulting in a corresponding increase in accuracy.

4.2 Clinical condition assessment and speed of analysis

These two performance criteria comprise aspects of determining patients' conditions from records. The most obvious feature to affect such criteria would be a computerised reporting application that encouraged staff to report on certain orders and make (via a VDU) pertinent observations. However, the systems at Exeter and Birmingham do not as yet have such an application. Nevertheless, it is hypothesised that the increase in the completeness and accuracy of the nursing order section of the record would enable nursing staff to assess a patient's clinical condition far more readily and quickly.

Because of the amount of effort necessary these two criteria were measured only in Birmingham. The method adopted to measure them was a peer audit using a pre-determined checklist. A random selection of the records gathered during the completeness/accuracy survey was used as an information base. From this base, two records (one a pre-computer, the other a post-computer record) were given to each of the nursing staff participating in the audit. The nurse was asked to scrutinise the record (consisting of a nursing report from admission to a certain day, plus the orders section for that day) and write down on the checklist provided a series of answers relating to condition and treatment. The time taken to complete the task for each of the records was noted, having ensured that half the participants started with a pre-computer record and half with a post-computer one. The checklists completed by participants were checked against the actual patients' condition (which had been established in 4.1) to determine what proportion of items of care had been gleaned from the written record. The results of the exercise are displayed in Table II below.

Table II: Clinical condition assessment and speed of analysis

Criterion	Manual		Computer		Significance
	Sample size	Mean	Sample size	Mean	
Clinical condition assessment	273 items	61%	273 items	74%	99.5% (z = 3.26)
Speed of analysis	20 nursing staff	18.3 min	20 nursing staff	15.3 min	n.s. (t = 0.37)

The results suggest, perhaps surprisingly, that despite the fact that no reporting application is operational and that reporting on orders has not changed due to computerisation, the more complete nursing orders section of the record does enable nursing staff to get a more complete picture of patients' clinical condition when used with the nursing report section. There is also evidence to suggest that, although not statistically significant, the time needed to assess a patient's condition from the partly computerised record is less than with a manual one.

4.3 Abbreviations

This criterion is defined as the extent to which abbreviations in the record are misunderstood. When examined closely this definition comprises two aspects: that of usage of abbreviations and that of interpretation of, or rather failure to interpret, an abbreviation correctly.

The use (and abuse) of abbreviations in nursing records is largely dependent on management policy. For instance before the introduction of the computer an official list of approved abbreviations was in existence at Birmingham and this list was utilised when the phrases comprising the computer-held nursing orders were compiled. No approved abbreviations existed officially at Exeter but as the computer-held file of nursing orders phrases does contain some abbreviations (such as Rt for right, GA for general anaesthetic and a few others) the management policy of having no abbreviations has perhaps been somewhat less rigid in practice.

In order to be able to guage the effect of the computer by using the figures from both locations attention has been focused only on non-approved abbreviations present in nursing orders.

Under the computer system nurses make up an order for a patient by selecting the appropriate phrases from the VDU screen. As these computer-held phrases do not contain any non-approved abbreviations the only way a non-approved abbreviation can appear in the nursing orders is by the use of the "free-text" facility on the VDU, or by writing on the hard copy of nursing orders (or nursing care list in the Birmingham case). It was therefore reasonable to expect that the proportion of orders containing non-approved abbreviations would decrease with the introduction of computer, a fact which is demonstrated in Table III below.

Table III: Proportion of orders containing non-approved abbreviations.

	Manual	Computer
Birmingham	17.9%	0.7%
Exeter	17.4%	0%

As the results show, computerisation means a dramatic decrease in the proportion of orders containing abbreviations. To judge the implications of this decrease attention must be turned to the other aspect of this criterion, viz the rate of misinterpretation.

Although the usage of abbreviations depends on what system of nursing record keeping is in operation, failure to interpret abbreviations is independent of whether the system is computerised or not. To obtain an insight into the consequences of the use of abbreviations it was not necessary to measure this rate at both sites and both before and after the introduction of the computer. It was sufficient to perform this part of the study only in Birmingham where it was found that the failure rate to interpret non-approved abbreviations was 44%, ie in almost half of the cases the abbreviations were not correctly understood.

A great deal of care should be taken when making use of this figure. Failure to interpret an abbreviation correctly does not necessarily imply that the patient in question would have received wrong treatment. In most instances where a nurse did not know the correct meaning no attempt was usually made to interpret, and presumably, in the ward situation advice would have been sought. However, there was a number of abbreviations that were interpreted in several different ways - each of them seemingly logical. Their use is obviously more likely to lead to patients receiving incorrect treatment. At any rate from comments received from the participants in this exercise and from the general attitude of nursing staff using the system it is clear that the nurses feel that the fewer abbreviations used the better. By virtually eliminating the use of non-approved abbreviations computerisation brings about a marked decrease in the total use of abbreviations and it is reasonable to assume that any problems caused by abbreviating nursing orders have been alleviated by the computer system.

4.4 Record maintenance time

This performance criterion is defined as the time taken to maintain the necessary information in the nursing orders and the nursing reports sections of the nursing record. At Exeter all contacts made with nursing records in a general surgical ward were studied for two hours at a time distributed randomly between 0800 and 2100 hours on 7 consecutive days. At Birmingham activities associated with the update of orders and reporting were measured by continuous observation after the introduction of the computer. In the pre-computer stage a simplified study was performed where only the time necessary for the daily batch update of orders in the nursing care list was investigated. The results of these studies are summarised in the table below.

Table IV: Record maintenance (minutes per 8 hours of day shift)

	Manual		Computer	
	Exeter	Birmingham	Exeter	Birmingham
Orders update	16.0	14.6*	20.7	22.1
Reporting	51.3	NA	39.4	34.8

* includes only daily batch update time.

The figures seem to indicate that updating orders on the computer takes longer than used to be the case with nursing records that were kept manually. There are several reasons for this finding. Firstly, the cancellation of an order on the computer requires a positive action as opposed simply to not writing the order down in the Kardex or on the nursing care list. This increases clerical effort for all orders that are to be cancelled on the Exeter system, and for a proportion of such orders on the Birmingham system where some orders are cancelled automatically.

Furthermore, updating an existing order or adding a new order means that the user has to find the screen where the phrases corresponding to the order are displayed and indicate on this screen which phrases are to be selected. Although these activities are offset against the writing or typing of orders under the manual system, the overall effect is an increase in the required time.

The existence of a screen of orders that are most frequent on a given ward in the Birmingham system, and the ability to create an order by using shortcuts which allow to bypass the display of phrases for selection in Exeter, are two successful attempts at minimising the increase in the work effort. It must also be emphasised that the small increase in the time taken for updating the orders is more than compensated for by having nursing orders that are far more complete and accurate as has been demonstrated in 4.1. If a manually kept nursing record was to be maintained to a similar standard of completeness the effort required for this would probably be greater than with the computer.

Table IV above suggests that computerisation resulted in a decrease in the time that the nurses spend on reporting. Although computerisation of nursing orders has not changed reporting, which is still done manually, this finding is probably due to the fact that a more complete record of nursing orders enables the staff often to simply initial the order when it is completed rather than having to write a separate entry in the nursing report.

4.5 Costs

The following costing is based on an expected transfer of the nursing records system onto new equipment, which will shortly take place in Exeter. ICL ME29/45 with 768 kB of memory is thought to be sufficient to support a network of 16 local workstations (one per each of the 15 wards and another as a console) and 8 hard copy printers, as well as some 180 MB of backing store, a line printer and a magnetic tape unit. Total capital cost of equipment, including the installation charge and VAT at 15%, is some £150,370 which represents capital expenditure of approximately £10,000 per ward. At 1981 cost levels the annual revenue cost per ward is some £2,920 (including VAT at 15%).

It is assumed in the above that all operating staff are embedded in the existing management structure and no additional management costs are therefore incurred, and that they are backed for absence by nursing staff as appropriate. The machine will be housed in the hospital and no air conditioning is deemed necessary. No cabling cost has been considered but, on the other hand, neither has any discount on equipment been allowed. Maintenance will cover the hardware only during the prime shift.

The reader may find it surprising that in an age when a small business user can pick up off the shelf a variety of computer systems for less than £5,000, the projected capital cost of the nursing records system is at least twice as much. The extra cost can be partially explained by the fact that the proposed solution is a hospital based, rather than a ward based system which enables automatic collating of nursing management information for the whole hospital and provides for an interface with a patient administration system. The other reason for this comparatively high cost is the requirement to provide a computer system which is secure against accidental loss of data and confidential with respect to the access to patient information.

Finally, it should be remembered that nearly half the revenue cost is accounted for by salaries of operating staff. Although the nursing system must operate round the clock every day of the year the necessity of specialised staff to operate a modern "user-friendly" computer system has repeatedly been questioned. The true magnitude of this cost component will only be revealed when the system has been operational on new equipment for a length of time.

5. CONCLUSIONS

Although the two nursing record systems have been developed independently the evaluation results show a remarkable degree of agreement. This agreement has enabled the authors to draw conclusions about the effect of computerisation on the nursing record in general. The measures of performance reported in this paper illustrate that this effect has been considerable. The quality of the record in particular has improved at both sites. For nursing orders the measures show that the completeness and accuracy rate have increased substantially although this is offset marginally by a small increase in the number of superfluous orders being recorded; and the use of non-approved abbreviations in the orders section of the record has been reduced to a negligible level.

It has also been shown that the outcome of the above improvements to the quality of the record is to make the record as a whole more effective. It has enabled nurses to assess patients' clinical condition more readily and quickly and has considerably reduced the possibility of an order being misinterpreted. Whether or not these outcomes have led to better patient management and improved patient care has not been investigated - the authors have left that assessment to the judgement of nursing staff reading this paper.

There is evidence to support the hypothesis that the nursing orders on the computer system take slightly longer to maintain and update than the manual situation. However, it must be remembered that this small increase in update time is outweighed by the increase in the number of orders being recorded. Indeed, it seems that the effort required to maintain a manual record to the level of completeness and accuracy achieved by the computerised record would be greater than that required by the two computer systems. It seems that the time spent on reporting is decreased after computerisation.

Obviously the cost of achieving the above improvements is not inconsiderable and the report illustrates typical capital and revenue costs of computerising the nursing record.

6. REFERENCES

(1) Department of Health & Social Security, London, Performance Criteria Project Report, March 1978.

(2) Ashton C., A Nursing Record System, Symposium on Computers in Health Care, (Sperry Univac), 15-17 May 1979.

(3) Head A.E., Maintaining the Nursing Record with the Aid of a Computer, MEDCOMP 77, Berlin. ISBN 0 903796 16X, ONLINE 1977, Uxbridge, UK. pp 469-483.

(4) Department of Health & Social Security, London, Handbook on the Measurement of Performance Criteria, June 1979.

THE ROLE OF A COMPUTERISED INFORMATION SYSTEM

IN THE NURSING CARE OF THE ELDERLY

Sister E. Murray SRN.
Sister S. Curtis SRN.
Professor J. Anderson, Department of Medicine
Dr. M. Kataria, Geriatrician
Mr. J. Steif, Systems Analyst

King's College Hospital Group, Denmark Hill, London SE5.

Summary

A global descriptive view of the information system for the care of the elderly at St. Giles' Hospital of the King's College Hospital Group is presented. Nursing care information centres around the development of the nursing process of care and nursing care plans for the elderly. These plans are based on the individual patient care needs. These plans are implemented by a number of organised nursing care decisions. These nursing care decisions are recorded in the nursing care record as well as the patient's history and relevant psychological and social data both from the patient and relatives. A record of the delivery of care to meet the patient's need is kept so that nursing performance can be reviewed. Special discharge advice to hand over the patient to the community nurse is given to ensure continuity of care when the patient leaves hospital. The patient and relatives are kept informed by means of a patient diary reflecting important aspects of care that has been given. This enables the patient's relatives to participate in therapy as much as possible. The system is designed to implement participatory care of the elderly in all its aspects.

1. Introduction

Computer systems for recording general nursing orders and procedures and for keeping records of student nurses in training, have been developed in several centres in the United Kingdom and elsewhere.[1,2] Less attention has been given to the role that accurate and timely nursing data and information can play in the short and longer term care of the elderly. This is a demanding and special area of nursing activity, which requires as much information support as possible to all members of the health care team and to the patient, in order to respond adequately to the needs of the elderly for nursing care.

A careful analysis of the nursing information system objectives and procedures indicates the new and different views that are current about the nursing record and the team methods of implementation of agreed decisions are seen to be more critical than orders in the past. Also because of the wide range of care needs of the elderly covering not only the physical but the psychological and social aspects of of their lives, there is a need for a much more detailed nursing record. This must be supported by a standardised vocabulary describing both plans, decisions and procedures in all areas to ensure that the optimum decisions about care requirements are understood by all. It is important that there be information feed-back to the nursing team about the progress of care in order that effective care can be monitored. There is now more emphasis on care assessment both in hospital and in the community to ensure the continuity of care surveyance that is necessary. Thus the nursing record not only requires its specific vocabulary but also involves links to other members of the health care team and very effective communication for it to support its objectives.

2. Nursing Care Plan

Basic to the nursing care of the elderly is the development of appropriate individual nursing care plans for each patient. The decisions about care needs to meet the personal problems of the elderly patient are prepared as soon as the patient is admitted in relation to the physical aspects of care and in the next 24-48 hours to include all the problems of the elderly that can by then be recognised. These needs will embrace the psychological and social aspects of care as well as the physical disorders. The care needs often change rapidly at first but soon become fairly stable. There will be also medical, physiotherapy and social work input to the nursing care team so that a global therapeutic plan can be created. It is important that the patient can participate in his or her care and we have used a patient diary giving specific information about his care. In this way, he and his relatives can be kept informed by the information system as well as by personal communication with nursing and medical staff. It is essential for the nursing care record to be all embracing and it must reflect the data obtained from the patient's history and also psychological and social information derived both from the patient, relatives and friends.

These care plans are implemented by the actions of the health care team on the ward following the patient's admission. There are several key areas where the special needs of patients have to be considered. For example, social and administrative data are checked and especially the information provided by the general practitioner and the relatives and friends of the patient. The social history is useful documenting the social circumstances of the patient prior to admission and how they relate to his special needs. Psychological needs are also evaluated and assessed as well as attention given to physical care needs. This has necessitated the development of a special data dictionary fully specifying all the needs of the patient and linking these needs to nursing procedures and action automatically. This enables the care implementation to reflect the patient's needs. The system can respond to the senior nursing staff with suggestions about care which they can modify easily and up-date.

3. Nursing Care Action

The nursing team use a visual display unit and also printout to allow the nurse to know the decisions that are being implemented as part of the care plan. The implementation of the care plan leads to the acknowledgement of nursing action by the nursing team. Adjustments to care decisions are made by the sister or a senior member of the nursing team as the patient's condition changes. Thus the nursing actions are flexible and altered to meet the changing needs of the patient. Nursing decisions also involve therapy not only related to drugs, which is especially important in the elderly, but also to physiotherapy and social and occupational therapy. These basic care actions will also be reflected in the patient diary to keep the patient and the relatives informed. Naturally this diary will not be written in professional language.

4. Nursing Communication

Feedback of information about nursing actions completed and observations about clinical progress and communications from the different members of the care team by means of visual display units enables senior nursing personnel to monitor the patient's recovery and progress. It is also important to have records of interviews of relatives by nurses who have current knowledge of the patient's care needs ensuring that special care needs of patients are met. Thus nursing communication in relation to patient education and relative information is important and available for all those who need such information.

In the care of the elderly much attention has to be paid to nutrition and mobility and this is planned in the care plan and carried through by the appropriate nursing actions. The utility of an agreed set of flexible procedures and the establishment of appropriate data dictionaries in data base allows the computer system to adapt and change to meet the varying care needs of the patient as these progress during his stay. Communication is important between the different members of the health care team using computer systems for it enables them all to see how the agreed care needs are being met and to ensure that optimum care is provided including planning for the patient's discharge.

It is important, when the patient is about to be discharged, that the care team develop appropriate communication for the district nurse so that there can be continuity of care between the hospital and community. Such information should bring nurses in the community up to date with the information not only held in the medical, but in the nursing record and it should provide an assessment of the patient's state on discharge. Thus the hospital nurse can hand over to the community nurse a nursing summary without dictation and typing. This information is also useful to the general practitioner and his team. It promotes better communication in the community about the patient.

5. Nursing Performance and Review

As the nursing team reach agreement about care plans so they need to be kept informed by the information system of the progress of care and the changes required in the on-going plan. Implementation of nursing actions must be recorded as well as clinical data about the patient's progress and care. Thus acknowledgement of nursing actions when implemented through the visual display unit is necessary not only for nursing management but also for communication with patients and their relatives.

Measures of performance for nursing management have been agreed and are being implemented including information about the percentage of nursing decisions carried out and the care actions taken in relation to different nurse provision including by shift and by day. Naturally, such data will reflect the number of nurses available for care at a particular time. It should also enable judgments to be made about the clinical nursing load of all patients under the care of a particular nursing team. As it is important to adjust nursing time to the care load, it is important to develop indices to express these factors.

6. Planning Duty Rosters

One of the difficulties nursing sisters have is planning and amending duty rosters to meet the wishes of nursing staff and to ensure that patients are cared for adequately during all their stay. The information system can offer a method of allocation which is flexible and can be updated to meet changing demands and requirements.

7. Patient/Nurse Communication and the Patient Diary

During the development of the health care process we have emphasised that the patient should have a say in his treatment. This can be done by using a patient diary which records all the aspects of medical and nursing decisions which are implemented, so that the patient can have a greater awareness of what is about to happen to him. This will not only include basic data about his physical needs, but also data about investigation and therapy. It will emphasise to him that more time will be spent explaining the various nursing and clinical procedures to him so as to have his cooperation. In this way it is possible for patients to participate in their care especially when they know what kind of drugs they are taking and what they look like. It also enables the elderly patient with a poor memory to learn what is happening to him so he does not feel lost. It also helps communication with the patient's relatives to understand more about the care plan and to appreciate what nursing care is achieving. This is especially true in relation to drug therapy, to social work and physiotherapy.

8. Liaising with Doctors, Physiotherapists, Occupational Therapists and Social Workers.

It is important not to view hospital care in isolation and discharge advice ensures that communication continues between nurses inside and outside the hospital. We hope that the patient diary will eventually be exploited in the community. Community care workers also can learn from the care plans developed in hospitals. There also will be relationships with the medical record and special records of other departments which will also help in both patient investigation and care.

9. Conclusions

We believe that this planned system to meet the special needs of care of the elderly is necessary if we are to keep appropriate control of patient care through timely feedback. We have introduced the concept of a patient diary to help patients and their relatives understand care and its execution. The system also promotes better communication between care personnel within the hospital and district and the patient and his relatives.

REFERENCES

1. Head, A.E. (1977) pp. 469-83 Medcomp 77, Online London.

2. Collins, S.M., Cundy, A.D., Shah, A.R. (1979) pp. 230-43 Medical Informatics Berlin, Springer Verlag.

THE USE OF CLINFO AS A TEACHING TOOL TO INTRODUCE HEALTH CARE PERSONNEL TO COMPUTERS AND THEIR APPLICATIONS

Kathryn Erat,
Elizabeth Worcester,
Brigham & Women's Hospital
Boston, MA   02115   U.S.A.

SUMMARY

The introduction of medical and health care personnel to computers and their uses requires a computer course specifically tailored to their interests. The course must also operate within severe time constraints. The use of the CLINFO Data Management and Analysis System provides a suitable workstation environment for rapid introduction of students to the basic concepts of computer systems and the construction of relevant medical applications rapidly. The structure provided by a CLINFO learning situation is also compatible with Piaget's learning theory of data gathering, arranging, processing, system structuring, assimilation, and accommodation. CLINFO applications for dietary and nursing are detailed.

INTRODUCTION

For the past 17 years one of the authors (Erat) has conducted introductory computer courses for several different categories of health professionals: doctors, nurses, social workers, dietitians, researchers, etc.[1,2] Every course consists of the presentation of the fundamentals of computing: the components of a computer and their logical operations (arithmetic units, mass memory, input/output devices); organization and coding of data; an introduction to programming at machine, assembly, and higher language levels; the presentation of computing concepts represented by a 300-word vocabulary; and presentation of several medical applications of computers relevant to the participants' interests. Since every course is very limited in class time and relatively little can be demanded of the participants in out-of-class study, the classroom activity must be sufficiently complete to impart in a very short time an adequate appreciation of what computers can do and how they do it.

This work supported by U.S.P.H.S. grant #RR 00888-07. The development of CLINFO Data Management and Analysis System has been sponsored by the General Clinical Research Centers and Biotechnology Resources Branches of the Division of Research Resources, National Institutes of Health, Bethesda, MD.

The best teacher of computing is the actual programming of problems that illustrate computer fundamentals and that reflect the participants' fields of practical interest and need. However, two difficulties arise; (1) the inadequate amount of time for any lengthy programming that is really relevant to the students' medical interests, and (2) participants' frustration with the clerical idiosyncrasies of programming and input keying errors that can quickly eclipse their vision of the larger purpose. There is nothing more frustrating and de-energizing to a participant than to find her/his execution of programming is being thwarted by misplaced commas or unmatched parentheses. In a longer course these snags recede into subconscious detail but in a short course they imperil the student's assimilation of meaningful computing concepts and general perception of the relevance of computing to her/his professional activity.

LEARNING ENVIRONMENT

The ideal situation would be to place the participants in a friendly work-station environment where they could construct a useful or relevant medical exer-cise by doing meaningful operations on pertinent data. This first computer en-counter should allow them to enter data, edit data, analyze it, and receive output rather painlessly or at least by performing steps that seem intuitively sensible to them. It is this success that will spark their imagination to be creative con-cerning computer applications in their own areas of interest. Until recently, the friendly user workstation has not been readily available. However, with the de-velopment of the CLINFO Data Management and Analysis System which is a computer resource developed under the auspices of the U.S. Public Health Service (General Clinical Research Centers and Biotechnology Resources Branch of the Division of Research Resources of the National Institute of Health USA) specifically to sup-port clinical investigators in a research environment, a suitable tool is at hand for quick immersion of students into an environment where they can quickly build a data base of their own design; enter data; retrieve data; subset data; arithmeti-cally and logically manipulate and massage data; statistically analyze data; and obtain meaningful output in graphs, tables, and text reports.[3]

The added advantage of immersing the students in a friendly total system is that many computer system concepts are naturally encountered in a logical way as follows:

1. Logging on and off system, password, security
2. Response time, system load, priorities of applications
3. Preciseness of data coding, kinds of data coding, editing, error checking of data
4. Data base files, records, fields, storage sizing, utilization of storage, archiving, indexing, deletion of data

5. Organization of data logically and relative to ease of input, retrieval and analysis
6. Retrieving data, subsetting data, sorting and rearranging data
7. Executing boolean selections for retrieval of data
8. Using programs (principally statistical analysis including descriptive statistics, analysis of variance, chi-square, life table, linear regression, T-tests, nonparametric tests, etc.)
9. Developing mathematical programs to operate on data
10. Using very high-level-programming response files to facilitate repetitive input and system commands
11. Communications with other computer systems and languages (transfer of data)
12. Human factors relating to user interaction with system
    a. prompts
    b. response choices
    c. logical function pathways
    d. analogies between system commands available to user and logical functions
    e. repetitive keying requirements
    f. clarity of presentation on displays
    g. flexibility for presentation of data on displays and reports
    h. housekeeping burdens on user
    i. aids to overall management of user's activity of system
    j. system's simplicity/complexity and user's learning curve for use of system
    k. security measures
    l. system and data protection against unsophisticated user
    m. workstation physical arrangement
    n. relationship of frequency and duration of system use to user fatigue, accuracy, and memory retention of important system concepts
    o. cost in time and repetition of keying to user for mistakes and inefficient choice of system commands
    p. the relationship of response time to user efficiency and acceptance of system
11. Analysis of problem relative to system application
    a. protocol for problem/task
    b. protocol for data collection relative to problem/task
    c. broad concept flowchart of all activities related to data collection, storage, and analysis
    d. details of broad concepts
    e. desired output
12. System resource utilization and accounting
13. Real-time and time-sharing.

Given this approach one must ask is this a better practical introduction to computers than coding a short statistical program such as a chi-square in BASIC which is about all the programming time a very short course can accommodate. Granted, an immersion in a higher level workstation like CLINFO does mask the basic repertoire of programming constructs: loops, addressing concepts, branches, comparisons, data moving; and most basic of all, the reduction of all computer activity to sequences of arithmetic operations, data moves, and tests. Therefore, the course lectures still involve the exposition of the basic constructs, and one short BASIC program (a search or sort) is still introduced and programmed. However, for this group of health participants pedagogically it is sounder to whet the appetite and have interesting feedback. Also, it is important to avoid a course presentation that is not too closely allied to a mathematical approach in

order to assure success for students who are not comfortable with math. Therefore, a quick shift is made to CLINFO. However, when the shift is made to CLINFO,
it is important that the applications being worked on in CLINFO are relevant to
the participants. Two applications, one for dietary and one for the nursing department, will be detailed.

APPLICATION EXERCISES

1. Dietary.

A consistent need of clinical dietitians caring for patients whose nutritional states and needs are intimately related to their pathology/health is the
caloric, mineral, electrolyte, and nutrient totals for these patients per day.
Our institutional food list has 300 items. Each item has 18 nutrients that are of
immediate concern:

total calories	niacin mg	
carbohydrate gms	thiamine mg	water-soluble vitamins
protein gms	riboflavin mg	
fat gms	calcium mg	
cholesterol mg	phosphorus mg	bone matrix
sodium mg	Vitamin D I.U.D.	
potassium mg	Iron mg	
Vitamin A mg — fat-soluble	Folic acid mg	hematology matrix
Vitamin K I.U.D. — vitamins	Vitamin C mg	

To calculate these totals by hand, by consulting handbooks for values for each
food consumed by the patient and multiplying the values by the amount of each food
the patient consumed and then summing is a tedious, repetitive job which consumes
a considerable amount of dietitian time.[4,5] CLINFO is a very suitable tool for
the development of a food/nutrient data bank and a series of user commands that
the dietitian can execute on patient intake and output to calculate patient nutrient levels. The patients' data may be stored for the duration of the dietitians'
interest, and selected groups of patients may be analyzed for nutritional effects
of diseases and response to different therapies. Even the cost/benefit of different therapies can be analyzed in a limited amount of time. The ongoing addition
of patients to the data base makes it possible to rapidly detect trends with little user effort. The dietitian has thus been involved in developing a computer
aid that has immediate relevance to her dietetic responsibilities.

2. Nursing.

One of the currently required tasks for nurses is the initial and continuing assessment of the levels of care required for their patients.[6] These
assessments have many immediate and long-range uses as follows:

a. The assignment of staff to nursing units both in numbers and skills
b. Detection of epidemiological and care trends within the institution
c. The correlation of patient care mixes with hospital costs
d. The design of relevant inservice education.

One level-of-care assessment method involves clustering various patient conditions and care procedures; such as respiratory treatments, invasive vital signs monitoring, complex dressings, in groups that are representative of various levels of nursing care that patients require. The clusters and their relation to a level of care are usually developed by a committee. Each patient is then matched to the cluster which most adequately describes her/him. The assignment automatically indicates the patient's level of care. Another method is for a committee to assign weights to a list of patient conditions and care procedures. The patient is then matched against the list and the weights of the matched items are totaled. The final total determines the level of care. For example, a score of <25 might be level 1; a score of 26-50 might be level 2, etc. This assessment and the design and refinement of the method used is an ongoing activity that continually involves nursing. With CLINFO, class participants can build protocols for both methods of assessment, enter patient data and compare the two methods for ease of use, predictive accuracy, calculation of staffing plans, and trend analysis. With CLINFO the students can manipulate and refine the methods relatively easily and thus have an experience in using a decision support system to help them design a needed clinical/administrative tool. In other words, the nurses have access to a system which has not only enabled them to understand something about computing but readily helped them grasp the concepts of user implementation with a decision support system.

PSYCHOLOGY OF LEARNING

The above educational method is supported not only by student success, but is also supported by learning theory. The introduction of new concepts, systems, and procedures to students should incorporate cognitive support, behavioral support, and performance linkage. Piaget's theory of cognitive learning with its emphasis on ordering, classification, and grouping is akin to the activities one applies to assembling and analyzing data. "Piagets" theory suggests that the manner in which data is grouped (arranged hierarchically) and processed through a set of consistent strategies determines the scope and nature of the cognitive structure making up an individual's intellect."[7] Closely allied with these concepts are assimilation and accommodation. Assimilation incorporates new information into existing cognitive structures and accommodation rearranges or refines or develops new cognitive structures capable of interpreting new or contradictory input. The process is a continuous one aiming at an orderly system. Introducing a student to the concepts of programming, problem analysis, and solution synthesis via a CLINFO exercise markedly mimics Piaget's theory of learning. The student, in using CLINFO, assembles basic data and organizes it by applying a sequence of activities. The sequences of CLINFO commands or operations can form the bases for representation of abstract ideas. The commands and operations in CLINFO are at a sufficiently high level that the system's approach to problem analysis and solution synthesis is highlighted and reinforced. It is this rapport with modular approach to computer application that the CLINFO experience reinforces. It is important to remember in introducing students to computers that three things are being stressed:

1. What a computer is and how it works.
2. How can a computer be helpful to her/him in her/his field of interest.
3. How to construct a modular analysis/synthesis of a computer application.

It is this last item that is the most difficult to teach. It must be learned by doing, and here CLINFO is extremely supportive -- fortunately because the CLINFO process is so akin to the cognitive process.

Behavior support is an application of reinforcement theory: incremental learning, proceeding from simple to complex, immediate feedback, and frequent success. Again, CLINFO provides reinforcement. The student is on-line, her/his use of commands provides meaningful results, and sequences of commands provide more sophisticated results.

Performance is an outcome measure of the result of multiple behaviors. Performance linkage is the appropriate attribution of performance (success or failure) to fundamental causes. Because CLINFO use is modular and commands are high level, a student can rapidly correlate results with the appropriateness and inappropriateness of choice of a command. She/he can rapidly choose another command and reassess results and performance. There can easily be a progression of successes that alleviates the tendency to passivity in the presence of repeated failure that has been documented.

CONCLUSION

The versatility of the CLINFO system, its design for medical research, and its structural similarity to sound learning psychology make it an ideal tool for introducing health care personnel to computing.

BIBLIOGRAPHY

(1) Erat K, McGrath S. "Developing a teaching/learning experience for nurses in fundamentals of computer programming preliminary to nursing research." In Proceedings of NECC 1979 National Educational Computing Conference edited by D. Harris, The University of Iowa, Iowa City 1979; 316-325.

(2) Erat K, McGrath S. "A computer education experience for nurses in leadership roles." In MEDINFO 80, edited by D. Lindberg and S. Kaihara North-Holland Publishing Co, Amsterdam 1980; 362.

(3) Whitehead SF, Bilofsky HS. "CLINFO - a clinical research data management and analysis system." In Proceedings The Fourth Annual Symposium on Computer Applications in Medical Care edited by Joseph T. O'Neill, IEEE-Computer Society, Los Alamitos, CA 1980; 1286-1291.

(4) "Composition of Foods Handbook #8, 8-1 (1976) 8-2 (1977) 8-3 (1978) 8-4 (1979) 8-5 (1979)." Published by Dept. of Agricultural Research Service, U.S. Department of Agriculture, Superintendent of Documents U.S. Government Printing Office, Washington, DC.

(5) "Nutritive Value of American Foods in Common Units Agriculture Handbook #456." Published by Dept. of Agricultural Research Service, U.S. Department of Agriculture, Superintendent of Documents U.S. Government Printing Office, Washington, DC.

(6) Gebhardt AN, R.N. "Utilizing an on-line computer system for patient classification and staff determination." In press.

(7) Henderson JC, Martinko MJ. "Cognitive learning theory and the design of decision support systems." DSS-81 Transactions edited by Donovan Young and Peter G. W. Keen, Published by First International Conference on Decision Support Systems sponsored by Execucom Systems Corp. 1981; 45-50.

SIMULTANEOUS PHARMACY COMPUTERIZATION IN 3 UNIVERSITY HOSPITALS

H.B.J. NIEMAN

BAZIS, UNIVERSITY HOSPITAL LEYDEN

THE NETHERLANDS

Abstract

A great deal of the pharmacy functions lend themselves to computerization. Many
hospital pharmacies use batch type systems to support inventory management and
and drug-turnover monitoring. These systems generally are based on the needs of a
specific pharmacy. This paper reports on a joint effort of pharmacists of 3
university hospitals, cooperating in the specification and development of a real
time information system. The system should be applicable not only in the three organizations participating in the project, but also in many other (university) hospital
pharmacies. The scope and main functions of the system are described, as well as
the proceedings of the project. Although it is too early to indicate the operational
results, some experiences with regard to the initial implementation can be reported.

Introduction

From 1974, parts of an integrated information system (HIS) are operational in the
Leyden university hospital. At present the university hospitals of Groningen,
Rotterdam, Utrecht and Amsterdam and several other hospital organizations have im-
plemented already a great deal of the 40 subsystems of the Leyden-HIS. An organi-
zation,called BAZIS was founded for further development and support of the system.
This group cooperates with the data processing departments of the various hospitals.
In 1977 a project for the realization of a pharmacy system, embedded in the HIS,
started. Three university hospitals and BAZIS participate in the specification of
the system.
Characteristics of the Leyden-HIS:
At Leyden 1500 users communicate via 220 terminals with a half a million patient
databank. Every day the minicomputer configuration processes a workload of 250.000
messages, i.e. over a 1.3 million characters are typed in. The Leyden university
hospital has 900 beds divided over 40 wards. Daily 1200 outpatients visit the hospital, every year some 20.000 inpatients are admitted.

Scope of the pharmacy system

The type and volume of the pharmacy's operations can be characterized by:
   the central pharmacy in an university hospital stocks about 3500 different items,

not only drugs but also wound-dressings, disinfectants etc.
. Daily over 900 requests for drugs are sent to the pharmacy. These requests
  result in refilling the stock on the ward within 24 hours.
. The purchase department of the pharmacy orders daily 50 different drugs.
. The yearly turnover of the pharmacy is some 4 million US dollar.

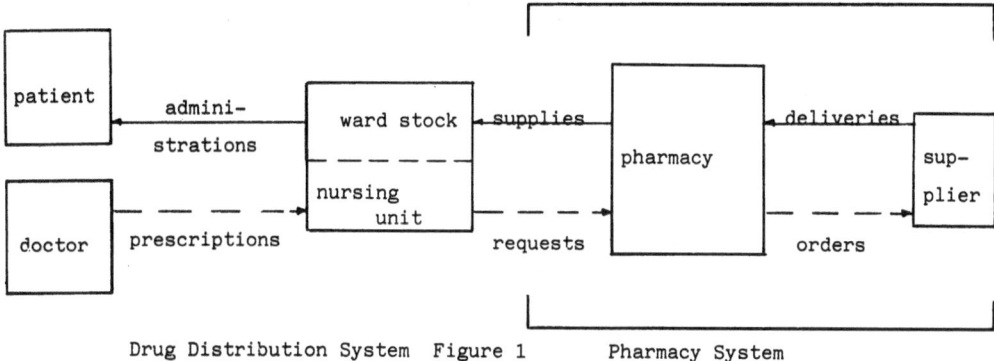

      Drug Distribution System Figure 1   Pharmacy System

The professional interest of the pharmacists is focused on patient oriented systems
for drug distribution and therapeutic monitoring. The Pharmacy system, however,
mainly supports drugs usage and turnover monitoring as well as the inventory management of the pharmacy itself. (Fig. 1). It was decided that an extensive drug
distribution system could not be realized until a pharmacy system had been introduced successfully. Computerization of the pharmacy should provide a solid basis
for future developments in the field of drug distribution.

Objectives

In 1978 one of the pharmacies used a manual system. The data processing facilities
of the other two pharmacies were rather poor. Batch type systems were used to keep
track of only 25% of the drug requests. Data entry and error correction were time
consuming activities, printed reports were available only every four weeks and
differences between actual stocks and stocks on paper turned out to be considerable.
The quality and quantity of the information produced by the systems left much to
be desired. The aim of the pharmacy project is to develop a real time system to
support inventory management and drug usage and turnover monitoring. The new system
should reduce clerical effort and it should support the pharmacy's daily operations.
The pharmacy system should allow stepwise implementation and it had to be transportable and acceptable to the 3 pharmacies participating in the project. The HIS set-up
guarantees a fast response, a sufficient storage capacity and a good availability .
These features have been discussed elsewhere.[1] To provide an adequate realtime
environment no special effort had to be made with regard to the pharmacy project.

Main functions of the system

In figure 2 an overview of the system is shown.

File creation and maintenance

The drug identification date are: a 6 digit number, the brand and generic name, the
dosage form, strength and route, and drug packing. Whenever one of these items
changes a new record is created in the drugfile. In this way a file of 20.000 records
with approximately 4000 different pharmaceutical substances is developed. Via drugnumber or 6 characters of the name, an online facility provides access to 5 terminal
screens with drug information,including: warnings for adminstration and storage instructions, purchase and inventory information, drug components, consumption and
formulary data. A special function is designed to fill 8 separate files with codes,
e.g. dosage forms and therapeutic groups. The files of the pharmacy system require
a storage capacity of 15 Mbytes.

Request registration

Pharmacy technicians register online the drugs requested by the wards. The data entry
technique is very simple and does not require any special skills. Identification of
patients is based on number or name and data of birth. The system searches the
patient database and census data, stored in an admission file. Every accepted request
immediately results in an update of the stock level. A message appears on the screen
in case of a shortage or out of stock situation. Reminders are displayed whenever
special attention has to be given to a drug request. Pointers in the drugfile
enable the system to suggest the supply of equivalent drugs.

Order registration

Order advises are generated automatically whenever stock falls below a minimum level,
which is either a fixed quantity or based on the average consumption of the drug
over the last 12 months. The daily order proposals include inventory, drug and usage
information as well as purchase history and the various packings and suppliers of
the drug. Drug orders and deliveries are registered online. The user identifies the
supplier and types in drugnumber and quantity.

Labels and forms

As a result of the online registration activities, delivery notes, receipt and order
forms are issued by printers at a speed of 180 characters per second. A delivery
note is a worksheet for gathering the drugs; the same form accompanies the distribution of the drugs to the wards. Labels are printed with the drug identification
data and special remarks e.g. storage recommendations and mode of use. A special
online function is designed to compose and produce multiple labels at any time.

Daily data processing

Figures on drug usage per ward and turnover per therapeutic code are updated daily,
according to the recorded drug supplies. Monthly a program automatically generates
input to the General Ledger system. These data processing functions are carried
out by a series of programs which operate under control of a software monitor.

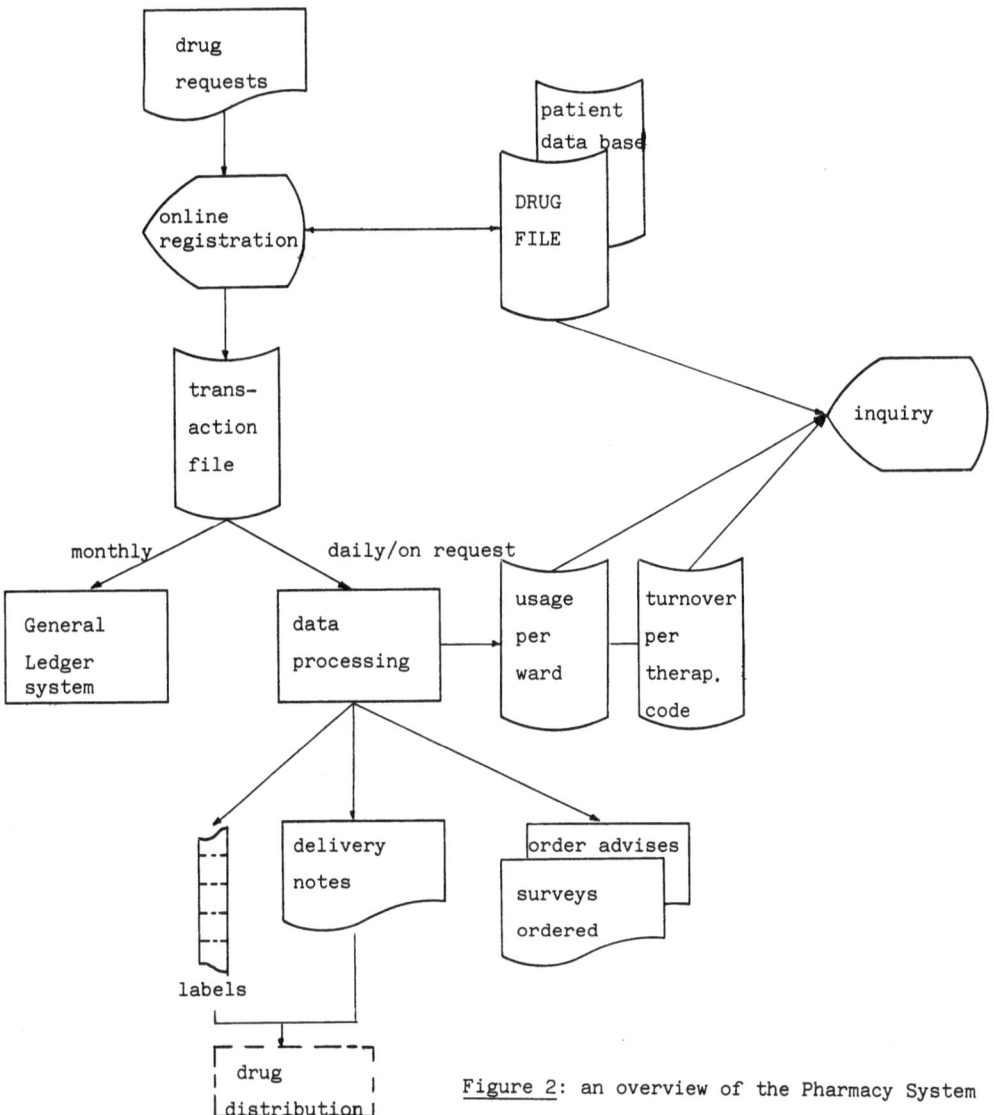

Figure 2: an overview of the Pharmacy System

Every day, the monitor determines which programs in what sequence have to run. A display with the selected menu offers the computercentre a prognosis of the workload, specified by the number of discaccesses and lines to be printed. A similar screen reports the user upon the surveys to be produced.

Output

With a special function the users can define and order selective reports on inventory and drug items. The online output definition includes the data to be selected, the sorting sequence and the desired layout of the survey. Daily a report generator is activated. This tool processes the relevant data and prints the surveys ordered. The output of the pharmacy system includes:

- turnover per ward per therapeutic code (and reversed)
- consumption statistics per ward, per drug (and reversed)

- outstanding order survey
- reports on file-updates
- summary of the pharmacy operations
- drug distribution per patient
- answers to spontaneous questions

- purchases per supplier
- formulary information
- stock per inventory unit
- drugs returned to the pharmacy

Project history

The pharmacy project started in November 1977. A projectteam was organized with representatives of the pharmacies and the data processing departments of three university hospitals. This team had to draw up the functional specifications of the system, considering the present and future requirements. The BAZIS-development group coordinated the activities. Since the pharmacists participated activily in the specification process, it took 20 meetings to discuss the major functions of the system. At the end of 1978 the specifications and the design of the system were completed. It was decided that the system should be developed and introduced stepwise. The development of the software started in the summer of 1979. The total software package was divided into so called 'versions',i.e. series of programs to perform specific functions. A version was discussed in the projectteam, developed, tested and sent to the hospitals. The first version was released in September 1979; the hospitals received every 3 months a new version. In February 1981, 7 versions were available, including programs for file creation, label printing, online registration, data processing and survey-production. In September 1981 the software development will be completed with the eight and final version. The total effort of the development group is 6 manyears. Specification and design of the system take about 17%, programming and testing 65% and the remainder concerns support and coordination activities. At present (June 1981) 55.000 fortran statements have been produced, including 20 interactive and some 30 batch programs. The pharmacies established their own committees, composed of the direct users, to coordinate and carry out the implementation activities. These activities include file creation, stock-taking, user training, physical rearrangement of the pharmacy, the introduction of new procedures and installation of the appropriate hardware. It was determined to start the inventory management, assisted by the pharmacy system, with a limited number of drugs. This way the feasibility of the software and the new procedures can be tested without an increase of the workload, while human or hardware failures do not affect the daily operations of the pharmacy. Based on feedback of operational results, refinements of the system can be specified and developed. In October 1980 the system became operational in the Groningen (500 inventory items) and Utrecht (100 narcotics) pharmacy. In January 1981 the Rotterdam pharmacy decided to implement some parts of the system to register the supply of drugs to third parties (2500 inventory items). Recently the pharmacy

of the Leyden university hospital started the planning of the introduction of the
system.

Experiences

Although the main functions of the participating pharmacies are similar, there are
considerable differences, in the way the daily operations are performed. The
request procedures, inventory management and drug distribution differ, as well as
the contacts with the nursing area. Consequently much attention had to be given
to the flexibility of the system. Some special features are developed to enable
the users to tailor the system to their requirements:

. A subsystem is incorporated for online output definition and the control of batch-
  runs.
. With a simple online facility, terminals and printers can be switched in case of
  hardware failures.
. An online function is available to indicate which messages should be displayed
  on screens and printed on labels and forms.
. The authorization of users with regard to storage and retrieval of data can be
  defined and checked on sub-function level.

Software testing took a lot of time because the various organizations had to be
simulated. The pharmacists designed in a joint effort the codes for dosage routes
and forms. The therapeutic code of the Royal Dutch Pharmaceutical Association was
adapted for the system by one of the pharmacists. These standardization activities
provide a base for mutual comparability of drug turnover and usage statistics.
As mentioned in the previous section, 7 versions of programs have been released
during the development phase. This approach facilitates a gradual implementation of
the system, it improves the contribution of the users in the further specification
of the system and it simplifies the planning of programming and user-oriented
activities. On the other hand when the projectteam does not specify the next version
in time, the pace of software development slows down. Unexpected interruptions, due
to problem reports from the data processing departments of the hospitals, disturbed
the development climate slightly. Retrieval of software errors has taken only 1%
of the total programming effort. Although the personnel of the pharmacy is in-
experienced with regard to data processing, it did not take much time to introduce
the online functions to the direct users. The interactive part of the system
appeared to be very userfriendly. Most users required only a few hours to become
comfortable with the online facilities. One of the pharmacies provided computer-
games to introduce and promote keyboard handling. The other implementation activities took considerably longer. Especially the creation of the drug file turned
out to be very time consuming, although the Farmodex database was used for initial
filling. The Farmodex foundation provides a magnetic tape with data of a great
deal of the pharmaceutical substances, available in the Netherlands. [2]

Nevertheless, the relevant drugs in the pharmacy's inventory had to be identified and stock and other supplementary data had to be entered in the system. When performed without extra staff these activities, together with the introduction of new procedures take at least one year.

Concluding remarks

It can be stated that the jointly effort to develop a realtime pharmacy system has been successful.The experiences obtained during the initial implementation, encourage the users to intensify the activities for further introduction of the system. The implementation in Leyden shows that the system is also applicable in a pharmacy that did not participate in the project.

References

[1] Bakker, A.R., Scope and limitations of a mini-based centralized hospital information system. Proc. Medinfo 80 p.505-509. North-Holland Amsterdam (1980).

[2] Hoelen, A.J., E. Dammers, H. Smits, De Farmodex, database voor geneesmiddelen. Proc. MIC 78 p. 227-230. Vrije Universiteit Amsterdam (1978).

THE ROLE OF CASE DOCUMENTATION IN POISON INFORMATION

C. Zink, H.-J. Christen, J. Apitzsch, Hj. Meyer and H.-G. Reinhardt
GSD Gesellschaft für Systemforschung und Dienstleistungen
im Gesundheitswesen mbH
Einemstraße 9, D-1000 Berlin (West) 30

SUMMARY

The systematic and standardized documentation of poisoning cases could facilitate information in cases of acute poisoning, but also the evaluation, update and completion of toxicological data bases. For this reason, case documentations are part of the information structure of an organizational model in West Berlin, integrating all institutions concerned with different aspects of poison control and prevention.

Standardized basic documentation of routine data - necessary for the observation of trends and new poisoning risks on a European scale - will be completed by more extensive documentations of the outcome of poisoning cases. A regular analysis of this data will then allow an evaluation and control of poison information and treatment strategies, and can be used to develop more efficient preventive activities.

1. INTRODUCTION

Along with an increasing number of toxic products appearing on the market, there is a rapidly growing need for toxicological information. This can also be shown by increasing poisoning morbidity-rates and an increasingly large number of calls to Poison Information Centers (1-3).

For this reason, the 'Institute for Systems Research in the Health Service' (GSD), a government-owned non-profit institute for applied systems research and data processing in the health service - particularly of West Berlin -, was charged by the West Berlin Government with the development of a toxicological information system integrating the different services involved in toxicology in this city. The main aim was to facilitate and effectivate information retrieval and update in all the institutions concerned (4).

This seemed to be all the more important, as West Berlin concentrates, to an extent reached nowhere else in the Federal Republic, institutions and services ensuring toxicological information, treatment, analysis, and, to some extent, drug monitoring and control. These institutions, including two Poison Information Centers, two hospital intensive-care units, an institution for toxicological analysis, a department of clinical pharmacology, an institute for medical factory supervision, and an institute of embryonal pharmacology, co-operate up to now only on a personal scale. From the informational point of view this implies that in each institution the basis for their work consists mainly of their own information systems and data bases, usually card index files compiled for their own specific purposes and according to their own need and experiences. There is no systematic exchange of information between these different services.

2.   INFORMATION STRUCTURE OF THE 'HUMAN TOXICOLOGY CENTER'

The most efficient way to improve this situation seems to be to unify the already existing institutions by creating a common information and documentation structure for all of them. The idea is not to build up a new service but to install only a small co-ordinating working group. This means to make, in the best possible form, individual knowledge of the different services available to all participating institutions by means of structural innovation only.

The advantages of such a system are obviously the following:

o   A common access of all institutions concerned to the same basic data will allow an intense connection between toxicological information, therapy, and research.

o   The systematic exchange of new information and experiences between the institutions will guarantee up-to-date information, also in the very complicated fields of embryonal, environmental and occupational toxicology.

These uncontestable benefits of an integrative model for poison information will be completed by a third aspect:

o   A coordinated documentation of cases will allow a rapid retrieval of earlier and similar poisoning case histories, not only of patients of the institution itself, but also of the other participating units. Particularly in poison information, where a growing number of rapidly changing toxic substances have to be observed, and where the effects of a certain toxic vary a lot according to characteristics of the patient in question (e.g. age-group), it is essential to have case histories readily available, as only experience may often show the adequate therapeutic procedure.

These case documentations can also be used for an evaluation of efficiency, and for epidemiological purposes, such as the early identification of new poisoning risks ('poison monitoring') and the planning of preventive activities. They will also facilitate organization and documentation in the different services.

The structure of this integrative model for toxicology information, documentation and control is represented in Figure 1: The toxicological database includes information from existing documentations, industrial and literature information. It is completed by case documentations with data on poison information, hospital treatment and laboratory analysis, together with clinical or other follow-up data. This data is in turn used to facilitate poison information, and to complete, update or correct the substance data available. The information system so works as a closed circle. – The co-ordinating working group assures a systematic evaluation of the collected data and screens their importance for epidemiological analysis and for the development of preventive strategies.

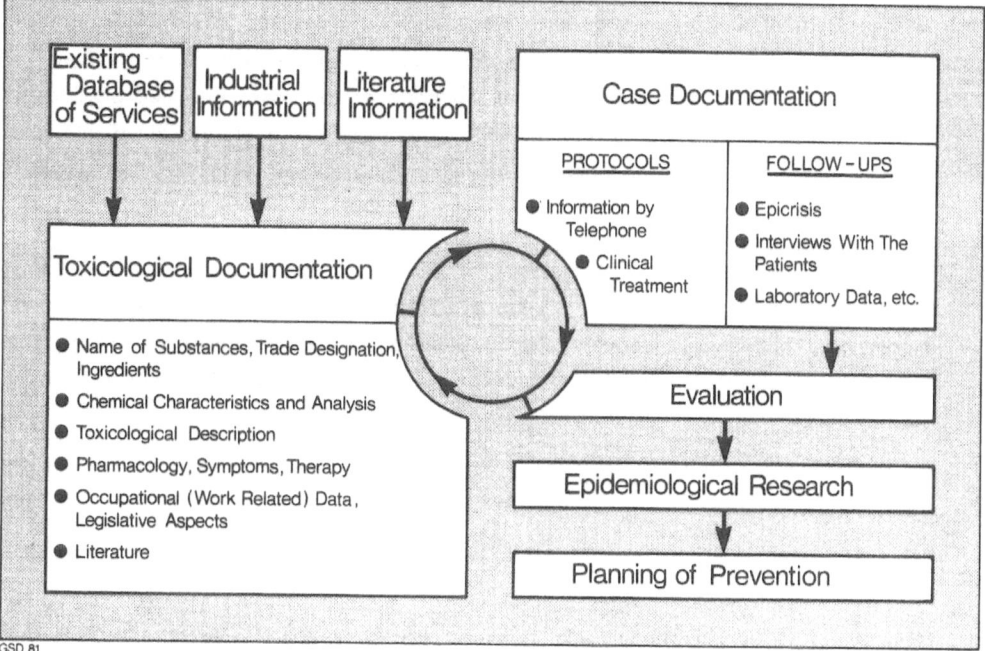

Fig. 1:   Human Toxicology Center: Information-flow

Substance information is presently compiled by the German Institute of Medical Documentation and Information in Cologne, and will be made accessible to a larger number of users as a toxicological data bank under the name of 'Giftpool'.

The development of such a data bank for substance information presents only minor difficulties, as most toxicologists and computer scientists agree on the necessary data structure (5,6). This, up to now, is not so much the case of case-documentations.

However, this second half of the information system is essential, since control and update of substance information is possible only on the base of thorough case follow-ups.

3. PRINCIPLES OF CASE DOCUMENTATION IN POISON CONTROL

Most Poison Control Centers in Europe use one or the other type of case documentation (2,6-10). Telephone calls to Poison Control Centers are generally documented on simple protocol sheets. They are followed-up usually only for very severe or rare types of poisoning. Hospital records on poisoning cases are generally compiled in a way which does not permit data processing procedures.

Some Poison Control Centers (and some hospitals) now develop case documentation systems which can be computerized, but which usually contain very large numbers of variables, so that a systematic and regular analysis of this data becomes practically unfeasible. This is why, on a European scale, the need for a standardized minimum structure for case documentation becomes increasingly apparent (11,12).

Case documentations in toxicology should fulfill the following general requirements:

o   Routine documentations should not be overloaded with information of secondary importance, but should concentrate on a small number of items describing the essentials of the poisoning case (or the telephone call to the Poison Control Center).

o   Routine documentations must simplify, never complicate, the task of the health personnel involved.

o   All case documentations should attain a level of standardization of classifications, definitions and categorizations allowing international comparisons.

o   Item structure and methodological approach must be specific for the purpose of the case documentation. This will above all mean a strict distinction between routine documentations and what could be called 'research documentations'.

Considering these general requirements, the following - certainly theoretical - systematics of poisoning case documentation can be defined: Information on poisoning cases may be collected - according to the general development of a poisoning case - at four different phases of the intoxication, and the obtained data consequently permits differently far-going analyses. Figure 2 illustrates this systematics:

o   The first phase is the poisoning event, with information to be collected on the case history, the circumstances of the intoxication and other background factors necessary to study the pathogenesis of poisonings.

o   The second phase is characterized by the use of a Poison Control Center or the hospital admission of a poisoned patient. Information to be collected at this moment concentrates on a short description of the poisoning event and more detailed data about the actual status of the patient.

o   The response of medical institutions constitutes a third phase: Information now usually results from an analysis of reports about the information given by the Poison Control Centers' personnel, or the type of first aid measures administered in the hospital.

o   The fourth phase – phase of restitution – allows the collection of data on the further development of the patient's status. Data is generally based on written reports from doctors, and on information given by the patients themselves or by their families.

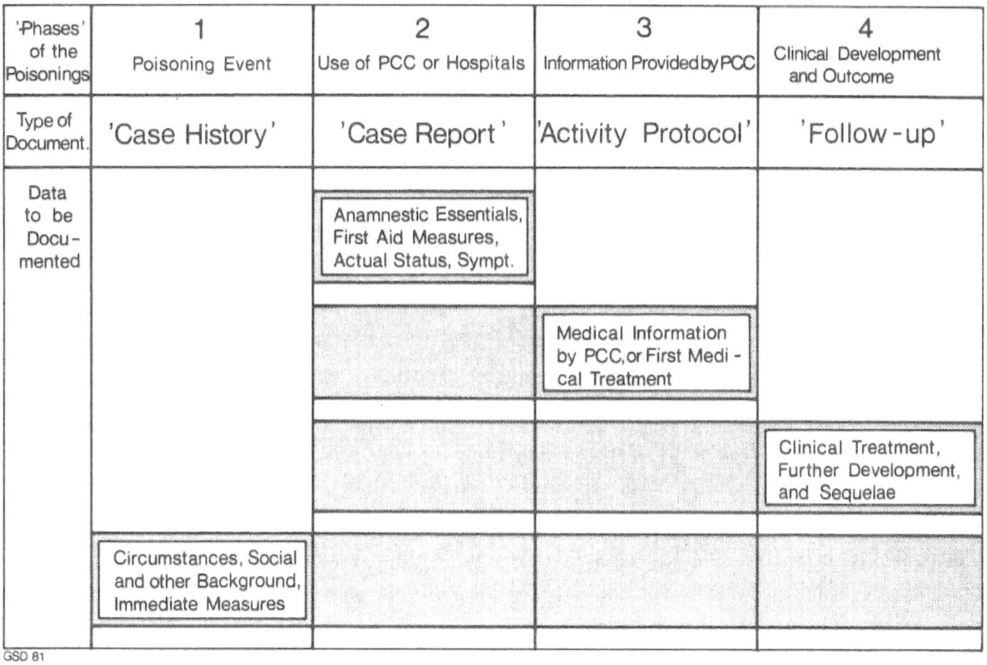

'Phases' of the Poisonings	1 Poisoning Event	2 Use of PCC or Hospitals	3 Information Provided by PCC	4 Clinical Development and Outcome
Type of Document.	'Case History'	'Case Report'	'Activity Protocol'	'Follow-up'
Data to be Documented		Anamnestic Essentials, First Aid Measures, Actual Status, Sympt.		
			Medical Information by PCC, or First Medical Treatment	
				Clinical Treatment, Further Development, and Sequelae
	Circumstances, Social and other Background, Immediate Measures			

GSD 81

Fig. 2: Types of documentation in Poison Control

In order to meet the different needs of case observation and documentation in toxicology, data from each of these four phases is necessary. The purposes for data-collection are different in each case, questions to be answered vary from one to the other. A general systematics of these aspects is given in Table I.

Table I: Characteristics and use of case documentations in Poison Control

Type of Documentation (Phase)	Documenting Person/ Institution	Characteristics of documentation	Use of the data, Research questions
Case Report (2)	Information specialists in PCC, Medical personnel in hospitals	Very few items, highly standardized structure	Structure of clientele, distribution of poisonings among certain populations
Activity Protocol (2,3)	Information specialists in PCC, Medical personnel in hospitals	Few items, standardized structure	Basis of medical reference for future calls or hospital treatments
Clinical or other Follow-Up (2-4)	Treating medical personnel, patients relatives	More ample questionnaires, applicable to all types of poisonings	Evaluation of effectiveness of poison information, questions in clinical toxicology
Case History (1-4)	Patients, relatives	Questionnaires, varied according to research purposes	Epidemiological questions, basis for planning of prevention

It becomes evident that there is no particular type of case documentation suitable to every purpose and need in poison control. On the contrary, it will be necessary to combine different types of documentation: A routine documentation for all cases – reduced to very few items – will be of the utmost importance for an efficient monitoring of noxious effects of drugs, poisons, chemicals, and particularly environmental chemical agents. – This routine documentation, however, will have to be complemented by intermittent epidemiological studies and analyses, in order to clarify more specific questions. Only such studies will allow a continuous evaluation of the effectiveness of the information provided. They will also allow to develop efficient, high-risk population centered preventive approaches (13).

4. CONCLUSIONS AND PERSPECTIVES

In the first place, a routine documentation should be developed according to the necessities of a short protocol of telephone calls in Poison Control Centers and of the information provided. This type of documentation should be as much standardized as possible. An international co-ordination in this respect should be given absolute priority, as it will allow to detect and to compare national and international trends in poisoning morbidity.

Besides these routine case documentations, outcome and background of the poisonings must be regularly analyzed. This means - in a second step - to develop routine follow-up procedures and specific anamnestic approaches for particular types of poisonings. Such approaches should be developed on a local or national scale, nevertheless using standardized classifications and definitions in order to obtain comparable results.

Case documentation in poison control thus means to allow, on the one hand, an efficient medical treatment of poisonings by improving the possibilities of rapid and up-to-date poison information. On the other hand, besides this pragmatic aspect, precise epidemiological knowledge and the development of specific measures will permit a more efficient monitoring of developments in order to prevent future poisonings.

REFERENCES

(1) Descotes J, Roux H, Ducloux B, Robert J, Vincent V: The Poison Control Center of Lyons - report of activity for 1975. Comparison of the reports of activity for 1965 and 1975. Acta Pharmacol Toxicol. 1977; 41 (Suppl.II): 572-576.

(2) Jouglard J, Michela G: Les Centres Anti-Poisons Francais et leur expérience en informatique. In: Roche L (Ed): Toxicovigilance, p.227-262. Paris (Masson), 1979.

(3) Temple AR, Veltri JC: One year's experience in a regional poison control center: The Intermountain Regional Poison Control Center. Clin Toxicol. 1978; 12: 277-289.

(4) Apitzsch J, Meyer Hj, Zink C: Verbund der an Beratung und Versorgung von Vergiftungen beteiligten Berliner Einrichtungen zum Humantoxikologischen Zentrum. Gutachten im Auftrag des Senators für Gesundheit und Umweltschutz Berlin. Berlin (GSD), 1981.

(5) v Clarmann M, Daunderer M, Mathes G: The EDV in the Munich poisons reference center. In: Roche L (Ed): Toxicovigilance, op. cit., p. 163-167.

(6) Moriarty RW, Barton FB: Computerization of patient data at Poison Control Centers. Bull Méd Légale, Urg Méd, CAP. 1977; 20: 282-291.

(7) Govaerts-Lepicard M: Traitement des données et utilisation des techniques informatiques. Centre Belge anti-poisons 1969-1978. In: Roche L (Ed): Toxicovigilance, op.cit., p.185-203.

(8) Krienke EG: Erfahrungen einer Beratungsstelle für Vergiftungserscheinungen im Kindesalter. Dtsch Med J. 1967; 18: 230-240.

(9) Lorent JP: Rôle et structure d'un centre d'information toxicologique.In: Roche L (Ed): Toxicovigilance, op.cit., p.271-278.

(10) Magalini SI, De Francisci G, De Giacomo M: Data storage, elaboration and retrieval by an electronic system in the Anti-Poison Centre of the Gemelli Hospital. Acta Pharmacol Toxicol. 1977; 41 (Suppl.II): 496-501.

(11) Wahba AHW: Some international aspects of poison control. In: Roche L (Ed): Toxicovigilance, op.cit., p.57-66.

(12) WHO-Regional Comittee For Europe: The organization and functioning of Poisons Information Centres. Summary report of a meeting held at Istanbul, 7-11 September, 1965. WHO-Regional Comittee for Europe (EUR/RC15/Techn. Disc./4), Copenhagen, 1965.

(13) Christen H-J, Karsten J, Korporal J, v Törne J, Zink A, Zink C: Accidental poisoning in children under eight years of age: Epidemiology - social risks. Méd Légale, Toxicol. 1980; 23: 654-661.

PHARMACY SYSTEM PLANNING AND ORGANIZATIONAL GROWTH

Adriaan J. HOELEN

Medical Information Services

Sint Radboud Hospital,

Catholic University,

Nijmegen, Netherlands.

1. OVERVIEW

In the early seventies the St. Radboudhospital saw many modifications
to the then existing drug distribution methods. Introduction of
computer assisted inventory and turnover management, a hospital-wide
formulary, unit-dose packaging, standard procedures for the recording of drug administrations and assistant-pharmacists for ward-
services were accompanied by improved procedures in the pharmacy and
expansion of pharmaceutical and pharmacological research.

The proposal for the development of the drug distribution system as
presented in 1976 projected
1) introduction of an on-line pharmacy inventory control system,
2) introduction of an on-line medication-order entry system with ward-
inventory control, 3) introduction of structures for direct unit-
dose distribution from the pharmacy to the patient. After acceptance
of phase 1 a commercially available program package was implemented
and adapted to the pharmacy's needs (IBM Health Care Support Pharmacy Inventory Control System). To the support of the drug database
a national drug-product information file service was developed with
the support of ten other hospitals, and subsequently transferred to
the independent FARMODEX-foundation.

A study of the fulfilment of the necessary conditions for the start
of phase 2 has now been completed. Standard procedures for written
medication orders and recording of drug administrations are operational on most wards. Medication-carts and other physical distribution means and procedures are generally accepted. Deliveries, returns
and inter-ward drugs exchanges are recorded on standard forms.
Assistent pharmacists check periodically the ward stock. The data for
a closed drug control system are thus available. Periodical feedback
of actual drug consumption (and loss of data) to the staff of several representative wards has shown to stimulate awareness and accuracy of drug handling. The feedback data, however, can only be produced routinely by an on-line system (1).

Disturbing factors such as use of fractions of tablets, multi flacons
and stat medication orders were easily detected and were brought in
discussion. By simulation of data-entry, computer algorithms and
output it was shown that an on-line drug comsumption and inventory
control system on the wards can work in practice. The study generated
considerable support by the pharmacy and nursing personnel for the
development and implementation of such a system. The broad support
will lead to better system specifications and faster implementation.
Thus the necessary conditions for minimizing the risk of the development in terms of return on investment are fulfilled.

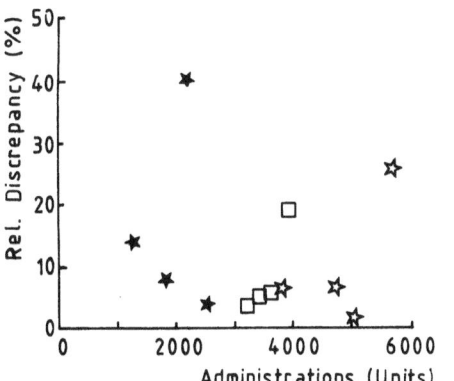

Figure 1. Relative discrepancy vs. total administrations on record. □=ward A, ★=ward B, ☆=ward C.

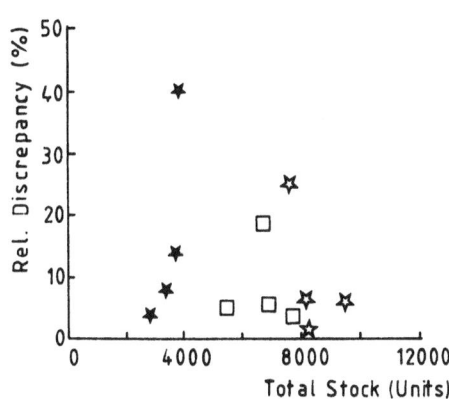

Figure 2. Relative discrepancy vs. average total stock on the ward.

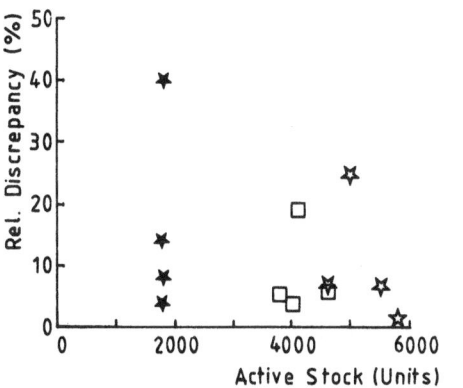

Figure 3. Relative discrepancy vs. average active stock.

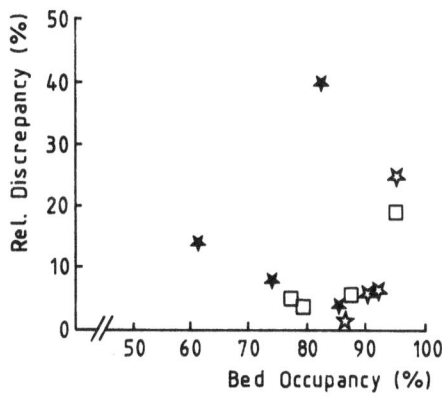

Figure 4. Relative discrepancy vs. bed occupancy.

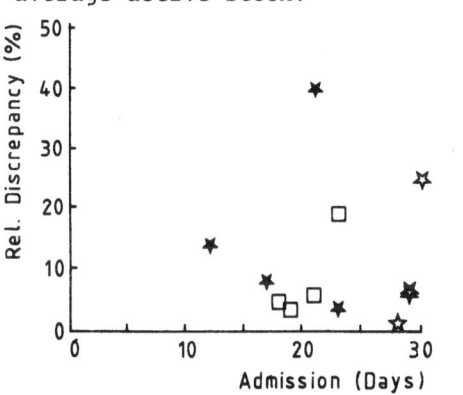

Figure 5. Relative discrepancy vs. average duration of hospitalisation.

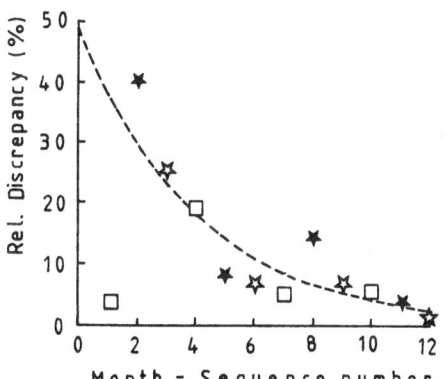

Figure 6. The effect of learning on accounting accuracy.
(--- = $48.e^{-j/4}$).

2. THE SIMULATION STUDY

2.1. Simulation and feedback as change agents

Existing litterature points to a variety of medication errors and to
resistance to on-line performance monitoring (2). Therefore, a measure for the quality of drug handling should be easily acceptable in
order to obtain co-operation. Doubtful therapy and the like should
be studied seperately. In addition the measure should reflect the
quality of the handling process in toto, rather than highlight errors
at a personal level. The manually simulated computation of such a
measure would meet little resistance. Feedback of the results could
be used as a change agent(3).

2.2. Measure of performance

In a cyclic pattern three wards participated in twelf substudies of
four weeks each. Per period the number of administrations per drug
was computed from the medication charts. At the end the clerical
stock was computed for each drug indexed by i as:
clerical stock = initial actual stock + deliveries to ward + borrows
from other wards - returns to pharmacy - loans to other wards - number of administrations.
The relative total discrepancy per period j was computed as:
$\delta_r(j) = 100.\sum |\{\text{clerical stock} - \text{actual final stock}\}_{i,j}|/N_j$ %
where Nj = total number of administrations in period j. The final
figure $\delta_r(j)$ and the underlying data were discussed in meetings of
nursing, pharmacy and administrative personnel. Corrective procedural actions were encouraged. However, reports to higher management
were delayed until after the study.
After the twelf substudies the correlations between relative discrepancies and total administrations, the average of total stock,
active stock, bed occupancy and duration of hospitalisation, and the
sequence number of the period were plotted (figures 1 through 6).

2.3. Results and conclusions

Significant relations between relative discrepancies in drug handling and the different measures of workload could not be demonstrated. The effect of feedback and evaluation, however, is distinct.
(figure 6).
A relative discrepancy below 2 % per month could easily be achieved.
Retrospective evelutation and feedback across wards can be a strong
motivator for the improvement of medication handling. Reflection on
possible causes of discrepancies out of the heat of immediate patient
care creates freedom to learn.

Litterature

1. Hoelen AJ etal·(1981). Progress in Clinical Pharmacy III. Elsevier-
   North Holland, Amsterdam pp 339 - 350.

2. Souder DE etal.(1979). Computer Aid to Drug Therapy and to Drug
   Monitoring. North Holland, Amsterdam, pp. 291-301.

3. Rogers CR (1969). Freedom to Learn. Merrill, Columbus, Ohio.

Joerg Hasford

Institut für Medizinische Informationsverarbeitung, Statistik und Biomathematik
(ISB) der Universität München (Vorstand: Prof. Dr. K. Überla)

Klinikum Großhadern

8000 München 70

Federal Republic of Germany

20 YEARS OF ADVERSE DRUG REACTION MONITORING: A REVIEW

Zusammenfassung:

Als Folge der Contergan Katastrophe wurden in den vergangenen 20 Jahren
spezielle Verfahren zur systematischen Suche, Erfassung und Auswertung
von unerwünschten Arzneimittelwirkungen entwickelt. Die wichtigsten
Ansätze wie Intensive Drug Monitoring, Medical Record Linkage,
Registered Release, Geweberegister und Spontanerfassung werden kurz
beschrieben. Anhand der Kriterien: Beobachtete Population, beobachtete
Medikamente, Art der erfaßten unerwünschten Reaktion, Beobachtungs-
dauer und Qualität der Daten wird eine Beurteilung der bisherigen
Leistungen dieser Verfahren versucht. Abschließend wird auf den Ein-
fluß der Arzneimittelüberwachung auf Verschreibungsgewohnheiten und
Patientenverhalten eingegangen.

Fairly exactly twenty years ago the Thalidomide-disaster made us realize the potential dangers of drug use. As a corollary systematic Adverse Drug Reaction Monitoring (ADRM) was born. Meanwhile this newborn
child has grown and time has come to think about the achievements and
failures of this young adult.
Methods developed specifically for the detection of Adverse Drug
Reactions (ADRs) will be shortly described first. Later some ideas
will be presented how to evaluate the given methods and structures
of ADRM.

Spontaneous Reporting (SR) is one of the oldest and most common ways
of collecting and analysing case reports of adverse events. Mostly
doctors working in outpatient care and, to a lesser degree, pharmacists inform the national registry or the pharmaceutical manufacturer
by mailing given questionnaires, e.g. yellow card. The questionnaire
contains demographic data, data on underlying diseases, the actual
medication, temporal sequence, and a description of the adverse event.

The registry analyses the report and, if necessary, further steps are taken. Many national registries cooperate with the WHO·SR-registry, containing about 215000 case reports in their files (1). SR requires an individual, who links an adverse event with a drug as causative factor.

This prerequisite forms the basis of the case report sections in medical journals like the BMJ, the Lancet and the N. Engl. J. Med. and of the Registry of Tissue Reactions to Drugs (TR) of the Armed Forces Institute of Pathology. There, tissue specimens of autopsies and biopsies of suspected ADRs are examined in order to assess the ADR as such and the probability of a true drug – adverse event relationship.

The tisues are to a great extent received from army – or VA-hospitals. About 4000 case have been investigated until now (2).

When patients are closely watched by nurses or doctors for eventually occurring adverse events, this is called Intensive Drug Monitoring (IDM). Usually all relevant data of every patient are collected: Anamnese, drug history, diagnoses and labtests, drug intake and all events according to the specific definition of the project. These data are analysed for frequencies and screened for associations; case-control and cohort studies can be done. IDM is preferably used in hospitals and its best known representative is the Boston Collaborative Drug Surveillance Program (3,4). There was at least one attempt to use the IDM procedure in outpatient care (5).

But as outpatients cannot be monitored as intensively as inpatients, the Kaiser Permanente Drug Reaction Monitoring System (KPDRMS) used the techniques of Medical Record Linkage (MRL) i.e. integrating medical data of individuals gathered from different sources (6) for analysing their data. For example: One links the data of a congenital malformation registry or of a cancer registry with the data of a prescription registry and looks for associations, which then have to be further investigated. A prerequisite is the identification of individuals in the linked registries by the same code e.g. the social security number. According to the data bases, in- or outpatients can be monitored, but usually at least one hospital fed registry is necessary. Prototypes of MRL are the Oxford Record Linkage Study (ORLS) (7) and the 'Finnish Case-Control Study on Breast Cancer and the Use of Rauwolfia' (8).

Questionnaires (SAQ) administered by the patients themselves have been used for ADRM of chronically sick people like diabetics, hypertonics and rheumatoid arthritics (9).

There are further methods for ADRM too, mainly for adhoc research resp. a single purpose: Case-control studies, analyses of morbidity and mortality (vital) statistics and studies about special drugs. These are the most common concepts for ADRM of the last 20 years. Monitored, Restricted, Recorded or Registered Release (RR) mean more or less the same and are among the very recent developments (10,11). The first consumers of newly marketed drugs get centrally registered to form a cohort, which can be followed-up prospectively to recognize adverse effects as early as possible. The registration is done either by the prescribing physician, the dispensing pharmacist or the patient himself. The cohort can be intensively monitored or only be used as an always accessible data base, if suddenly an alerting signal occurs. The limited experience with this approach is partly promising (12,13). A certain type of RR is the Prescription-Event Monitoring (PEM), which has just started its work, no results being available at present (14). Having all these tools of ADRM in mind one will be amazed that the opinions about the achieved level of 'drug safety' i.e. knowledge about the risks of drug use are quite contradictory (3,15) and that there are with few exceptions no attempts of a systematic evaluation of the present situation of ADRM (16,17).

I will concentrate now on the following questions, which seem to be appropriate for discussing the achieved level of ADRM:
1. What kind of drug consumers are surveyed ?
2. What kind of drugs are monitored ?
3. What kind of ADRs are looked for ?
4. How long are the observation periods ?
5. Which is the quality of the collected data ?
6. What kind of conclusions can be drawn from these data ?
7. Which is the institutional basis of ADRM-projects ?
8. What is the impact of ADRM on society ?

Of course more questions could be asked, but even these questions cannot be answered at length within the limits of this paper. Nevertheless my aim is to contribute to the evaluation of the achieved comprehensiveness of ADRM.

1. What kind of drug consumers are monitored ?

Basically there are three different kinds of drug consumers: Inpatients, outpatients and non-patients i.e. people who take drugs without contact to professional help. Non-patients are an important drug consumers group; in the FRG about every fourth DM spent on drugs is paid by non-patients. And one should not forget those people who take drugs prescribed for others. Most of the systematic ADRM schemes with huge data banks like IDM and MRL cover mainly inpatients as does TR.

Outpatients have only rarely been monitored with an IDM scheme like the KPDRMS. Apart from that, outpatients are covered by SR, RR, PEM and partly MRL, but these are the less accurate procedures. Lay drug consumption is not systematically monitored at all at present. To put it to an extreme, the larger the population the lesser is the intensity of ADRM.

Patients can be further differentiated according to their underlying medical condition. Going into details we would find important differences in the intensity of monitoring.

2. What kind of drugs are monitored ?

Dividing drugs in the groups of established, newly marketed, prescription and otc drugs, we will find that IDM covers mainly established and prescription drugs, which are used in hospitals. Prescription drugs are monitored by MRL, RR, PEM and the KPDRMS. RR and PEM have been developed mainly for newly marketed drugs, MRL preferably works with established drugs. SR covers all groups as long as the patient gets in contact with a professional. The most neglected groups are otc and newly marketed drugs, because RR is a single purpose approach and not in common use. Drugs can be more detailed differentiated according to their therapeutic properties, their use in diagnosis or therapy or their underlying concept like homeopathic drugs, the latter are not systematically monitored at all.

3. What kind of ADRs are looked for ?

There is no generally accepted definition of ADR. Each project works with its own definition. Mostly these definitions are linked with certain impacts on physician's behaviour like 'causes stop or change of the current medication'. As physicians dominate all ADRM projects, there will be a medical bias in observation and interpretation. IDM projects quite often use adverse event check lists, so implicitely one knows already beforehand what kind of ADRs one will find. IDM projects tend to find severe medical events and reactions detectable by diagnostic techniques. Additionally inpatients have a very restricted life style, so many ADRs connected with common daily living e.g. alcohol, work, food cannot be detected in a hospital setting. Generally spoken IDM, MRL and TR concentrate on more serious medical events. SR, SAQ, PEM and partly RR and MRL use broader definitions of ADRs: Medical, mental and behavioural, psychomotoric, minor and extraordinary effects (18) can be detected. The chance to detect therapeutic failures or previously unknown positive effects - both generally not included in the objectives of the projects - is greater with IDM.

4. How long are the observation periods ?

The time lag between drug intake and adverse reaction may vary considerably. An anaphylactoid reaction can start within seconds, whereas a carcinoma takes years or a whole generation to develop. Detecting immediate, visible reactions poses hardly any problem. IDM will find ADRs as long as the patient is in hospital, on the average about thirty days. This observation period is prolonged for the time the drug history is taken, or when the patient is in the same hospital more than once. SR could cover the whole latent period, but it is less likely that a doctor will link an adverse event with a drug intake a long time ago. MRL, RR and PEM can be used for long latent periods, but there is almost no experience with RR and PEM in this field.

5. How is the quality of the collected data ?

Given the premise that good quality of data in Drug Monitoring means
- exact recording of the drug intake of every observed person,
- exact recording of the ADR (temporal sequence, clinical symptoms etc.),
- exact recording of the underlying diseases of the patient,
the IDM data are of the relatively best quality. All relevant data are recorded, the hospital files are accessible and the data are collected for ADRM purposes. RR and PEM data will also be of quite good quality if they are collected properly. The data of MRL usually are of lower quality, mainly because these data have not been collected for ADRM purposes. The quality of SR data depends on the accuracy with which the questionnaires are filled in. But the quite common lack of accuracy can be compensated, as it is done in the UK, by reexamining the reported cases by specialists.

Is must be noted however that the quality of the data as defined here is of variable importance for the different methods.

6. What kind of conclusions can be drawn from the data ?

The data should allow at least
- an assessment of the probability of a true drug - adverse event relationship,
- an estimation of the incidence of the ADR, and
- a risk - benefit evaluation.

An assessment of a true drug - adverse event relationship is possible with IDM, MRL, RR and PEM by generally accepted epidemiological techniques, it is still very difficult with SR. IDM, MRL, RR and PEM can be used to generate and to prove hypotheses, SR serving as an early warning system only for generating hypotheses. Incidence data can be expected by IDM, MRL, RR and PEM but not by SR. The reason is the

lack of a denominator and unquantifiable underreporting. Consequently
SR data are not well qualified for risk-benefit assessments.

7. Which is the institutional basis of ADRM-projects ?

The drug laws of most countries do not provide ADRM as a compulsory
part of drug marketing. The majority of IDM, MRL, RR and PEM schemes
are research projects financed by grants for a more of less limited
time. Among other disadvantages this insecure position creates problems
for the recruitment of qualified manpower and it endangers independence
from the financing body and its interests. More than one promising ADRM
project had to close for a lack of money. ADRM still depends largely on
the economic situation and is not an accepted necessity of responsible
drug use.

Only SR as a pretty cheap scheme is in a relatively secure position.
This weak institutional basis of ADRM is one reason for the fact an
integrated ADRM program covering all relevant fields is lacking. Quite
often the different projects work on their own, being uncoordinated as
to their objectives.

8. What is the impact of ADRM on society ?

There are four target groups of ARDM findings:

- Regulatory agencies,

- pharmaceutical manufacturers,

- physicians and

- consumers.

Till today regulatory agencies tend to overestimate the benefit of
premarketing safety tests. There is an abundance of official guidelines for animal tests but almost none for ADRM. Only some regulatory
agencies do ADRM themselves, but a lot of them support them financially.
Once severe ADRs did occur the rationale of the agencies' decisions
are not always transparent. One gets the impression that the chance
of withdrawal is greater for newley marketed drugs than for established
drugs. 'Oldtimers' demonstrate sometimes a remarkable resistance as in
the FRG Chloramphenicol, Metamizol and Phenacetin are still marketed.
As far as physicians' prescription and peoples' consumption behaviour
is concerned serious doubts about a positive impact of ADRM findings
exist. The number of drug prescriptions is increasing and as case
studies demonstrate even proven ADRs do not sufficiently influence
physician's prescribing, even when there are adequate therapeutic
alternatives (19). Of course prescription habits can be changed by
continued education, but in many countries an independent continued
education scheme i.e. not funded by the pharmaceutical industry does
not exist. There is not much information about lay drug consumption

habits, but there are clues that even in spite of the well known risks of drug intake during pregnancy there is still an enormous drug intake even for minor ailments (20).

Conclusion

There has been made considerable progress in the development of suitable methods for ADRM in the last years, however a comprehensive system, covering all fields of potential drug risks, does not exist anywhere. But at least in some western countries ADRM of established drugs works well with inpatients, especially for ADRs with an onset within short time. The situation of ADRs with a long latent period, ADRs with a low incidence and of ADRs similar to spontaneously occuring events is less satisfying. The state of hardly recognizable ADRs, of drugs with low sales figures, of nonpatients and of otc drugs is even worse.
The legal status of ADRM should be strengthened. Education of researchers interested in ADRM should be started.
Finally, I think, assessing the risks of postmarketing drug use is a responsibility of the pharmaceutical manufacturer, who should have ADRM done by an independent institution.

References:

1. Dunne, J.F.: World Health Organisation. In: Monitoring for Drug Safety, Inman, W.H.W., (ed.),pp. 133 Lancaster: MTP Press Ltd. 1980

2. Irey, N.S.: Adverse Drug Reactions and Death: A Review of 827 Cases. JAMA 236,575 (1976).

3. Jick, H.: In-Hospital Monitoring of Drug Effects - Past Accomplishments and Future Needs. In: Computer Aid to Drug Therapy and to Drug Monitoring, Ducrot, H., Goldberg, M., Hoigné, R., Middleton, P., (eds.), pp.3, Amsterdam- New York- Oxford: North Holland PC 1978.

4. Lawson, D.H.: Hospital-based Intensive Drug Monitoring. In: Drug Monitoring, Gross, F.H., Inman. W.H.W. (eds.), pp. 27, London: Academic Press 1977.

5. Friedman, G.D., Collen, M.F., Harris, L.E., Van Brunt, E.E., Davis L.S.: Experience in Monitoring Drug Reactions in Outpatients: The Kaiser Permanente Drug Monitoring System. JAMA 271,567 (1971).

6. Acheson, E.D.: Linkage of Medical Records. Br. Med. Bull. 24, 206 (1968).

7. Skegg, D.C.G.: Medical Record Linkage. In: Monitoring for Drug Safety, Inman, W.H.W. (ed.), pp. 337 Lancaster: MTP Press Ltd. 1980.

8. Aromaa, A., Hakama, M., Hakulinen, T., Saxen, E., Teppo, L., Heikkilä, J.: Breast Cancer and Use of Rauwolfia and other Antihypertensive Agents in Hypertensive Patients: A Nationwide Case-Control Study in Finland. Int. J. Cancer 18, 727 (1976).

9. Bulpitt, C.J., Dollery, C.T.: Evalution of the Symptoms of treated hypertensive Patients. Meth. Inform. Med. 18, 36 (1979).

10. Dollery, C.T., Rawlins, M.D.: Monitoring adverse reactions to drugs. Br. Med. J. I, 96 (1977).

11. Lawson, D.H., Henry, H.A.: Monitoring adverse reactions to new drugs: "restricted release" or "monitored release"? Br. Med. J. I, 691 (1977).

12. Überla, K.K.: Statistische Gesichtspunkte zur Überwachung unerwünschter Nebenwirkungen zugelassener Medikamente. Vortrag am Methformin-Symposium, Wien 7.3.1980.

13. Wardell, W.M., Tsianco, M.C., Anavekar, S.N., Davis, H.T.: Postmarketing Surveillance of New Drugs: I. Review of Objectives and Methodology. II. Case Studies. I. J. Clin. Pharmacol. 19, 85 (1979). II. J. Clin. Pharmacol. 19, 169 (1979).

14. Inman,W.H.W.: Postmarketing surveillance of adverse drug reactions in general practice. II. Prescription-event monitoring at the University of Southampton. Br. Med. J. 282, 1216 (1981).

15. Karch, F., Lasagna, L.: Adverse Drug Reactions in the US. MIPI (Medicine in the public interest) Washington DC 1974.

16. Joint Commission of Prescription Drug Use: Report of Joint Commission on Prescription Drug Use - Final Report. Rockville 1980.

17. Hasford, J.: Drug Monitoring - State of the Art. Erweitertes Vortragsmanuskript, ISB München 1980.

18. Skegg, D.C.G., Richard, S.M., Doll. R.: Minor tranquillisers and road accidents. Br. Med. J. I, 917 (1979).

19. Stewart, D.J.: Prevalence of Tetracyclines in Children's Teeth - Study II: A Resurvey after Five Years. Br. Med. J. 3, 320 (1973).

20. Deutsche Forschungsgemeinschaft (Hrsg.): Schwangerschaftsverlauf und Kindesentwicklung- Forschungsbericht. Boppard: Harald Bold (1977).

USING A MICRO-COMPUTER FOR DRUG MONITORING
IN GENERAL PRACTICE

M. G. Sheldon
Senior Lecturer in General Practice
Department of Community Health
Nottingham University Medical School
Nottingham.   NG7 2UH
England

SUMMARY

A Z80 based microcomputer system was installed in a busy health centre serving 12,000 patients. Problems arose with the choice of computer hardware and operating system, methods of data collection, entry and verification, file structure and production of output. An encounter form was designed to collect information. These problems are discussed and some of the solutions used are described.

INTRODUCTION

Many general practitioners in Great Britain are now experimenting with computers in their practices. Mostly they are engaged in routine administrative tasks such as maintaining practice registers, organising recall systems and running repeat prescription systems. If computer systems are going to play a part in the clinical care of patients it must first be demonstrated that accurate clinical information can be routinely collected by the general practitioner and his staff.

Several difficulties have been encountered with a computer system installed two years ago in a busy health centre serving 12,000 patients. The main problem areas have been the choice of computer hardware and operating systems, data collection, data entry and verification, and the file structure and output.

The first step in a successful implementation is for the doctors and the systems analyst to spend a lengthy gestation period discussing the aims and practicalities of the system. Only by combining computer expertise and clinical expertise can a reliable, efficient and effective computer system be produced where the benefits accruing may outweigh the difficulties and problems which are bound to occur.

COMPUTER HARDWARE

An Equinox series 8000 8 bit microcomputer, (Z80 based) with 64K memory, was installed using the FAMOS operating system. First attempts to use floppy discs and then a Winchester disc were abandoned in favour of a 16 Mb fixed and 16 Mb exchangable disc unit. Both the quantity of information collected, and the need for rapid copying for security purposes, necessitated the fixed and exchangable hard disc unit although the initial cost was higher.

Using the FAMOS operating system we have found this installation barely sufficient to run two VDU's, with unacceptable delays in accessing files because the basic data files have to be searched on each occasion when any file is to be interrogated. Other operating systems (such as CP/M) also have drawbacks and at present we probably have to accept that multi-users on the cheaper microcomputers leaves much to be desired. As is always the case in computing, the models becoming available just after the purchase of one's own system are so much superior. Hopefully, future users with 16 bit microprocessors and improved operating systems will by-pass the problems we experienced - and probably discover other problems at present undreamt of!

DATA COLLECTION

A major problem in the creation of a G.P. information system is the decision concerning which information to collect and which to omit. This problem is heightened if more than one doctor is involved, mainly because no-one has a clear idea of what to do with the information once it has been entered into the computer. The most useful starting point is for the doctors to commit to paper the aims and objectives of the system. The relevant portion of our aims were:-

Information will be collected so that we may:-

AUDIT the process of clinical care, particularly the medications used on prescriptions;

ANALYSE the practice workload;

MONITOR DRUG THERAPY by event recording.

In order to achieve these aims we realised that data collection must be continuous, comprehensive and correct.

CONTINUOUS: The method of data capture must fit into the practice routine and not involve the doctor in extra work or significantly alter his method of working.

COMPREHENSIVE: Clinical information is generated in a variety of ways. Face to face consultations take place in the surgery, the home and even the street. Then there are telephone consultations, repeat prescriptions and letters and reports about patients. The patient may also be seen by other health workers in the practice and the

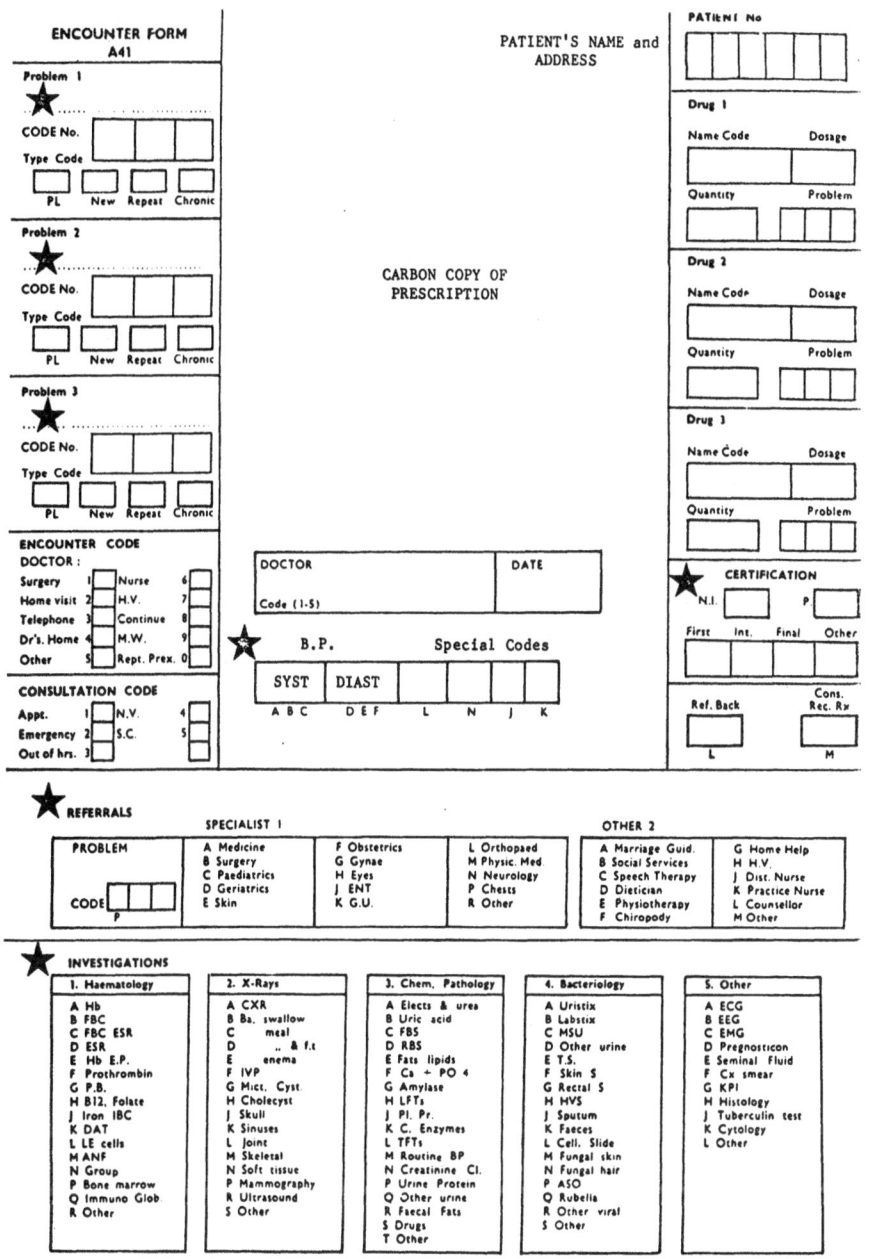

FIG. 1 - A sample of A4 sized encounter form used to collect data in the practice. A prescription is pinned over the form as indicated and the patient identifying data, doctor and date automatically recorded. The GP fills in the data indicated by a star. Coding is done separately by a trained member of the practice staff.

method of data collection must cope with all these factors.

CORRECT: Data verification is usually ignored in general practice. It was decided to put all data entry into the hands of trained ancillary staff and allow the G.P. to verify the data by producing a print-out of each patient's record, placing it in the patient's record to be seen by the doctor at each future consultation. This procedure raised further problems in the volume of paper produced and the time required for filing. At the present, these seems to be no ideal way for the doctor to verify the data, although with complete replacement of the medical record, the G.P. should be able to edit using the VDU screen during the consultation. (1)

To meet these requirements for data collection an ENCOUNTER FORM was designed (Fig. 1) This form was used mainly by the doctor during a consultation, but also served as the common data collection vehicle in the practice. Using action paper a carbon copy of any prescription issued is automatically taken and if the practice receptionist adds the patient identification data all the doctor needs to add are the problems encountered and any other important clinical notes or decisions taken. This form is completed in addition to maintaining the written records, so must be as simple as possible for the doctor to complete. Extensive experience with this type of form has indicated that it is practical and easy to use. (2,3).

DATA ENTRY

At this stage in the use of computers it is probably unrealistic to expect doctors to code information or learn to type accurately enough to enter data into a computer system. A secretary is best trained to code drugs and diagnoses, enter the information and run the computer. We have found that a practice of four doctors will require approximately one full-time ancillary worker to cope with all the extra work generated. In a practice of 12,000 patients it was found that two VDU's were needed for access of information, but with the operating system used this caused considerable problems with delay in accessing information and 'locking' of terminals when both tried to access the basic patient data file at the same time.

FILE STRUCTURE

An indexed file structure was used using the patient number as the key. All associated records were linked together by the key and a date for each encounter record. A counter on the basic data file was used which meant that this file had to be accessed each time the encounter file was to be searched. This dramatically

slowed the whole process. Other serious flaws in the system used were lack of
duplicate keys and lack of multiple indexes. Again, the effect was to slow
access and reduce multi-user effectiveness.

ORGANISATION OF OUTPUT

As with many first-time users all the effort and energy went into designing the
system to allow easy input and very little thought was given to what output would be
needed. We would recommend that as much thought is given to the final uses of the
information as to how to collect it. Two of the main uses of the output for this
system were for drug monitoring using event recording and analysis of prescriptions

---

PRIMARY CARE COMPUTERS LTD.   PATIENT RECORDS SYSTEM   DATE : 23-06-80

                                      PATIENT EVENT DATA   SEX : MALE

PATIENT NUMBER : 110001   NAME : BLOGGS FRED   TITLE : MR   DOCTOR : M S HARVEY

DATE : 01-04-80   ENCOUNTER NO   : 0001   ENCOUNTER CODE : SURGERY   CONSULTATION CODE : APPT

                   CERTIFICATION : 1A   ENCOUNTER DR   : P WILLIAMS

                   INVESTIGATIONS : 1A   3D

                   NOTES   : 1   1   5   0   9   5   *   *   *   *   *   *

                   ---REFERRALS---   ---------DIAGNOSES----------   ----------------DRUGS----------------
                   PROB   CODE   DESCRIPTION   TYPE   DESCRIPTION   DOSE PROB QTY

                    1   2K   ACUTE TONSILLITIS   A   AMOXIL 125MG/5ML SYR   B   1   100
                    2   1K   URETHRITIS   A   CHLORAMPHNN.EYEDROPS   D   1   90
                                   OBS.&CARE O.HIGHRISK PTS. B   PROPRANOLOL160MGSA T   K   1   50

DATE : 01-05-80   ENCOUNTER NO   : 0002   ENCOUNTER CODE : HOME VISIT   CONSULTATION CODE : APPT

                   CERTIFICATION : 1A   ENCOUNTER DR   : M R NEWBY

                   INVESTIGATIONS : 4C

                   NOTES   : *   *   *   *   *   *   *   *   *   *   *   Y

                   ---REFERRALS---   ---------DIAGNOSES----------   ----------------DRUGS----------------
                   PROB   CODE   DESCRIPTION   TYPE   DESCRIPTION   DOSE PROB QTY

                                   CONTACT WITH V.D.   A   PIRITON 4MG. TABS.   D   1   100
                                   IATROGENIC DISEASE   D   PENICILLIN V 250MG T   D   1   50
                                   RASH&O.NONSPEC.SKIN ERUPT G

FIG. 2 - Sample of patient event record produced by the computer. Several
           entries can be condensed onto one sheet and provide a summary of all
           events for each patient.

384

issued.

Event Recording

By collecting information on diagnosis, therapy and referral for every encounter a picture can be built up of the events occurring after the use of a new drug. This method of collecting data has been recommended as one of the best ways of post-marketing surveillance for new drugs (4), and the use of an encounter form and encounter record (Fig. 2) are convenient ways of achieving such surveillance.

		Patient Records System				Page 2		
		Print Morbidity Register				Date 01-02-81		

Morbidity Register for the quarter 01-10-80 to 31-12-80

Diagnosis------- Description	Patient Number	Encounter Date	Dr	Date of Birth	Sex	Drug	Type	Qty
	113393	291080	1	190716	Male	Frusemide 20mg. Tab	1	40
						Slow-K Tabs.	1	40
						Stilboestrol 1mg.Tab	3	120
Hypertension,on Treatment	112582	111280	1	110629	Male	Hydrallazine 50mg.T.	4	120
						Tenormin 100mg. Tab.	1	30
	112582	121180	1	110629	Male	Tenormin 100mg. Tab.	1	30
						Bendrofluazide 5mg.T	1	30
						Hydrallazine 50mg.T.	4	120
	112582	011080	1	110629	Male	Bendrofluazide 5mg.T	1	30
						Hydrallazine 50mg.T.	4	120
						Tenormin 100mg. Tab.	1	30
	112732	241180	1	040325	Male	Inderal 80mg Tabs.	4	120
						Hydrallazine 50mg.T.	4	120
						Navidrex K. Tabs.	1	30
	112732	271080	1	040325	Male	Inderal 80mg Tabs.	4	120
						Hydrallazine 50mg.T.	4	120
						Navidrex K. Tabs.	1	30
	112732	311280	1	040325	Male	Inderal 80mg Tabs.	4	120
						Hydrallazine 50mg.T.	4	120
						Navidrex K. Tabs.	1	30
	112737	231280	1	040806	Male	Trasicor 40mg.Tabs.	2	60
						Apresoline 25mg Tabs	2	60
	112779	291280	1	241110	Male	Aldomet 250mg. Tab	3	90
	112809	061180	1	310142	Male	Inderal L A 160mg.C.	1	30
						Hydrallazine 25mg.T.	4	120
						Bendrofluazide 5mg.T	1	30

FIG. 3 - Sample of the morbidity register showing some of the hypertensive patients, the number of encounters and therapy given.

Prescription Analysis

This system allows information to be displayed either under the drugs used or the diagnoses made. Fig. 3 is a sample of the print-out of patients on treatment for hypertension indicating the number of times they were seen and the drug therapy used. These tables can be used to audit the process of care or to provide an analysis of the therapeutic armamentarium of the doctors in the practice.

CONCLUSION

Before embarking on a computer installation in general practice thought should be given to data capture, entry and verification. The output and uses to which the information is to be put must be agreed and a sufficient amount of cash made available to purchase a suitable computer and software package. It is probably unrealistic to expect a computer system to make a significant contribution to clinical care in the practice for an outlay of less than 50p per patient per annum.

REFERENCES

1. GRUMMITT, A. (1977) "Real-time record management in general practice". Int. J. Bio-Medical Computing, 8, 131 - 150.

2. HAMLEY, J. G., BROWN, S. V., CROOKS, J. et al (1981) "Prescribing in General Practice and the Provision of Drug Information". Journal of the Royal College of General Practitioners 31, 654-660.

3. SHELDON, M. G. (1979) "Self-Audit of Prescribing Habits and Clinical Care in General Practice". Journal of the Royal College of General Practitioners 29, 703 - 711.

4. SKEGG, D. C. G. (1977) "Possible methods of monitoring adverse reactions to drugs in general practice" in 'Drug Monitoring'. Ed. Gross, F. H. and Inman, V. H. W. Academic Press 1977.

THE DEVELOPMENT OF INTEGRATED COMPUTER

FACILITIES WITHIN A DISTRICT HEALTH AUTHORITY

J. Roberts, S. Brook, K. Broadey
Lancaster District Health Authority
Lancaster LA1 4RP

SUMMARY

The Health District considered in this paper in the North of England
has within its sphere of responsibility many of the facets of the
Health Care services faced in any location, without the additional
benefits which may accrue from Teaching Hospital bases in the area.
The brief of the Management structure is to make the most efficient
use of Management resources - be they nursing, clinical, technical,
auxillary, personnel or equipment available. The overview provided
by a District Computer Applications Committee shows the advantages of
cooperation and communication in the best use of limited facilities.

1. INTRODUCTION

Computing power is becoming of more widespread use in the Health Care
field. In the light of the growth of projects requiring the high
speed facilities offered by our mini computer at the Royal Lancaster
Infirmary, a District Computer Working Party was set up in 1979.
Initially used as a communication channel to keep interested parties
up to date with developments, it has now expanded to be a technical
advisory body for the District Management Team and has changed its
title to Computer Applications Advisory Group.

The Lancaster Health District serves a resident population of 125,000
extended by those patients on the periphery and in remote areas who
chose to visit Lancaster for their prime care, giving an estimated
permanent catchment population of 200,000 patients. The population
is quite well defined, "The captive market," a factor which, incidentally assists in the monitoring of the Casualty Activity Profiles
for the prime acute hospital in the District. (1,2,3,4,5). The
Health Care usage is weighted by an influx of holiday makers to the
resorts on the coast and in the Lake District and the proximity of
heavily used motorway and rail links between England and Scotland.
Detailed figures of the use made of facilities is available retrospectively from the Hospital Activity Analysis System. We are working

towards a real-time management information system which will be responsive to and give data for the rapidly altering local situation.

Financial limits are placed on the procurement of equipment for
various purposes locally before Area/Regional agreement is required.
A limit of fifty thousand pounds for total project development would,
up to five years ago, preclude the purchase of viable 'systems' hardware at local level. This is no longer the case, as a processor
(notionally called a microcomputer!) with a 64K of working space,
machine code and high level facilities, and a large amount of backing
storage on floppy or hard discs can now be purchased for around £2,000.
(In the past a number of computers were bought and not used produc-
tively).

2. STRATEGY

The philosophy adhered to in the Lancaster District is to develop
systems in a phased way. Attempts are made to keep in mind the possibility of future extensions to computer-aided systems and the integration into use by or communication between other health care practice
areas. The minimization of duplication of facilities is a foremost
aim. The production of 'tools' to release trained specialists in
particular fields from tedious tasks is also an asset acknowledged as
useful by our administrative and clinical hierarchies locally.

For the credibility of computer services and the justification of the
money put into project development, efforts must be seen to be productive in as short a time as possible and also must be considered of
benefit to the subsequent users. A considerable effort put into a
project with a long time scale which produces little results in the
short term is damaging to the image of Health Care computer personnel.
It also leads to future reticence for other projects.

Successfully implemented computer-aided systems are never achieved
without trauma. Only projects with significant consequences are
particularly noted the others integrate into common use without
further acknowledgement.

3. DEVELOPMENT

The developments carried out in our District involve the design,
implementation and proving of subsystems before integration into
larger projects. For example, the proving of the Delphi-Phoenix
Pathology Data base philosophy on the Ferranti Argus equipment was

carried out in the Biochemistry discipline before progression into
Haematology. Examination of the 'system' in detail has resulted in
the following conclusions. It has been recognized that input/output
requirements of any clinical specialty cannot be generalized to apply
across a number of hospitals. In no way can any 'system' be implemented overnight with completely new equipment. It has been seen that
in for example Biochemistry no two hospitals operate with the same
analytic equipment or have the same operating criteria (and constraints). All laboratories have some established procedures both in
operation of the laboratory and in their reporting techniques which
cannot be terminated instantaneously and for practical reasons cannot
be replaced immediately with efficiently operational "British Standard
Analyzers and Technicians."

The 'core procedures' to collect raw data, turn it into information,
efficiently store, manipulate and secure it, can be provided (6).The
'building blocks' of programs and interfaces required by the particular location can be selected after due consideration from an available
menu of proven working computer 'tools.'

Applying the above principles it is felt that we can offer serviceable
'tools' to, for example radiography, microbiology from the proven
basic working programs in the Phoenix suite.

By looking at ideas and requirements this way it is felt that the
limited computer programming resources can be directed into tailoring
the 'Core systems' to the particular idiosyncracies of the User Department.

Communication at the frequent District Computer Applications Advisory
Committee meetings has resulted in coordination in the multiple use of
facilities in other specialties and areas.

Facilities such as VDU's are installed in a location in response to
the needs of one particular system, but the District Committee has the
opportunity to stand back and review what other demands are potential
from the health care practitioners in operation in that area. An
access device can offer in-house shop-floor teaching aids based on
proven clinical computer aided projects. In our own case a VDU
installed as an Enquiry Terminal for the Pathology system also gives
access to Chemotherapy, Intravenous feeding and other toxic drug calculation programs.

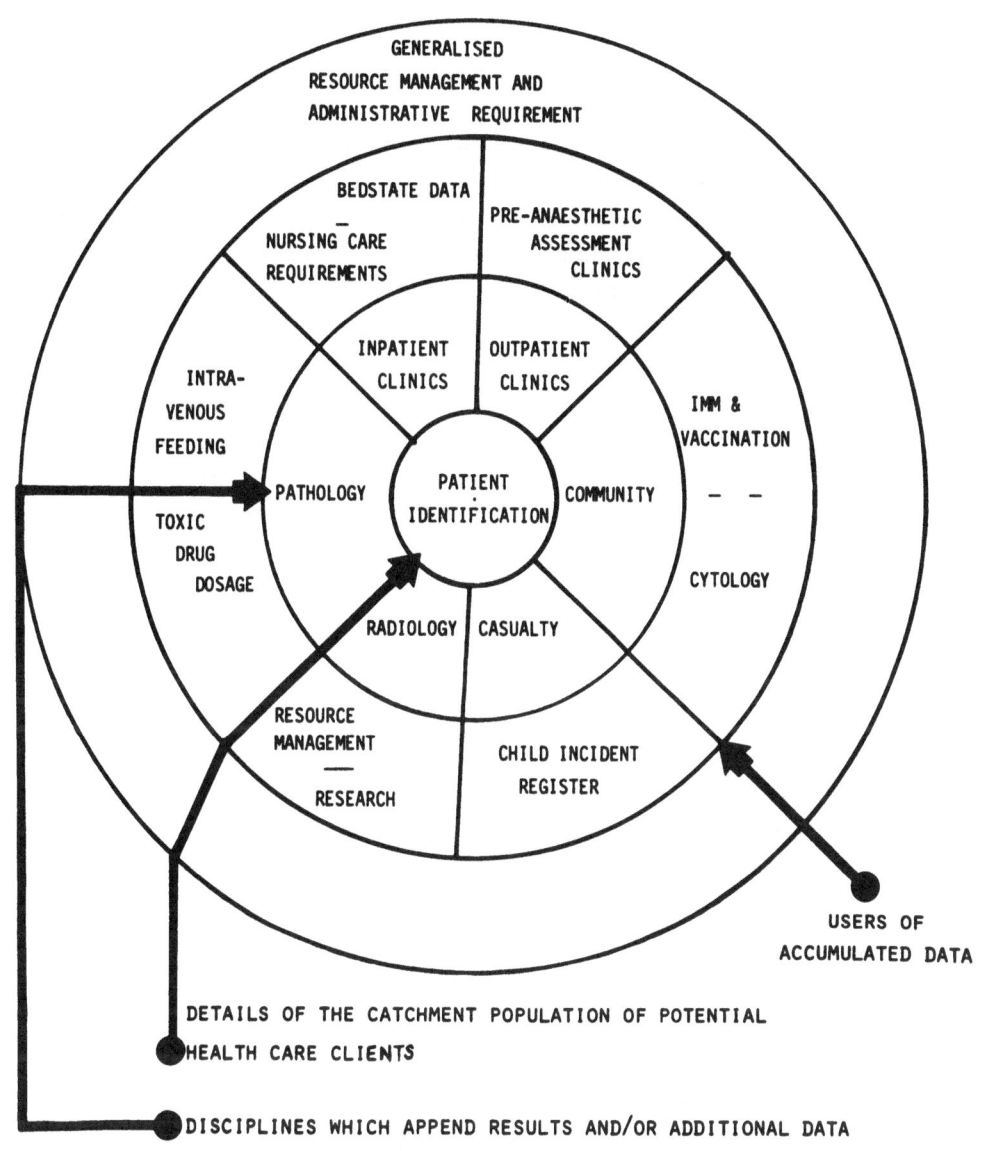

FIGURE 1.

EXAMPLE OF THE INFORMATION REQUIREMENT IN THE DISTRICT

4. EXTENSION

Awareness of the potential use of computer facilities is growing.
There is still a lack of communications between disciplines and locations but the energetic dissemination of material by the B.C.S.,
I.E.E.T.E., and various technical publications such as Medical Informatics and Health and Social Services Journal should ease the problem
IF originators and developers of projects are prepared to declare and/
or publish on their work. Dietetics, Nursing, Occupational Health,
and Electromyography are some of the departments whose computing requirement is becoming more loudly proclaimed. Basically any procedures
that involve data capture, storage and routine analysis may be helped
by the high speed moronic computer. What must be stressed is that
the thought of the introduction of computer facilities will not solve
all problems. Detailed assessment of the current system may highlight
significant areas for improvement without resorting to capital outlay
on computer facilities.

The Computer Committee in a District, as a corporate body of diverse
constituents, exerts an unbiased view on potential gains of project
implementation. This hypothesis has been operated successfully in
our District. Whilst certain bids for immediate project assistance
have been suspended until resources are availabe, the decision has
been accepted as it came from within the 'peer group.'

This idea can be projected upwards in the Health Care hierarchy, but
it is felt necessary to retain a close affinity to the basic activity
of patient care (7). We are well aware that, as in any business we
must make Management Information available,but it must also be of the
right sort at the right level at the right time and only to the right
people.

The U.K. Steering Group on Health Services Information has considered
the information requirements of operational managers and the mechanics of the patient information system. The Report produced (8)
states that data provided must be relevant and timely and the costs
of acquiring such data must be considered. Linkages between sources
of data and users are highlighted without dismissing the controls
required for confidentiality. Our District Computer Policy (9)
appears to be in line with these requirements. In setting up any
Information System on computer it has been found that the data input
devices such as Data Loggers, Bar Code Scanners and Optical Mark and
character readers are considered as tools for the whole range of data
capture requirements in the District. The D.C.A.A.C. can assess a

request for expensive devices in the light of future identified areas of need rather than in isolation. As well as considering the multiplicity of roles for V.D.U.'s and other input/output peripherals, the Committee is conscious that systems can share information such as patient identification details (P.I.D) which perhaps in previous non-related autonomous Health Care systems needed to be kept in duplicate in each of the individual specialties. In this point the D.C.A.A.C. review body is able to allocate facilities by usage and not by emotive 'empire building' demands.

5. PORTABILITY

Every hospital environment is different - all have particular operational constraints and requirements. In designing systems within a District Service, we become not only tolerant of and sensitive to particular Health Care criteria but we aim, through an assessment of the repeated use of basic procedures, protocols and definitions to make our system transferable to other (inter and intra) Regional locations.

It is hoped that communication between ourselves and others at District, Region and D.H.S.S. level will result (a) in other places avoiding the pitfalls we fell into (and got out of eventually!) and that (b) the feedback is cyclic and we are able to benefit from other people's experience in project areas new to us, in order for us to reach efficient service computing functions with as cost-effective use of resources as possible.

6. CONCLUSION

In conclusion it is felt that the coordination of the thoughts of specialists in health care fields, with a particular interest in seeing efficient use of computer facilities, results in better overall deployment of scarce resources and the use of equipment in the areas of greatest need. Constructive criticism by fully informed 'Devils Advocates' amongst one's own Health Care colleagues results in the formulation of more reasoned, logical and hopefully effective proposals for computer assistance in work, be it day-to-day clinical practice, research or health care administration.

The philosophy of a multi-disciplinary team operating as a cohesive force could also be applied to non-computer assisted areas in the Health Care professions. The substantiation of specialized projects in a general forum of informed parties results in an effective end product - that of better Health Care practices.

7. REFERENCES

(1) Harvey P.W., Farrer J.A. Investigation of the Work of the
    Casualty Department by Analysis of a Sample of the Case Notes
    MEDINFO 1974 North Holland Publishing Company 1974 p.523-527.

(2) Roberts J.M., Harvey P.W., Farrer J.A., The Use of a Computer
    System in the Study of the Attendance Profile in a District
    General Hospital Casualty Department Computers in Biomedicine
    1977 Vol.7 No.4 p.291-299.

(3) Roberts J.M., Farrer J.A., Harvey P.W. A Progressive Study of
    the Emergency Room Demands by the Community Medicial Inform.
    1977 Vol.2 No.3 p.197-201.

(4) Dyer J., Farrer J.A., Harvey P.W., Roberts J.M. The Demands made
    on Emergency Room Facilities by an Urban Population Public
    Health 1978 Vol. 92 p.79-85.

(5) Farrer J.A., Harvey P.W., Roberts J.M. Dyer J. A Study of the
    Demands made on Casualty Services by the Population of Socially
    Deprived Urban Areas Medical Informatics Europe 1978
    Springer Verlag Berlin 1978 p. 597-603.

(6) Delphi-Phoenix System - Computer Based Data Handling for
    Pathology Laboratories Ferranti Computer Systems Limited/
    D.H.S.S. Feb. 1980.

(7) Harvey P.W., Roberts J.M. The Problems of Transfering Software:
    a medical case history Medical Inform. 1979 Vol.4 No.4
    p.219-223.

(8) The Steering Group on Health Services Information. Chairman -
    Ms E. Korner Consultative Document N.H.S./D.H.S.S. London.

(9) Computer Applications Working Group - Policy Statement concerning
    the Application of Computers in the Lancaster Health District
    (Internal Document KB/BB/34) March 1981.

A real time system for patient data administration in university
hospitals with distributed processing

T. Landersdorfer, B.-A. Meyer-Bender, R. Greiller
Rechenzentrum der Ludwig-Maximilians-Universität München für die
Medizinische Fakultät, 8000 München 70, Germany

Summary

At the Ludwig-Maximilians-University in Munich the system for patient
data administration is at present being converted from batch processing
to real time processing. This has several important advantages. Processing occurs under the eyes of the administrative personell, that
can thus easier understand and correct errors that might occur. Furthermore, restart facilities have been incorporated.

1. Introduction

In the past 8 years, the computing centre for the medical school of
the Ludwig-Maximilians-University in Munich (RZM) has gained comprehensive experience using batch techniques for patient administration in a large centralized hospital (1).

In 1977 the Universities of the state of Bavaria developed a mutual
plan to install similar EDP-systems in all of the state's medical
schools, the incentive to this venture having been given by
Bavaria's Ministry for Education and Culture. The RZM having by far
the most experience in this field, it was designated to carry the
main burden in planning and implementing the new system.
As opposed to the large centralized hospital of Munich University
- Klinikum Grosshadern - that had so far been the main field of
activity in the RZM, the other medical schools have quite diverse
structures, in general consisting of many small decentralized
hospitals.
Thus, it was imperative to redesign the previous system to enable
real time processing in dialog mode, allowing for both data-acquisition and printout at the seperate local sites. In the course of
this task we took the opportunity to tackle the main difficulties
encountered in the past.

2. Problems encountered in the past

It is possible to divide the most serious problems caused or
furthered by the former batch system into three classes:

- The behaviour of users confronted with logical errors

  Working in batch mode, logical errors - such as demanding a X-Ray
  examination for a patient already dismissed - is not recognized
  until long after acquisition of the erroneous data. Errors of
  this kind lead to the transaction being rejected and a message
  being printed in a comprehensive listing. The resulting delay is
  a considerable nuisance to the terminal operator, being forced to
  review a process he believed long settled. In addition it is
  quite probable that he will have to repeat further transactions,
  initiated after the erroneous one, and rejected on account of the
  resulting incomplete state of data, in spite of their commonly
  being correct.

- The rigid time schedule inposed on unrelated functions

  In a batch system all functions of a certain type have to be
  processed together, and different functions must be executed in a
  serial manner, if there is a possibility that one may be dependant
  on the results of another. However, it is quite common for one
  sequence of batch programs to only execute a single function for
  most cases (patient-records) involved, so that no real interdependance exists. In spite of this factual independance, batch
  processing cannot allow separately processing single cases of high
  priority.

- System behaviour in case of technical failures

  If a batch process is interrupted, it is often impossible, or
  extremely ineffective, to pinpoint the state of progress reached
  so far. As a result, the complete procedure has to be rerun. This
  is quite feasible in an environment using separate input and output files, but using data bases it is very ineffective to execute
  a partial backup and prevent real or fictitious errors caused by
  repetition of functions. It is much easier to rebuild the data
  base from the latest security copy and rerun the complete batch
  sequence. However, this causes a further delay, that can in the
  worst case completely disarrange the user's organzation.

3. Possible solutions

In our oppinion, these difficulties can be overcome by a procedure having the following properties:

- real time transaction processing

    Each user must be able to start any transaction at any time, without regard to the behaviour of other users, and having it processed immediately.

- functional decomposition into data acquisition with checking for formal errors and processing of transactions after performance of logical error checks

    Errors can be classified as belonging to one of two types:

    o formal errors, such as entering an illegal number (check-digit), can easily be discovered and rejected

    o logical errors, needing a comparision between acquired and stored data for detection, call for execution of a considerable part of the process before the check can be made.

    We will show that separation of these functions increases efficiency and safety of the overall system.

- Immediate notification of detection of errors and online correction

    As opposed to the batch processes described above, not only formal errors must be immediately reported and corrected; in fact the possibility of correcting logical errors online is of prime importance. The immediate rejection of logicaly inconsistant data facilitates finding the cause of errors and thus promotes the correctness of data with minimum time lag.

- Enquiry system taylored to the user's needs

    Quite commonly, logical errors can only be analyzed and corrected by the terminal operator after comparision with data previously stored - in fact the error may have been made at an earlier stage and have been detected by the attempt to process a subsequent correct transaction. In the previous system it was necessary to have data base experts to analyze these cases; in the new system the user can request information about the data presently stored, without leaving the momentary mode of performance and employing an enquiry system taylored to his needs. This enquiry mode can, of course, be envoked at any time, not only in case of errors.

4. Implementation

The RZM has a network of computers at its disposal that, as far as patient administration is concerned, consists of a central computer and two preprocessors (2). However, the preprocessors are run in a stand-by mode to enhance availability of vital processes in the hospital, so that only one of them needs be taken into consideration. The terminals for data acquisition and the peripheral printers, both situated in the distributed hospitals or clinics, are attached on-line to the preprocessor. The patient data bases and other mass data, however, are stored in the more powerful central system. This struc-ture reflects the decomposition of task afore mentioned:

- data acquisition and formal checks are carried out on the pre-processor;

- logical checking and processing of transactions - if correct - are executed on the central computer.

Although this structure seems simple at first sight, it actually calls for some software measures that surpass the possibilities of a common data communication system (v. figure 1).

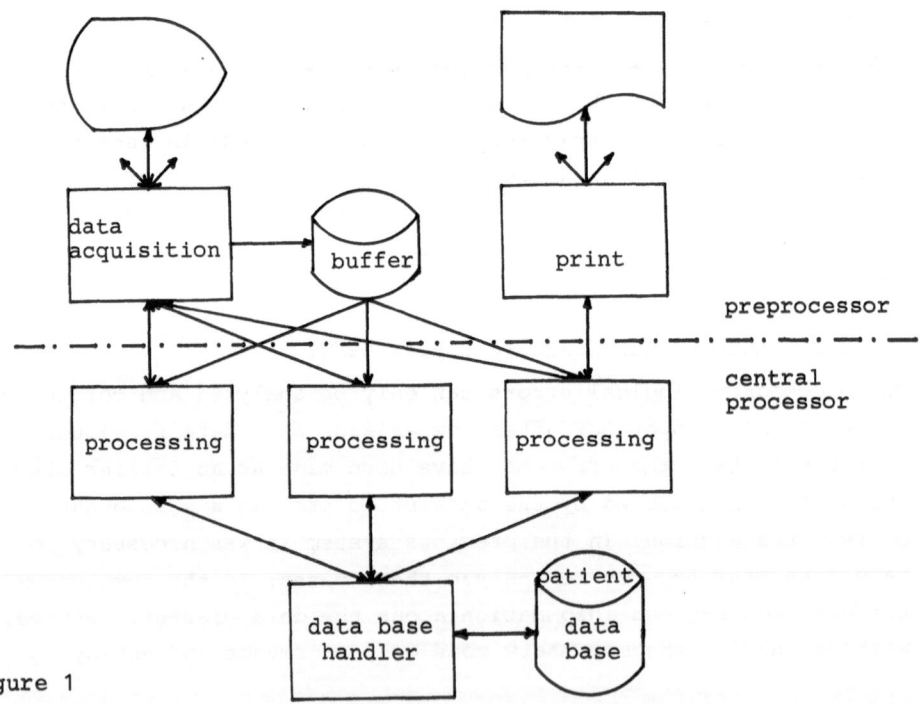

figure 1

- Synchronization of data acquisition and processing

  As far as the user is concerned, a transaction is a single process, although in fact both processors are involved. However, the
  processing of data in the main system occurs in an environment
  and in a time scale different to the user's interface; it is
  therefore imperative, to restore synchronism of messages returned
  to the data acquisition process in the preprocessor.

- Distribution of function of several processes

  The fact that a multitude of diverse transactions are triggered
  by many users at a time, entails the danger of a long queue forming at the entry of the process in the main computer, leading to
  intolerable response times. In order to prevent this, the processing functions are distributed among several jobs running
  simultaneously on the central system. The association of different
  functions to the seperate jobs can be varied according to practical experience, thus enabling optimization of performance; however
  logicaly interdependant functions must be processed in a single
  job.

- Continuation of data acquisition in case of main system failure

  It is very important to prevent the technical state of apparatus
  influencing the organization of the user's time schedule too much.
  The dialog process of data acquisition must therefore be kept in
  action, even if the main computer doing the actual processing
  fails. Of course this implies that for a certain period only
  formal checks can be made, and that the data must be buffered
  until normal work can be resumed.

- Automatic processing of buffered information at restart of the
  main system

  As soon as processing functions are available after restart of the
  main system, the information buffered during the inactive period
  is processed with high priority, in order to maintain the correct
  logical sequence of interdependant data.

- Insertion of messages caused by logical errors detected during
  restart procedures

  The delayed processing after systems restart described above, can,
  of course, detect logical errors, reject execution of the transaction involved, and send error messages to the preprocessor.

Taking into account, what was said about user behaviour in a batch environment, it does not seem appropriate to take the easy way and just print the messages produced in a quasi-batch mode. On the other hand, the terminal operator who initiated the trans- action will at this time almost certainly be working on different data, if he has not left the terminal all together. Thus it is not feasible to relay these messages to the terminal operator in a more or less indiscriminate manner. On the contrary, these messages, having been sent to the preprocessor, must be sorted out into a multitude of queues, each corresponding to a type of function and a set of users (hospital or such). In subsequence the real time process in the preprocessor can see to it, that new terminal activities are prevented until there errors have been corrected, if there is a possibility of interdependance with data newly acquired.

5. Conclusion

The system we have discribed is a great improvement on the previous batch solution. Working in a real time mode, it is adaptable to the user's organization and time schedule, thus noticeably increasing overall acceptance of the system. The terminal operators are much more willing to acquire data correctly and to check the results. The outcome is a marked improvement in correctness and availability of stored data, all errors being detected and corrected at the first moment possible. Furthermore the new programs are less sensivitive to technical failures; the immediate processing of all data entered renders it unnecessary to back all files up to a state secured long before. Only the transaction active at the moment of failure has to be checked and somtimes reentered.

The advantages we have shown in this paper have not yet been proven in productive work, implementation still being in process. At pre- sent the first parts of the system are being integrated into a test version.
However, one property of our new system was a great advantage even during the implementation phase:
In spite of distributed data acquisition and output, we were able to maintain centralized data storage. This saved us a multitude of problems concerning data safety, privacy and global evaluation of distributed data.

Bibliography

(1) SELBMANN, ÜBERLA, GREILLER:
Alternativen medizinischer Datenverarbeitung,
Medizinische Informatik und Statistik, Springer-Verlag, 1976

(2) Autorenteam München, Erlangen, Würzburg:
Datenverarbeitung an den bayerischen Universitätskliniken
data report 16 (1981) Heft 2

The DP-supported Appointment and Control System SARA (Scheduling and Resource Allocation)

Ellsaesser, K.-H., Koehler, C.O., Vosseler, C.

From the Tumor Center Heidelberg/Mannheim (President: Prof. Dr. Dr. h.c. mult. F. Linder) and the German Cancer Research Center, Institute for Documentation, Information and Statistics (Director: Prof. Dr. G. Wagner), Department Central Data Processing (Head Dr.: C.O. Koehler)

SARA (Scheduling And Resource Allocation) is a generator for an appointment and flow control system for outpatients of a hospital in which also inpatients have to be treated in the different laboratories. SARA is part of KRAZTUR, a system for a documentation and information system containing generators for data acquisition, printing, data evaluation and data presentation. SARA can be implemented by only defining the specific parameters for each clinic or hospital in a dialog mode. The user needs not to have DP-knowledge.

1. Introduction

The use of computers in hospitals requires a systematic analysis of organizational structures and events in clinical institutions. On the basis of such a system analysis standardized modules can be developed which can then be adapted to the individual requirements and needs of the respective users by variable parameters.

This technique of software development leads to a system consisting of several modules from which the user selects those that are relevant for him. Such a system is the software and generator system KRAZTUR which is being used at the Tumor Center Heidelberg/Mannheim in a computer network.

In the course of the development of this system an appointment system (appointment and flow control) was also developed; in this paper we want to report on this subsystem.

An effective appointment system fulfils several purposes:
- Punctual and orderly information transfer to the hospitals and service stations to be visited by the patient,
- Lists of patients and appointments for the staff,
- Realistic staff assignment and constantly use of resources,
- Complete monitoring of patients who have to undergo follow-up,
- Shortening of waiting time for patients and thus more rational routine work in the hospital (no waiting queues, smaller waiting rooms) and improvement of the atmosphere of treatment as well as the decrease of wasted working-time for the patients.

2. Tumor Center Heidelberg/Mannheim

The Tumor Center Heidelberg/Mannheim is a pool of hospitals and research institutions in the area Heidelberg/Mannheim for the purpose of coordinating cancer research and cancer control.

In the Tumor Center the generator system KRAZTUR (minicomputer-supported general documentation system with additional text and retrieval functions) - written in MUMPS - is used with the aim of setting up a complete and standardized patient documentation and of rendering assistance for a complete follow-up of tumor patients.

As the hospitals connected to the Tumor Center are scattered throughout a wide area, data processing is realized in a computer network in the form of a star with a central computer (PDP11/60) and four nodes (PDP11/34) (see Fig. 1).

With the aid of KRAZTUR different types of datasets (item carriers) can be processed which may be logically interconnected. The items of all kinds of datasets are fixed in the database description. They form the basis for all activities.

The "dialog generator" permits the setting up of data acquisition functions adaptable to special wishes of the user in a simple manner (plausibility checks, conditional branches, default values).

The "printing generator" generates letters, lists or tables according to the principle of data-directed word processing.

With the function "retrieval" any datafile can be searched for different queries.

As normally personal data will be processed by KRAZTUR, protective functions are included in accordance with the regulations of the law on data protection.

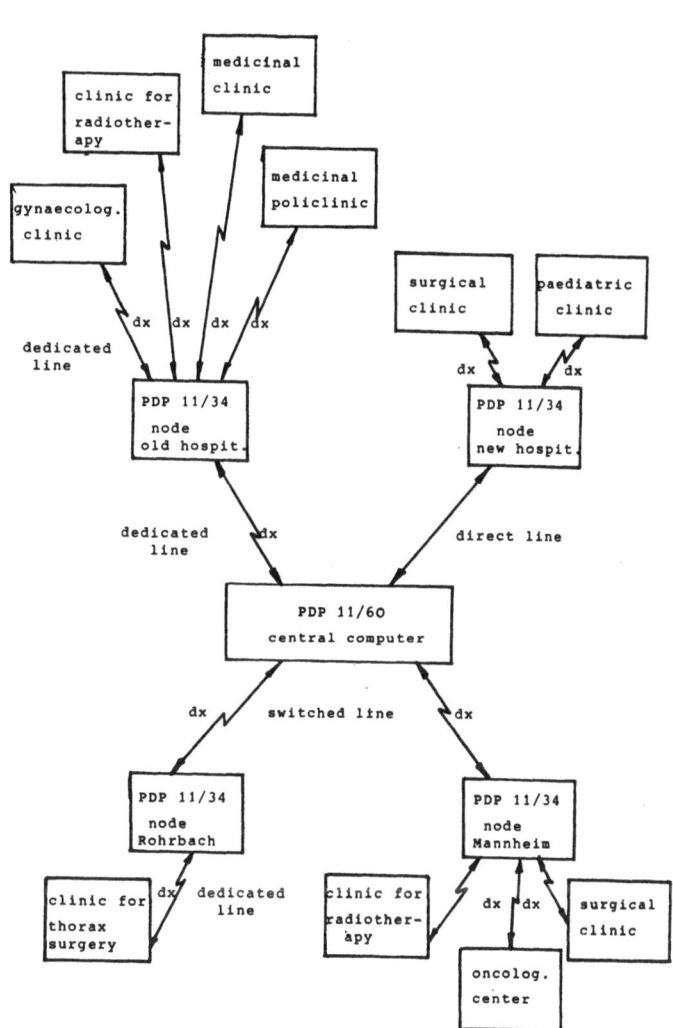

Fig. 1: Computer network

3. Description of SARA

Considering the specific routine structures and problems of a follow-up institution as well as the demanded width of application, this appointment system was conceived as a generator and incorporated into the KRAZTUR system.

It solves any tasks demanded for an appointment and flow control system.

SARA is divided into five components:

1. Parameter input,
2. Patient selection,
3. Setting of priorities,
4. Planning of appointments and assignment of patients,
5. Printed output.

3.1 Parameter Input

The manifestations of the parameters form the basis for generating the hospital-specific appointment system. Via a KRAZTUR acquisition dialog every hospital is able to assign values to the parameters according to its individual requirements for its follow-up consulting hours.

The establishment of parameter values has to be based on a careful analysis of conditions prevailing in the hospital and requires extensive statistical investigations. The values are subject to continuous control and modification and will adapt to reality as time goes on.

3.1.1 Description of the parameters

Tumor consulting hours: Every patient is assigned to tumor consulting hours held in the hospital by the competent physician(s) on the basis of his tumor localization. The manifestation is stored in the patient's follow-up data.

Follow-up program y/n: If "yes" is fed in, the input of the follow-up program goes on with the next two parameters; otherwise these are skipped.

Interval p.o. (p.o. = postoperative): Statement of time in months depending on the primary therapy according to follow-up program.

Service stations: The service stations belonging to the prestated interval are enumerated according to the follow-up program.

Duration of consulting hours (from - to): On the basis of the duration of consulting hours the number of patients who can be examined and treated during this time is calculated.

Breaks: This parameter is only indicated if a break is to be planned for all service points at the same time; during this time no appointments are made.

Number of walk-in patients: This figure should be estimated at the lower level because otherwise unnecessary time is wasted for planned capacities for walk-ins. Moreover, the number of patients having appointments is reduced if too many walk-ins are estimated.

Number of physicians: Statement of the number of physicians in the outpatient department available for the physical examination.

First examination: The first examination is either the physical examination by the physician or the examination in a service station. The appointment interval, i.e. the interval between patient appointments, depends on the duration of the first examination.

Duration of treatment/physician: Statement of time in minutes on the estimated or calculated mean for the duration of the physical examination.

Service station: A maximum of four service stations are considered in the planning. They are processed in the order indicated; the mode of processing follows from the planning algorithm.

Examination: Indication of examination to be carried out at the service station previously stated.

Duration of treatment / service station: Statement of time in minutes on the estimated or calculated mean for the examination at the service station.

Empty stomach y/n: Indication if the patient will have to turn up sober for this examination.

Planning algorithm: Covering the number and arranging of the service stations. With four service stations to be considered, there are eleven different possibilities coded as follows:

AO   physical examination only,
                        no service station

B1 B2 B3 B4   fixed arrangement of 1,2,3,4
                        service stations

C2 C3 C4   variable arrangement of 2,3,4
                        service stations

D3 D4   fixed and variable arrangement,
                        1 fixed is followed by 2,3
                        variable service stations

E4   fixed and variable arrangement,
                        2 fixed are followed by 2
                        variable service stations

3.1.2 Planning algorithms

On account of the problems in connection with mathematical approaches and the high abstraction content of possible solutions, the planning algorithms were developed on a heuristic basis.

The general rule for the service stations to be considered is:

The more service stations will be included in the planning, the more difficult the optimal planning will be.

The   patients will get an   appointment at time   intervals dependent on
the duration of the first examination.

By taking the B-algorithms the order of the service stations is fixed;
therefore,there can be no optimal planning; waiting times for patients
and waste of time at the service points must be anticipated.

By taking the C-algorithms the service stations can be planned in a
variable order. An algorithm was designed assigning the service
stations to the patients according to the criteria of waiting-time
minimization and wasted time minimization.

3.2. Selection of patients

The patients having an appointment are selected via the retrieval
function in KRAZTUR.
The patients which are within the planning period are chosen from the
database via the feature "next examination". In addition, there are
those patients who missed their last appointment and will have to be
appointed once more. Patients whose final investigation (i.e.
elimination from the follow-up) is covered are excluded from patient
scheduling.

Through the retrieval run a set of results is obtained containing the
patients which are considered for the planning.

3.3 Setting priorities

The follow-up interval is calculated for all patients of the set of
results. It follows from the difference between the scheduling date
and the date of the last follow-up. Depending on the follow-up
interval the the patients are assigned the corresponding priority.

Follow-up interval	Priority
< 5 weeks	1
>4 and <13 weeks	2
>12 and <25 weeks	3
>24 and <50 weeks	4
>49 weeks	5

The number of patients to be scheduled per date follows from the
values of the parameter input. It is calculated as follows:

Duration of consulting time
--------------------------- - break - number of walk-ins
longest time of treatment

Principally, all patients with priority 1 are scheduled for the next
date, even if this means that the number of patients to be scheduled
is exceeded. If the number of patients to be scheduled is larger than
the number of patients with priority 1, patients with lower priorities
(2 to 5) can be scheduled. Every time the scheduling is planned, the
priority of those patients not yet considered is lowered by 1.

3.4 Scheduling and patient assignment

On the basis of the planning algorithms chosen, the consultations with the physician and necessary visits to the service stations are calculated. In order to take into account certain influence factors, such as nationality and age of the patient, patient-specific prolongations are added to the mean treatment time:

with respect to nationality for all foreigners,
with respect to age for patients over 65 or under 5 years.

The order of patient scheduling depends on the place of residence. All patients residing near the hospital are given early dates. In case of consulting hours with follow-up program those patients who have to come with an empty stomach are also given early morning appoinments. If the date coincides with the patient's birthday, it is postponed.

The walk-ins are fitted in as follows: Three or four of them are fitted in after a group of patients, the others at the end of all invited patients. Thus a varying number of walk-ins disturbs the scheduling of the other patients the least.

3.5. Printed output

Following the scheduling program, notifications for patients and/or their familiy doctors are printed and various lists set up:

List 1 is a list of patients for the outpatient clinic. It contains the patients' names, the tsarting time of their appointment and the service stations to be visited (see Fig. 2).

List 2 is the appointment list for the physician. It contains the patients' names and the service points which the patient has already visited or will have to visit (see Fig 3).

List 3 is set up for every service station. It contains the times of start and end of the examination, the patients' names and the examination to be performed (see Fig. 4).

List 4 is a patient control slip. It contains the starting times at the service stations for every patient (see Fig. 5).

Patient list for the outpatient department
Date: Wednesday 8-5-81

Time	Patient Name	Service Station
10.00	Hoen Elke	radioscopy-lab.-physician
10.15	Gobli Christa	radioscopy-lab.-physician
10.25	Goebel Wolfgang	lab.-radioscopy-physician
10.30	Steiner Fritz	radioscopy-lab.-physician
10.45	--free--	lab.-radioscopy-physician
11.05	Siegler Fritz	lab.-radioscopy-physician

Fig. 2: Patient list

```
Appointment list for the physician
Date: Wednesday 8-5-81

Time            Patient Name            Service Station

10.45           Hoen Elke               radioscopy-lab.
11.00           Gobli Christa           radioscopy-lab.
11.15           Goebel Wolfgang         lab.-radioscopy
11.30           Steiner Fritz           radioscopy-lab.
11.50           --free--                lab.-radioscopy
12.05           Siegler Fritz           lab.-radioscopy
```

Fig. 3: Appointment list for the physician


```
Appointment list for the laboratory
Date: Wednesday 8-5-81

Time              Patient Name            Examination

10.00 - 10.25     Hoen Elke               blood test
10.25 - 10.35     Goebel Wolfgang         blood test
10.35 - 10.45     Gobli Christa           blood test
10.45 - 10.55     --free--                blood test
10.55 - 11.05     Steiner Fritz           blood test
11.05 - 11.15     Siegler Fritz           blood test
```

Fig. 4: Appointment list for the laboratory


```
Patient control slips
Date: Wednesday 8-5-81

Patient Name          Time            Service Station

Hoen Elke             10.00           radioscopy
                      10.15           laboratory
                      10.45           physician

Gobli Christa         10.15           radioscopy
                      10.35           laboratory
                      11.00           physician

Goebel Wolfgang       10.25           laboratory
                      10.50           radioscopy
                      11.15           physician
```

Fig. 5: Patient control slips

4. References

1. Bailey, N.T.J., Welch, J.D.:
   Appointment System in Hospital-Out-Patient Departments Lancet
   1952, I: 1105-1108
2. Bailey, N.J.T.:
   A Note on Equalising the Mean Waiting Times of Successive
   Customers in a Finite Queue. J. roy. statist. Soc., Ser.B 17
   (1955) 262-263
3. Cederlund, C.:
   Termin- und Arbeitsplanung in einem Krankenhaus in Schweden.
   In Datenverarbeitung und Medizin, IBM-Seminar, Bad Liebenzell
   1970, S.131-139, IBM Form K12-1012-0.
4. Christl, H.L.:
   Some Methods of Operations Research Applied to Patient
   Schedulings Problems.
   Med. Progr. Technol. 2 (1973) 19-27.
5. Dusberger, W., Henn, M., Koehler, C.O., Meinzer, H.P.,
   Schaefer, D.O.:
   Analyse der Durchgangszeiten einer Ambulanz und
   Roentgenabteilung einer medizinischen Klinik In Wagner, G.,
   Koehler, C.O. (Hrsg.): Interaktive Datenverarbeitung in der
   Medizin - Mensch-Maschine-Dialog (Seite 331-337). Stuttgart -
   New York, Schattauer 1979.
6. Ellsaesser, K.-H., Koehler, C.O.:
   Einbestellsystem fuer eine onkologische Nachsorge-Ambulanz
   In Jesdinsky, H.J., (Hrsg.): Modelle der Medizin, S.
   242-248 Berlin - Heidelberg - New York, Springer 1980
7. Ellsaesser, K.-H., Koehler, C.O., Wagner, G.:
   KRAZTUR - A Generator for Medical Documentation and Information
   Systems. Meth.Inform.Med. 20 (1981) S. 191-195
8. Fetter, R.B., Thompson, J.D.:
   Patients 'Waiting Time and Doctors' Idle Time in Outpatient
   Setting.
   Hlth Serv. Res. 1 (1966) 66-90
9. Koehler, C.O.:
   Integriertes Krankenhaus-Informationssystem -Zielbestimmung und
   Rahmenmodell-. Meisenheim, Hain 1973
10. Ohrt, W.:
    Patientenbestellsysteme in ambulanten Einrichtungen des
    Gesundheitswesens.
    Z. aerztl. Fortb. (Jena) 68 (1974) 308-312.
11. Ohrt, W.:
    Wartezeiten in ambulanten Einrichtungen des Gesundheitswesens.
    Z. aerztl. Fortb. (Jena) 66 (1972) 30-35.
12. Rourke, T.A., Roger, A.C.N., Chow, M.C., McFadden,
    E.T.,Nikodem, D.:
    Computer-assisted Scheduling of Elective Admissions,
    Meth.Inform.Med. 18 (1979), S. 146-151
13. Vosseler, C.:
    SARA - Scheduling and Resource Allocation. Ein Einbestell- und
    Durchlaufsteuerungssystem fuer eine Krebsnachsorge - Einrichtung
    am Tumorzentrum Heidelberg/Mannheim. (Diplomarbeit, Fachbereich
    Medizinische Informatik) Universitaet Heidelberg, Fachhochschule
    Heilbronn, 1981

TOREN, A TOOL OF MANAGEMENT.

W.J. Hofdijk

Leyden University Hospital — Bazis

ABSTRACT.

Within the Hospital Information System as developed by the Bazis group in the Leyden University Hospital millions of data are being recorded by more than 40 different subsystems.
These data offer the possibility to monitor closely both the treatment process of the patients and the use of the facilities of the hospital by aggregating the production data. The last part is the objective of the so called TOREN subsystem.

THE USE OF THE HOSPITAL FACILITIES.

The control of the hospital facilities is a topic for most hospital managers espe- cially in these days of short falling financial possibilities. To this extent the Leyden Hospital Information System offers a lot of useful subsystems. From the very start subsystems were operational recording activities like laboratory and radio- logical tests etc.
At the end of 1976 the development was started to create a centralised subsystem with the aim to collect production data in order to gain control over the use of the scarce funds of the hospital.
This meant the creation of the TOREN subsystem, Total Output Registration En(and) Nota's(Billing).
This subsystem has two main objectives:
1) Registration of all activities and procedures undertaken in connection with the treatment of patients.
2) The execution of the main administrative functions like charging and billing as well as production and turnover statistics.
The development of this subsystem had administrative and dataprocessing aspects , which had to be looked after to the same extent.
A first investigation learned that daily 16.000 medical activities and procedures take place in the Leyden University Hospital. From this amount already 9000 were recorded by other HIS subsystems. By creating a standard protocol these data could be easily transferred from the primary registering subsystems to TOREN.
The other 8000created a managerial problem as the frequency of the informationflow varied from daily to once a year. The TOREN Steering Committee decided to aim at a routine and continous information flow.

A pair of pilot studies were started to gain experience how to organize the datacollection on a routine base. Both an internal and a surgical specialism was chosen, the Pediatrics and the Oto-laryngology.

The pilotstudies produced some interesting results. On the one hand the registering of procedures of the in- and outpatients was rather underdeveloped. On the other hand the conclusion had to be made that the existing codesystems were not able to cover all procedures and other medical activities.

The codesystems were originally derived from the ICD code system, but they face two main problems; they are not up to date and they differ to some extent. This led to the decision to create an own TOREN codesystem, which should have the potential to register all medical activities and procedures from the clinical as well as from the ancillary departments. This decision was supported by all University Hospitals. The problem was also nationally brought to the attention of the Classification and Coding Commission of the Ministry of Health and has lead to the setup of a group aiming at the uniforming of the procedure codesystem.

In cooperation with the other in BAZIS participating Univerity Hospitals the specification of the TOREN subsystem was worked out and the development was started in Leyden. In the beginning of 1978 the system became operational and the data gathered within the pilotstudies were processed. In the course of the same year the facilities for charging and billing of outpatients and for the processing of the statistics were implemented.

The last days of 1978 were memorable when the actual linkup with the laboratoy and radiological subsystems was succesfully made. The daily production rose to about 9000 and grew steadily to around 14.000 in 1981.

The charging and billing function kept pace with this development, especially since the inpatient billing function became operational in the beginning of 1981.

The implementation of the TOREN subsystem by the other University Hospitals is delayed by some interesting facts.

Most University Hospitals worked together in developing the specifications of the TOREN subsystem.

Some of them already had an operational billing subsystem. The main feature of the TOREN subsystem is to record all production data and subsequently handle the charging and billing activities as these are rather complex. The development was spread over a period of three years. For some hospitals the implementation of the TOREN subsystem was related to the completion of the charging and billing facilities, while other hospitals started with the production recording and will implement the charging and billing in a subsequent phase. The planning provides that after the summer of 1982 all participating hospitals will be on the same level.

MANAGEMENT INFORMATION.

The TOREN subsystem supplies regular statistical surveys about the production and turnover of the hospital, based on the production data gathered from the subsystems that are linked up with TOREN and from the manual input.The turnover data are derived from the charging process embedded in the TOREN system.

This means the realisation of one of the main objectives of this system namely to present to the original suppliers of production data as soon as possible the aggregated production to give an instrument for controlling their activities.

Analysis showed that the ancillary departments are very keen on the periodic surveys (monthly,quarterly and yearly).The fact that the production data are split to a high level of detail, procedure, producer, applicant and patient category,is used as an instrument to control their own production.

The information flow from the in- and outpatient clinics about their activities was rather slow when the TOREN project started. To let this flow swell to reach the equivalent of the total output of the hospital, the so called data collection program was initiated. Originally started in Leyden, soon a national approach was adopted to setup and coordinate the programs to investigate the activities of the different specialisms and to improve the existing information flow. The coordination of these activities was also placed within the scope of the TOREN-project.

The two main objectives of the clinical departments to support these programs were the facility to register more information about the treatment of patients in the database giving an easier instrument for research. On the other hand to gather information which could be usefull for the departmentwise budgetting program to be implemented within some years.

In Leyden, for about 30% of the specialisms the datacollection activities have been finished so far and the target is to complete these programs nationally within three years. By this approach the base is provided for sound and useful management information that can be mutually compared. But it is very clear that only when all productive activities are recorded in the HIS and processed by the TOREN subsystem, real management information can be provided.

Till then, the information must be treated with care and the interpretation must be authorised by the original suppliers before it can be used for managerial purposes.

The existence of one centralised subsystem, producing management information already proved to be worthwhile,although the finalizing will take quite some time.

SOME STATISTICAL RESULTS.

The TOREN subsystem is implemented in the University Hospitals of Leyden, Rotterdam, Groningen and Utrecht.

The last two became operational in the course of 1981, Rotterdam in 1980 and Leyden in 1978.

In the first years the increase of the production is mainly caused by the number of subsystems and producers connected with the TOREN subsystem.

The statistics from Leyden reflect the growth of the TOREN production in the last three years. (figure 1)

TOREN output in Leyden   Figure 1

Year	Number of producers	Procedures	Total TOREN production
1978	9	258	75.000
1979	49	938	250.000
1980	59	1110	3.000.000
1981 1e half year	73	1229	1.900.000

The quarterly figures show an interesting "picture" of the seasonal influence of the medical activities. Figure 2 gives some indications about the quarterly growth, showing that the highest production is recorded in the last quarter of the year.

The quarterly index is computed with the corresponding quarter of 1979 as base.

The influence of the growing number of participating producers must be kept in mind before drawing real conclusions.

The turnover statistics are more and more used to give a specification of the yield-accounts of the general ledger.

This proves to be an useful instrument to explain the trends within the income statement.

QUARTER I	1979	1980	1981
Total Production	638.789	713.502	906.978
Year Percentage	25.1	23.1	-
Quarterly Index	100	111	141
QUARTER II			
Total Production	629.352	698.619	940.228
Year Percentage	24.7	22.6	-
Quarterly Index	100	111	149
QUARTER III			
Total Production	623.502	825.672	1.237.075
Year Percentage	24.5	26.7	-
Quarterly Index	100	132	198
QUARTER IV			
Total Production	656.885	853.140	
Year Percentage	25.8	27.6	
Quarterly Index	100	129	

Conclusion:

The experience of nearly four TOREN years has learned that a centralised approach
of the gathering and recording of production data is feasible as well as worthwhile.
The implementation of this subsystem requires a multidiscipinal   approach, it is
necessary that managers, controllers, EDP people and medical specialists are
involved to cover all aspects of the hospital process in the "output" field.
This demands highly motivated top management, thus guaranteing realistic total
output registration. Only then the sound base for real management information is
built, not only within but also between hospitals.
Thus providing a real Health Care control instrument.

"STRUCTURED" TECHNIQUES FOR DESIGN -
EXPERIENCES IN THEIR USE FOR AN EXTENSIVE HOSPITAL COMPUTER SYSTEM

A R Wills
The John Ellicott Centre
The London Hospital
Whitechapel, London. E1 1BB

1. INTRODUCTION

Faced with the task of re-writing a massive collection of real-time computer services, and at the same time adapting them to operate at a number of additional hospitals, what modern techniques and aids are available, and how effective are they?

The question has been tackled at The London Hospital by selecting a combination of Structured Systems Analysis and Design techniques, and powerful computer software which is designed to enable services to be written, tested and modified with considerably less effort than has previously been required for systems of similar scale.

The 10-year-old computer system has demonstrated the value of real-time services in the wards, as well as in service centres, and now embraces the three larger Clinical Laboratory departments, X-ray and Nursing Records applications in addition to Patient Administration and numerous smaller applications (1 to 13). Currently two hospital sites have ward level services, with limited services at two further sites.

2. TECHNIQUES

The conventions and rules adopted at The London Hospital are derived from the "Stradis Methodology" (14). This "methodology" sets out to combine structured design and structured programming techniques into an integrated planning and project management discipline. The methodology covers all activities from the first investigation of requests for a new service, through to the implementation of a fully functioning system of services. Many parallels are drawn between a properly formulated development plan and that needed when developing a piece of civil engineering, where the product cannot be properly demonstrated other than in model form until it has been finally constructed.

The object of using such a methodology is:

To identify properly what is required, before work starts on producing it.

To concentrate effort into the design processes, using structured techniques, so that the systems produced are versatile, easy to amend, and as far as possible error-free.

To control the design, writing, testing and implementing of the services, so that any problems of integration, interfaces, basic concepts, etc come to light early on in the development, not at System Testing time.

3. "DATA FLOW DIAGRAMS"

These diagrams are a key feature of the methodology. They are designed to summarise the flow of data between transactions, which by analysis are found to describe what happens in the real world when a set of useful tasks is performed.

The diagrams may be used to "talk through" how a set of tasks operate in practice, when the Analyst is checking with the Users that the activity is correctly perceived in the system design process. The diagrams feature in the official documents produced as part of the design methodology, which define the design for the computer services. Such diagrams may also be used to define non-computer tasks.

When anyone tries to draw a system-wide data flow diagram, it is surprising how many questions emerge about how things are done and who does them. The initial benefit is thus to draw attention to one's detailed understanding of a department's activities, and if the questions are not side-stepped, a very complete picture can be built up naturally.

The second step is to examine the data flows, particularly those into and out of the computer data stores. From this, a preliminary design of the computer data files, and the methods of access to the individual records, proceeds.

The internal activities of each transaction are then examined. This is the stage where all the variations and exceptions which have to be coped with are identified. This analysis of the transaction results in a "detail-level data flow diagram" describing the component computer processes, and the data which flows between them. Additional accesses to data stores may come to light from this work. From the distinct "processes" discovered by this design action, the foundations for structuring the computer programs themselves is laid. Defining the common routines used in different transactions becomes straightforward, and all the complexity can be kept within the low-level processes. This aids the production of computer programs which are easy to understand and straightforward to test and alter.

4. PLANNING THE DEVELOPMENT OF COMPUTER SERVICES

In this activity, even the best tools in the world cannot guarantee success; they can only lay down a good discipline which encourages the early integration of services. The evolution of the preliminary design, based on the above summary of activities, certainly helps one to discern sensible and appropriate computer services; the next stage is to sort out how to provide an appropriate phasing for the introduction of services.

When computer services are being introduced into new areas, when real-time services are replacing batch services, or when the various services all operate quite independently of each other, then it is possible to phase the introduction of services.

The recommended approach is to provide limited services which cover all the main stages of activity; for instance in our X-ray department, the first phase was to provide requesting, work management and reporting, but not including casualty examinations. To have attempted to implement services covering all types of report without the benefit of requesting would have created substantial extra work in the department during that interim phase. Subsequent phases then consisted of adding further types of X-ray investigation and new services such as statistics analysis and an archive of film references.

It is vital to design all major aspects before the first phase of programming begins; this is why one starts with the system-wide diagrams, followed by the evolution of the structure of all the component transactions, before selecting the phases.

In the case of the Tower Hamlets Health District, where the new services are to replace equivalent services on an older computer, it is technically unrealistic to phase the changeover of the real-time services. How can one be reasonably confident that everything will work at switch-over day?

The approach adopted is to implement live services in Newham District first, for Medical Records and Patient Administration activities. Within that area of work, a number of stages has been defined, whereby a limited-scale system test is used to demonstrate the successful linkage of all component transactions at the earliest stage possible, including operation at more than one hospital. The objective is to obtain a complete set of all services which create or modify information held in the computer, plus the crucial ones which display data, before programming all the variations that need to be handled by the system. However, all such variations must have been specified beforehand, so that the programs contain the structure for dealing with them, and dummy routines (or "stubs") can be substituted for the full code needed in the final system.

This approach avoids on the one hand, producing a pilot scheme which cannot cope with a full scale operation, and on the other hand a full solution, of which only isolated components can be demonstrated before final system testing, when any problems will inevitably produce major delays in the introduction of the services.

5.   APPROPRIATE SOFTWARE FACILITIES, DEVELOPMENT TIMESCALE

Very few software products yet provide a data dictionary fully integrated with both screen handling and data file accessing, and also enable a large number of terminals to work intensively on the same database, with response times short enough for use by busy hospital staff. One such product is SYSTEL (15), developed by Systime Limited of Leeds, for VAX and PDP-11 computers.

Analysis of the source code of operational programs at The London Hospital indicated that development effort would be halved by using SYSTEL.

The other major resource needed in developing a working system is the time taken to test and amend the programs, individually and in the form of groups of transactions. Limited memory on the old system forced each development group to take it in turn to have a testing session on the computer. On the VAX 11/780 computers with four Megabytes of memory, a number of individuals and groups can be working concurrently on the computer, hence alleviating that limitation.

Whilst most programming systems can be made to pool commonly used routines, and a "modular" design of programs, this is not always straightforward or efficient in operation. The "structured" approach described here actively encourages modular programming, and SYSTEL has been extended to enable this approach to be handled effectively.

These effects combine to enable the full set of services to be re-designed, written and tested in less than 3 years, after taking 10 years for the original development, using the same number of staff. Completion is planned for November, 1983.

6. FURTHER BENEFITS

The method of work described in this paper puts off the start of programming until the designs are drafted in considerable detail for the system as a whole. Staff also need to be educated in the conventions and activities involved. This may be seen as introducing delay into the overall timescale, but there are important compensations.

Firstly, this method of defining and designing systems has enabled staff of a wide range of experience to contribute to these tasks. Previously, there was always a bottleneck when the project team leaders and experienced staff were doing all the design and specification work, sometimes resulting in superficial and incomplete specification of the programs, and changes to the early specifications as design work proceeded. Other benefits from the new situation are the greater knowledge of the application in those producing the programs, no hiatus for the programmers while specification is being done, and good team spirit amongst the staff.

Secondly, the designs are recorded in a form which all other groups can quickly assimilate. This makes it feasible to expect each group to review each other's work at a number of stages. It is anticipated that far fewer problems will arise from the cross-links between application areas than occurred beforehand.

Should any problems in design get past this mutual scrutiny, they should emerge about one third of the way through the development activity, when the effects of change are limited, rather than near the end of the activity. This should result in much less re-working and re-testing of proven programs than happened before.

Thirdly, the "structured" approach provides clear landmarks, aiding the control of the whole project. The early documentation identifies the areas of change to the users compared with their previous facilities, and aspects of the new design can be easily talked through, based on the documents.

7. PORTABILITY

In order to reproduce computer services for another hospital, even on identical hard-ware, it is essential to recognise that superficially similar hospital activities at different sites may be based on significantly different management structures, and what may be a terrible problem at one place may be quite satisfactory under different conditions. In order for computer services to be sufficiently adaptable to fit into such situations effectively, they must be derived from a fundamentally correct analysis of the objectives and activities at more than one type of hospital. Structured design techniques used by health service computer professionals are more likely to achieve this than most alternatives.

A second pre-requisite for success is an appropriate level of parameterisation of the services, so that they can be adapted to fulfil the differing user requirements, without becoming excessively complex to develop and maintain, or extravagant on computing resources in operation.

Some attempts to re-write a successful and portable design for different computers have foundered (eg variants of the Hammersmith PHOENIX laboratory system). It is essential to assess the appropriateness of the file accessing software and the computer languages to be used, as well as the computer hardware, when choosing the computer for an active, multi-user application. With the methodology outlined in this paper, the oddities of the computer and its software are contained within the latter stages of program specification. It should therefore be much easier to re-write programs for a different computer from such specifications, than from a high-level, unstructured system description of the usual form.

8. CONCLUSIONS

Much useful good practice can be learnt from books such as Reference 14, which is exceedingly important to anyone who is considering the application of a computer, or even just seeking to review the organisation of their department. It is true that data flow diagrams need to be re-drawn several times as one learns the techniques and refines one's understanding of the procedures. Even a small system based on a microcomputer can take a while to get right, so such techniques are still of value here.

With larger projects, the need to communicate design decisions between groups working in parallel, and to establish all cross-application interfaces as early as possible, give further emphasis to the need for a "structured methodology", as is bourne out in the City and East London Area Project.

REFERENCES

(1)   Barber B. The Place of the Computer in the Delivery of Health Care.
      Univac symposium, Moscow, February 1975. Sperry Univac, Sperry Univac Centre,
      Stonebridge Park, N. Circular Road, London. NW10, UK.

(2)   Abbott WC. Planning and Implementation of the London Hospital Project.
      Univac symposium, Moscow, February 1975. Sperry Univac, Sperry Univac Centre,
      Stonebridge Park, N. Circular Road, London. NW10, UK.

(3)   Barber B, Cohen RD, et al. Some problems in Confidentiality in Medical Ethics.
      J. Medical Ethics June 1976 Vol 2(2) 71-73. Society for the study of Medical
      Ethics, London, UK.

(4)   Scholes M. The Role of Computers in Nursing.
      Nursing Mirror, September 1976.

(5)   Abbott WC. The Regional Computing Service Subsequent to the National Health
      Service Re-organisation. Proc MEDCOMP '77: 279-288. Online Conferences Ltd,
      Uxbridge, England, UK; 1977.

(6)   Scholes M, Forster KV, Gregg T. Continuing Education of Health Service Staff
      in Computing. Proc MEDCOMP '77: 639-648. Online Conferences Ltd,
      Uxbridge, England, UK; 1977.

(7)   Wills AR. A Computer Requesting and Reporting System for a Variety of
      Clinical Laboratories. Proc MEDCOMP '77: 151-164. Online Conferences Ltd,
      Uxbridge, England, UK; 1977.

(8)   Rowson JEM. Computerised Pathology Services at The London Hospital.
      Proc Univac Users Association (Europe), November 1977. Sperry Univac,
      Sperry Univac Centre, Stonebridge Park, N. Circular Road, London. NW10, UK.

(9)   Wills AR. Replicable Multi-purpose Patient Index Systems - an Analysis of
      some necessary features. Lecture notes in Medical Informatics, Vol 1. Proc
      MIE '78: 797-811. Springer-Verlag, Berlin, Heidelberg; 1978.

(10) Mace DR. A common approach to a variety of Clinical Laboratories. Lecture
      notes in Medical Informatics, Vol 1. Proc MIE '78: 509-519. Springer-Verlag,
      Berlin, Heidelberg; 1978.

(11) Real-Time Lab System at The London Hospital.
      Systems International magazine, January 1979.

(12) Rowson JEM. Ward Requesting and Reporting Systems.
      Univac Symposium, Nice, May 1979. Sperry Univac, Sperry Univac Centre,
      Stonebridge Park, N. Circular Road, London. NW10, UK.

(13) Mace DR. A Real-Time Nursing Manpower System. Annals of the World Association
      for Medical Informatics Vol 1(1) 23-28 May 1981. WAMI, 74 rue de la Colonie,
      75013 Paris, France.

(14) Gane C, Sarson T. Structured Systems Analysis: tools and techniques.
      IST Databooks. Imp Sys Tech SA, PO Box 118, 1196 Gland, Switzerland;
      published July 1977.

(15) An Introduction to SYSTEL (and associated manuals). Systime Limited,
      Concourse Computer Centre, 432 Dewsbury Road, Leeds. LS11 7DE.

IMPLEMENTATION OF A COMPUTER SYSTEM

DURING THE COMMISSIONING

OF A NEW PRIVATE HOSPITAL

R.A. Chown B.Sc., A.C.M.A.
Financial Controller
The Cromwell Hospital,
Cromwell Road,
LONDON

Introduction

It is not often that the opportunity arises to install a computer information system
during the commissioning stages of a new hospital. Such was the case with the
Cromwell Hospital, a 128 bed private hospital in the centre of London. We were
looking for a completely integrated hospital information system which could not only
provide internal communications and patient administration but would also handle
all the financial management applications for the hospital.

The aim of this paper is to comment on the experience of installing a computer system
in a new hospital, outlining the advantages, some of the problems encountered and the
lessons that were learned in the process. Around the time of writing there were
several announcements in the press of new hospital developments with an estimated
50 million pounds being invested. In the light of this the theme of this paper
should be particularly relevant.

Many of the advantages and some of the problems arose from what would be called the
 clean sheet' syndrome, the effect of which was evident in four areas each of which
are covered in subsequent sections of this paper, namely: the initial decision to
proceed with a computer system; the timing of the computer installation; the obvious
impact on staff and finally the potentially detrimental environment of the building
site.

The Decision

In a hospital which already has well-established manual information systems and
procedures it is possible to estimate the effect of computerisation in terms of e.g.
clerical staff savings, reducing time spent by nurses on administrative work, improving drug stock control, expediting ordering and reporting of laboratory tests etc.
However, in the commissioning stages of a new hospital there is no such operational
data or experience against which to gauge the cost-effectiveness of computerisation.

There was some evidence available from elsewhere of realisable savings. HAI's own
research in the USA indicated a potential 1-2% saving on the paramedical revenue

account resulting from the avoidance of lost charges. It was estimated that this would amount to around £75,000 p.a. We were also able to define a lower establishment than would otherwise have been required to handle the equivalent manual systems. Finally we felt that better management of patients and beds would result in improved occupancy. An increase of even 1% in bed occupancy would have marked financial consequences.

Such arguments were used in discussion with the financial backers. On the medical side several of the consultants had already seen such integrated computer information systems in the USA and were convinced that the quality of patient care could be improved by having correct information available in the right place at the right time.

Timing

Once the decision to go-ahead had been taken plans for the system could be drawn up. At the Cromwell it was a condition that the computer system should be operational on the opening date. Planning of the system started only six months beforehand so there was little time to draw up a detailed functional specification before going to tender. With such a tight deadline we looked for a vendor who could provide a turn-key solution, evidence of substantial experience in hospital systems and who could provide full support at all stages of the installation. At this stage there should be as many visits as possible to other hospitals which already have computer systems in operation. At the time the Cromwell was commissioned there were no hospitals in the UK with integrated financial and administrative computer systems.

Ironically the opening date was inevitably postponed several times with consequent need to synchronise computer hardware installation with the continually revised building schedules. This meant that hardware delivery dates were no problem and fortuitously enabled hardware to be fully tested in the vendor s offices before installation in the hospital thus minimising the risks of hardware teething troubles.

Staff

Designing and installing the system necessarily required a great deal of commitment, imagination and enthusiasm from staff concerned. All these were available because we were in a new hospital prior to opening. Each prospective employee was informed at the interview stage that his job would include working with a computer system, so anyone with qualms could back down at this stage. Hence there was virtually a total acceptance of the concepts of computerisation and those who joined the hospital were committed to making the system work most effectively. Staff had sufficient time available to contribute more effectively; thus there was the opportunity to develop and implement a completely integrated hospital system more smoothly, quickly and effectively than in a hospital where departments already had their own, independent procedures which would need to be amalgamated into an agreed format. The computer system provided a certain discipline for people's design activities. Having to go into some detail for the system design proved a useful learning experience for deciding the type of systems the hospital required. Without the computer to act as a catalyst this task would have been considerably more difficult. However, imagination needed to be curbed occassionally since ideas were sometimes over-ambitious or impractical and because of the 'clean sheet syndrome' there was obviously no opportunity to test out new, and possibly conflicting, ideas on a manual basis beforehand.

The Environment

Installing the system whilst building was taking place, brought its own challenges. Allowances for computing facilities are not automatically included in architect's or builder's plans. Workmen often found it hard to appreciate how stringent were the requirements for dust-free conditions around the computer. A room which would be technically complete in the definition of the building trade could still be sufficiently dirty to wreak havoc on the innards of a computer.

Conversely, it was of immense value to have a civil engineer on site to advise and respond instantly if changes in the building plans were required resulting from any alterations to the hardware configuration. A detailed physical specification for the system should be drawn up as early as possible to take fullest advantage of the obvious cost savings of being able to include all physical aspects of the installation (e.g. cable routing, designing the computer room etc.) into the building plan as well as in avoiding the disruption to both staff and patients that would otherwise have occurred if the hospital were operational.

Conclusions

Based on my experience at the Cromwell I would not hesitate in installing a computer system again during the commissioning stages of a hospital rather than wait until the hospital has been operational for some time. Installation can be much smoother during the commissioning period because of the amount of time, enthusiasm and commitment people can give to it. It should provide a convenient focus for systems design and should also allow time to test the systems rigorously without affecting the day-to-day routine of a hospital which is operational. Such features far outweigh any of the problems which may be encountered.

"INFORMATION SYSTEMS PLANNING FOR A REGIONAL HEALTH BOARD

Authors :   Donal O'Shea,   Terry Neill,

               North Western Health Board   Arthur Andersen & Co.
               Ireland.   Ireland.

SUMMARY

        In 1979, the North Western Health Board prepared an administrative
organisation and computer systems development plan, setting out the objectives,
priorities and resource requirements for the development of a practical range
of manual and computer systems in the areas of finance, personnel, patient
administration and community care management. The Board embarked upon the plan
when it was published and to early 1982 it has continued largely to meet the
targets set out in the plan.
        This paper describes the preparation of the plan, the benefits
flowing from its preparation and its impact on the Board's administration over
the two/three years.

BACKGROUND

        Ireland's eight regional health boards were set up in the early
1970's. Each board is responsible for planning, building and managing general
and special hospitals. The community care programme of each board covers a
very broad range of community health and social services - including home
support and income maintenance, and services to the handicapped.
        The North Western Health Board is responsible for the health services
for the counties of Donegal, Leitrim and Sligo - which are in the north west of
the Republic of Ireland. The Board employs some 4,000 personnel and is
responsible for two major general hospitals, two major psychiatric hospitals,
three geriatric, several local and district hospitals and for the community
care services of the three counties.
        In 1978, the management team decided to prepare a five-year computer
and manual systems development plan and engaged the services of management
consultants to assist in the process.

FUNCTION OF THE SYSTEMS PLAN

        Systems planning is not an exact science. The plan aimed to provide
a general context in which priorities for investment could be set in the light
of the economic or other implications for particular developments envisaged in
the planning period.
        This meant that systems and record keeping requirements had to be
defined to a level of detail which would allow reasonably accurate estimates
of: - volumes of transactions; file contents, sizes and numbers; service levels to
        users (turnaround times, response times, accuracy etc.); systems
        interrelationships and shared data, files and processing; personnel numbers,
        training and experience requirements; equipment and other non-pay
        implications
        The systems plan also provided guideposts for the acquisition and use
of computer hardware - though the detailed work required to select particular
equipment had to await the technical design of the initial systems.

GENERAL OBJECTIVES OF THE SYSTEMS PLAN

        The function of the Board is to plan and deliver a comprehensive
range of hospital and community care services - in line with statute,
government policy and Board and management team policy - within the constraints
of the resources available. Simplistically, the Health Board takes resources,
converts them into activities and applies them to patients, recipients, target
groups or particular problems.
        It was agreed that there were four essential elements of the Board's
ability to administer health services effectively:
-       a realistic and comprehensive policy and policy development
        framework
-       a sound organisation structure at all levels
-       talented, trained, well-motivated people
-       comprehensive, efficient, effective systems for record keeping and
        providing information.

Efficiency and Effectiveness

The efficiency of the Board is judged by how well it converts resources into activities. (It might be measured by cost statistics, service level performance against target, coverage and waiting list statistics or personnel performance measures. Efficiency relates essentially to inputs and their disposition).

The effectiveness of the Board would be judged by how well it changes patients or target groups "for the better" or maintains patients or target groups despite worsening environments. The development of effectiveness measures or comparisons is particularly difficult in health care because of the complexity and range of problems addressed.

For the purpose of the period covered by the Board's systems plan it was agreed that effectiveness measures must be judgemental and based on professional inputs. It was felt that, in general, it was not practical to include measurements of effectiveness in the information systems to be developed in the relatively short period covered by the plan.

The Board's Systems Development Philosophy

In 1979 the discussions leading to the publishing of the plan agreed that the main thrust of systems (and organisation) development should concentrate on building an appropriate structure for converting resources into activities to support the health and illness needs of the populations of Donegal, Leitrim and Sligo. The concept of "foundation systems" and "building block" approach was developed.

The building analogy was agreed to be realistic and was used to suggest that:

- basic foundation systems must be built first to support not only specific needs such as accounting, but also summaries and analyses for higher levels of management
- management reporting systems should be integrated and have the same bases and sources as transaction and record keeping systems, so that management decisions would be based on actual performance information
- a comprehensive picture of most systems requirements should be mapped out (in a systems plan)
    - to ensure as far as possible that individual systems (ie "building blocks") contribute to a coherent whole and
    - resource requirments - such as computers or trained support staff - should be identified for all the developments in the plan

It was the feeling of the management team that particular emphasis should be placed on the development of systems and reporting concepts in the community care programme, since this was - and continues to be - a complex and growing area which has been relatively unexplored in the past.

CONTENTS OF THE SYSTEMS PLAN

The systems plan - in two volumes - was set out under four main headings: - Community Care; Hospitals; Finance; Personnel

The systems requirements were summarised and set against the scope, costs and benefits in a management summary (volume 1) and a detailed description of each requirement comprised the whole of volume 2 of the plan.

The main systems projects were as follows:
(*indicates a computer system)

Community Care

- Financial and statistical reporting - enhancements from basic system *
- Allowance and welfare services
- Health professional activities
    - Phase 1 - develop formal policy manual and improve community procedures
    - Phase 2 - systems for trend reporting and for monitoring preventive services
- Medical card registration *
- Community index, registers and recordkeeping *
- Workshop business systems
- Community nursing units procedures
- Health inspectors' records *

-   Financial and statistical reporting - further
    enhancements *

Hospitals
-   Financial and statistical reporting systems - enhancements
    from basic system *
-   Radiology systems
-   Laboratory systems
-   Medical records location systems
-   Case notes procedures
-   Medical records clerical support systems
-   Pharmacy cost control *
-   Ward office administration
-   Patient master index *
-   Pharmacy service systems *
-   Maintenance scheduling
-   Financial and statistical reporting - further enhancements *

Finance
-   Design and install comprehensive statistics, general accounting and
    budgetary control system for all cost and sub-cost centres throughout
    the Board *
-   Design and install materials management, purchasing and stores system *
-   Design and install system for farmers' health contributions *
-   Budget development programme
-   Internal controls, internal audit and source paperwork programme
-   Integration of general accounting systems with stores system, and
    developments in the hospitals and community care programs *
-   General accounting/expenditure reporting - enhancements *
-   Fixed asset register *
-   Format of annual accounts mechanisation *
-   General accounting/expenditure reporting - further enhancements *

Personnel
-   Personnel record keeping systems - design and installation*
-   Staff and management training plans
-   Training programme development

Other aspects of the systems plan
Having defined and agreed the systems scope and priorities for the
five year period, the project team:
-   set out the main personnel/organisation issues which accrued from the
    review work
-   set out a series of recommendations for the development of
    personnel/organisation in the administrative and systems support
    areas. This included a recommended organisation structure for a new
    systems support unit whose role would be to support computer and
    manual systems development in the Board and whose personnel could
    include individuals with nursing or other professional training
-   set down a computer hardware strategy
-   set down a computer software strategy and
-   summarised the economic implications of the plan - as a basis for
    management approval.

PROGRESS TO DATE
The Board began the organisation development and systems work set out
in the plan in early 1979. It was agreed that the Board's main high volume
transaction systems (payroll, payments, general accounting and statistical
reporting) would continue to be processed on the government computer centre's
IBM 370/158 in Dublin. It was also agreed to be appropriate that the Board
should acquire their own minicomputer which - because the Board did not have a
technical computer group - should be as "user friendly" as possible and require
a relatively low level of technical support.

Management Information and Service Improvement

In 1979 the Board, with consultant help, designed and installed a comprehensive financial and statistical reporting system for all aspects of the Board's activities. Each month, the system reports budget performance, commitments, expenditure and budget variations for all sub-cost centres - and takes information from the payroll system and the general payments system. The hospital programme reports include statistical information on occupancy and length of stay by speciality; outpatient statistics (including new and return); support services statistics. (In each case prior year comparisons are also reported). In 1979 a system for invoicing and collecting farmers' health contributions was designed and installed, and a series of short (non computer) projects were undertaken in the areas of:

- cost control and improved service in community care offices
- improved eligibility assessment and client service in community care
- the development of improved internal communication systems in the Board's two general hospitals.

Computer Acquisition

In early 1980 the Board took delivery of its own minicomputer - an IBM System/34. The computer is at the Board's headquarters in Manorhamilton with data entry stations and VDU's in Sligo and Letterkenny.

In 1980/81 there were the following computer developments:

- enhancement of the general accounting and financial reporting systems
- the design and installation of a materials management system - integrated with the general accounting system
- the installation of communications facilities to allow the Board's own computer to act as an RJE terminal to the mainframe at the government computer centre.

Community Care Index

In 1981 work was begun on a major custom designed system to maintain index information for the approximately 200,000 individuals to whom the Board provides community care services. Information needs were specified through discussions with professionals and administrators throughout the community care programme and, following a review of application software, it was decided that the system should be custom designed. The main objective of the community index system is to move record keeping from "service based" systems to "patient/recipient" based systems providing a more integrated basis for co-ordinating the work of the different health and social services professionals.

Personnel Information

Also in 1981 the Board approved a substantial project to design and install the first phase of a personnel records and information system for the all the Board's employees.

MAIN BENEFITS

The benefits of the work are under several headings:

Overcoming the "frustration gap"

It is important that organisation changes and developments be supported by parallel development of people and support systems. Otherwise - at the simplest level - individuals are equipped with new job titles without the support to enable them to act differently in fact. (This has been particularly true of the health services re-organisations of the the early '70's). Even if these important systems and other developments are set in train at the time of a re-organisation, their implementation usually lags months or years behind because of the effort involved in the design and implementation of large scale computer systems.

This period is sometimes called "the frustration gap" - the period when new jobs are set up and filled but adequate information support is still not available to their incumbents. The systems plan has allowed the setting of accurate lead times and user expectations - and has, to some extent, addressed this issue.

A vehicle for having staff examine their roles and relationships with fellow providers of services

The work involved in the development of the plan has encouraged staff - especially in community care - to think carefully about their roles, responsibilities and relationships through the process of defining information needs.

A framework for setting management team responsibilities

The comprehensiveness of the systems plan has given the management team a realistic framework in which to set priorities - because they are able to discuss the "trade-offs" and costs and benefits of pursuing one system or organisation investment as opposed to another.

A clear picture of resource requirements

Computer systems in organisations as large as health boards or hospitals, require substantial investments of people, money and other resources. The systems plan provided realistic cost and effort estimates - so as to provide the management team with a sound understanding of the resource implications of the plan to which they were committing.

Developing integrated systems

The development of integrated systems - where information is input once and passed to other systems for summarisation or reformatting, provides economic, efficient systems. Because systems have been planned several years ahead - the initial systems could be designed on a "building block" basis with a clear indication as to how they might integrate with future systems developments.

Development of systems disciplines

The management team, by involving itself and its personnel in systems developments, has begun to disseminate a sound understanding of the disciplines required for the effective exploitation of the computer. A systems support group has now been set up - and its members are formally involved in each of the systems projects that the Board is undertaking.

The use of a proven methodology

The systems plan and the systems design and installation projects following it have used Arthur Andersen & Co.'s standard systems methodology ("Method/1"). This has brought substantial benefits in terms of consistency of approach, standards for design and installation work, effective project team communications and comprehensive documentation.

427

MANAGEMENT DATA SYSTEM IN INTENSIVE CARE

J.Villalobos, J.L.Manzano.
Intensive Care Unit, R.S.Ntra.Sra. del Pino
Las Palmas de Gran Canaria, SPAIN, Canary Islands.
J.L.Bozal, J.Huguet
I-Cuatro S.A. Madrid, SPAIN.

SUMMARY.

To solve the problem of data management, a Digital Computer was introduced in our intensive care unit (I.C.U.) in 1977. Data are manually entered at the bedside alpha-numeric Keyboard and two beds are directly connected to the computer. The user's application programs were developed in our I.C.U. in collaboration with the electronic firm I-Cuatro S.A.(Spain). The main objectives,to organize data acquisition, to perform complex computations for information not normally available, to automate our problem oriented records, to suggest possible diagnosis and therapeutic interventions, and to facilitate statistics in order to derive prognostic indicators.

Since 1977 we have computerized 3000 patients and our conclusions are: data management and communication have improved thus allowing nurses more time for direct patient care; teaching of residents and nurses has been facilitated, minimising the effects of their different experience; it has led to a more systematic approach to patient care; it has permitted the continuous utilization by the less experienced personnel of the experience of those who wrote the protocols according to which the computer analyzes data to suggest decisions.

INTRODUCTION.

To manage the increasing flow of generated data that requires immediate evaluation, in order to make it useful for an effective and efficient treatment of the patients, digital computers were introduced in the I.C.U. during the 1960's (1). Their principal objectives were: to accelerate the acquisition, processing, and presentation of data; to generate new data not normally available, and to reduce the work load of nurses and doctors. Based on their capability to analyse data relative to protocols, computers began being used in decision-making (2,3).

With these objectives in mind, a computerized system of data management was introduced in the I.C.U. Our aims were the complete control of the patients' records, the utilization of the computer as an alarm system and the derivation of prognostic scores based on the empirical and statistic scoring of each of the patient's problems. After defining clinical needs, the authors selected the necessary hardware and gradually developed the software. Since 1977, over 3000 patients have been managed using data generated by the computer. The purpose of this paper is to review this experience (4).

MATERIALS AND METHODS.

The actual hardware used is a PDP 11/35 Central Processor unit with a core memory of 96 Kwords(16 bits),3 Moving head disks with a store capacity of 1.2 Mwords --
each,9 alpha-numeric displays with with attached keyboards,2 line printers and a 16
channel analogical digital convertor (AR-11).

A Real Time Multiprogramming System(RSX/11/D) was used,and the programs were -
written in fortran and digital assembler.A tree overlayed program with 25.000 lines
and a mean response time of 0.3 sec was used.

The displays are located at the bedside,and the data of each patient can be -
managed from any of the displays.

The original idea was to manage the patients with the help of the computer.To
accomplish this,the software developed to manage the patients in the I.C.U. was the
following:

State of the Unit.- This allows one to know which beds are occupied or vacant;
after selecting one of them,one has access to the different functions of the system
through special function keys.

Admission and discharge.- All the identification data are entered in the system through this program;when the patient is discharged,the computer checks whether
the patient's record is complete and if it is so,the printer automatically produces
a hard-copy of the patient's history to be included in the hospital record and a file storing for statistical purpose.Other options of this program are-change of bed-
and-hard copy of all the patients records.

Free text.- Through this function,and from the bedside alpha-numeric keyboards
doctors and nurses can enter or display information in a free text form.On the display screens it is posible to correct,modify,annul or add complete lines of text.

Physical examination.- This function allows a systematic physical examination -
in codified form.Some of the physical signs are automatically included by the computer in the list of problems and when these signs are not longer present,the problem
is automatically closed.Different options of the program allow to annul,change,dis-
play or obtain, through the printer,the last or all the examinations performed.

Variables.- All the cardiorespiratory measurements may be manually emtered and
displayed.From the monitors of two specific beds,directly connected to the computer,
the cardiorespiratory variables may be automatically obtained.When these direct values are entered,the computer derives new data from standard formulae.In a single -
display the last values reflect the overall status of the patient.When one wants to
examine trends,the measurements may be presented in tabulated or graphic form.When
some of the entered values are outside certain specified limits,defined according -
to the clinical condition,the computer gives an alarm.There are options that allow
correction of the errors previously entered manually or automatically.The variables
of all the patients are stored in the computer for any length of time that they --

stay in the I.C.U.

Problems.- Our records are problem oriented and these problems constitute the - working objectives on which the care of the patients is based (5,6).The problems de- rived from the physical examination,variables,medical orders,techniques,fluids and - laboratory are automatically opened and closed(Figure I).

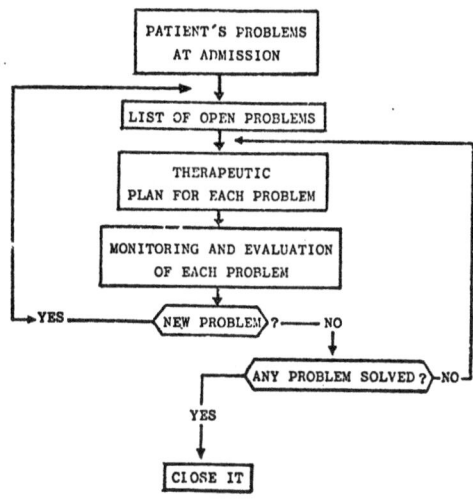

FIGURE I. Management of Patient's Problems.

Those derived from clinical diagnosis are manually managed by doctor and nurses. The options of this program are:open,annul,close display and printer.Doctors and nur- ses can review and revise the opened problems,or all the problems of any patient at - any time and from any of the displays.(FIGURE II).

Physician orders.- All the doctors orders and nursing care plans are manually - introduced in the computer system and oriented to the existing problems.The standard orders are entered in codified form and the computer calculates doses based on the - patient's weight.Protocol treatments are also codified,in order to facilitate their - entry in the list or orders(FIGURE III).The options of this program are;open(an order) accomplish,discontinue,annul,display and hard copy.The orders that have not been in- terrupted at the end of a medical day,are automatically included in the list of or- ders of the following day.

BED N°7 NAME: A.S.   SEX: M   H.N.: 1.989
WEIGHT/KG: 95   HEIGHT/CMS: 170   B.S./m²:2.06
DIAGNOSIS: A.M.I.   ADMISSION: 2-1-1.980

DATE: 2-1-1.980

PROBLEMS

TIME OPEN	TIME RESOLVED	PROBLEM
2-1-80(19h.)		0- GROUP A
2-1-80(19h.)		1- A.M.I.
2-1-80(19h.)	3-1-80(4h.)	2- COMPLETE A-V BLOCK
2-1-80(19,30h.)	5-1-80(12h.)	3- TRANSIT. PACEMAKER
2-1-80(20h.)		4- CARDIOMEGALY
2-1-80(22h.)	4-1-80(10h.)	5- HYPERTENSION
2-1-80(23h.)	3-1-80(20h.)	6- BACKWARD FAILURE
2-1-80(23h.)	3-1-80(3h.)	7- OLIGURIA
2-1-80(24h.)		8- DIGITALISATION
3-1-80(2h.)	5-1-80(12h.)	9- IPPR-PEEP
3-1-80(3h.)	3-1-80(4h.)	10- NEUMOTHORAX
3-1-80(3,15h.)	4-1-80(20h.)	11- PLEURAL DRAINAGE
3-1-80(16h.)	3-1-80(23h.)	12- COMPLETE A-V BLOCK

BED N°7   NAME: A. S.   SEX: M   H. N.: 1.989
WEIGHT/KG: 95   HEIGHT/CM.: 170   B.S.: 2.06
DIAGNOSIS: A.M.I.   ADMISSION: 2-1-1.980

DATE: 5-1-1.980

TREATMENT

DATE	ORDER	DOSE/VIA	TIME (HOURS)
5-1-80(9h.)	**NUTRITION		
"	Dextrose 50%	1000cc/IV	Continuous
"	Aminosol 10%	1000cc/IV	Continuous
"	Na	100 mEq/IV	Continuous
"	K	120 mEq/IV	Continuous
	**NEUMONIA		
"	Keflin	2 grs. /IV	6-12-18-24
"	Gentamycin	80 mg. /IV	6-14-22
"	IPPR-PEEP	---------	Continuous
"	**GENERAL		
"	Heparin	75 mg. /SC	12-24
"	Xr	---------	10
"	**HYPERTENSION		
"	Hyperstad	300 mg./IV	12
"	Furosemide	10 m. /IV	12-20

FIGURE II.List of Patient's Problems.   FIGURE III. Physician orders display.

Fluid and blood balance.Through this program the computer calculates the fluid and bood balance hourly.If they are outside predetermined limits,a diagnostic and the rapentic message is displayed.Doctors and nurses may review the fluid-blood balance - of the last 4-8-24 hours and the total balance from the time of admission.

Decision tables.- These constitute the clinical algorithms for the management of fluid,electrolytes and acid-based balance,shock,renal and respiratory failure,blood - transfusión and cardiac performance in the postoperative patient(7, 8,9) When the — monitored variables and laboratory measurements of any patient combine according to - the clinical algorithms,the computer generates a diagnostic and therapentic message. The number of this patient is shown on all the displays and the screens of the diffe- rent programs.Doctors and nurses may check the message and know the conditions on — which it was generated through the "Messages" function.

Scoring systems.- These are based on the score of the problems that each group of patients present during their stay in I.C.The value of each problem was derived - empirically and through the application of χ^2 test after knowing its incidence on - the patients of each group an its incidence on mortality .When the statistic scoring was calculated problems with $p > 0.02$ were not considered.The total number of pro— blems, the number of specific problems,and the empirical and statistical score of — each patient were calculated in several group of patients and the scoring separated the surviving from the non-surviving.

DISCUSSION.

Data produced by intensive care patients are difficult to manage with the necce-
sary speed and this may result in useless information that doctors and nurses are -
not able to interpret properly.Trainig might eliminate these problems,but the difficulty probably lies in the doctor's intrinsic limit as a processor of information and
for this reason it is thought that computers may be of value.

The computer has improved data adquisition and processing and we think that the
aplication of decision tables has helped less experience personel in the interpreta-
tation of the collected data in the selection of the appropiate treatment.Other bene-
ficts obtained from computer analysis of data,according to rules of logic,have been -
the standardization of diagnostic and therapeutic criteria and the reduction of the -
adverse effects due to the varying experience of the medical staff.The limitation has
been our own limitations to develop adequate protocols and our lack of understanding
of the pathophysiologic organ interactions in the critically ill patients(10,11).

A complete understanding of the role of the computer and its flexbility are essential in I.C.The system must meet the needs of the unit and when its output is unfamiliar to nurses and doctors,our experience is that most often it will not be ac-
cepted-by them.In this unit,doctors and nurses paiticipated in the development of the
computer programs and since their introduction,the nurses have been relieved from many of their monotonous duties.The system's capability to display diagnostic and therapeutic recommendations has decreased their anxieties about failure to appreciate -
important information(12).

We have now developed scoring systems in several groups of patients(Craneal trau
ma,thoracic trauma,hyaline membrane,meconium aspiration,memingococal sepsis)and these
have helped us in the clasification of our patients in the I.C.U.The scoring have -
appropriately separated the surviving from the non-surviving and this has facilitated
our decisions to withdraw therapy and the selection of patients to be admitted or dis
charged.We think that if different units work on the development of these scoring sys
tems their working standards could be determined and their effectivity imporved.

For these computerized systems to be useful,they must be accepted by all person-
nel.Because of this,the authors think that their introduction must be gradual.During
the training period,special attention must be given to emphasize their advantages as
well as their limitations.

Each person must understand that the computer does not substitute any one and -
that it is only a mechanical device that improves efficiency,increases the information base and helps interpret it with extreme rapidity.

BIBLIOGRAPHY.

1.- Weil M.N.,Shubin H.,Rand W.:Experience with a digital computer for study and improved management of the critically ill.Jama 198:147,1.966.

2.- Sheppard L.C.,Kirklin J.W. and kouchoukos N.T. Computer controlled interventions for the acutelly ill patient.Comput.Biomed.Res. 4:135,1.974.

3.- Sheppard L.C. and Kouchoukos N.T.:Computers as monitors.Anaesthesiology 45:250, 1.976.

4.- Manzano J.L.,Villalobos J.,Church A.,Manzano J.J.Computierized information system for I.C.U. patient management. Crit.Care Med. 8:745,1.980.

5.- Weed L.Medical Records that guide and teach.N.Engl.J.Med. 278:593,1.968.

6.- Villalobos J.,Manzano J.L.Manejo de pacientes según sus problemas en Medicina Intensiva.4:201,1.980.

7.- Manzano J.L.,Villalobos J.,Quintana J.Cuidados Postoperatorios Cardiacos con ayuda del Ordenador.Medicina Intensiva,4:139,1.980.

8.- Sheppard L.C.The computer in the care of critically ill patient.Proceeding IEEE. 67:1300,1.979.

9.- Robiseck F.,Masters T.N.,Reichertz P.L.,Dangherty H.R. and Cook J.W.Three years experience with computer based intensive care patients following agen heart and major vascular surgery.Surgery 81:12,1.977.

10.- Phillips G.D.,Austin R.L.Intensive Care Data-II:A new unit's first two years. Anaesth.Intens.Care 7:329,1.979.

11.- Johson J.H.,Gianneth R.A.The reliability of diagnosis by technician,computer and algorithm. .J.Cl.Psych 36:448,1.980.

12.- Cullin D.J.,Teplick R.The role of computers in the future of Intensive Care.Proc. IEE, 67:9,1.979.

A DISTRIBUTED SYSTEMS APPROACH TO PATIENT MONITORING

AND MEDICAL DATA MANAGEMENT

M. Michael Shabot, M.D., Assistant Professor of Surgery,
Paul C. Carlton, M.D., Resident in Anesthesia,
and Michael Laks, M.D., Professor of Medicine

Harbor/UCLA Medical Center, 1000 West Carson Street,
Torrance, California 90509/USA

Computer-based patient monitoring and medical data management systems are expanding at a rapid rate. Advances in hardware capabilities, coupled with tumbling price structures, have facilitated the introduction of computer systems in clinical areas of the hospital including intensive care units, the clinical laboratory and the pharmacy (1,2). To a lesser extent these systems have been used for hospital-wide data retrieval and medical data management. Existing systems have been described on hardware ranging from mainframe to microprocessor in size (3,4). Software has varied from purchased "turnkey" software to entirely user written code. Relatively little effort has been expended on building networks of computer systems for monitoring and medical data management. We have developed a comprehensive hospital-wide network of distributed mini-computers for clinical data entry and retrieval, using commercially available systems and applications software whenever possible.

METHODS

The Harbor/UCLA Medical Center System consists of five distributed minicomputers and associated software (Figure 1). Two networked Hewlett-Packard 1000 MX-E computers with 512 kilobytes of memory and 100 megabytes of disc storage are dedicated to real-time monitoring of 64 patients in eight intensive care units and one operating room (Figure 2). Twenty-three terminals and thirteen line printers are attached to the patient monitoring computers for data entry and results retrieval. These computers operate under the RTE-IV Real Time Executive operating system and modified HP 78706 Patient Data Management System (PDMS) software for analog-to-digital data conversions, patient database organization and physiologic data displays. RTE and PDMS software readily allows the addition and incorporation of user written code; we have made many modifications to the PDMS system. We have added distributed systems (DS) applications software to link two blood gas laboratories to printers in eight intensive care units. Standard DS/1000 software and hardware was utilized for computer-to-computer communications. Fortran and Ratfor were used as our programming languages on the monitoring computers.

The two patient monitoring computers are networked to a Hewlett-Packard 3000/44 computer system and two HP 1000 MX-F ECG management systems. The 3000/44 system has one megabyte of semiconductor memory and 240 megabytes of disc storage (Figure 3). This sixteen bit minicomputer features a virtual, stack oriented operating system which handles up to 96 on-line terminals. The 3000/44 is used for medical data entry and retrieval from the Blood Bank, the Emergency Laboratory, Radiology, Nuclear Medicine, Ultrasound, and the Computerized Axial Tomography areas. Printed reports are generated for each data entry site with the exception of the Blood Bank. Twenty-one cathode ray terminals in ward, clinic and emergency room areas are attached to the HP 3000/44 for data retrieval. A built-in printer in each HP 2624A terminal allows for convenient hardcopy of all displayed data. We have developed custom data entry and retrieval software for our attached terminals, interfacing with the HP VIEW/3000 block mode screen handling package and the IMAGE/3000 data base management package. VIEW/3000 facilitates rapid development of block mode forms and configurable data validation protocols. Erroneous data entry fields are automatically highlighted by VIEW/3000, and the applications programmer can ensure that only error-free data sets are entered into the data base. For similar reasons we used IMAGE/3000 as our data base management system. IMAGE files are readily configured and system data base code is isolated from program code. Use of VIEW and IMAGE markedly speeded software development and allowed us to write relatively modest amounts of program code to accomplish our goals. Compiled Basic was used as the programming language on the 3000/44.

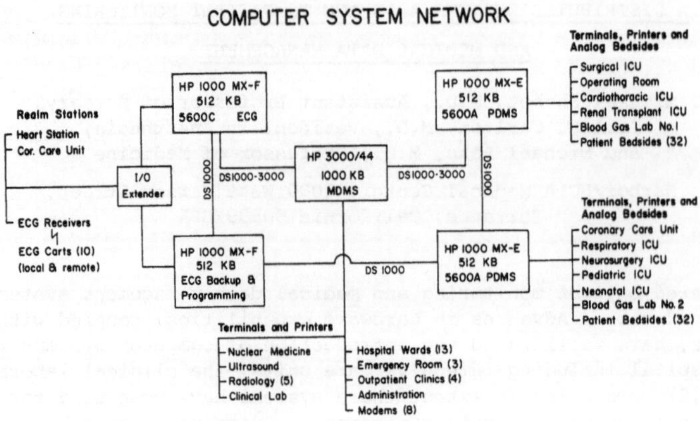

COMPUTER SYSTEM NETWORK

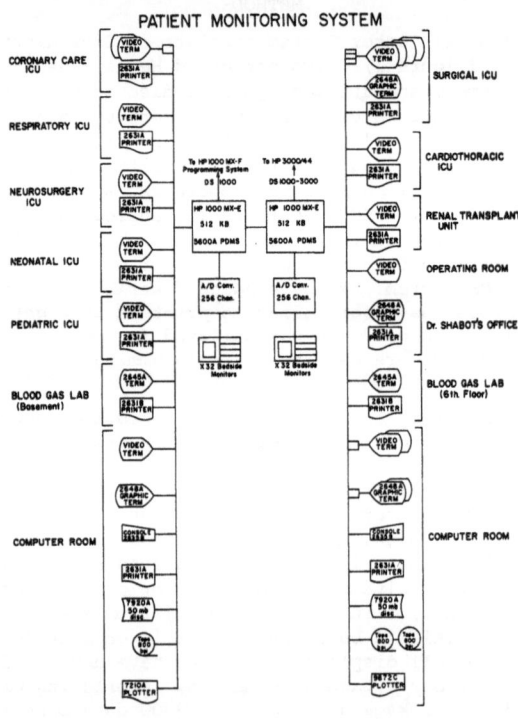

Figure 1. Distributed Systems Diagram

Figure 2. Patient Monitoring System Diagram

MEDICAL DATA MANAGEMENT SYSTEM

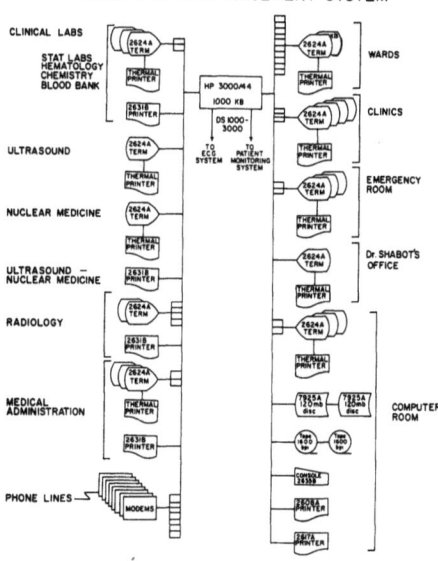

Figure 3. Medical Data Management System Diagram

Two ECG analysis systems run on HP 1000 MX-F computers which operate under RTE-IV and modified HP 5600C ECG Analysis software. These computers have 512 kilobyte semiconductor memories and share 375 megabytes of disc (Figure 4). Hardware redundancy is provided to ensure continuous operation. The spare CPU is used as a programming system. These computers receive approximately 3000 sets of 12 lead ECG's per month over local hospital and long distance phone lines, and prepare full computerized diagnostic interpretation in approximately 20 seconds per ECG. All in-hospital ECG's are over-read by staff cardiologists, with a final integrated waveform and printed report returned to the chart within 24 hours. We have developed an ECG computer language, a pediatric ECG analysis program and an ECG statistical evaluation report. We are in the process of linking these systems to the 3000/44 and the patient monitoring systems so that computer-generated ECG diagnoses may be accessed in real time. Fortran is used as the programming language on the ECG system.

<u>RESULTS</u>

All systems operate 24 hours per day except for servicing or data base backup to magnetic tape. Each system will be described separately.

I. <u>Patient Monitoring Systems</u>

The two patient monitoring systems sample approximately 500 analog signal lines from 64 beds at a rate of once per second. Periodically this data is stored to disc. Lab data is stored to disc in patient files managed by the HP 78706 PDMS software. We have added software to enter, compute and display cardiorespiratory data for critically ill patients (5). We have written a graphics compiler for creation of graphic displays configured with an English language command table. Figures 5 and 6 show typical graphic displays of cardiorespiratory and acid-base data. Comprehensive but compact printed reports are available in each intensive care unit (Figure 7). This printed report subsystem was written at Harbor and also features an English language command file. Printed reports are added or modified by simple editing of a command file rather than program code.

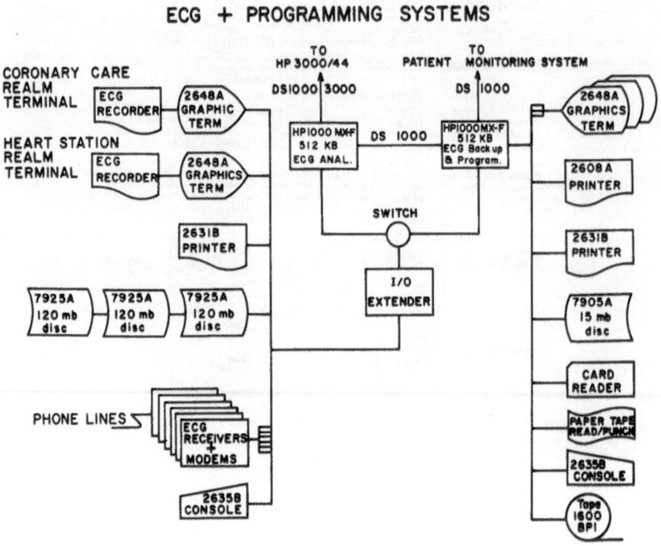

ECG + PROGRAMMING SYSTEMS

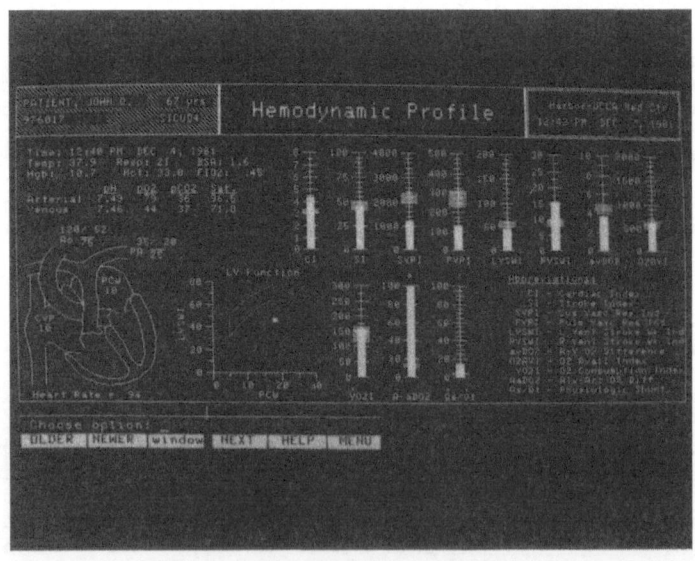

Figure 4.   ECG + Programming Systems Diagram

Figure 5.   Hemodynamic Profile Video Screen

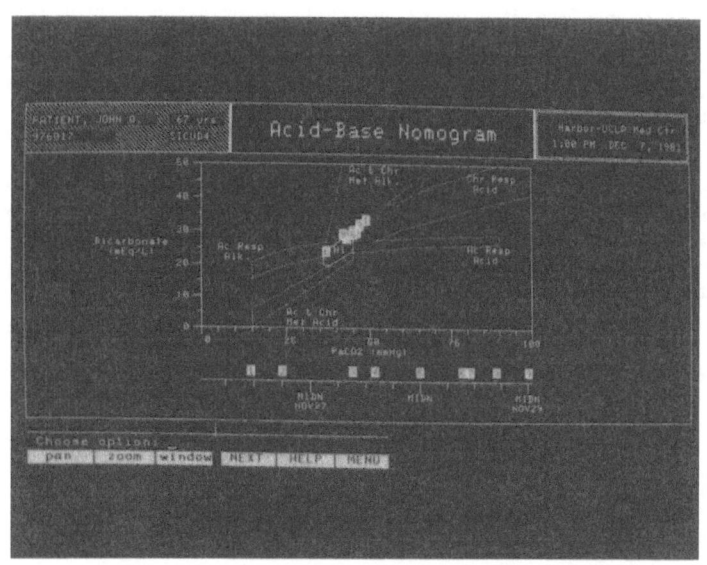

Figure 6. Acid-Base Nomogram Video Screen

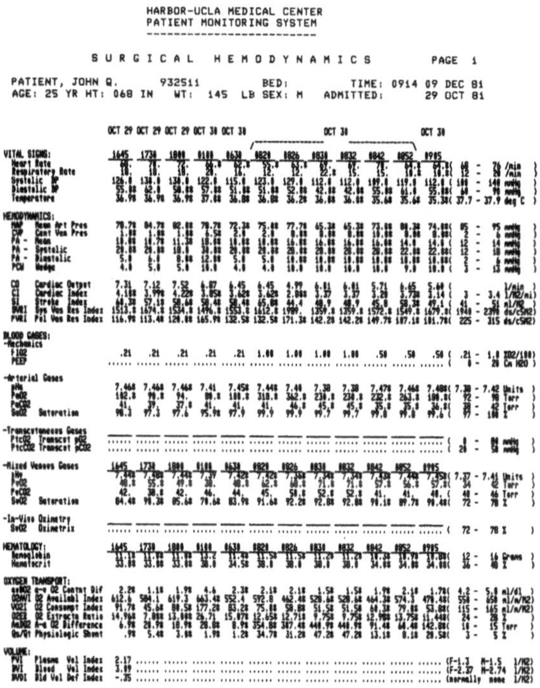

HARBOR-UCLA MEDICAL CENTER
PATIENT MONITORING SYSTEM

S U R G I C A L   H E M O D Y N A M I C S   PAGE 1

PATIENT, JOHN Q.   932511   BED: TIME: 0914 09 DEC 81
AGE: 25 YR HT: 068 IN   WT: 145 LB SEX: M   ADMITTED: 29 OCT 81

Figure 7. Hemodynamic Summary Printed Report

438

Custom data entry and printed report software was written for two blood gas laboratories to ensure error-free data entry and reliable printing of stat reports directly in the intensive care areas. The blood gas laboratory technician is automatically notified if the computers cannot immediately deliver or print a stat report due to hardware, software, data link or printer problems. The blood gas data entry terminals operate in block mode rather than character-by-character transmission (Figure 8). We have utilized block mode exclusively for data entry for several reasons:

(1) Block mode provides a familiar "form" for technicians to view and complete.
(2) Erroneous or out-of-range data fields may be checked by the terminal or computer and then highlighted with inverse video or blinking. The technician's attention is readily drawn to the erroneous field.
(3) Terminal-to-computer communication overhead is very low using this technique.

Block mode transmission requires an "intelligent" terminal with its own microprocessor; this distributed intelligence markedly reduces main central processing unit (CPU) overhead.

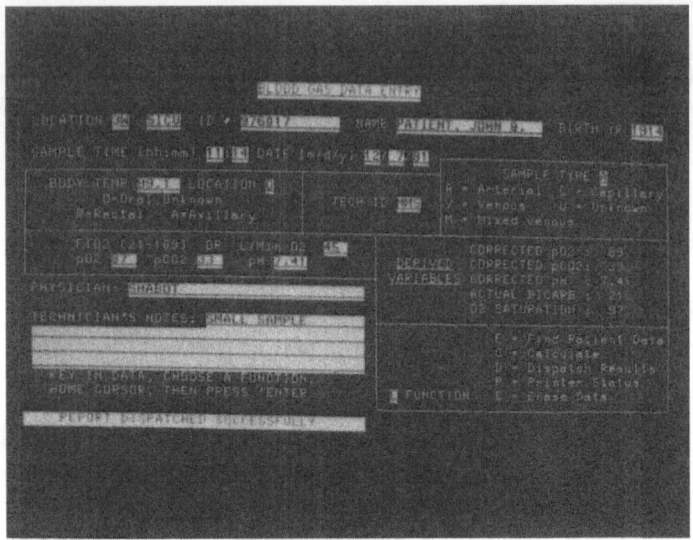

Figure 8. Blood Gas Lab Data Entry Video Screen

DS/1000 hardware and software was used to link the two patient monitoring systems in a manner transparent to the blood gas technicians. Lab terminal software treats the two computers as one; blood gas technicians have no knowledge of which computer manages a particular patient's data file or remote printer.

II. Emergency Lab/X-Ray/Blood Bank Reporting System

This system resides on the HP 3000/44 computer. We have written data entry and results retrieval software for the Emergency Lab, the Blood Bank, General Radiology, Nuclear Medicine, and Ultrasound-Computerized Axial Tomography areas. All entry and retrieval terminals run in block mode using VIEW/3000 software package.

All data entry and retrieval terminals are automatically initialized and started upon system boot-up. We developed a monitor program which checks each terminal every two minutes and restarts the appropriate entry or retrieval program if for some reason it is not running at that time.

The Emergency Chemistry lab entry form features several types of validity checking (Figure 9). Lab values outside the normal range are automatically "tagged" with a single asterisk. If a value is in a dangerously abnormal range the software tags it with two asterisks. If the entered result is outside the physiologic range, the field is brightly inversed and an error message appears. Our software will not allow storage of truly erroneous data. A final report is printed daily for the patient's chart (Figure 10).

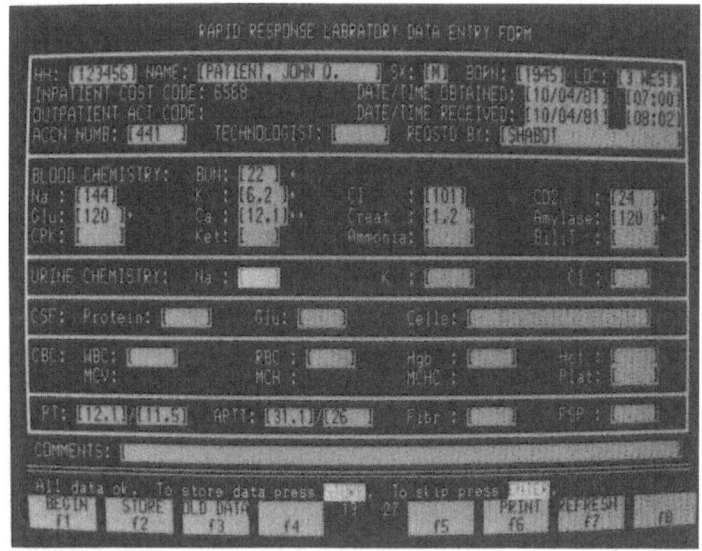

Figure 9.   Emergency Laboratory Data Entry Video Screen

The Blood Bank subsystem allows hospital personnel to determine instantly the blood products available for any patient (Figure 11). The entry and retrieval forms differ only in that a technologist identification code is required to enter or alter data (the retrieval form is shown here). Update of an existing blood bank record usually only requires two or three keystrokes. Room is provided on the form for a "global" Blood Bank message as well as a message unique for each patient, if needed.

Radiology reporting software was written for entry terminals in the General Radiology, Nuclear Medicine and Ultrasound-CAT scan areas. This software is table driven from lists of approximately 225 types of examinations and 750 diagnostic comments. Exam type and results are entered by number and the computer responds with the corresponding English language statements (Figure 12). Seven lines for free form text is provided so that word processing for a computer generated report can be performed by the system.

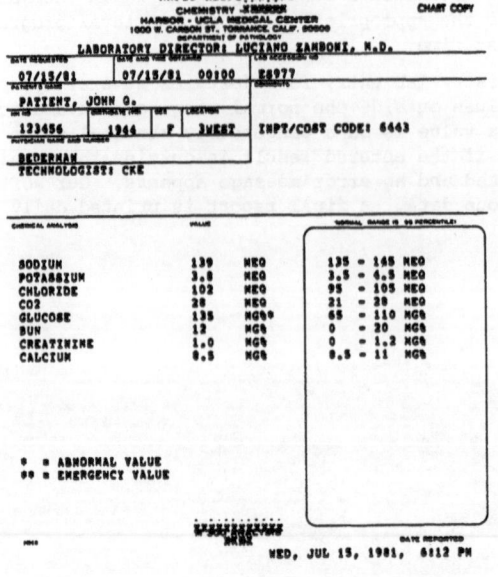

Figure 10. Rapid Response Laboratory Printed Report

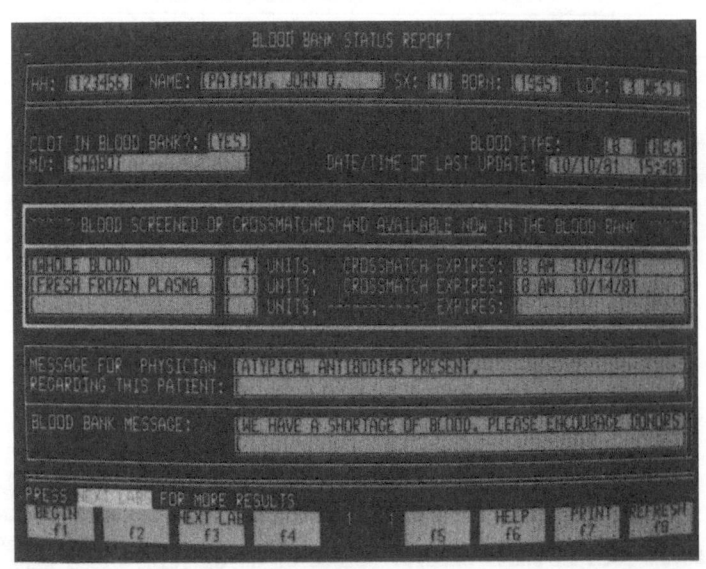

Figure 11. Blood Bank Status Video Screen

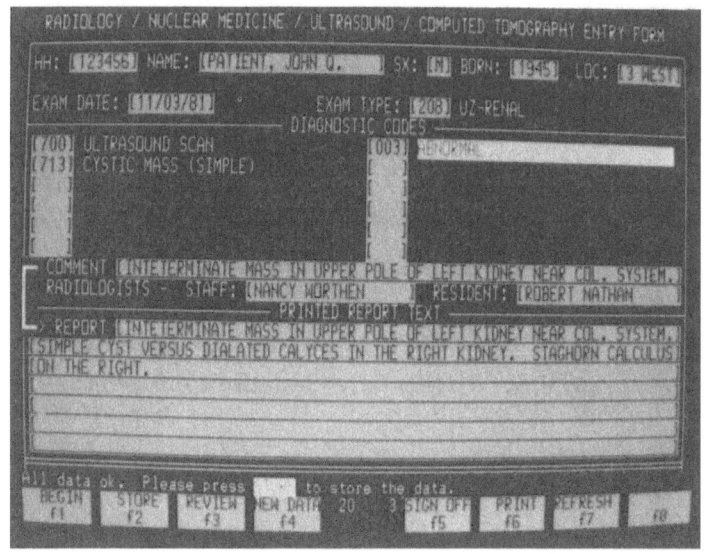

Figure 12. Radiologic Data Entry Video Screen

All twenty-one lab data retrieval terminals run the same program. Data is selected for retrieval in the most simple manner possible. The physician or nurse has only to type in the patient's identification number and "X" boxes corresponding to the data needed (Figure 13). Note that most user interaction with the terminal is accomplished with eight "soft" function keys labeled at the bottom of the video screen and physically located at the top of the keyboard. Supplementary user assistance is available at each stage with the f6 "HELP" soft key.

Typical data retrieval forms for Chemistry and Radiology results are shown in Figures 14 and 15. Data is always displayed in reverse chronological order, regardless of the time it was entered into the data base. Abnormal or "emergency" values are displayed tagged with one or two asterisks, respectively. The user may rapidly obtain a printed copy of any screen by pressing the f7 "PRINT" soft key. A built-in 120 character per second thermal printer produces a screen copy in seconds. Similar report screens are available for CSF Chemistry, Urine Chemistry, Hematology, Spinal Fluid Cell count, Coagulation, Blood Gas and Blood Bank studies.

III. Electrocardiogram (ECG) Analysis Systems

These systems provide automatic ECG diagnoses for Harbor/UCLA Medical Center, several other Los Angeles County hospitals and a number of remote hospitals served by long distance lines. ECG analysis takes about 20 seconds and diagnoses may be returned directly to ECG carts equipped with remote printers (Figure 16). All ECG data is digitized, compressed and stored in long-term disc files. Serial comparisons are automatically performed by the system and may be printed at the Realm Stations.

We have written an ECG Statistical evaluation report which records every time a diagnosis is confirmed, added, deleted or modified by the overreading cardiologist (6,7). When significant differences between the ECG program's and the overreading cardiologist's diagnoses are noted, the ECG program may be modified, if appropriate. By continually improving our program's diagnostic criteria, we have raised the program's statement accuracy rate to about 91%.

We have also developed a pediatric ECG computer program with diagnostic criteria configured for patients newborn to 15 years of age (8). The ECG technician enters

442

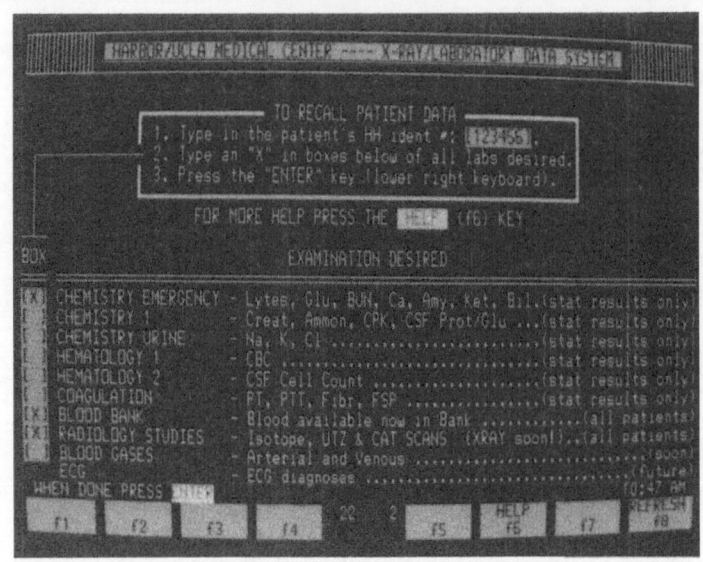

Figure 13. Data Recall Selection Video Screen

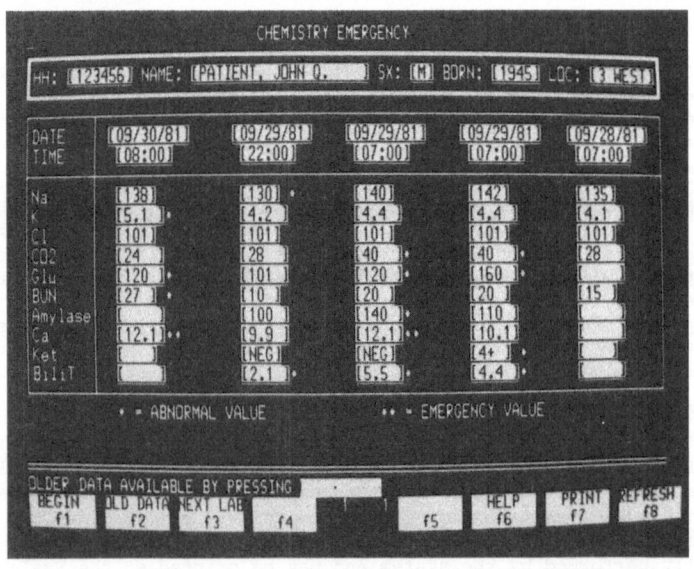

Figure 14. Emergency Chemistry Recall Video Screen

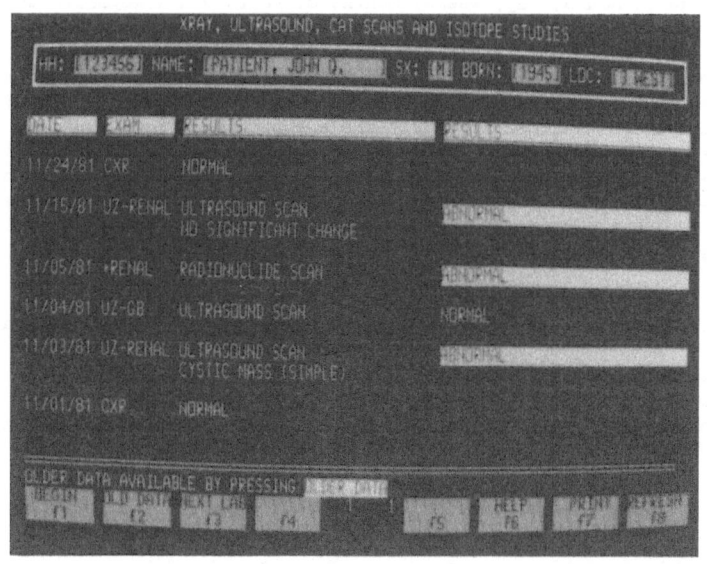

Figure 15. Radiology Data Recall Video Screen

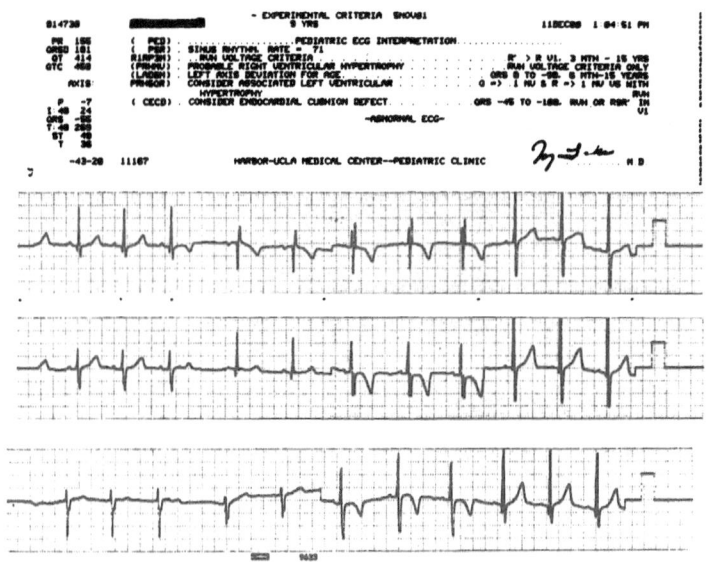

Figure 16. Pediatric Electrocardiogram Report

the patient's age in hours, day, weeks, months or years via a keyboard on the ECG cart; the computer selects the diagnostic criteria appropriate for the patient's age. Since pediatric electrocardiographic criteria are complex and change with the patient's age, an electrocardiographer cannot easily remember all the possible variations of normal but must himself refer to a published table for appropriate criteria. The program was written so that detailed criteria are printed (Figure 16) and electro-cardiographers are spared the time that may be required to look for specific criteria. In addition, since the computer has a quality control program informing the technician of the technical quality of the tracing, the quality of the ECG record has markedly improved. Lastly, since pediatric cardiologists are few and poorly distributed, proper reading of the pediatric ECG is available for more physicians.

DISCUSSION

Computerized clinical information systems for hospitals are about ten years old (9). There have likely been more failures than successes (10). A number of individuals have described special data base systems for clinical data (11,12). Relatively few reports concern computerizing Blood Bank data. Clayton and coworkers have described a radiology data entry and reporting system based on most likely diagnoses (13). By far the most attention has been afforded to clinical laboratory data systems (14,15).

We have described a comprehensive patient monitoring and medical data management system based on distributed minicomputers coupled to intelligent terminals. Our thrust has been to link on-line systems for physiologic ICU monitoring with other on-line systems for lab, radiology, blood bank and ECG data management. Our system currently comprises five distributed central processing units, 57 terminals, 19 line printers and other associated equipment.

Unlike Begtrup (15) we do not yet have data demonstrating a reduction in operating expenses in the computer system. There is relatively wide-spread appreciation that our computers vastly outperform the manual systems they replaced. The addition of computerized word processing for the Radiology, Nuclear Medicine and Ultrasound-CAT scan areas may soon provide solid evidence of cost containment and reduction.

Distributing systems for patient monitoring and medical data management provides an efficient means to achieve the goals of rapid response times for widely varying medical and computational needs. Distributed systems software and hardware provides a common pathway for data to be shared among specialized systems which could otherwise serve only a limited number of hospital users and locations.

BIBLIOGRAPHY

(1) Duboid, RM. Clinical information systems: Current trends and outlook for the 80's. Computers in Hospitals 1981; 2(1): 38-47.

(2) Crist, ER. Laboratory computers: Where we are today. Computers in Hospitals 1981; 2(2): 22-29.

(3) Whitcomb, CC, Vogt, CC and Wilbur, NM. Clinical laboratory data processing with a central hospital computer. Computers in Biol and Med 1978; 8: 197-206.

(4) Biese, LP. The laboratory eprom: Normal values and histograms. Phys Microcomputer Report 1979; 2(1): 28-36.

(5) Shabot, MM, Bland, R, Shoemaker, WC, et al. Computerized on-line hemodynamic analysis and predictive indices for critically ill surgical patients. In Rechnergestutzte Intensivpflege, Stuttgart, Georg Thieme Verlag publishers, 1981.

(6) Hamilton, KK, Clifton, JG, Laks, MM. A real-time approach to performance evaluation of EKG interpretative programs. Proceed of an Engineering Foundation Conference, Computerized Interpretation of the Electrocardiog 1975, Rindge, New Hampshire, U.S. Dept. Health Educ and Welfare (Ed.) 1976, 145-191.

(7) Laks, MM. Computer systems for the processing of diagnostic electrocardiography. Proc of Computers in Cardiol 1978, published in IEEE Jo, 1980; 80: 186-210.

(8) Hamilton, D, Clifton, J, Laks, MM. Computerized pediatric ECG interpretative review of the first year of life. Proceed Engineer Foundation Conf - Computerized Interpretation of the ECG IV, 1979; 239-312.

(9) Cook, M, Fleming, JJ and Buchanan, NS. El Camino Hospital: Ten Years Later. Computers in Hospitals 1981; 2(4): 22-25.

(10) Covvey, H, Dominic and McAlister, NH. Medical computing: Promise and peril, In Computers in the Practice of Medicine, Vol. I, Addison-Wesley Publishing Co, Reading, Massachusetts, 1980: 4-13.

(11) Ludwig, H. Specifications for an interactive retrieval system: CUPID. In Computer Applications and Techniques in Clinical Medicine, John Wiley & Sons, New York, 1974: 136-164.

(12) Leavitt, MB and Leinbach, RC. A generalized system for corroborative on-line data collection. Computers & Biomed Res 1977; 10:413-421.

(13) Clayton, PD, Ostler, DB, Gennaro, SS, et al. A radiology reporting system based on most likely diagnoses. Computers & Biomed Res 180; 13: 258-270.

(14) Hamilton, WF and Raymond S. ECLIPS: An extended clinical laboratory information processing system. Computers in Biol & Med 1973; 3: 3-12.

(15) Begtrup, H. Running a clinical-chemistry laboratory with and without the help of a computer. Med Informatics 1981; 6: 137-140.

A REGISTRATION SYSTEM IN AN INTENSIVE CARE UNIT.

Lis Dragsted, Qvist J., Janstrup F, Johansen SH.
Department of Anesthesia, Herlev Hospital, 2730 Herlev, Denmark and
Danish Institute for Clinical Epidemiology, Svanemøllevey 25,
2100 Copenhagen, Denmark.

SUMMARY.

A simple registration system is presented that gives information on
long term and short term outcome from intensive therapy, on the activity level or life quality after discharge and an evaluation of the
function of various organ systems. The system makes comparisons of
outcome from therapy in different units possible. The system can be
used in a continuous "production" control and can be of help in establishing criterias for selecting patient categories for treatment in
the ICU.

During the last thirty years intensive therapy has been developed
and intensive care units (ICU) are found in almost all hospitals with
acute care.

Though many lives have been saved and the number of units have
increased, the ICU's have remained under almost constant scrutiny and
criticism. There have been published several papers (1,2,3) concerning
the outcome of intensive therapy, each using their own classification
system to measure the success of treatment. It is necessary to compare
the outcome for different patient categories treated in different ICU's,
this can only be done if all the units use the same registration system.

In the intensive care unit at Herlev Hospital we have in cooperation with the Danish Institute for Clinical Epidemiology developed a
patient registration system that fulfils the needs we have for evaluation
of the effects of intensive therapy. The system is designed for data
processing and used with specific processing programmes presents the
outcome in terms of mortality compared to the expected mortality of a
normal population, besides the other informations we gain.

The informations gained are:

A: Results of treatment

B: "Prognostic indicators"

C: Life quality

A: Results of treatment are presented as

    1) Demographic data (age, sex, number, origin)

    2) Disease categories

    3) In-unit and in-hospital outcome

With these data we are able from one year to another to compare our
patients according to the demographic data, disease categories and the
short term outcome, that is in-unit and in-hospital mortality.

B: Prognostic indicators expressed by

    1) The need for ventilatory assistance with a high inspiratory
       oxygen content.

    2) Parenchymal involvement (kidney, lung, liver)

    3) Immunocompetence (test for anergy)

The most common cause of death in the ICU is multiorgan failure and
the early identification of symptoms showing involvement of different
organ systems is very important.   In the study on extracorporal
membrane oxygenation (ECMO-study) (4) it was demonstrated that patients
on ventilators demanding 50% or more oxygen during the first 24 hours
had a significantly higher mortality than those patients who required
a lower oxygen content.   Fry et al (1980) (5) found a mortality of
41% in patients with uncomplicated acute respiratory failure, if it
was accompanied by renal failure the mortality was 85%.   If 4 or more
organ systems failed the mortality was 100%.   In our system we get an
evaluation of the renal, the liver and the pulmonary function shortly
after the patients admission.   MacLean et al (1975) and Meakins et al
(1979) (6,7) showed that skintesting for anergy was a reliable method
to identify a group of patients in high risk of developing sepsis with
a high mortality after elective surgery.   Skintesting for anergy in
the ICU during the first 24 hours after admission, reflects the patients
immunocompetence (the host defense mechanism) and can be used in
identification of high risk patients at an early stage of their disease.

C: Life quality expressed as

    1) Patients activity level after discharge.

    2) Mortality after discharge.

The short term outcome has our interest because it serves as a kind of
immediate production control, but we are very interested in the patients
activity after discharge from the hospital, because it is to us a
better measure of success from intensive therapy.   After discharge
the patients at regular intervals receive a questionnaire concerning
their activity level, if they are back in normal activity, in limited
activity or still under care.   We have found that one year after
admission to the ICU 45% of the patients have died, 27% are back in
normal activity, 24% in limited and the rest are still under care.
These results are in accordance with those from other studies (8,9).

        Through the National Register we get information concerning the
mortality after discharge and the Danish Institute for Clinical

Epidemiology can by special processing programmes calculate the expected mortality for a normal population of same age and sex distribution and thereby we get a comparison between our patients' mortality and the expected mortality, the results are presented in graphic form.   Like-wise we can compare the long term outcome for patients with a specific diagnosis to a normal population and to the long term outcome for patients with the same diagnosis treated in another ICU.

All the informations we gain through our registration system can be used as
A) a continuous production control on our therapy - and in combination with the search for reliable, early identified prognostic indicators.
B) it contributes to the continued effort of establishing improved criterias for which patients should be selected for intensive therapy with all its ensuing consequences.

REFERENCES.
1. Shoemaker WC, Chang P, Czer L et al.   Cardiorespiratory monitoring in postoperative patients I. Prediction of outcome and severity of illness.   Crit Care Med 1979;   7:237.
2. Cullen DJ, Ferrara LC, Gilbert J, Briggs BA, Walker PF.   Indicators of intensive care in critically ill patients. Crit Care Med 1977; 5: 173.
3. Cullen DJ, Civetta JM, Briggs BA, Ferrara LC.   Therapeutic intervention scoring system: a method for quantitative comparison of patient care.   Crit Care Med 1974;   2:57.
4. Rie MA, Zapol WM, Stabile J, Pontoppidan H.   High mortality of ventilatory assistance for 24 hours with FiO_2 > 0.5.   Am Rev Resp Dis 1976;   154.
5. Fry DE, Garrison N, Heitsch RC, Calhoun K, Polk HC.   Determinants of death in patients with intraabdominal abcesses.   Surgery 1980;   517.
6. Meakins JL, Christau NV, Shizgal HM, Maclean LD.   Therapeutic Approaches to Anergy in Surgical patients.   Ann Surg 1979;   286.
7. MacLean LD, Meakins JL, Taguchi K et al.   Host resistance in sepsis and trauma.   Ann Surg 1975;   182:207.
8. Cullen DJ, Ferrara LC, Briggs BA, Walker PF, Gilbert I.   Survival, hospitalization charges and follow-up results in critically ill patients.   N Eng J Med 1976;   294:982.
9. LeGall JR, Latournerie J, Plevin D, Trunet P, Candau P.   Evaluation de l'etat de sante avant et apres hospitalisation en reanimation (1981).   In: Medical Informatics Europe 81. Editors: F.Grémy, P. Degoulet, B. Barber and R. Salamon.   Springer Verlag, Berlin-Heidelberg-New York 1981.

Electronic Records in Accident & Emergency

By

I AHMAD
Consultant in Charge
Accident & Emergency Department
Corbett Hospital, Stourbridge, West Midlands, England

Introduction

Corbett Hospital, Stourbridge and Guest Hospital, Dudley are general hospitals, each with a busy A & E Department. They are about 7 miles apart and are managed by the Dudley Area Health Authority of the West Midlands Regional Health Authority of the National Health Service of Great Britain.

The combined number of new patients seen in the 2 A & E Departments during 1979 was 67,165, follow-up patients numbered 19,790 for Corbett and 34,066 for Guest. This makes a grand total of 121,021 patient attendances through the A & E services of Dudley Area Health Authority. When these figures are translated into medical record keeping activity, the result is a hectic chaos.

The new district hospital is expected to be commissioned in 1983. It will be situated about 5 miles from Corbett Hospital. The Guest Hospital A & E Department at that stage will close and Corbett Hospital A & E Department will become a 9 am to 5 pm follow-up unit. The new district hospital A & E Department is planned for an attendance of about 70,000 new patients a year.

The Present Record System - Its Difficulties

Patient records are kept on 7" x 5" cards. With 70,000 new records being created every year, a massive storage problem already exists. Space required for storage has to be in or near the Departments, which not only makes it expensive, but also self-limiting over a long period. Both the hospitals ran out of space for storage 2 - 3 years ago. Since then records have been stored in the department corridors, in the basement and in another hospital some miles away. This has resulted in a retrieval problem which occupies considerable staff time, as it is slow and not always successful.

The bare minimum of information is collected about each patient; this is un-satisfactory from the professional point of view and does not permit the production of statistics.

The most important drawback is the inability to write promptly to a patient's own doctor in order to inform him of the circumstances. The reason is quite simply that too many typists would be required in order to write the necessary 200 or more letters every day, in addition to their other duties.

The result of this inability to write to doctors promptly is that many patients - about 75% - come back to the hospital for minor follow-up, which in turn means that space and time are taken up which would be better used for new patients.

One further problem is that it is very difficult to keep track of such things as non-accidental injuries, hospital-hoppers, drug overdosages and addicts.

Objectives of an Electronic System

I set 3 main objectives for a system:

1. To capture much more information about a patient.

2. To minimise the space requirement and yet make records more easily accessable.

3. To reduce the number of follow-up patients by referring them promptly to their own doctors.

Research

I had had several years' experience of a main-frame-computer-based record system at a hospital in the south of England.[1] This fulfilled our first objective but neither the second or the third; furthermore, the compilation of statistics took a long time.

I considered that the third objective was the one which would produce a tangible cost saving because it would enable us to contain the number of nursing staff and to cope with the present examination area.

It seemed logical, therefore, to look for a system which could combine the patient information and the diagnosis/treatment reports into letters written in good English and of good appearance. In addition, I wanted to be able to compile statistics. A system which might perform all these functions seemed likely to be an information-processing machine.

After much investigation, trials, consideration and lengthy procurement procedures at West Midlands Regional Health Authority, I was able to select an information-processor.

The heart of the system installed at Corbett Hospital as a pilot scheme is the IBM System 6 with daisy-wheel printer (model 6/452). This is supported by an MC96 Magnetic Card Typewriter in the Reception Office and another in the secretaries' office. The daisy wheel printer was chosen (in preference to the inkjet) because of the several difficult types of stationery to be used (letterhead, plain, forms, labels). The MC96 operates very much like a normal typewriter and has lift-off error correction.

The IBM System 6 is a high-level information processing machine with a display screen; its main storage medium is a floppy disk and it will handle magnetic cards. It has, in addition, a very advanced programme for the manipulation of records - maintenance, selection, sorting, printing and merging with text. Furthermore - and this is crucial - the particular piece or pieces of text appropriate to a given record can be indicated by number in that record and the system will select the text from its library and merge it with the required 'fields' for the record in order to produce, for example, a letter. This means that records can be prepared in advance and all documents can be printed in batch. Complete formatting and printing instructions are stored on disks and called up as needed.

The result is that complicated operations can be easily performed by secretaries without any technical knowledge. The operating programme is built into System 6 as a 'firmware'. As a result, there was no extra cost for programming and the system was put into operation immediately.

Operator training was carried out by means of a set of training disks and manuals supplied with the machine and supported by IBM staff.

Procedure

When a patient arrives, the receptionist takes a new record sheet (2-fold) and a punch-clock entres the date and time and a sequential registration number. She then puts the sheet into the MC96 typewriter and enters the patient information as it is given to her. The MC96 captures this data and stores it on a magnetic card. The record sheet accompanies the patient into the examination area and the magnetic card is later collected by a secretary.

The examining doctor writes his history, examination and treatment on the duplicate of the record sheet, which is later collected by a secretary. The secretary matches the record sheet with the magnetic card, puts both into her MC96 and types out the doctor's writing, thus combining the report with the data originally collected in Reception to form the patient record.

Either at this stage or later (when the record has been transferred to the System 6) the secretary adds the appropriate reference numbers (as determined by the treatment prescribed) and also the codes defining such things as where injury occurred, its duration, the type of road accident. Also entered are the International Classification of Diseases[2] primary and secondary codes defining the injury or ailment. This means that the statistical information is nationally or internationallly exchangable. At various times during the day, the magnetic cards containing the patient records are transferred to a diskette on the System 6 and all the documents pertaining to these records are printed in a batch.

The system will also extract and print lists, for example, of those patients who are to attend a Fracture Clinic or a complete alphabetical list cross-referenced against the registration number.

Finally, the system is able to produce statisics - full lists or numbers only - by selecting rcords which qualify under criteria entered by the operator. If a list is required, the system will also sort the selected records into alpha. or numerical order and print only those fields which are required.

Communications

The System 6 machines are fitted with bisynchronous communications adaptors so that they can exchange data over the public telephone system. This will be very useful when the district general hospital is commissioned and all new patients are seen there and those from Stourbridge later followed up at Corbett Hospital. A link to a central computer for the Patient Administration System for Dudley Area is being investigated.

Benefits Gained

By the use of this system, we are able to write to the doctor of every new patient within 24 hours of the patient's visit. This applies equally to patients who are admitted to the hospital - previously, the doctor often did not know of the admission until after the patient had been discharged or until relatives telephoned to enquire.

As a result of this improved communication with the doctors, the number of follow-up visits for minor reasons - removal of sutures, change of dressings -is being reduced dramatically, which in turn means:-

a. that we have more time to deal with new patients.

b. that our space restriction is not so onerous.

c. that we shall be able to avoid increasing our staff.

Retrieval of records has been made much easier. The records sheet (written) will be retained locally for a maximum of 2 years and will then be removed to a remote archive. The disks - one per week - are retained locally and records are retrieved via a comprehensive cross-index produced by the system itself. As a result, far less time is wasted in retrieval - this was previously done by nurses, which was particularly unsatisfactory. Furthermore, the space required for storage has been vastly reduced - a whole year's records on disk occupy about 30 cms of shelf space.

Lastly, because we are now collecting full information on each patient, we have begun compiling statistics. ICD^2 primary and secondary codes are entred in each record, but in addition we have developed a simple coding system of our own to denote such things as:-

-Where the accident/injury occurred - home, work, sport, etc.

-How the patient was brought in.

-Time elapsed.

-Disposal - discharged, out-patient, admitted, died.

-If admitted, to which speciality.

-In the case of a traffic accident, whether the patient was a pedestrian, cyclist, front passenger or driver, with or without a seat-belt.

I hope the result will be that we have ready access to information about such things as non-accidental injuries, poisoning, habitual attenders under false pretences, missing persons and that we shall be able, for example, to pin-point places at which road accidents frequently occur. Research projects should be greatly assisted.

Conclusion

The system I have described has only been recently installed but is already proving its worth. We shall continue to develop it and expect to see it define the Accident & Emergency record keeping activity precisely and then perhaps become a standard in the Region.

REFERENCES

1. Mason, A. A. (1975) "Accident Records on Computer", Hospital and Social Services Journal, p. 708.

2. World Health Organisation. International Classification of Diseases. Geneva: WHO (9th Revision) 1977.

ACKNOWLEDGEMENTS

1. Over, Julian. IBM (United Kingdom).

2. Mason, A. A. District Patient Services Information Officer, Frenchay Health District, Bristol.

INFORMATION ANALYSIS OF AN EMERGENCY UNIT AND OF A PREDIAGNOSIS UNIT

HUET B.[*], ROLLAND C.[**], MARTIN J.[***]

[*] Univ. Paris XIII, UER de Médecine – Informatique Médicale, 74, rue Marcel Cachin, 93012 BOBIGNY CEDEX (France)

[**] Univ. Paris I, Dépt. d'Informatique, 12, Place du Panthéon, 75231 PARIS CEDEX (France)

[***] Univ. NANCY I, UER de Médecine, Informatique Médicale, Groupe INSERM U 115 (France)

ABSTRACT

Most of the information analysis methodologies, do not analyze the dynamical aspects of organizations. The concepts presented here, allow analysis on two aspects : a statical one (based on CODD relational works) and a dynamical one (based on the concepts of operators and events). They constitute the first part of this paper. In the second part the concepts are applied to the analysis of an emergency unit, and of a prediagnosis unit in a Parisian hospital (France). Several conclusions are drawn from these analysis : 1) reduction of the number of relations ; 2) better understanding of the hospital information ; 3) clear definition of the I/O interfaces ; 4) shows the phases which can be easily automated. The last part discusses about 3 poles : 1) impact of such a method on the implementation of a whole Hospital Information System ; 2) Advantages and disadvantages of decentralized Hospital Information System ; 3) Feasibility of decentralized Hospital Information System.

INTRODUCTION

Our first work presented in MONTREAL (1) had for objective to present a conceptual tool allowing to analyse complex situations met in a hospital. This tool is able to analyse the static part (relational approach) and the dynamic aspect of an H.I.S.

1. The conceptual modelling

1-1. Principle

To model the functionning of the emergency unit in its all generality, we propose to build a drawing, of the perceived reality, in terms of types (i.e. categories) independent of any technical factor.

This modelling leads to a conceptual super schema which covers the conceptual schema in the sense of the ANSI-SPARC (2) and extend it to a drawing of the dynamic. This super schema, which is constituted in two parts the static one and the dynamic one, is a relational one (3). It was theoretically defined in. (4) (5).

1-2. The concepts

In a real system, three categories of phenomena are observed : OBJECT, OPERATION, EVENT. Those three categories are interconnected. All the links are represented by three categories of associations : MODIFY (operation-object). ASCERTAIN (object-event). TRIGGER (event-operation).

From this analysis, results the following definitions :

An OBJECT is a concrete or abstract component of the organization that can be particularized, for example : the patient Smith, the bed number 2 in the ward 538. An OPERATION is an action that can be executed alone, at a given time, within the organization and that induces state changes on one or more objects, for example : clinical examination of a patient is an operation which can lead to diagnosis. An EVENT is the ascertainning of a remarkable change of state of one or several objects, which triggers the execution of one or several operations, for example : the arrival of a patient for consulting in pneumology is an event which triggers the operation of clinical examination.

To go from the descriptive step to a rigorous modelling, it is necessary to use a formalism. We chose a relational formalism (6) and prescribed the following rules :

1) any phenomenon is represented by one or several relationships ;

2) to recognize the category of a phenomenon, we introduced types of designated relations C. OB (C. Object) C. OP (C. Operation), C. EV (C. event) ;

3) for modelling the parameter time and resulting on a minimal conceptual schema (in the meaning of DELOBEL (7) we introduced a normalized from called "permanent relation".

The classes of real objects, real operations, real events are respectively represented by several relations : C.OB type, C.OP type, C.EV type. The modelling is normalized (6) (8).

1-3.   Let us define quickly each component

Relation "C. OB" : a relation C. OB type represents a particular aspect of a class of real objects.

Relation "C. OP" type. A relation C. OP type represents an elementary aspect of a class of real operations.

Relation "C. EV" type : a relation C. EV type represents an elementary aspect of a class of real events and several C. EV relations are necessary to describe the class.

2.   Static and dynamic information analysis of an emergency unit and of a prediagnosis unit

2-1.   The analysis of the emergency unit of the hospital Avicenne 93000 - PARIS-NORD - France) led to the following results.

2-1.1.   Statical schema :

2-1.1.1. Objects relative to the reception and the sort of patients between medical emergency and surgical emergency

OB 1 : Reception (Nr receptionnist, date, mean of transportation) ;

OB 2 : Identity (Nr patient, name, christian name, adress, date birth, profession, person to call) ;

OB 3 : call doctor (Nr arrival, hour call, n type doctor) ;

OB 4 : Arrival doctor (Hour arrival doctor, nr doctor, nr arrival) ;

OB 5 : Moving (Nr patient, date, Nr place (origin), Nr place (destination) ;

2–1.1.2. Objects relative to the clinicians methodology to result to a diagnosis and/or a medical therapy and/or a surgical therapy

      OB 6 : Subregion information (Nr patient, date, Nr subregion, result) ;

      OB 7 : Region information (Nr patient, date, Nr region, result) ;

      OB 8 : Global result on patient information (Nr patient, date, synthesis result) ;

      OB 9 : Diagnosis (Nr patient, date, Nr dor, Nr diagnosis) ;

      OB 10 : Medical therapy (Nr patient, date, Nr doctor, Nr medicine, Nr posology) ;

      OB 11 : Surgical therapy (Nr patient, date, Nr surgeon, Nr intervention) ;

2–1.1.3. Objectifs relative to exchanged information between a prescribing department and an excuting department (laboratory).

2–1.1.4. Asking for a complementary test :

      OB 12 : patient's complementary (Nr test, Nr sample) ;

      OB 13 : sample (Nr sample, date Nr patient, Nr sampler, Nr place) ;

2–1.1.5. Transfer of result :

      OB 14 : Result complementary test (Nr test, date result, Nr result, checking) ;

      OB 15 : Interpretation result (Nr test, date interpretation, Nr interpretation, Nr interpreter) ;

      OB 16 : Aid to diagnosis result (Nr test, Nr patient, date, Nr proposition, Nr person) ;

      OB 17 : Call for a new sample (Nr call, Nr test) ;

2–1.1.6. Object relative to an appointment in a clinical or surgical or biological department :

      OB 18 : Rendez-vous (Nr Rendez-vous, Nr call, state of Rendez-vous).

2–1.1.7. General objects :

      OB 19 : Receptionnist (Nr receptionnist, name) ;

      OB 20 : Transportation (Nr code, mean) ;

      OB 21 : Doctor (Nr type doctor, name) ;

      OB 22 : Place (Nr place, place) ;

      OB 23 : Subregion (Nr subregion, wording) ;

      OB 24 : Region (Nr region, wording) ;

      OB 25 : Diagnosis (Nr diagnosis, wording) ;

      OB 26 : Medicine (Nr medicine, wording) ;

2–1.2. **Dynamical schema :**

2–1.2.1. Operations :

      OP 1 : Interview of the patient to know some administrative information ;

      OP 2 : Call for the doctor after external examination ;

      OP 3 : Delay-waiting for the doctor ;

      OP 4 : Acquisition of an elementary clinical information (clinical examination) ;

      OP 5 : Acquisition of a regional clinical information (clinical examination) ;

OP 6 : A destination is given to the patient if C_1 ;

OP 7 : Processing of clinical information ;

OP 8 : Elaboration of a conclusion about diagnosis ;

OP 9 : Writing out of a prescription of C_3 and C_4 ;

OP 10 : Action for surgical therapy if C3 and C4 and C5 ;

OP 11 : Elaboration of a call for a complementary test if C2 ;

OP 12 : Identification of the complementary test if C2 ;

OP 13 : New global synthesis on the state of the patient after come back of a complementary test result ;

OP 14 : New global synthesis on the state of the patient after come back of an interpretation result ;

OP 15 : New global synthesis on the state of the patient after come back of an aid to diagnosis result ;

OP 16 : A new sample is asked for the laboratory ;

OP 17 : Ask for appointment ;

2-1.2.2. Events :

EV 1 : Arrival of the patient in emergency ;

EV 2 : Calling for the surgical doctor or medical doctor ;

EV 3 : Arrival of the doctor ;

EV 4 : Clinical examination is over ;

EV 5 : Patient data processing by clinician is over ;

2-1.2.3. Conditions :

C 1 : The patient needs hospitalization in another hospital ;

C 2 : The clinician decides to ask for complementary tests ;

C 3 : The clinician is able to organize a therapy ;

C 4 : Those is no counter indication ;

C 5 : The patient agrees for a surgical therapy ;

2-2. Analysis of the prediagnostic unit

2-2.1. Statical schema :

The occurencies created along the study of the patient in UPUC will be made from the C-objects defined in analysis of the emergency unit. The objects which serve for model to create occurencies are : OB 5, OB 6, OB 7, OB 8, OB 9, OB 10, OB 12, OB 13, OB 14, OB 15, OB 16, OB 17, OB 18, OB 22, OB 23, OB 24, OB 25, OB 26.

2-2.2. Dynamical schema :

2-2.2.1. Operations :

The operations involved correspond to the ones defined in the emergency analysis because same events happen and they lead to the generation of the same occurencies OP 4, OP 5, OP 6, OP 7, OP 8, OP 9, OP 10, OP 11, OP 12, OP 13, OP 14, OP 15, OP 16, OP 17.

2–2.1.2. Events :

The events were already defined they are the following ones :

EV 3 : Arrival in the unit ;

EV 4 : Clinical examination is over ;

EV 5 : Patient data processing by the clinician is over ;

2–2.1.3. Conditions :

The conditions are the same ones as those defined in the analysis of the emergency unit.

DISCUSSION

This discussion will run around 3 principal poles :

1. Impact of the conceptual schema on the implementation of computerized systems

1–1. Interest for a whole hospital information system :

The existence of a bijective correspondance between the conceptual schema and the described organization leads to implement a better adapted computerized system.

1–2. Interest by decreasing semantical redundancy observed in large computerized systems :

This decrease in semantical redundancy was shown by the study of the whole hospital in which various sorts of objects were studied ; in this manner there whill be a minimal number of relationships to describe static and dynamic aspects of the hospital.

1–3. Interest for communication between departments :

This information analysis has put in evidence the objects, generated in the system and the I/0 objects.

1–4. Implementation of an information analysis :

To implement a decentralized hospital information system corresponding to information analysis is to build local work stations fitted with local data banks and local programs bank (for decentralized data and programs) connected with a central work station fitted with a centralized data bank and centralized programs bank.

2. Advantages/Disadvantages of decentralized hospital information systems

2–1. Advantages

2–1.1. Conceptual advantages :

Our information analysis was extended to the whole hospital, several conclusions can be deduced from this work :

– Existence of common conceptual subschemas in departments ;

– Existence of clearly defined interfaces between departments ;

This leads to a necessarily integrated study of information semantics and explains the difficulties met in realization of big hospital information systems (MATRIX (9)...) which were lacking of a global view from the beginning of implementation.

BAKKER (10) has the same judgement, he recommands a definition of data independently of computerized systems.

2-1.2. Advantages on operational system : I/O facilities ; I/O have to be done in clinical departments and laboratories, this is easier and more effective with private programs banks and data banks especially with new individual works stations which will be soon presented in Bureautics (11). Advantages are especially on :
- Availability ;
- Data protection : (12) (13) Farer than those classical measures, many researches on system architectures for distributed data base security are led today (14).

2-2. Disadvantages :
They are cited by BAKKER (10) They concern data storage and costs.

3. **Feasibility of decentralized hospital information systems** :
The computerized implementation of decentralized hospital information systems implies independent units linked by coherent relationships ; on this approach is built the most recent local computer network : the DANUBE (Donau) network included in the project pilot KAYAK supported by INRIA (15) (16).

CONCLUSION
The role of information analysis is to put in evidence a certain structure in the organization, based on semantical analysis.
Computerized hospital information systems have to integrate this semantical analysis during their implementation to result to well-adapted information systems.

REFERENCES
(1)   ROLLAND D., HUET B. : "Une approche structurée pour la conception des systèmes d'Information Médicaux". IInd International congress on system Science in Health Care. Proc. Montreal. 13-17 July 1980.
(2)   ANSI/X3/S PARC (1977) : Report in data base management system. Final Report. Washington.
(3)   CODD E.F. : A relational model for large shared data banks. Com. A.C.D. 13 (6), 377-387 (1970).
(4)   ROLLAND C., FOUCAUT O. : Concepts for the design of an information system conceptuals schema and its utilization in the REMORA project. Proc. IVth International Conference VLDB – Berlin 1978.
(5)   ROLLAND C., LEIFERT S., RICHARD C. : Tools for information systems dynamics management. Proc. Vth International Conference VLDB – Rio de Janeiro 1979.
(6)   CODD E.F. : Further normalization of the data base relational model data base systems. Prentice Hall – New York (1972).

(7)   DELOBEL C. : Contribution théorique à la conception et à l'évaluation d'un système informatique appliqué à la gestion. Thèse Docteur ès-Science – Grenoble 1973.

(8)   BEERI C., BERNSTEIN A., GOODMAN N. : A sophisticated introduction to data base normalization theory. Proc. IVth International Conference VLDB Berlin 1978.

(9)   SNEIDER R.M., BOYAR R.E., TAPELLA C.A. : The MATRIX data base management system. Computer, Nov. 28-31, 1979.

(10)   BAKKER A.R. : Centralized versus decentralized hospital information system. Proc. MEDINFO 77 – North Holland 895-899.

(11)   SCHEURER B., BIARNAUD M.L., MANTAOUX G., BERBER D., QUERARD B. : Le buroviseur, poste de travail dans le bureau du futur. Bull. Liaison Rech. Inform. Autom. (1981) Juin, n° 70, 7-8.

(12)   BAKKER A.R. : Centralization and decentralization aspects in hospital Information systems. Proc. IIIrd Congress Medical Information Europe 1981. 9-13 March, 41-49, Springer-Verlag.

(13)   BAKKER A.R. : Scope and limitations of a minibased centralized hospital Information System. Proc. MEDINFO 80 – North Holland, 504-509.

(14)   HARTSON H. Rex : Data base security. System architectures. Inform. Systems (1981), vol. 6, n° 1, 1-22.

(15)   MARTIN M., MERCEIER-MARUENT C., NAFFAH N., SCHEURER B. : Les réseaux locaux : définition et exemple de réalisation (Danube). Bull. Liaison Rech. Inform. Autom. (1981), Juin n° 70, 8-12.

(16)   GODEFROY E., ROCHE P., BOWLES S., LARGILLIERE D. : Méthodologie de développement de logiciel dans Kayak. Bull. Liaison Rech. Autom. (1981), Juin, n° 70, 13-15.

SIMULTANEOUS STUDIES OF INTRACRANIAL PRESSURE AND ELECTROENCEPHALOGRAM.

P. BIXIO-SALORT, J.-D. GUIEU, M. JOMIN, F. LESOIN

Service d'Explorations Fonctionnelles Neuro-Chirurgicales -

Centre Hospitalier Régional et Universitaire - 59037-LILLE-Cédex - France.

1- INTRODUCTION

Numerous studies have been carried out separately on Intracranial Pressure (ICP) and Electroencephalogram (EEG), to evaluate the central nervous system functions, in patients with head injuries. These studies were done, either in real time, making use of elementary methods, or off line, using elaborate methods that needed larger computer systems.

Recent papers have stressed the importance of a simultaneous study of the ICP and EEG, but in most cases, they do not go beyond the observation of clinical cases.

In patients with impaired conciousness (i.e. cranial trauma) we did the two monitorings simultaneously (2 channels of EEG, 1 channel of ICP for 2 beds). They can be operated by a practician or a nurse, since they do not require knowledge of data processing. After entering the parameters, at the begining, no manual intervention is needed. The last 25 minutes of the ICP and EEG are continuously computed and displayed which allows the practician to immediately see the evolution of the patient. All the results are stored for a more detailed study at the end of the monitoring period.

2- MATERIAL USED AND PROGRAM CONCEPTION

For the acquisition and preliminary analysis, we made use of readily available material. The signals obtained were transfered to a portable mini-computer placed at the patients bedside. The computer was equipped with an analog-digital conversion module, a semi-graphic video display and a keyboard, two floppydisks, and a printer-plotter connected through an IEEE bus.

Using the keyboard, the first step of the program consists of entering identification parameters of the patients, followed by the choice of control parameters. Eventually a calibration is carried out in order to restitute the ICP scale. All these steps can be carried out within two minutes.

The real time program is then started. A first subroutine is meant for the acquisition of the ICP and the computation and storage of its trend. The interrupt subroutine is entered at regular intervals for the acquisition of the EEG.

During 15 seconds, the second subroutine stores the morphology of ICP and computes the peak to peak difference and first derivative of the rising edge, in each cycle and stores them. The analysis of the EEG then proceeds, one bed after the other. It consists of the computation and storage of power spectra using 8 seconds of signal, several times.

Then the program reverts to the first ICP subroutine and, bed after bed, adds the display of the trend of ICP for the last 25 minutes and the spectra corresponding to the last 2 interruptions.

At the end of the monitoring process, an interrupt starts a subroutine to print out on a plotter :

     - patient's identification

     - results for ICP :

         . morphology of the ICP and the mean of the peak to peak differences and of the rising edges, just before EEG interruption

         . trend of the ICP during entire monitoring period

     - results for EEG :

         . representation of the EEG's after taking the mean over the spectra of each sequence, by frequency bands ; the more important frequency is represented in each band with its value

         . the calculation of the ratio $\alpha + \beta / \Delta + \Theta$

         . the difference between right and left.

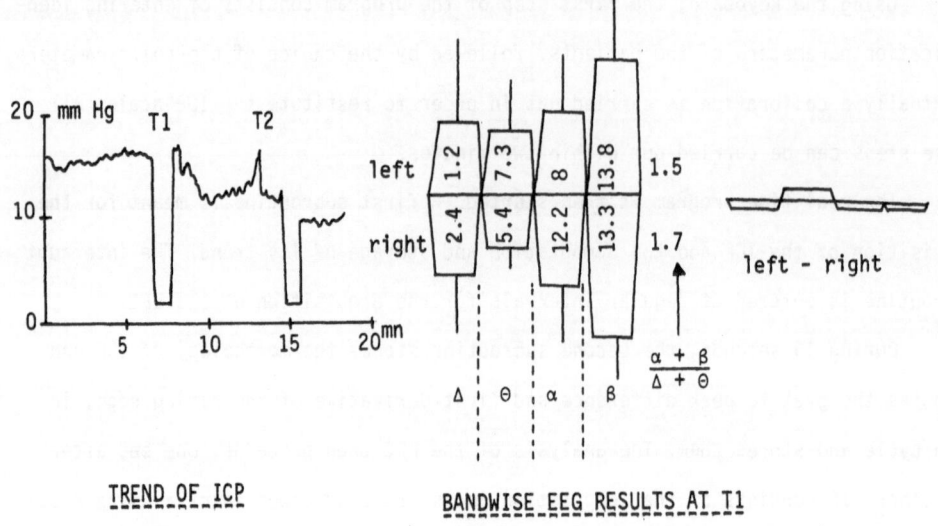

TREND OF ICP   BANDWISE EEG RESULTS AT T1

3- CONCLUSIONS

  This monitoring process, in its present state has been used, in a neurosurgical ward, and has proved to be satisfactory.

  The first step allows, the clinician to follow continuously, the evolution of the ICP and EEG during the last 25 minutes.

  The graphic representation carried out at the end of the monitoring period is readily interpreted by the practician, since it brings out visually correlations between ICP and EEG.

  These investigations will be enlarged in the future, by more detailed studies, leading to improvement in the monitoring process and, we hope finally to the definition of a microprocessing device extended to several patients.

A Microcomputer System for patient data management in the Intensive Care Unit.

Timothy Stafford and Michael Slazenger,
Formerly of The Anaesthetic Research Department,
The Royal College of Surgeons of England,
Lincoln's Inn Fields,
London WC2,
England.

Current Addresses

Timothy Stafford,   Michael Slazenger,
279 Beacon Street,   St.Vincent's Hospital,
Boston,   Elm Park,
U.S.A.   Dublin 4,
                                     Ireland.

The recent advances in microcomputer technology have resulted in a dramatic increase in the power and reliability of computing and a hugh reduction in the cost.   This had made computing available to many people who would not otherwise consider the use of computers. Unfortunately the same cannot be said for the software.   This deficiency is particularly evident in the medical field.   There have been a few worthy efforts in the general medical field but in the area of intensive care data collection and management there is very little software written for the new microcomputer systems.   The current generation of medical specialists are not familiar with computer systems and tend to be intimidated by them.   We felt that it was necessary to offer a system that would not require any computer expertise by the user but would nevertheless be of low cost.

Initially it was thought that one could simply write a program to run on one of the microcomputer systems already available. Unfortunately it became apparent that this would not work because of the intimidating effect of the computer keyboard where the function of the various keys was not self evident.   The decision to use a micro-computer system was made primarily because of the low cost of such a system.   Existing systems are very expensive.   They also suffer from the further disadvantage that if there is a system failure one loses access to all the data during the period of the breakdown.   By having a complete micro-computer system for each patient this risk is reduced to minimal proportions particularly as data is stored on magnetic media as soon as it is acquired.   Because of the low cost it is feasible to have a spare system in the event of breakdown into which can be loaded the data from the failed system.   This obviates the need for an expensive service contract.

The system is designed to manage all the data gathered concerning the patient during the stay in ICU. Although the bulk of the data is entered manually many variables can be entered automatically. The equipment is provided with a standard serial interface for accepting data from peripheral measuring equipment such as automated blood gas analyzers and "ion-selective membrane" measuring equipment for determining serum sodium and potassium which are now being used in ICU. As well as this sort of data the output from blood pressure monitors and ECG equipment can be sampled. For equipment that does not have digital output of data there are 8 analogue channels for data collection. They can be used as well as the digital channels.

The data is stored and the program is designed in such a way that any desired variables can be displayed either graphically with respect to time or as single values in tabular form. Both numeric and graphical values can be displayed on the screen at the same time. Fluid balance can be displayed graphically as a cumulative display or numerically in the conventional tabular form. These displays are accessed by the minimum number of keystrokes consistent with ease of operation. In addition to the screen display it is possible to get a print out of any of the information displayed on the screen at any time.

It is intended that one system can store in memory all the data concerning one patient for their entire stay in the ICU. If the nature of the ICU work is such that one anticipates very long stays then it may be necessary to reduce the variety of variables recorded. It is feasible to hold approximately 7500 values in memory. Although there is a comments page for free text, excessive use of this facility could result in reduction of the space available for storing numeric values. In practice we have not found this to be a problem.

In addition to having ready access to data concerning the patient one also has all the patient data stored in a computer readable form for statistical analysis. We are at present working on the design of a central station which will hold all the data for all the patients. This will be held on a hard disk system and searches of the database thus generated will be easy to perform at incredibly low cost compared to current costs for research projects involving the search of ICU records. In addition the data is likely to be much more accurate than at present.

Since medicine is very much an information dependent art/science any improvement in the way information is handled must result in improved patient care.

A DRUG INFUSION CALCULATOR FOR THE ADMINISTRATION
OF CONTINUOUS IV DRUGS

M. Michael Shabot, M.D., Assistant Professor of Surgery,
and Paul Carlton, M.D., Resident in Anesthesia
Harbor/UCLA Medical Center,
1000 West Carson Street
Torrance, California 90509/USA

Computation of the rate parameters involved in the administration of intravenous drugs via infusion pump is an essential and frequently performed calculation in the ICU environment. Nurses and physicians are aware of the difficulty of reliably performing this seemingly simple computation. The arithmetic problem of converting among the various dosage unit systems involved is compounded by the pressures of a busy clinical environment. A pocket calculator does not appreciably alleviate the problem of unit conversions, and introduces an additional source of operator error.

We have developed an interactive program that assists the user in computation of parameters for the administration of continuous IV drugs. The program is implemented on a commercially available patient monitoring computer system, the Hewlett-Packard 5600A. Design of the program emphasizes a simple user interface, informative data display, and flexibility to accommodate changes in drug usage. User interaction with the program occurs on a cathode ray terminal (CRT) via fixed-format data entry form unique to each of 14 different drugs (Figure 1).

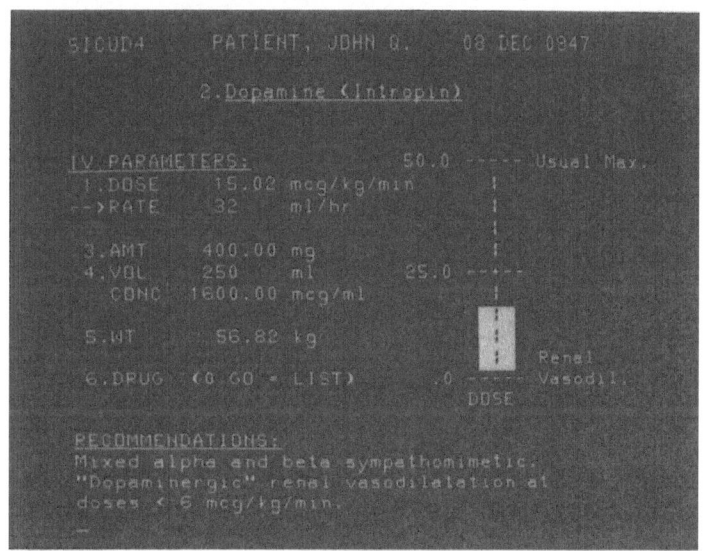

Figure 1. Video display for dopamine administered
with a standard pharmacy concentration.

Appropriate default values consistent with local pharmacy preparations are provided to streamline the data entry process. If non-standard drug concentrations are required, these are inputted and the resultant change in administration rate is displayed immediately (Figure 2). Comparison of the current administration rate to pharmacologic norms is aided by displaying the dose graphically on an annotated "dose meter". A "Recommendations" area of the display is provided to remind the user of important drug-specific information. The program is largely table-driven to allow customization to a wide range of clinical environments. The tables are created by a configuration program whose input is conversational commands. The configuration program facilitates easy modification of existing drug frames and rapid addition of new drugs.

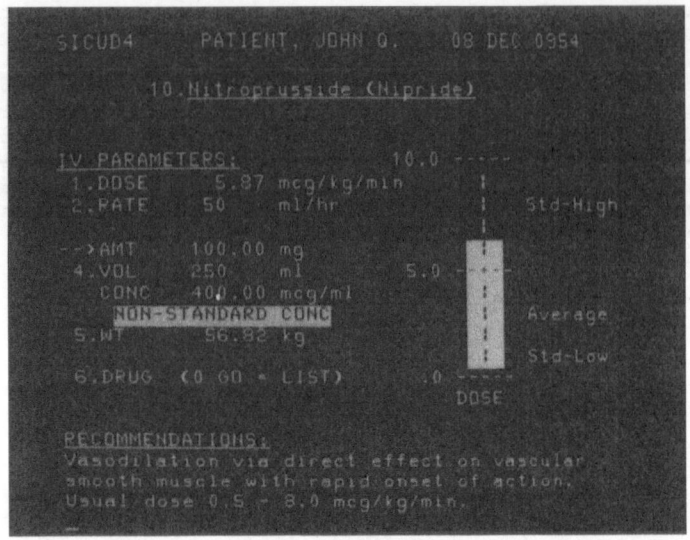

Figure 2. Video display for nitroprusside administered in a non-standard concentration.

ON THE DEVELOPMENT OF A COMPUTER-ASSISTED

DIAGNOSTIC STRATEGY

H.Sator, W.Vogt and D.Nagel

Institut für klinische Chemie am Klinikum Großhadern

der Ludwig-Maximilians-Universität

Postfach 701260, 8000 München 70, GFR

ABSTRACT

One of the obligations of clinical chemistry is to help the clinician to find a correct diagnosis. How can this task be fullfilled most effectively? There exist some models, which are suited to support the clinician in interpreting the results of the clinical chemical tests. All these methods, however, have serious drawbacks, which induced us to look for an alternative.
In a first step we used cluster analysis to find groupings of similar patients. These clusters found are the actual carriers of information. In a second step a strategy was developed, to assign a patient to a cluster with a certain probability. This strategy is a sequential process, which determines the next clinical chemical parameter to be measured depending on the values of the previously measured parameters. The advantage of this strategy is, that it is simple, quick, individual for every patient, generally applicable and efficient.

1. INTRODUCTION

The diagnostic process consists of rational and intuitive elements which contribute to the decision with different and variable weight depending on the individuality of the physician and the nature of the disease. Despite of this interlacement of ponderable and inponderable components the diagnostic procedure can be analyzed and systemized (1).

How can clinical chemistry with its comprehensive diagnostic tools support the clinician most effectively? As a first step, can computerized procedures be found to reduce data, while increasing the utilizable information content? Secondly, can diagnostic strategy models be formulated for applying clinical chemical tests stepwise and thus using them in an economical way? On classification by cluster analysis we have published recently (2, 3). The subject of this presentation is a new strategy model.

The development of such a model proceeds usually in two steps: First, the information content of the clinical chemical parameters, single and in combination, has to be estimated. Then based on this a strategy has to be formulated, which establishes the stepwise diagnostic procedure by which a patient can be assigned to a defined group with an acceptable probability.

To estimate the information content and the separating performance of the individual parameters, discriminating, mathematical procedures are suited, like the discriminant analysis. Using it the information content of individual parameters can be determined and a sequence can be defind, on which sequential procedure is based.

Discriminant analysis, however, has a very important drawback. An optimal separation can be achieved only if the parameters within the groupings to be separated are distributed normally. In practice for groups of patients this is nearly never the case.

Once the information content of individual parameters is estimated, the conversion into a stepwise procedure follows next. For this purpose a dichotomous branching structure is commonly used.

A disadvantage of this procedure, however, is, that quantitative values are transformed to a qualitative binary Yes- or No-answer. Such a model seemed not suited to our concept, that as far as possible the full information content of quantitative data should be conserved.

Continuing from our previous results (2,3) the goal of our studies was to replace discriminant analysis and parallel procedure used up to now by another economically more advantageous, sequential strategy. It should avoid the just mentioned disadvantages of the other procedures.

2. METHODS AND MATERIAL

2.1. Characterisation of the sampled group of patients and acquisition of data.

In our prospective study the sample consisted of 592 outpatients with the tentative diagnosis of thyroid disease. As clinical chemical parameters total thyroxine (T4), triiodothyronine (T3), T3-up take (TBI), thyroxine binding globulin (TBG) and TSH before and after stimulation with TRH (200 µg i.v.) were measured quantitatively and the difference Δ TSH was calculated. More detailed information on the data basis can be found in ref. (3).

2.2. Classification and reclassification

After a transformation and normalization of these seven parameters the patients data were subjected to a cluster analysis. The decision on the number of clusters was independent of clinical symptoms and signs and especially of the final diagnosis. The methods used for clustering were the sift- and shift-algorithm (4) and the method of Ward (5,6). The former algorithm also was used to reclassify the patients. The object of it is to minimize the following function,

$$y = \sum_{j=1}^{n_c} \sum_{i=1}^{n_j} ||x_{ij} - \bar{x}_j||^2 = \sum_{j=1}^{n_c} \frac{1}{n_j} \sum_{k=1}^{n_j} \sum_{i=1}^{k-1} ||x_{ij} - x_{kj}||^2$$

where n_c = number of clusters, n_j = number of elements in cluster j, x_{ij} = element i in cluster j and $\bar{x}_j = \frac{1}{n_j} \cdot \sum_{i=1}^{n_j} x_{ij}$ = centroid in cluster j.

471

This way the sum of the variances within the clusters is minimized. To assign one patient x to a cluster, the term $\|x - \bar{x}_j\|^2 \cdot n_j / (n_j+1)$ has to be computed for all clusters. The cluster with the smallest value for this term is then chosen.

2.3. Strategy algorithm

The strategy algorithm also is based on the sift- and shift-algorithm described above.

3.   RESULTS AND DISCUSSION

3.1. Classification and reclassification

Before deciding on suited algorithms for clustering and reclassifying the patients, we had to take into account four important points:

1. Because the distributions of the measurements of the single parameters cannot be assumed to be normally distributed, the reclassification algorithm must be non-parametric.

2. To determine the contents of information the reclassification method must allow to reclassify patients also with less than all seven parameters.

3. To use the model effectively in the daily routine, the computing time and storage capabilities must be small, as mentioned above.

4. The methods of classification and reclassification must be compatible, i.e. all patients defining the clusters must be reclassified by the reclassification method to their original clusters.

A method, which fulfills all these demands, and which can be used both for clustering as well as for reclassifying is the sift- and shift-algorithm, also known under the name KMEANS (4). Before starting the algorithm requires the number of clusters to be defined and arbitrary preliminary clusters. Therefore we used the hierarchical cluster algorithm recommended by Ward (5), which also minimizes the variances within the clusters. In this way we received a reasonable number of clusters and a nearly optimal starting-configuration.

3.2. Strategy algorithm

We had three requirements for the strategy algorithm:

1. In every step it should be possible to assign a patient to one of the total number of clusters. A hierarchical structure would not allow this and narrow down the theoretically possible number of clusters to which a patient could be assigned by a stepwise procedure.

2. The path should not be rigid, but dependent on the results of the

parameters already determined. In this way the path can be different for various patients.

3. It should be possible to choose the criterion of termination. We decided to use a probability of correct classification of ≥ 0.9.
   This agrees with the predictive value of the positive (7).

To estimate the contribution of information of the single parameters with respect to the single clusters the patients were assigned to the established clusters by the sift- and shift-algorithm with all possible combinations of the parameters. The results are $\sum_{i=1}^{m-1} \frac{m!}{i! \cdot (m-i)!}$ reclassification matrices (m = number of parameters). Following probabilities can be estimated with the help of these matrices shown on an example of 4 clusters in figure 1.

$p_j^{a_1' \cdots a_n}(I)$ is the probability, that a patient, who is assigned to cluster j after the determination of parameters $a_1, \ldots a_n$ belongs to cluster i. $p_I^{a_1' \cdots a_n}(j)$ is the probability, that a patient, who belongs to cluster i is assigned to cluster j after the determination of parameters $a_1, \ldots a_n$.

The probability $p_i^{a_1' \cdots a_n}(I)$ agrees with the predictive value of the positive.

Pat. assigned to

Pat. belonging to	1	2	3	4	Σ
1	1	2	1		4
2		4	1	1	6
3	2		1	2	5
4			3	2	5
Σ	3	6	6	5	20

Figure 1:
Reclassification matrix
of clin.chem.param. a

$$p_I^a(i) = \frac{1}{3}, \quad p_i^a(J) = \frac{2}{3}, \quad p_i^a(I) = \frac{1}{4}$$

$I \equiv i = 1, J = 3$

Now we can define a matrix A, where the lines correspond to all possible combinations of the parameters, and the columns to the various clusters. The values of the elements of A are the $p_i^{a_1' \cdots a_n}(I)$. In principle this matrix A can be reduced to a binary matrix, if a threshold for finishing the algorithm has been chosen, because it is needed only as a criterion for termination. In addition there are other ways possible for computing the elements, e.g. the predictive value of the negative.

Since the decision to measure next the parameter a_{n+1} is determined by the aim to maximize the probability $p_i^{a_1' \cdots a_{n+1}}(I)$ for a correct assignment, following condition is imposed,

$$\sum_{I \equiv i=1}^{n_c} (p_j^{a_1' \cdots a_{n+1}}(I))^k \cdot p_j^{a_1' \cdots a_n}(I) \cdot p_I^{a_1' \cdots a_{n+1}}(i) = \text{max !} \qquad (1)$$

where n_c means the number of clusters, j means the cluster, to which the patient was assigned with the known parameters $a_1, \ldots a_n$, and $k \geq 1$ is a constant, which can be used to weigh higher values of $p_i^{a_1' \cdots a_n}(I)$ app-

ropriately. Obviously the term $p_j^{a_1,\ldots,a_n}(I) \cdot p_I^{a_1,\ldots,a_{n+1}}(i)$ is the probability that a patient belongs to cluster i and is assigned to cluster i.
This can be verified as follows: The term

$$p^{a_1,\ldots,a_{n+1}}(iI) = p_I^{a_1,\ldots,a_{n+1}}(i) \cdot p(I)$$

is the definition of the constitional probability. If the patient is
assigned to cluster j after the determination of parameters $a_1,\ldots a_n$
then $p^{a_1,\ldots,a_n}(j) = 1$ holds. It follows, that $p(I) = p_j^{a_1,\ldots,a_n}(I)$.QED.
To find the path in our strategy model we define a second matrix B with
the same lines and columns. The elements, however, are the parameters,
which maximize the condition (1).

With these two matrices we can define our strategy algorithm in a very
simple way requiring very little computing time:

1. Take a fixed parameter or select one arbitrarily. Usually that one
   is chosen, which promises most information on the average, if nothing
   is known about the patient.

2. Measure the value of this parameter.

3. Classify the patient by the sift- and shift-algorithm with the up to
   now measured parameters.

4. Take the corresponding element of matrix A and finish if necessary
   the algorithm.

5. Take the corresponding element of matrix B. This is the next parameter to be measured. Go to 2.

3.3. Analysis of the reclassification process

The number of the parameters needed to classify the patients into the
clusters with the probability of ≥ 0.9 for the single clusters of our
example is shown in figure 2. The mean for all clusters is 5.3 parameters to be determined to classify a patient. Here it is shown, that the
proposed method is suited to reduce the parameters needed for classifying.
The patients in clusters 11 and 12 are classified at an early step, similarly in cluster 16, which includes only manifest hyperthyroid patients.
Cluster 5 is special; in the best case only one parameter is needed, in
the worst case all seven. To show the distribution of the number of the
parameters needed in detail, we have selected 4 clusters (figure 3).Nearly
90 % of the patients of cluster 2 can be reclassified by 4 parameters.
In cluster 5 the correct classification is reached mostly by determining
5 and 6 parameters. Clusters 2 and 16 are examples, where a very small

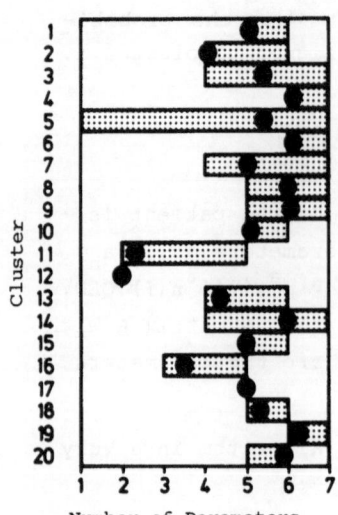

Figure 2:
Number of parameters needed to
reclassify the patients

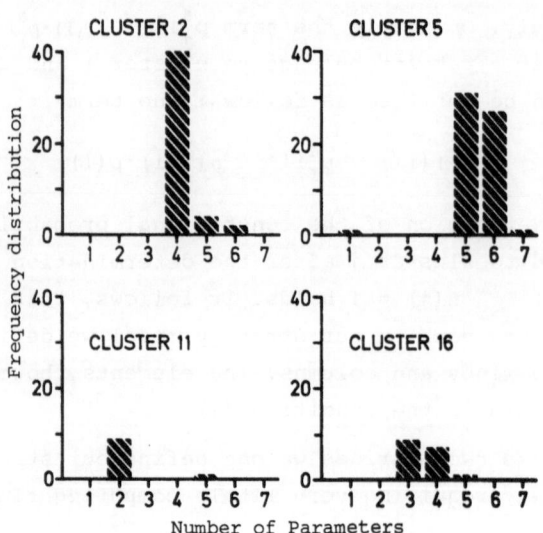

Figure 3:
Frequency distribution of the number of parameters needed to reclassify the patients.

number of parameters is needed to classify patients.

3.4. Criticsm

The advantage of this model is, that it is simple, quick, individual for
every patient, generally applicable and efficient. In our example of 20
clusters was shown, that the average number of parameters needed to classify a patient can be reduced. This reduction, however, could be maxi-
mized by an optimal and non arbitrary choice of the number of clusters.
Furthermore following objection can be raised against this model.
A certain collective of patients is the basis of this model. The clusters
obtained depend only on these patients. Possibly the patients are not a
representative profile or only a representative profile in a certain region, or for a certain hospital and so on. In addition the representative
profile can change during the years. It is therefore necessary to develop
a model, which adapts the clusters to the existent reality. Furthermore
a procedure is necessary to recognize outliers, e.g. if a certain rare
disease was not represented by patients defining the clusters.

REFERENCES

1. Sackett DL. The physician`s logic in making a decision. In, Clinician and chemist (Young DS, Nipper H, Udding D, Hicks J, King JS eds.), The American Association for Clinical Chemistry, Washington. 1979; 23 - 30.

2. Sandel P, Vogt W. A comparison of discriminant methods. In, Computing in clinical laboratories (Siemaszko F. ed.), Pitman Medical Publ., London. 1978; 272 - 282.

3. Vogt W, Sandel P, Schwarzfischer P, Braun SL, Langfelder C, Knedel M. Cluster-orientied discriminant analysis; taxonomic classification of the thyroid function. Clin Chem Acta. 1981; 112: 213 - 223.

4. Späth H. Cluster-Analyse-Algorithmen zur Objektklassifizierung und Datenreduktion. R.Oldenbourg Verlag, München-Wien. 1977; 68 - 113.

5. Ward JH. Hierarchical grouping to optimize an objective function. J Am Stat Ass. 1963; 58: 236 - 244.

6. Wishart D. CLUSTAN User maual, 3rd edition, Program library unit. Edinburgh University. 1978.

7. Veccio TJ. Predictive value of a single diagnostic test in unselected populations. New Engl J Med. 1976; 274: 1171 - 1173.

A TOOL FOR DECISION MAKING ASSISTANCE : SPHINX

M. FIESCHI - M. JOUBERT - D. FIESCHI - M. ROUX

Service Universitaire de Biomathématiques

Faculté de Médecine - 13385 Marseille Cedex 5

France

SUMMARY

This paper presents a system for medical aided-diagnosis, the SPHINX system, based on methods of inference and pattern-matching used in Artificial Intelligence and on various heuristic features : fuzzy heuristics in relation with the suggestion power of the signs and heuristics based on the costs of complementary investigations. The first application was achieved in the diagnosis of epigastric pain. Its results are presented and discussed in the paper.

INTRODUCTION

Among many systems of computer aided diagnosis, the Bayes theorem and derived techniques are very popular but they are not always currently used by physicians.

In a recent paper, Fox and al. [3] explore the problem of medical decision making and explain that the mathematical justification of such methods is hard to assimilate and that the algorithms remain opaque for the physician. In conclusion, Fox suggests that the approach to aided-diagnosis methods should match human reasoning more closely.

It is therefore useful to develop other methods where the executed algorithms should correspond to the user's reasoning. For this reason, it is necessary to analyse the logic of the diagnosis process, to define its general rules and to explain the mechanisms which determine the use of such rules in aided-diagnosis.

A number of authors have been working in this way for 10 years. They have studied the structure of medical knowledge and the processes through which it is manipulated. Several systems have been designed, among which we would like to mention the best known : MYCIN [5], CASNET [8], INTERNIST [4], and the works of Pauker [9], and Gorry [10].

Diagnosis concepts may be viewed as a special class of "recognition" problems, by the use of Artificial Intelligence methods and by the presentation of the medical diagnosis system with a set of symptoms, signs, paraclinical results. The procedure allows the identification of one or several diseases whose signs match more or less closely the patient's state.

I. BACKGROUND

For some years now, we already considered the problem of aided-diagnosis [1] [2] and this research has enabled us to design the SPHINX system with a first application to the field of epigastric pain.

The user is connected with a module called DIALOGUE provided with a specified knowledge in order to solve all the problems relevant to the coherence of the discourse of the user and to set up the information needed in the module of decision making. The connection between the DIALOGUE module and the DECISION module described here is activated via the monitor according to the state of the system (fig. 1).

The DECISION module inputs consist of two types of information concerning the patient : data provided by the patient's complaint and information it asks.

Two components are involved in the problem of decision making :

- A static component : a set of inference rules, each one representing a part of clinical medical knowledge.

Application of these rules according to the usual Modus Ponens schema in logic is the basic pattern of human reasoning the system uses.

- A dynamic component : the control process which activates and selects the inference rules.

Note that the description of the medical knowledge in the framework of inference rules offers a modularity which facilitates the understanding of the system's chain reasoning in the man-machine interactions.

The rules and the set of signs are determined in relation to the predicate calculus which allows a finer analysis of the signs. For instance, if a patient complains of epigastric pain, it is important to determine some attributes of this pain such as : irradiation, intensity, type, periodicity, which constitute the arguments of a predicate called pain.

It is obvious that the organisation of the diagnostic processing is neither entirely probabilistic nor entirely logical. In fact, the physician attitude varies during his search of diagnosis. In a first time, he remains inactive, listening to the patient who describes his signs.

We think that during this time the physician refers to an orientation knowledge which we call the "suggestion power" of the signs. For that we use a process of approximate reasoning power likely to suggest a number of diagnostic orientations. It is not used to establish diagnoses. Then, it is necessary to compare these orientations, in logical reasoning, with the suggestive signs.

Diagnoses will be made after complementary results required by the knwoledge rules to identify the diseases just like physicians require complementary examinations.

II. SPHINX : A TOOL FOR DECISION MAKING ASSISTANCE

1. Basic concepts

Our system is a member of the class of "Pattern Directed Inference Systems" [7] which are conceived from a very high and simple basic notion : a data-driven program strategy that makes the program reacting to each change in its environment.

In the system SPHINX, patterns are organized as tree structures. In our application each one of the trees corresponds to one of the syndromes related to the epigastric pain. For instance : syndrome of intoxication, angina, infectious syndrome, cholostatic syndrome... The rules connected to each node include complementary signs and data that must be or can be required for the accuracy of a diagnosis.

The executive which controls the selection and the activation of the rules is explicitly carried out by means of several heuristics or metarules. They serve to schedule the ways of search.

2. The structure of knowledge : Patterns

a - Trees

The static part of medical knowledge is structured in trees whose subtrees correspond to pathological units or to different clinical conditions of diseases. The farther nodes (not necessarily the leaves) are labelled as diagnosis nodes while intermediate nodes correspond to clinical states characterizing syndrome based on clinical signs, at upper levels, and paraclinical results, at lower levels. Terminal nodes can stand for etiologic diagnoses and intermediate nodes can represent class diagnoses. "Successful" nodes are all the nodes labelled "diagnosis". So that the diagnosis is more accurate if it reaches a terminal node.

For instance :

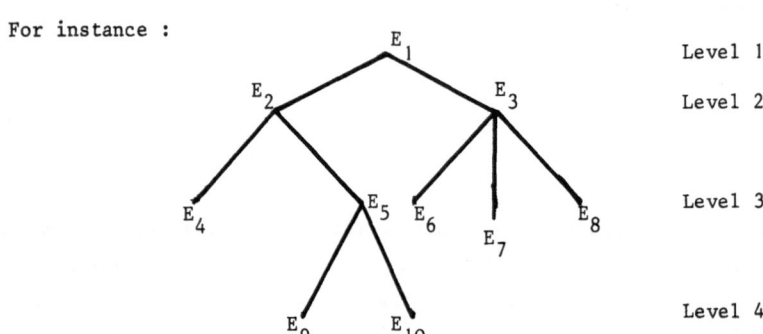

	Level 1
	Level 2
	Level 3
	Level 4

Each state E_i is determined by, at least, one set of signs $\$_i$: $\$_i \to E_i . E_i$ can be inferred from several sets : $\$_j \to E_i$ or $\$_k \to E_i$. Each $\$_i$ is a conjunction of predicates the patient's data should match in order to identify the associated state.

For instance Level 1 will refer to the signs and the data provided by the patient, Level 2 will refer to the data collected through clinical examination while Levels 3 and 4 will be the paraclinical examinations necessary for the diagnosis. Transition from an identified state E_2 to a lower Level E_5 is realized only if the conditions expressed by the predicates $\$_5$ are satisfied.

b - Suggestion power - Rejection power

For a better choice of the branching (that is the set of rules) likely to yield a solution to the problem of diagnosis, the system is organized with reference to metarules of the clinical content of the patient data and to choice a direction in diagnostic search.

Metarules are used to determine the range of diagnostic orientations and eventually to minimize the search space. New data are provided by examinations that physicians would ask in such clinical situations.

Numerical values,ranging from 0 to 1,are given to the signs in order to suggest orientations of search. Thus, depending on its attribute-values (locations, irradiation, intensity, circumstances, type of a pain), some pain will determine a suggestion value different for trees connected with diagnosis of myocardial infarction, benign gastro-duodenal ulcer, acute pancreatitis,volvulus of stomach, etc...

In the same way, the absence of some signs entails the rejection on some diagnoses by means of what is called the rejection power which takes values in the unit interval, too. For instance the absence of signs inferred from a state of shock is a strong element of rejection towards a diagnostic search of some clinical conditions of myocardial infarction or perforated ulcer.

The setting of rejection and suggestion values of clinical signs is an application of extended Modus Ponens and extended Modus Tollens used in fuzzy logic [6].

c – Heuristic features

During the diagnosis search two heuristic features are taken into account : they are the costs of examinations and the numbers of successfull branchings.

These elements are examined by heuristics activated at the farther levels of the branches of explored trees. To each examination required by the SPHINX system corresponds a cost in relation with the pretium doloris and the period of time necessary to obtain the results. Whenever a success is reached through a node, this success is taken into account. So that the system maintains an heuristic feature based on the frequency of diagnoses.

These elements produce a heuristic method dealing with the more frequently identified states and with the costs of complementary examinations for their identification.

3. Control process

The control is explicitly performed by specific metaknowledge associated to each step of the system processing. In the initial step, the heuristic implication of suggestion and rejection values is systematically activated to evaluate the context. During the other steps, the control process activates a "cost-success" heuristic and uses a depth-first or breadth-first strategy according to the context. For example, to assert the etiology of pericarditis, the control selects a cost-success heuristic, while in case of emergency, the patient's situation will be processed by a breadth-first search. Our system does not mention any hypothesis on diagnoses and does not imply that diagnoses are exclusive. The diagnostic search is carried out within the orientations determined by suggestion and rejection values.

III. USE OF SPHINX

The processing of SPHINX is composed of three steps :

1/ Record the patient's context ;

2/ Determine the set of syndromes of which the signs presented by the patient could be manifestations, and determine the range of the various diagnostic orientations ;

3/ Require complementary investigations when they are necessary to identify the suggested diseases.

In the decision program, four procedures are activated as shown in fig. 2 :

- SUGGESTS which evaluates the data and designs the diagnostic search strategy ;

- DEMMU which tries to satisfy the conditions expressed by the rules without external help. It allows the calculation of the costs of alternative too and detects invalid assertions according to the data base ;

- CHOICE which gives the best branching in function of specific heuristic features ;

- DEMP which tries to satisfy the conditions expressed by the rules and can ask questions to the user (by means of a procedure, called DIALOGUE, that will be described in a forthcoming paper).

Moreover, the SPHINX system can provide the user with a listing of the signs connected to a diagnosis or, on the contrary, a listing of the signs rejecting a diagnosis. Complementary data are also available through a procedure DOCUM (bibliography and special comments). The time of response ranges within a few seconds and allows a conversational use.

These procedures have been written in FORTRAN for a mini-computer. All the SPHINX program requires 30 K bytes of memory for instructions.

IV. RESULTS AND DISCUSSION

This paper reports the results obtained through the processing of an evaluation achieved with a SPHINX prototype. These results will certainly be improved in the future.

The evaluation of such a system can be based on various scales of interest and utility : the reliability of the advice expressed by the system, its teaching function and its use by the physicians. It is too soon to assess the teaching function of the system SPHINX but we must say that it was one of our purposes in the conception and organization of SPHINX. Moreover, it is difficult to discuss this aspect since the system has not yet been validated and it is not yet available for students.

On the contrary, all the discussion we had with experts in our attempt to give a definition of medical knowledge, showed that they were interested in this research and that they have certainly modified their attitude as regards to the problem of diagnosis.

We have tried to measure the degree of accuracy of the diagnostic classification processed by the system. It must be pointed out that the study deals with records of in-patients, that is will a complex context concerning the problem of diagnosis as

481

well as the intrication of pathologic causes of the hospitalization. Fig. 3 reports the results obtained in 50 cases chosen at random.

This table shows 15 out of the 28 diagnoses recorded in the SPHINX system up to now. Number 16 represents the particulary complex cases concerning a large intricacy of possible diagnoses. These cases presented an accident of pulmonary embolism associated with cholecystitis and a case of liver cyrrhosis associated with a cancer of liver. The last case only was correctly diagnosed by SPHINX, the two others were classified in the "?" column, indicating the absence of diagnosis.

By now, SPHINX allows a diagnosis in 80 to 85 per cent of the cases. The results are satisfactory for two reasons. First, it will be easy to improve the results by the addition of extra knowledge rules. A research is carried out in this field. Second the assessment of diagnoses by SPHINX was a cheaper procedure than the conventional procedure which requires a great number of examinations and tests. Of course complementary data are required in different contexts according as the patient is present or his file only. But the processings of the computer act as an "auditing" device which makes the physician more critical towards himself and towards the computer.

AKNOWLEDGMENTS

We are grateful to Prof. J.L. SAN MARCO, Dr G. BOTTI *and* Dr D. MONCHARMONT *for their helpful comments.*

REFERENCES

[1] FIESCHI M., JOUBERT M. - Application d'une méthode logique à l'aide à la décision en médecine. La méthode de Davis et Putnam en logique propositionnelle - IIe Congrès AFCET-IRIA, Reconnaissance Formes Intell. Artific., Toulouse (France) Sept 1979.

[2] FIESCHI M., JOUBERT M., ROUX M. - Sur un modèle de représentation de la connaissance médicale en logique symbolique en vue de l'aide à la décision en médecine - Jour. Informat. Medic., Toulouse (France), Mai 1980.

[3] FOX J., BARBER D., BARDHAN K.D. - Aleternative to Bayes ? A quantitative comparison with rule-based diagnostic inference - Meth. Inform. Med. 19 (1980), pp 210-215.

[4] POPLE H.E. Jr., MYERS J.D., MILLER R.A. - DIALOG : A model of diagnostic logic for internal medicine - Proc. 4th IJCAI (1975), Tbilissi (USSR), pp 848-855.

[5] SHORTLIFFE E.H. - Computer based medical consultations:MYCIN - (American Elsevier : New York 1976).

[6] SOULA G. - Aide à la décision en logique floue. Application en médecine - Thèse B.H. Faculté Médecine Marseille,1981.

[7] WATERMAN D.A., HAYES-ROTH F. - Pattern directed inference systems - Academic Press, New York 1978).

[8] WEISS S., KULISOWSKI C.A., SAFIR A. - Glaucoma consultation by computer - Comput. Biol. Med. 8(1978), pp 25-40.

[9] PAUKER S.G., SZOLOVITS P. - Analyzing and simulating taking the history of the present illness : context formation -- Comput. Linguistics in Medicine. Schneider Sagvall Hein eds. North Holland 1977., pp 109-118.

[10]GORRY G.A. - Computer-Assisted clinical decision making - Meth. Inform. Med. Vol. 12.1, 1973.

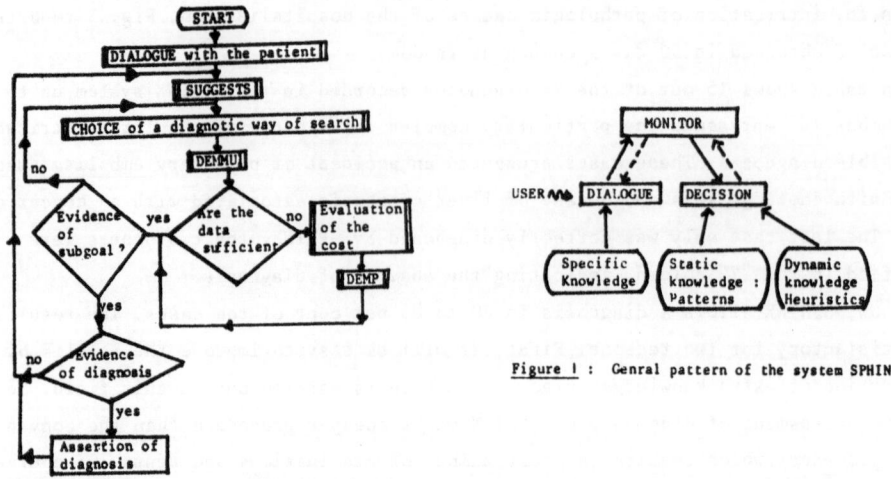

Figure 1 : Genral pattern of the system SPHINX

Figure 2 : Flowchart of the DECISION process.

True Diagnosis \ Diagnosis of SPHINX	1	2	3	4	5	6	7	8	9	10	11	12	13	14	15	16	?
1	3																1
2		2															
3			1														1
4				5													
5					2												1
6						6											
7							1										
8								1									
9									7								
10										3							
11											2						
12												1					
13													3				
14														6			
15															0		1
16																1	2

Diagnosis

1 : cancer of lever
2 : cancer of biliarytracts
5 : chronic pancreatitis
7 : cancer of oesophagus
9 : gastro duodenal ulcer
11 : occlusion
13 : angor
15 : very complex diagnoses

2 : cholecystitis
4 : biliary lithiasis
6 : cancer of stomach
8 : hiatal hernia
10 : perfored ulcer
12 : infections hepatitis
14 : myocardial infarction
16 : very complex diagnoses

Figure 3 : First results on 50 cases.

DECISION SUPPORTING SYSTEM FOR SCREENING PATIENTS FOR CERTAIN RHEUMATIC DISORDERS

Vladimir Srdanović, Center for Multidisciplinary Studies,
University of Belgrade
Branko Limić, M.D., Institute of Rheumatology of SR Serbia,
University of Belgrade

Summary

A system for computer assisted decision making in rheumatology at general practitioner level is proposed, planned to be directed mainly towards screening of rheumatic patients suffering from ankylosing spondilitis and various degenerative rheumatic disorders. The knowledge base employs accumulated medical expert experience as well as results obtained after analysing the data collected.

The system was employed for screening two pilot groups, and the results obtained were satisfactory.

Introduction

Since the first study on the computer assisted medical diagnosis, more than 20 years ago (1), many approaches to the subject were investigated, including purely statistical ones on one hand (2), pattern recognition (3), theory of information, as well as the purely logical ones on another. What they all have in common is that decision process is carried out in rather inflexible, rough and unrealistic formal frameworks. Excellent reviews of the past accomplishments, as well as of the entire research area, may be found in the papers presented by Pople (4), and Szolovits and Pauker (5).

Present goals

An array of the diseases and conditions may be manifested by the symp-

toms and signs within the locomotory apparatus and/or visceral organs,
indicating systemic disease of the connective tissue (alterations in
joints in the course of malignant haemopathies, congenital disorders
of the connective tissue development, occult tumor metastases in various
skeletal segments, specific and nonspecific arthritis and spondylo-
arthritis, etc.). The physician in charge is frequently faced with the
problem of differential diagnosis between the rheumatic and pararheumatic
process. Therefore, the aim of this work is to test the possibility of
patients screening based upon the existing symptoms and signs, in order
to direct them to an expert consultation for establishing definite diagnosis.

Accordingly, at the first stage, using medical documentation available
at the Institute of Rheumatology regarding in-patients only, a data base
has been created. It consists of patients suffering from ankylosing
spondilitis (AS), as well as those suffering from various degenerative
rheumatic disorders (DRD).

System approach

The fact is that experts are able to solve complex problems in their
domains much better and faster than a computer. Medical experts, undoubtedly, to a certain degree employ the elements of probability in addition
to categoric reasoning; but their capability to determine a proper ratio
of the former to the latter, and to restructure their knowledge in order
to apply it in a given situation and in the best manner, is even more
important (5,6).

Bearing in mind that categorical medical statements and decision rules
derive from the previously accumulated facts, the reason why computer
assisted diagnostic procedures are ever more inclined to such approach
is quite obvious.Present diagnostic programmes employ new methods, so
called artificial intelligence methods, which are to assume the reasoning
of medical experts.Their aim is to make the best use of logic and statistics, knowledge and experience (7,8,9,10).

Material and methods

Data collected in the population observed and expert knowledge were used in the process of the knowledge base formation.

The Clinical Information System (KIS), developed at the University of Belgrade Center for Multidisciplinary Studies (11), was used in data collection and analysis, allowing the expert to define data required, and set up the questionnaire in the natural language, thus avoiding the need for programmer´s help.

Following the questionnaire design (based upon theoretical criteria and practice unanimously accepted by rheumatologists), data were entered for the population of several hundreds of patients. The groups were as follows: 316 AS patients hospitally treated at the Institute of Rheumatology in the period from 1965 till 1980 whose cases were thoroughly reviewed and diagnoses confirmed, and 100 out-patients with DRD, mainly affecting spine.

Questionnaire data are naturally divided into several groups: general, symptoms and signs, laboratory and additional medical findings.

The further step was data processing with the purpose of evaluating frequency and the significance of the particular clinical features. Selection of more important features produced key information to be used as the basis for screening procedure of diseases encountered.

When the consulting help is needed, after initial data about the patient are entered, the system takes on and makes a choice of further questions to be asked about the patient. Questions that discriminate the most among alternative diagnoses are asked first. The less "costly" questions (those requiring less time to collect data, noninvasive and less expensive analyses) are asked first, too.

Each answer (manifestation) is related to each of disease categories considered, and this is expressed by a number between 0 and 10 (0 meaning that manifestation does not occur with the particular disease and 10 that it is pathognomonic for the disease).

The data are than evaluated and scores are formed for each disease category considered. The system terminates consultation by suggesting the most likely diagnosis when data provide sufficient evidence for it (score above predetermined treshold). Otherwise, or in cases when no single diagnosis can be reached by a predetermined margin, the system would suggest performance of the additional, more complex tests (but also more or less pathognomonic to the disease considered) and eventually, if the decision still cannot be made, it will ask for help from the expert specialist.

Results

The system described was applied to two control groups.

The group of 100 AS patients in hospital treated at the Institute of Rheumatology comprised the first one. In the first step, the system classified 86 patients as AS ones, none of them as DRD, and 14 patients required additional examinations. After processing the additional data, the system has classified 13 of the remaining patients, the final result being 99 patients diagnosed as AS, and one still not classified due to the lack of available medical documentation.

The second group consisted of 100 unselected out-patients encountered at the Institute during 1981. In the first step 68 patients were classified as DRD, 6 as AS, and 26 required additional examinations. Finally, 80 patients were classified as DRD, 6 as AS, and 14 patients were still unclassified, one of them suggesting AS and 13 DRD. Expert diagnosis versus computer assisted diagnosis in these 100 patients was as follows: 98 DRD patients and 2 AS patients. It is worth noting that these 2 AS patients were correctly classified by the system already in the first step.

Conclusions

Based upon medical documentation of hospitalized patients at the Institute of Rheumatology in Belgrade, and the experience of the medical expert, the knowledge base was formed as described in the paper. It has been evaluated by existing cases for which the diagnoses were confirmed.

Authors share the opinion that the system should be extended to include other rheumatic diseases from the group of seronegative arthropaties (HLA, B-27 positive arthropaties), and tested against the "average" population of rheumatic patients.

The results thus obtained shall contribute to the evaluation of the system as a possible screening procedure in the everyday rheumatology practice, as well as a supplementary mean in the training of medical students.

References

1. Ledley, R.S., Lusted, L.B., Reasoning Foundation of Medical Diagnosis: Symbolic Logic, Probability and Value Theory and our Understanding of How Physicians Reason, Science, 130:9, 1959.

2. Gorry, G.A., Barnett, G.O., Experience with a Model of Sequential Diagnosis, Comput. Biomed. Res. 1, 490-507, 1968.

3. Kulikowski, C.A., Pattern Recognition Approach to Medical Diagnosis, Proc. of the IEEE-SSCG Conference, IEEE Trans. of SSCG, 173-178, 1970.

4. Pople, H.E., Technology Aided Diagnosis, presented at CAS Seminar, Technology in the Health Care System, Dubrovnik, 1978.

5. Szolovits, P., Pauker, S.G., Categorical and Probabilistic Reasoning in Medical Diagnosis, AI, 11, 115-144, 1978.

6. Swanson, D.B., Fetlovich, P.J., Johnson, P.E., Psychological Analysis of Physician Expertise: Implications for Design of Decision Support Systems, Proc. of the MEDINFO 77 Conf., IFIP 1977.

7. Shortliffe, E., Computer-based Medical Consultations: MYCIN, Elsevier, New York, 1976.

8. Weiss, S.M., Kulikowski, C.A., Safir, A., A Model Based Consultation System for the Long-term Management of Glaucoma, Proc. IJCAI-5, 826-832, Boston, 1977.

9. Pople, H.E., The Formation of Composite Hypothesis in Diagnostic Problem Solving: An Exercise in Synthetic Reasoning, Proc. IJCAI-5, Boston, 1977.

10. Pauker, S.G., Gorry, G.A., Kassirer, J.P., Schwartz, W.B., Toward the Simulation of Clinical Cognition: Taking a Present Illness by Computer, AJM, Vol. 60, 981-995, 1976.

11. Radanović, L., Elementi kliničkog informacionog sistema realizovani na programskom sistemu "MUMPS", presented at the Symposium on Multi-disciplinary Sciences and their Role in the Scientific and Technical Progress, Belgrade, 1980.

A NON-STATIONARY MARKOV MODEL APPLIED TO THE FOLLOW-UP
OF PATIENTS TREATED FOR THYROTOXICOSIS

by D. Commenges[*], M. Commenges-Ducos[**], P. Barberger-Gateau[*]

[*] Département Informatique, Prof. R. SALAMON, Université de Bordeaux II
146, rue léo Saignat, 33075 BORDEAUX CEDEX (France)
[**] Service d'Endocrinologie, Prof. J.L. LATAPIE, Hôpital du Haut-Lévèque,
Avenue Magellan, 33604 PESSAC (France)

Abstract

In the course of their treatment, hyperthyroïd patients can evolve between three
different states : hyperthyroïdism, euthyroïdism and hypothyroïdism. We analyse the
follow-up of 195 patients by a method based on the notion of state which is a generalization of the actuarial estimate for survival data. While conventional methods
consider only two states -life and death- the method presented here can be applied
to problems involving an arbitrary number of transient states.

Key-words : failure time data analysis - multi-state problems - thyrotoxicosis

1 - Introduction

Treatment of dynamic data requiresmethods able to use the information contained in
censored observations. This has given rise to the development of specific methods
for failure time data analysis (1,2). In particular it is possible to estimate the
survivor function, which is useful to summarize the survival experience of given
groups of patients.

However conventional methods are inadequate for describing the evolution of hyperthyroïd patients. These can be cured, become permanantly or temporarily hypothyroïd
or revert to hyperthyroïdism after a period of hypo or euthyroïdism. Thus this problem requires more sophisticated methods than the conventional ones since a great
number of different events can occur.

There exist some generalizations of the survivor function (2, ch 7) for multiple
failures. However these methods are still based on the notion of event. We propose
a method based on the notion of state (Markov model) which seems more appropriate
here. Three states can easily be defined : hyperthyroïdism, euthyroïdism and hypothyroïdism. It is possible to estimate a "multivariate survivor function" via the
estimation of the transition probabilities from one state to another.

Conventional failure time data can be viewed as a particular case of this approach
in the following manner : only two states exist - life and death - and only one
irreversible evolution is possible. This can be represented by the graph :

$$ L \longrightarrow D $$

On the other hand the graph relative to our problem is much more complex :

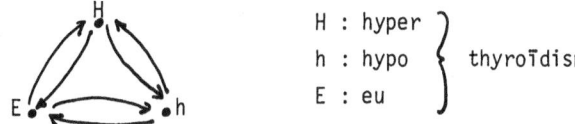

H : hyper ⎫
h : hypo ⎬ thyroīdism
E : eu ⎭

Weiss and Zelen (3) were the first to propose a semi-Markov model for medical data
but their method did not accomodate censoring. Lagakos, Sommer and Zelen (4) proposed a semi-Markov model with non-parametric survivor functions which offers one generalization of the Kaplan-Meīer estimator. But their model is not completely satisfactory since transition probabilities and survivor functions are time-invariant.
We present here a non-stationary discrete-time Markov model and we focus on the
estimation of the probability of being in state i at step k. We apply this model to
the follow-up of patients suffering from thyrotoxicosis treated by radioactive
iodine (RA^{131}I therapy)

2 - Mathematical development

2.1 The model

For greater simplicity we present here a discrete-time model. We first suppose that
we know the transition probabilities a step k $t_{ij}(k)$ for all i, j, k : $t_{ij}(k)$ is the
probability that the system be in state i at step k knowing that it is in state j at
step k-1. Using Bayes theorem we can compute the probability that the system be in
state i at step k if we know the probabilities $p_j(k-1)$ that the system be in state
j, for all j, at step k-1 :

$$p_i(k) = \sum_j p_j(k-1) \, t_{ij}(k)$$

which can be writen in matrix notation :

$$P(k) = T(k) \, P(k-1)$$

where P(k) is the m-vector $(p_i(k))$
and T(k) is the m x m matrix $(t_{ij}(k))$, m being the number of states.
Thus if we know the state at time zero we know P(o) and we can compute P(n) by :

$$P(n) = \prod_{k=1}^{n} T(k) \, P(o)$$

which is a conventional result of Markov chain theory.

2.2 Estimation of $p_i(k)$

In practice however we do not know the transition probabilities so, the actual problem is to find an estimator of P(k) and evaluate its variance. An approximate result , conditional   on the observations can easily be obtained. We propose to estimate P(n) by :

$$\hat{P}(n) = \prod_{k=1}^{n} \hat{T}(k) \, P_0$$

where $\hat{T}(k)$ are the estimated transition matrices ($\hat{t}_{ij}$ (k)); $\hat{t}_{ij}(k)$ is the conventional unbiased estimator of the parameter of a binomial law :

$$\hat{t}_{ij}(k) = \frac{n_{ij}(k)}{N_j(k-1) - D_j(k-1)}$$

where $n_{ij}(k)$ is the number of observations in state j at step k-1 and in state i at step k.

$N_j(k-1)$ is the number of observations in state j at step k-1.

$D_j(k-1)$ is the number of observations censored after step k-1.

Conditional on the observations $\hat{p}(k-1)$ and $\hat{t}_{ij}(k)$ are independant : it follows that if $\hat{P}(k-1)$ is unbiased so is $\hat{P}(k)$ for :

$$E\ (\hat{p}_i(k)) = E\ [\ \Sigma\ \hat{t}_{ij}(k)\ \hat{p}_j(k-1)\ ]$$

$$= \Sigma\ E\ [\ \hat{t}_{ij}(k)\ ]\ E\ [\ \hat{p}_j(k-1)\ ]$$

$$= \Sigma\ t_{ij}(k)\ p_j(k-1)$$

$$= p_i(k)$$

since P(o) is known, $\hat{P}(n)$ is unbiased.

2.3 Recursive formula for the variance

Using the same arguments we obtain a recursive formula for the covariance matrix.
We have :

$$v_{ij}(k) = E\ [\ \hat{p}_i(k)\ \hat{p}_j(k)\ ] = E\ [\ \Sigma\ \hat{t}_{i1}\ \hat{p}_1(k-1)\ \Sigma\ \hat{t}_{jm}\ \hat{p}_m(k-1)\ ]$$

$$= \Sigma\ \Sigma\ E\ [\ \hat{t}_{i1}(k)\ \hat{t}_{jm}(k)\ ]\ E\ [\ \hat{p}_1(k-1)\ \hat{p}_m(k-1)\ ]$$

For $1 \neq m$ $E\ [\ \hat{t}_{i1}\ \hat{t}_{jm}\ ] = t_{i1}\ t_{jm}$

For l=m and $j \neq i$ $E\ [\ \hat{t}_{i1}\ \hat{t}_{j1}\ ] = t_{i1}\ t_{j1} - t_{i1}\ t_{j1/n1}$

where $n_1 = N_1 - D_1$

For l=m and j=i $E\ [\ \hat{t}_{i1}^2\ ] = \dfrac{t_{i1}(1-t_{i1})}{n_1} + t_{i1}^2$

$$= t_{i1}^2 - t_{i1}^2/n1 + t_{i1/n1}$$

Let $V(k) = (v_{ij}(k))$

If we call D(V(k-1)) the diagonal matrix with diagonal terms : $v_{11}(k-1)/n1$ it can be seen that :

$V(k) = T(k)\ [\ V(k-1) - D(V(k-1))\ ]\ T'(k) + R(k)$

where R(k) is defined by : $r_{ij}(k) = o$ if $i \neq j$

$$r_{ii}(k) = \Sigma\ t_{i1}(k)\ v_{11}(k-1)/n1$$

3 - Application

3.1 Material

We apply the method to the follow-up of patients suffering from Graves' disease (except those presenting toxic nodular goiters) receiving $RA^{131}I$ therapy. The diagnoses were made on conventional clinical and biological (T3 and T4, RIA) criteria. Young patients (under 35) in whom the disease had recently appeared and who presented no ocular symptoms were treated by antithyroïd drugs and so do not enter the population studied here. All other patients initially received ^{131}I therapy and surgical treatment was undertaken where this failed (5 cases). These patients are included in the population and are considered to be suffering from Graves' disease until the last examination.

The sample analysed is constituted by all the patients receiving ^{131}I therapy in Pr. Latapie's Service at Haut-Leveque Hospital in Bordeaux between 1975 and 1980 : 196 patients (35 men and 161 women).

The patients received small iterative doses (2 or 3 mCi) of ^{131}I. Clinical and biological follow-up was carried out approximately every three months for the first year and then every year. The treatment and the frequency of examinations was adapted for each patient.

3.2 Application of the method

We sought to estimate the probability for a patient belonging to the population and receiving the ^{131}I therapy in the way described above, to be in one of the three states - (i) hyperthyroïdism, (ii) euthyroïdism, (iii) hypothyroïdism - at any time after the beginning of the treatment. The point of departure is the moment when the patient received the first iodine dose. We divided the time scale into equal intervals of three months. We considered that this was a case of non informative censoring. A program in FORTRAN IV was written to process the data.

3.3 Results

Results are given in Figure (1) where the three curves represent the estimation of the probability of being in one of the three states at time t. We have represented the estimated standard deviations by vertical segments of corresponding length. Since the moments of states changes are not precisely known we joined the points to obtain continuous curves. Although this is not rigorous it gives a more readable representation, especially when three curves have to be drawn on the same figure. The standart deviations grow as the number of patients decreases. They are reasonably small for the first three years. The conclusions of the study are roughly the same as in a work done on similar (but different) data which used the actuarial estimate (5). The recovery time is relatively long (35 % of patients are still hyperthyroïd after one year) and the probability of hypothyroïdism tends to increase after three years.

The method presented here allows us to take account of transient hypothyroïdism which occurs in the first two years, as well as relapses in hyperthyroïdism.

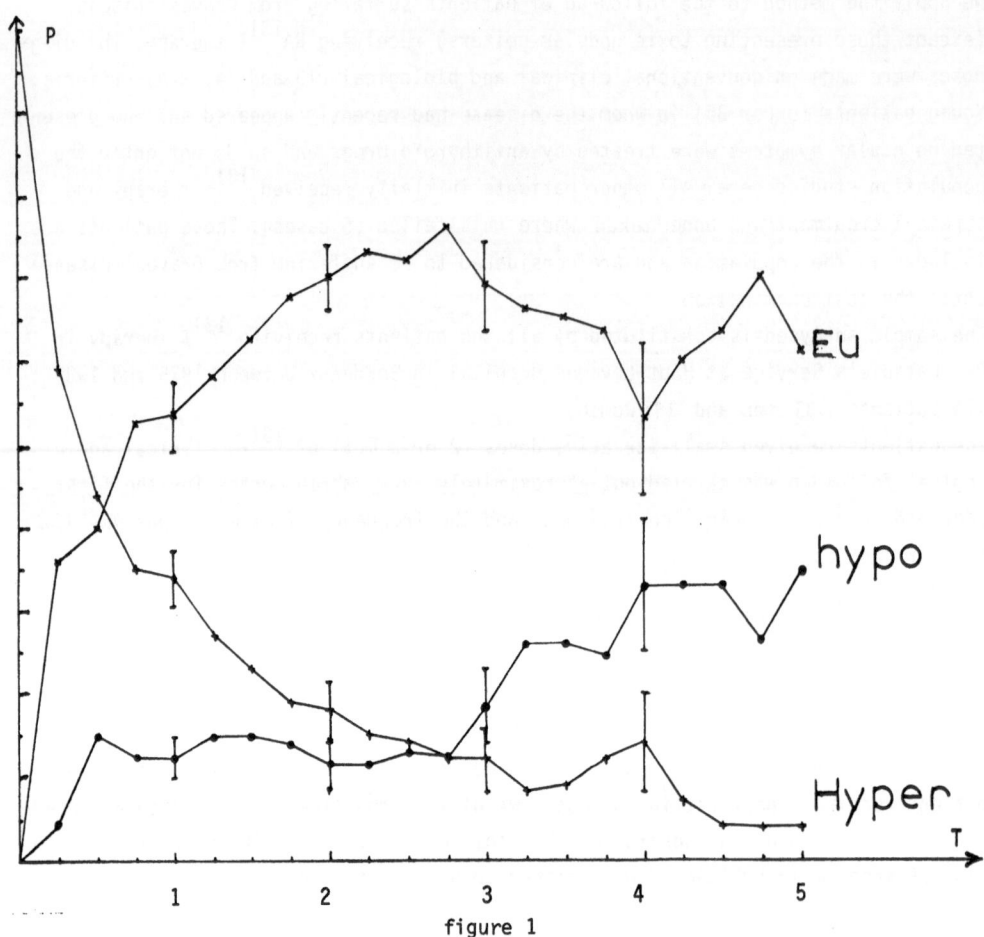

figure 1

4 - Conclusion

We have developed a method generalizing the actuarial estimate to problems involving an arbitrary number of states. It allowed us to analyse a censored sample of patients suffering from Graves'disease for which conventional methods were inadequate. We think that this method should prove useful in many other medical situations involving distinct changes of states. The approach should also be extended to clinical trials, and include explanatory variables.

References

(1) Kaplan EL, Meier P. Non parametric estimation from incomplete observations. J Am Stat Assoc. 1958; 53:457-481.

(2) Kalbfleish JD and Prentice RL. The statistical analysis of failure time data. 1980; Wiley, NY.

(3) Weiss GH and Zelen M. A semi-Markov model for clinical trials. 1965; J Appl Prob: 2, 269-85.

(4) Lagakos SW, Sommer CJ and Zelen M. Semi-Markov models for partially censored data. 1978; Biometrika : 65, 2, 311-7.

(5) Latapie JL, Lefort G, Commenges M, Roger P, Riviere LJ, Mauriac L. Traitement de la maladie de Basedow par petites doses repetees d'iode 131. 1980; An d'Endocrinologie : 41, 601-605.

CADIAG 1: A COMPUTER-ASSISTED DIAGNOSTIC SYSTEM ON THE BASIS OF SYMBOLIC LOGIC AND ITS APPLICATION IN INTERNAL MEDICINE.

K.-P. Adlaßnig[*], G. Kolarz[+], F. Lipomersky[*], I. Gröger[*], G. Grabner[*]

[*] Department of Medical Computer Sciences
(Director: Prof.Dr. G.Grabner), University of Vienna, A-1090 Vienna
and
[+] Ludwig Boltzmann Institute for Rheumatology and Focal Diseases
(Director: Prof.Dr. F.Endler and Prof.Dr. N.Thumb) A-2500 Baden

SUMMARY

Given a patient's symptom pattern, the computer-assisted diagnostic system is able to deduce medical diagnoses logically and to explain them. Not only proven or excluded diagnoses are presented but also diagnostic hypotheses attached to proposals for further examinations of the patient. At present, an extended application in rheumatology involving 1.500 cases with 2.000 symptoms, signs and test results of 200 diseases is being tested.

1. Presentation of medical knowledge

Medical knowledge is presented in form of relationships between medical entities (symptoms, symptom combinations, diseases) (see also /1,2/. The documentation of the relationships is carried out by a team of medical specialists.

1.1. Relationships between symptoms and diseases

The following relationships have been defined:

a) Symptom-disease relationships (see Figure 1)

OP: A symptom is obligatory and, if it occurs, proves the presence of a disease.

FP: A symptom is facultative and, if it occurs, proves the presence of a disease.

ON: A symptom is obligatory for a particular diagnosis but does not prove it.

FN: A symptom is facultative and does not prove the presence of a disease.

E: A symptom <u>excludes</u> a disease.

S: The symptom indicates a <u>second</u> <u>disease</u>.

-: The symptom-disease relationship is <u>unknown</u> or <u>unspecific</u>.

b) Symptom-symptom and disease-disease relationships OP, FP, ON, E and -.

SYMPTOMS	DISEASES GOUT	MIXED CONN. TISSUE DIS.	RHEUMATOID ARTHRITIS	PSORIATIC ARTHRITIS
PRESENT COMPLAINTS, OMALGIA, LEFT	FN	FN	FN	FN
GOT, SERUM, NORMAL	FN	FN	FN	FN
CREATINE,URINE, INCREASED		FN		
PUNCTURE, JOINT, URIC ACID CRYSTALS,INTRACELL.	FP	S	S	S
X-RAY, JOINT, ARTHRITIS MUTILANS			E	FN
BIOPSY , LYMPH NODES SARCOIDOSIS				

Figure 1: Section of the Symptom-Disease-Matrix.

1.2. <u>Relationships between symptom combinations and diseases</u> OP, FP, ON, E and -.

To formulate symptom combinations, <u>context-free languages</u> are presented (Table I). The definition of symptom combinations is carried out in two steps:

The first step consists in combining detailed symptoms or signs (e.g. tenderness on pressure, phalanx, distal 1; tenderness on pressure, phalanx, distal 2;...; tenderness on pressure, phalanx, proximal 5) to higher level symptoms or signs (e.g. tenderness on pressure of at

least one phalanx). These combinations are called symptom combinations I [1]. In a second step, the symptom combinations I form the
variables of the symptom combinations II. Only the category of symptom
combinations II is then related to diseases. Introducing a two
step procedure is necessary to carry out the transition from the
documentary level of symptoms (patient's record) to the diagnostic
level of symptoms (physician's use of symptom terms to characterize
a disease).

Table I: Rules of the Context-Free Languages that Define the
        Syntactical Structures of Symptom Combinations I and II.

RULES		REMARKS
⟨SYMPTOM COMBINATION PRIMARY⟩	::=⟨IDENTIFIER PRIMARY⟩=⟨EXPRESSION PRIMARY⟩;	
⟨IDENTIFIER PRIMARY⟩	::=A⟨INTEGER⟩	⟸MAPPING IN A THESAURUS OF SYMPTOM COMBINATIONS PRIMARY
⟨EXPRESSION PRIMARY⟩	::=⟨FACTOR PRIMARY⟩{∧⟨FACTOR PRIMARY⟩|∨⟨FACTOR PRIMARY⟩}*	
⟨FACTOR PRIMARY⟩	::=[~]⟨VARIABLE PRIMARY⟩	
⟨VARIABLE PRIMARY⟩	::=⟨SYMPTOM⟩|⟨DIAGNOSIS⟩|(⟨EXPRESSION PRIMARY⟩)| ⟨MINMAX-TERM PRIMARY⟩	
⟨SYMPTOM⟩	::=S⟨INTEGER⟩	⟸MAPPING IN A SYMPTOM THESAURUS
⟨DIAGNOSIS⟩	::=D⟨INTEGER⟩	⟸MAPPING IN A DIAGNOSIS THESAURUS
⟨MINMAX-TERM PRIMARY⟩	::={MIN|MAX}+⟨INTEGER⟩/⟨INTEGER⟩:⟨VARIABLE LIST PRIMARY⟩	⟸"LEFT" INTEGER ≦ "RIGHT" INTEGER=NUMBER OF EXPRESSIONS PRIMARY IN VARIABLE LIST PRIMARY
⟨VARIABLE LIST PRIMARY⟩	::=⟨EXPRESSION PRIMARY⟩;{⟨VARIABLE LIST PRIMARY⟩}*	
⟨INTEGER⟩	::=⟨DIGIT⟩[⟨INTEGER⟩]	
⟨DIGIT⟩	::=0|1|2|3|4|5|6|7|8|9	
⟨SYMPTOM COMBINATION SECONDARY⟩::=⟨IDENTIFIER SECONDARY⟩=⟨EXPRESSION SECONDARY⟩;		
⟨IDENTIFIER SECONDARY⟩	::=B⟨INTEGER⟩	⟸MAPPING IN A THESAURUS OF SYMPTOM COMBINATIONS SECONDARY
⟨EXPRESSION SECONDARY⟩	::=⟨FACTOR SECONDARY⟩{∧⟨FACTOR SECONDARY⟩|∨⟨FACTOR SECONDARY⟩}*	
⟨FACTOR SECONDARY⟩	::=[~]⟨VARIABLE SECONDARY⟩	
⟨VARIABLE SECONDARY⟩	::=⟨IDENTIFIER PRIMARY⟩|(⟨EXPRESSION SECONDARY⟩)| ⟨MINMAX-TERM SECONDARY⟩	
⟨MINMAX-TERM SECONDARY⟩	::={MIN|MAX}+⟨INTEGER⟩/⟨INTEGER⟩:⟨VARIABLE LIST SECONDARY⟩	⟸"LEFT" INTEGER ≦ "RIGHT" INTEGER=NUMBER OF EXPRESSIONS SECONDARY IN VARIABLE LIST SECONDARY
⟨VARIABLE LIST SECONDARY⟩	::=⟨EXPRESSION SECONDARY⟩;{⟨VARIABLE LIST SECONDARY⟩}*	

---

[1] In rheumatology, symptom combinations I are used to establish
    for instance major and minor manifestations for rheumatoid
    arthritis /16/ and rheumatic fever /4/ (see also /11/). WEISS et
    al. /22/ and LINDBERG et al. /12/ call those combinations
    "intermediate hypotheses".

1.3. Symbolic presentation of the defined relationships

The above mentioned relationships can be interpreted in different ways:

a) In terms of propositional logic /10/ (3-valued system of KLEENE /15/). Symptoms S_i and diseases D_j are considered to be logical variables (Table II). The relationships are regarded as logical operations (Table III).

Table II: Symptoms S_i and diseases D_j as logical variables.

logical variable	S_i	D_j
0	not present	not present (excluded)
$\frac{1}{2}$	not investigated	possible (hypothesis)
1	present	present (proven)

b) In terms of predicate logic (first-order predicate logic /18/). Symptoms S_i and diseases D_j establish unary predicates (property predicates of patient p) (Table III).

c) In terms of IF-THEN statements /5,6,21/. Medical knowledge is presented in IF "premise" THEN "conclusion" statements (Table III).

Table III: Symbolic Presentation of the Medical Relationships.

	OP	FP	ON	FN	E	S
PROPOSITIONAL LOGIC:	$S_i \Leftrightarrow D_j$ EQUIVALENCE	$S_i \Rightarrow D_j$ IMPLICATION	$S_i \Leftarrow D_j$ $\equiv$ $\neg S_i \Rightarrow \neg D_j$	$S_i \oslash D_j$ TAUTOLOGY $\equiv$ $(S_i \Rightarrow D_j) \lor (S_i \Rightarrow \neg D_j)$	$S_i \Rightarrow \neg D_j$ $\equiv$ $\neg(S_i \land D_j)$ NAND	$(S_1 \land D_1) \Rightarrow$ $D_2 \lor \ldots \lor D_N$ N+1-ARY OPERATION
PREDICATE LOGIC:	$\forall p[S_i(p) \Leftrightarrow D_j(p)]$ OR $\forall p[D_j(p) \Leftrightarrow S_i(p)]$	$\forall p[S_i(p) \Rightarrow D_j(p)]$	$\forall p[D_j(p) \Rightarrow S_i(p)]$ OR $\forall p[\neg S_i(p) \Rightarrow \neg D_j(p)]$	$\forall p[(S_i(p) \Rightarrow D_j(p)]$ $\lor(S_i(p) \Rightarrow \neg D_j(p))]$	$\forall p[S_i(p) \Rightarrow \neg D_j(p)]$ OR $\forall p[\neg (S_i(p) \land D_j(p))]$	$\forall p[(S_1(p) \land D_1(p)) \Rightarrow$ $D_2(p) \lor \ldots \lor D_N(p)]$
IF-THEN-STATEMENTS:	IF S_i THEN D_j, AND IF D_j THEN S_i.	IF S_i THEN D_j.	IF D_j THEN S_i, OR IF NOT S_i THEN NOT D_j.	IF S_i THEN "D_j WITH CERTAINTY x". $0 < x < 1$	IF S_i THEN NOT D_j.	IF $S_1 \land D_1$ THEN "SEARCH FOR D_j ". $2 \leq j \leq N$

498

d) As a semantic network /14,17/. Medical knowledge can be presented
as a semantic network. Symptoms, symptom combinations and diseases
form the nodes, and the relationships act as the edges of the net
(Figure 2).

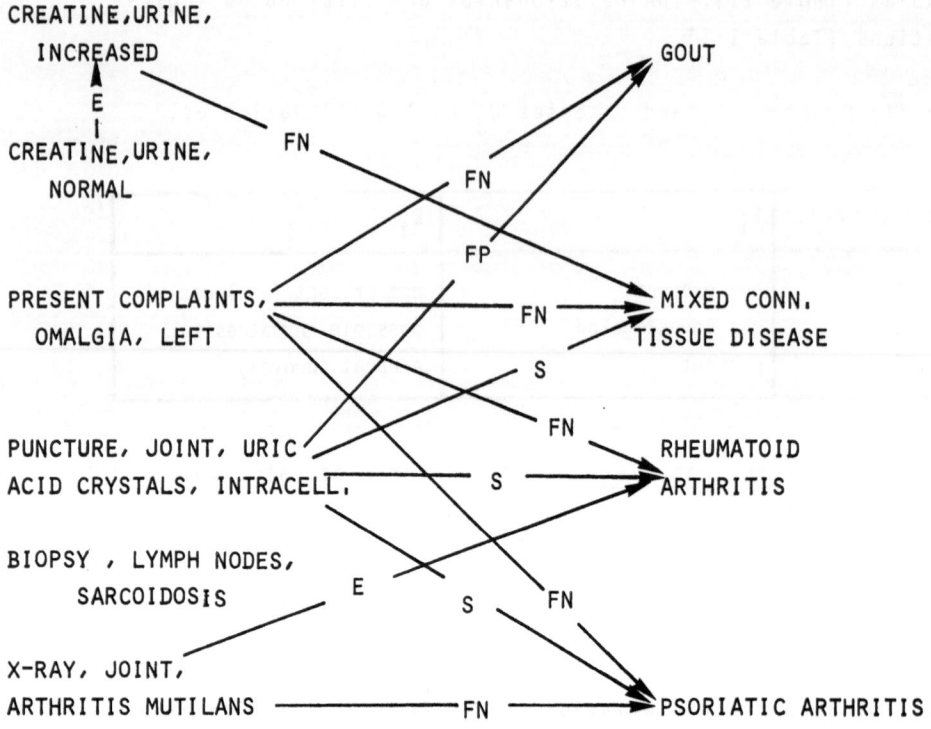

Figure 2: Section of the Semantic Network.

e) There are further similar symbolic presentations of the above
mentioned medical knowledge:

- Boolean matrices ("obligatory"matrix, "proving"matrix, "excluding"
  matrix). The diagnostic process is considered as a series of Boolean
  sum-product compositions (see also /19,20/).

- Fuzzy subsets (symptom S_i and diseases D_j), fuzzy expressions
  (symptom combinations) and fuzzy relationships between medical
  entities (occurrence and confirmability relations). Then the
  diagnostic process consists in performing fuzzy compositions /3,19/.

2. Computer-assisted diagnostic process

2.1. Preliminary work

In order to prepare the medical diagnostic process, the frequency of
the FN relationships of every symptom S_i in the symptom-disease
matrix is calculated and called the degree of frequency DF_i of the
symptom S_i. Symptoms with a low degree of frequency are used to
establish unique symptom patterns in the matrix. So, e.g., the
combination of arthritis mutilans osteolysis (DF_i=6), ileosacral-
arthritis (DF_i=7) and MENELL handgrip, positive (DF=8) forms a unique
symptom pattern for the diagnosis psoriatic arthritis.

2.2. Process of computer-assisted diagnosis

Figure 3 shows the process of the computer-assisted medical diagnosis.

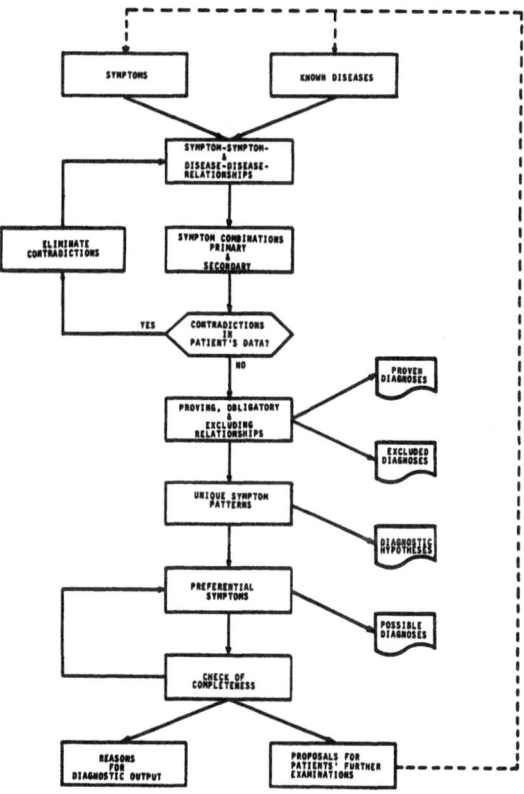

Figure 3: Computer-Assisted Medical Diagnostic Process of CADIAG 1.

Given a certain symptom pattern, proven diagnoses DP, excluded diagnoses DE, diagnostic hypotheses DH, and possible diagnoses DS are calculated. Proven diagnoses are obtained from symptoms present with OP or FP relationships. Excluded diagnoses are obtained from symptoms present with E relationships and from definitely absent symptoms with OP or ON relationships. Diagnostic hypotheses are calculated by means of unique symptom patterns. Possible diagnoses are established on the basis of selected preferential symptoms with FN relationships.

The output of reasons for the diagnostic results displayed as DP, DE, DH and DS diagnoses makes the diagnostic process comprehensible. The output of proposals for further examinations of the patient and subsequent input of the results of these examinations enables the physician to perform the diagnostic process step by step or to confirm or eliminate specific diagnostic hypotheses or possible diagnoses one after the other.

3. Application

a) Medical documentation of relationships
Medical documentation compiled as yet is shown in Table IV.

b) Acquisition of patients' data
Patients' symptoms and signs are gathered with the help of the documentary system of the Vienna Medical Information system WAMIS /7,8,9/. The lab test results are put in the laboratory information system of WAMIS /13/.

c) Evaluation of the system
Diagnoses are made automatically for patients suffering from one or more rheumatological diseases.

Table IV: Medical Documentation of Relationships (compiled as yet).

		R	L	H
SYMPTOMS		1.315	374	1.090
DISEASES		211	74	27
SYMPTOM COMBINATIONS PRIMARY		138	--	--
SYMPTOM COMBINATIONS SECONDARY		12	--	--
SYMPTOM-DISEASE RELATIONSHIPS		34.776	4.483	735
OF THESE	OP	18	1	9
	FP	45	13	2
	ON	199	113	76
	FN	30.010	4.302	598
	E	1.924	54	50
	H	2.580	--	--
SYMPTOM-SYMPTOM RELATIONSHIPS		1.063	111	589
OF THESE	OP	--	--	--
	FP	87	3	18
	ON	87	3	18
	E	889	105	553
DISEASE-DISEASE RELATIONSHIPS		1.532	--	--
OF THESE	OP	--	--	--
	FP	54	--	--
	ON	54	--	--
	E	1.424	--	--
RELATIONSHIPS BETWEEN SYMPTOM COMBINATIONS SECONDARY AND DISEASES		12	--	--
OF THESE	FP	11	--	--
	ON	1	--	--
UNIQUE SYMPTOM PATTERNS		1.452	820	77

R: RHEUMATOLOGICAL DISEASES
L: LIVER DISEASES
H: HEMATOLOGICAL DISEASES

Patients' data consists of

1. Physical examination
   (513 binary positions in   ==>   282 binary symptoms
   documentary system   in CADIAG 1)

2. Rheumatological history
   (372 binary positions in   ==>   158 binary symptoms
   documentary system   in CADIAG 1)

3. Rheumatological examination
   (1.227 binary positions in ==>   453 binary symptoms
   documentary system   in CADIAG 1)

4. Laboratory tests
   (80 lab tests   ==>   305 binary symptoms
                                       in CADIAG 1)

5. X-ray findings   (78 binary symptoms in CADIAG 1)

6. Histological findings   (75 binary symptoms in CADIAG 1)

— —

7. Final rheumatological diagnoses
   confirmed by the rheumatologist
   at the moment of patient's
   discharge   (211 rheumatological diagnoses)

By comparison with the documented final diagnoses confirmed by
physicians, the diagnostic results provided by CADIAG 1 can be
checked, and the accuracy of the method can be calculated. The
connection of CADIAG 1 to the medical data base of the hospital
information system WAMIS has been realized. The CADIAG 1 - data base
interface includes the calculation of binary symptoms from given
numerical lab test results and the evaluation of logical combinations
(similar to symptom combinations I) for simplest documentary data.

CADIAG 1 is at present being tested in retrospective mode to
evaluate and improve the medical knowledge system; it is planned
to be used in prospective mode to optimize the number of necessary
lab tests, X-ray checks, punctures, etc.

Furthermore, CADIAG 1 provides a deep insight into the physician's
mental diagnostic process because of its explanation and
substantiation capabilities and is highly suitable in medical
diagnostic training.

4. Implementation

The online consultation program of CADIAG 1 was written in APL and
runs in a 320 kByte workspace. During the consultation, the APL
functions communicate with the frame and rule based medical knowledge
of CADIAG 1.

REFERENCES

/1/ ADLASSNIG, K.-P., G. GRABNER: The Viennese Computer-Assisted
    Diagnostic System. Its Principles and Values. AUTOMEDICA 3 (1980),
    141-150.

/2/ ADLASSNIG, K.-P., G. GRABNER: Approaches to Computer-Assisted
    Diagnosis in Gastroenterology. EDV in Medizin und Biologie 11
    (1980), 74-80.

/3/ ADLASSNIG, K.-P.: A Fuzzy Logical Model of Computer-Assisted
     Medical Diagnosis. Meth.Inform.Med. 19 (1980), 141-148.

/4/ American Heart Association, Rheumatic Fever Committee of the
     Council on Rheumatic Fever and Congenital Heart Diseases
     Circulation 43 (1971), 983-988.

/5/ BUTTON, K.F.: Laboratory Diagnosis by Computer. Comput. Biol.
     Med. 3 (1973), 131-136.

/6/ GIESZL, L.R.: An Interactive Intelligence System for Medical
     Decision Aids. In LINDBERG, D.A.B., S. KAIHARA (Eds.): MEDINFO
     80. North-Holland Publishing Company Amsterdam-New York-Oxford
     1980, 809-814.

/7/ GRABNER, G., H. GRABNER: The Viennese General Medical Information
     System. Proceedings of MEDIS'75 TOKYO, Kansai Institute of
     Information Systems 1975, 156-163.

/8/ GRABNER, H., J. LEJHANEC: Das universelle Dokumentationssystem
     im Rahmen des Informationssystems WAMIS. EDV in Medizin und
     Biologie 2 (1976), 53-56.

/9/ GRABNER, H., G. GRABNER: Aims and Structure of the Vienna
     General Medical Information System WAMIS. In ANDERSON, J.,
     J.M. FORSYTHE (Eds.): MEDINFO 74. North-Holland Publishing
     Company Amsterdam-New York-Oxford 1974, 375-397.

/10/ KLAUS, G.: Moderne Logik. VEB Deutscher Verlag der Wissen-
     schaften, Berlin 1973.

/11/ KOLARZ, G.: Diagnosekriterien entzündlich rheumatischer
     Erkrankungen. In SINGER, F. (Hrsg.): Entzündlich-rheumatolo-
     gische Erkrankungen - ihre Bedeutung für den praktizierenden
     Arzt. Pensionsversicherungsanstalt der Arbeiter, 1977, 39-42.

/12/ LINDBERG, D.A.B., G.C. SHARP, L.C. KINGSLAND, III, J.H. ESTHER:
     Design of Criteria-Based Rheumatology Consulting System for
     a Microcomputer. In LINDBERG, D.A.B., S. KAIHARA (Eds.):
     MEDINFO 80. North-Holland Publishing Company Amsterdam-New York-
     Oxford, 1980, 1316-1320.

/13/ MARKSTEINER, A.: Prerequisits and Programs for On-line Data
     Acquisition in Clinical Laboratories, Connected with the Medical
     Information System WAMIS. EDV in Medizin und Biologie 4 (1974),
     106-110.

/14/ PEREZ-OJEDA, A.: Medical Knowledge Network: A Database for
     Computer-Aided Diagnosis. Masterthesis, Department of Industrial
     Engineering, Toronto 1976.

/15/ RESCHER, N.: Many-valued logic. Mc Graw-Hill Book Company,
     New York 1969.

/16/ ROPES, M.W., G.A. BENNETT, S. COBB, R. JACOX, R.A. GESSAR:
     1958 Revision of Diagnostic Criteria for Rheumatoid Arthritis.
     Arthr. Rheum. 2 (1959), 16-20.

/17/ ROUSSOPOULOS, N., J. MYLOPOULOS: Using Semantic Networks for
     Data Base Management.

/18/ SADEGH-ZADEH, K.: Grundlagenprobleme einer Theorie der klinischen Praxis, Teil 1: Explikation des medizinischen Diagnosebegriffs. METAMED 1 (1977), 76-102.

/19/ SANCHEZ, E.: Medical Diagnosis and Composite Fuzzy Relations. In GUPTA, M.M., R.K. RAGADE, R.R. YAGER (Eds.): Advances in Fuzzy Set Theory and Applications. North-Holland Publishing Company Amsterdam-New York-Oxford, 1979, 437-444.

/20/ SANCHEZ, E.: Compositions of Fuzzy Relations. In GUPTA, M.M., R.K. RAGADE, R.R. YAGER (Eds.): Advances in Fuzzy Set Theory and Applications. North-Holland Publishing Company Amsterdam-New York-Oxford, 1979, 421-433.

/21/ SHORTLIFFE, E.H.: Computer-Based Medical Consultations: MYCIN. Elsevier, New York-Oxford-Amsterdam 1976.

/22/ WEISS, S.M., K.B. KERN, C.A. KULIKOWSKI, M.F. USCHOLD: A Guide to the Use od the EXPERT Consultion System. Technical Report CBM-TR-94, Rutgers University, 1981.

A STUDY OF THE AGREEMENT OF MEDICAL INFORMATION APPLICATION TO HISTOLOGICAL SLIDE READINGS IN CHRONIC LYMPHOCYTIC LEUKEMIA

F. PLOYART*, M. RAPHAEL**, A. AUQUIER*, J. DIEBOLD[1], N. BROUSSE[2],

J. BRIERE[3], G. CHOMETTE[4], T. CAULET[5], S. MAYER[6], M. IMBERT[7],

H. JOUAULT[7], G. DELSOL[8], R. LAUMONIER[9], E. HALKIN[9], G. ANTIN[10],

Cl. SULTAN[7], Cl. CHASTANG*, J.L. BINET**, F. GREMY*

* Groupe INSERM U 88 : Méthodologie Informatique et Statistique en Médecine
CHU Pitié-Salpétrière - 91, Bld de l'Hôpital - 75634 PARIS Cedex 13

** Département d'Hématologie - Hôpital Pitié-Salpétrière
47, Bld de l'Hôpital - 75651 PARIS Cedex 13 FRANCE

- Département d'Anatomo-pathologie :
1 : Hôtel-Dieu, 2 : Beaujon PARIS, 3 : BREST, 4 : Pitié-Salpétrière PARIS, 5 : REIMS
6 : STRASBOURG, 7 : Henri-Mondor CRETEIL, 8 : TOULOUSE, 9 : ROUEN
10 : Antoine Béclère CLAMART

SUMMARY :   When searching for histological prognostic factors in Chronic Lymphocytic Leukemia (CLL) we focused on one aspect of the quality of the data, the agreement of slide readings between pathologists. A preliminary study allowed us to define a set of 10 useful items in the histology of CLL. The results of the main study which concerned 228 slides read by 12 anatomopathologists, were twofold : the items were lacking in information and/or not in agreement. These negative results and the difficulties encountered suggest recommandations for future agreement studies : selection of slides on the basis of technical quality selection of items rich in information, planning of such studies in different phases, centralized management of slides.

The continuous increasing amount of medical information, the more and more questioning on the practical use of this information suggests a study of the information quality as much as the increasing of health costs leads the funding of such studies to become more hesitant. The required qualities of any medical information are numerous : sensibility, specificity, reproductibility (agreement between readers), low cost in general... We will limit ourselves to one of the qualities mentioned above, the agreement of medical information between several pathologists. The interest of this quality is obvious and the maintaining of a good agreement between pathologists should be a criterion of quality control in the health system.

It is true that the nature of medical information constitutes a major difficulty in the realization of such studies : the instability of the information and the ethical problems can prevent such studies.

The study described concerns a very favorable situation : histological study where it is possible to fix the information and to transmit it easily. It is this particular domain which has been the most simple undertaking for such a project of agreement study. Such histologic studies have already been performed in gastroenterology (1) and in pneumology (2). This agreement study concerns Chronic Lymphocytic Leukemia (CLL). Its realization was possible thanks to the existence of the CLL cooperative group of the French Society of Hemathology created in 1974. In this disease, the interest of histo-pathological diagnosis (bone marrow biopsy) is :

- to confirm the bone marrow lymphocytosis, which is essential in types without lymph nodes and/or with discret peripheral blood lymphocytosis (3).

- to establish correlations between the anatomo-pathological and clinical patterns (4) (5) - (61) and to eventually point out new prognostic factors.

- to permit during the evolution, the evaluation of the bone marrow lymphocytosis and the positive diagnosis of a complete recovery.

This study of agreement has been suggested to us by the distributions of the histological diagnosis between centers which seemed to imply differences between pathologists. Moreover, the pathologists themselves were conscious of a probable disagreement among them whenever they were meeting. A protocol was therefore put into effect, including the physicians of the CLL group, the anatomopathologists and the statisticians. The results of the study were presented in June 1981 at the annual meeting of the CLL group. :group of the French Society of Hematology. More than the analysis of the results, we present here the different phases of the study, the difficulties encountered in its realization and its consequences in relation to the strategy when dealing with such projects.

I. PROTOCOL OF THE STUDY

From the beginning two phases were planned. When one tries to agree, it is indeed important to first agree on definitions of typical cases and then, agree on the classification of any case. To this effet, the first phase, a pre-study, was aimed at identifying the pertinent information and at defining a common language to be used between pathologists. Eight pathologists participated in this first phase consisting in an independent reading of 10 slides. The 10 slides were selected by an outside pathologist on the basis of a good technical quality and a good representivity of CLL patterns. The questionnaire was established by a single pathologist. Then two meetings permitted discussion of the results and the preparation of a second questionnaire. The objective of the second phase, the core of the study, was threefold : agreement study between the participating pathologists on the items of the questionnaire; study of the anatomo-clinical correlations; and finally a prognostic study.

The material used in this second phase was composed of the slides taken from the CLL 76 clinical trial, the first one initiated by the French CLL cooperative group. The participants in this study were the pathologists of different medical centers, each one wishing to take part in this first cooperative work in pathology of the CLL group : in fact, until recently the group was limited to clinicians and methodologists.

The first phase started in March 1980 and it was expected that the result of the study would be presented in June 1981.

2.a- First phase :

- This phase allowed to list the useful histopathology concepts in CLL and to establish common definitions of them. Meanwhile the reading of the 10 slides by the participants showed an important disagreement, sometimes a complete disagreement (as regards all the categories of a variable), sometimes partial (as regards some categories of a variable, for example, the pattern of infiltration). Therefore, this first phase resulted in a rediscussion of the usefulness of each item followed by a redefinition in a precise manner of those retained. It ended with the elaboration of a new questionnaire, which was completed by a reference iconography. Because of an apparently good common understanding of the new definitions, this first phase left a very favorable outlook for the second.

2.b- Second phase :

- Among the 220 initial bone marrow biopsies drawn from the computed records, only 154 were located. 9 boxes of slides were created on November 1980 and circulated among the 12 pathologists. It was planned that they would have 6 months to read these slides independently. Table 1 shows that this objective had not been reached. Several times, the boxes of slides had been left waiting in different laboratories. The fixed deadline (June 1981) forced us to make the analysis of these data in May 1981, even though all the pathologists had not yet viewed the complete set of slides.

TABLE 1 : STATUS OF THE READING IN THE GROUP ON MAY 20, 1981.

Boxes / Readers	I (23)	II (24)	III (17)	IV (19)	V (14)	VI (15)	VII (25)	VIII (17)
A (154)	X	X	X	X	X	X	X	X
B (154)	X	X	X	X	X	X	X	X
C (93)	X	X			X	X		X
D (113)	X		X	X	X	X	X	
E (92)			X	X	X	X		X
F (129)	X	X	X	X	X	X		X
G (50)			X	X	X			
H (17)			X					
I (64)	X	X	X					
J (40)						X	X	
K (62)	X				X		X	
L (41)		X						X

- At the first reading we were forced to reject 45 slides out of 154 (29% of the slides) because of bad technical quality recognized by all the readers.

- Statistical analysis was only feasible on 109 slides, studied for 10 criteria by only 6 pathologists (A, B, C, D, E, F) (the contribution of the other readers was judged two weak to be used for statistical purpose).

- 8 among the 10 criteria appeared as having no variance (e.g. the same response appeared in 90% of the slides). For such criteria, one would need a very large number of slides to detect disagreement between readers. For the two remaining ones, with variance in the response, the disagreement was high. Tables II and III show the agreement tables and the Kappa values concerning these criteria for two readers on 93 and 85 slides respectively.

TABLE II : PATTERNS OF INFILTRATION : AGREEEMENT TABLE FOR READERS A AND B.

Reader A / Reader B	Nodular (15)	Interstitial (10)	Mixed (47)	Diffuse (19)	Others (2)
Nodular (5)	2	-	2	1	-
Interstitial (25)	5	10	10	-	-
Mixed (43)	8	-	32	2	1
Diffuse (20)	-	-	3	16	1
Others	-	-	-	-	0

Kappa = 0,49

TABLE III : RETICULE FIBERS : AGREEMENT TABLE FOR READERS A AND B (85 SLIDES)

Reader A / Reader B	Normal (42)	Weak (36)	Moderate (4)	Important (3)
Normal (29)	23	6	-	-
Weak (45)	17	24	3	1
Moderate (11)	2	6	1	2
Important (0)	-	-	-	0

Kappa = 0,27

2.c- Histo-pathological conclusions :

The histo-pathological criteria such as they are used, even after an attempt to standardize them, (first phase) lacking in information and/or, are not in agreement.

This result implies the necessity to make the definition of the existing criteria more precisely and to effectively used these definitions. Also, it will be necessary to find new criteria. For this purpose, the definition of quantitative criteria seems promising. In particular, the morphometry would permit the testing of new histo-pathological criteria which would then be the object of a confrontation with a classic reading associated with a study of agreement.

III. WHAT THIS STUDY HAS BROUGHT AS FAR AS THE METHODOLOGY IS CONCERNED IN THE AGREEMENT STUDY ?.

Despite these apparently negative results, this study appears useful to define a better strategy in future agreement studies.

Schematically, we will make the greatest effort to avoid committing the following errors :

1/. Non selection of slides in the second phase, while it appeared that a large proportion (29%) was of poor quality and thereby useless. This attitude has two explanations : first there was a lack of agreement on the judgement of quality and the coordinator of the study was reluctant to select a subset of adequate slides; second the proportion of bad slides was totally underestimated. Therefore, it seems necessary to define precise minimum standards of quality which, when reached, must lead to the rejection of the concerned slide.

2/. Large acceptability of the potential readers from the very beginning of the study. This democratic attitude raised some organizational difficulties due to long stops in boxes rotation. In fact, it seems more efficient to distinguish two phases and possibly a third one :

a. Agreement study : aiming to identify the information in agreement and to point out the disagreements. A motivated small group of readers should take over this study. This group could be composed of readers considered as experts by potentiel readers. This study   must allow us to define the future information to look for.

b. Agreement test : this procedure allows us to validate previously defined information for the whole set of readers of the group. It involves the reading of an ad-hoc sample containing different profiles with a more or less easy characterization. This phase is nothing but a quality control procedure for the whole set of histo-pathologists.

c. Depending on the results of the agreement test, one could, in the best case, make a periodic agreement test on the whole set of readers to check that the agreement holds on and have any new reader tested against an old one; in the worst case (disagreement should read all the future slides in order to improve the agreement by giving better definitions, better classifications, etc...

3. <u>Non standardization of the techniques</u> : the important percentage of rejected slides points out the necessity of standardizing the techniques used for sampling and preparation, event in the absence of agreement study. Such procedures appear necessary to improve the quality of medical information.

4. <u>Absence of slide centralization</u> : the difficulties encountered to collect the slides, however recent, and the important failure rate (74 of 228 slides) lead us to suggest the early use of a centralized structutre of slide collection. We can imagine that each anatomo-pathological laboratory prepares, for the patients included in a study, some supplementary slides immediately addressed to the re-reading commitee secretary.

5. <u>Use of two many items with rare incidence</u> : it turned out indeed that most questions had the same answer for the majority of slides (more than 90%). Detecting disagreement for such items would require very large samples of slides. Therefore, such questions should be avoided in small or medium size agreement studies.

CONCLUSION :

The results of this study are not negative at all concerning the histological aspect as well as the methodological aspect. It is useful to know the discordant character of an information to be used and try to do the best to improve this information. As regards the methodological aspect, in addition to the consequences previously pointed out for the strategy of such studies, we have to emphasize the following points :

- This study is an example of the difficulty of obtaining a medical information of good quality; similar results were obtained in other medical domains (Karnofsky (8), Coronanography (9) Psychiatry (10), Respiratory System (11)).

- This study shows the interest of procedures of standardization, evaluation and quality control.

- Such studies are possible only if cooperative groups exist and their number is regrettably small presently in France.

- Any agreement study requires a careful planning and a strategy adapted to its aim, as detailed in the previous section.

- Such studies are time consuming from the organizers standpoint (planning, management), as well as from the readers standpoint (at least 10 minutes for each slide).

- The relative failure of the first phase which aimed to define homogeneous concepts, shows the difficulties of this approach in the medical field. This difficulty is related to the nature of the medical information and to the rigidity of habits and language as well, which must incite us to increase our pedagogical efforts in the adoption of new definitions sometimes in contradiction with the previous uses.

BIBLIOGRAPHY

(1) Theodessi A, Skene AM, Portmann B, Knill-Jones RP. Observer variation in assessment of liver biopsies including analysis by Kappa statistics. Gastroenterology 1980, 79, 232-241.

(2) Feinstein AR, Gelfman NA, Yesner R. Observer variability in the histopathologic diagnosis of lung cancer. Am Rev Respiratory Disease. 1970; 101 : 671.

(3) Gray JL, Jacobs A, Block M. Bone marrow and peripheral blood lymphocytosis in the prognosis of chronic lymphocytic leukemia. Cancer 1974; 33 : 1169-1178.

(4) Carbone A, Santuro A, Pilotti S, Rilke F. Bone marrow patterns and clinical staging in Chronic Lymphocytic Leukemia. Lancet 1978; 606.

(5) Charron D, Dighiero C, Raphael M, Binet JL. Bone marrow patterns and clinical staging in Chronic Lymphocytic Leukemia. Lancet 1977; 819.

(6) Hernandez-Nieto L, Montserrat-Costa E, Muncunill J, Rozman C. Bone marrow patterns and clinical staging in Chronic Lymphocytic Leukemia. Lancet 1977 b; 1269.

(7) Cohen J. A coefficient of agreement for nominal scales. Educ. and Psychol. Meas. 1960; 20 : 37-46.

(8) Hutchinson TA, Boyd NF, Feinstein AR. Scientific problems in clinical scales as demonstrated in the Karnofsky index of performance status. J of Chron. Diseases 1979; 32 : 661-666.

(9) Timothy A, Derouen PH D, John A, Murray MD, William Owen AB. Variability in the Analysis of Coronary arteriograms. Circulation 1977; 55, 2 : 324-328.

(10) Spitzer R, Fleiss J. Are analysis of the reliability of psychiatric diagnosis ?Brit J Psychiatric 1974; 125, 324.

(11) Smyllie HD, Blendis LM, Armitage P. Observer disagreement in physical signs of the respiratory system. Lancet 1965; 2 : 412.

512

ACQUIRING DATA THE LOGICAL WAY.

Dr.H.R.A. Townsend,
The National Hospital,
Queen Square,
London.

Many applications of Medical Computing are primarily concerned with
acquiring data.   There are significant advantages in using a simple
keyboard and some form of visual display, instead of requiring the
patient (or doctor) to "fill in a form".

In the first place the questions to be asked can be determined by
the responses (it is, for instance, unnecessarily embarrassing to ask
certain questions about gynaecological problems of a male respondent,
and vice versa).

In the second place the answers to questions can be checked as
the data collection is proceeding and the same question may be asked
in different ways with further explanations being offered where the
respondent's replies are inconsistent suggesting that there is some
misunderstanding or other difficulty.

Such "Intelligent Data Acquisition" programs are often difficult
to construct.   This communication described the use of the programming language PROLOG for this task.

A PROLOG program consists of a collection of logical statements.
Each statement is complete in itself, and therefore individual statements may be added to or deleted from the program as required, making
the total system relatively easy to modify and extend as experience
is gained.

PROLOG statements have the form:-

A :- B , C , D ;

which may be read as

"A" implies "B" and "C" and "D"

for example:-

Sex (female):- USE(gynae-questionnaire);

The statements of the language are simply logical propositions,
written in a particular symbolic form (strictly a PROLOG statement has
the structure of a Horn clause in symbolic logic).

These logical statements make it particularly easy to write down
formally the constraints and relations which must apply if the data
is to "make sense".

For example, if we wish to exclude paediatric and geriatric cases we would wish the following general rule to apply:-

"If X is the age of the patient (in years) then this implies
that X lies in the range 12 to 70 (X>12,X<70)"

in PROLOG this becomes

Age (X) :- X>12 , X<70;

A demonstration will be presented of a system being developed to
help train doctors to describe EEG records. Details of some of the
procedures will be examined and discussed in detail.

SUBJECTIVE HEALTH STATUS COMPONENTS IN A GENERAL POPULATION SURVEY

P.Potthoff

Gesellschaft für Strahlen- und Umweltforschung München (GSF)
Institut für Medizinische Informatik und Systemforschung (MEDIS)

Ingolstädter Landstr. 1
D-8042 Neuherberg

SUMMARY
A Functional Limitation Scale (FLS) and a Common Complaints Scale
(CCS) are presented as components of a health status measure that
indicates disease impacts on the quality of life. Distributions of
scale values and their relations to age, sex, utilization of medical
services and self-ratings of health and illness are reported on the
basis of a general health survey of 1384 inhabitants of the city of
Munich, Bavaria. Advantages and shortcomings of the health status
measures are discussed.

1. INTRODUCTION

Health status measures can be used as instruments for the evaluation
of health related activities like effectiveness-measurement of medical programs or estimation of the need for health care services.
Health indicators may be orientated towards mortality, the prevalence of certain diseases , or the effects of diseases on the quality of life (1,2). In this paper we shall be concerned with the
third variety of health status measures which indicates reductions
of the quality of life due to the occurence of incapacitation, limitations in the capacity to perform usual daily activities, or the
experience of pain and discomfort in the course of a disease.

Health status indicators that measure disease-impacts on the quality
of life have been constructed from various conceptualizations and
components: e.g. days of restricted activities, amount of functional
limitations, number of symptoms and complaints, mental, emotional or
social well-being. In the last decade numerous health status indicators have been devised that select some of these components and
combine them to synthetic indices that are supposed to scale the
continuum between complete well-being and death into successive
levels of health. Prominent examples are the Index of Well-Being (3)
or the Sickness Impact Profile (4).

Our approach to construct and validate health status indicators for
the application in German health services research started with a
multi-component concept of individual health status, that incorporated functional limitations, amount of common complaints, emotional
balance, and social integration. We call this concept "subjective
health" because it reflects subjectively experienced impacts of disease on life from a patient or consumer orientated viewpoint. In
this paper we report results concerning the scalability and validity
of two of the health status components, namely functional limitations and common complaints, in a general population survey.

2. METHODS

2.1 Sample
The data to be presented are based on a survey of the population of
the city of Munich, Bavaria, that was conducted from October 1980 to
February 1981. A random sample of the civilian population of German
nationality living in households was drawn from the municipal register. The initial sample included 2002 persons in the age between
20 and 65. 1384 persons responded to the questionnaire, which means
a response rate of 72% of the pool of correct addresses. The age,
sex, income and occupational characteristics of the respondents corresponded closely to those of the comparable Munich population(5) so
that there is no evidence for a systematic bias due to non-response.

2.2 Health Survey Questionnaire
A health survey questionnaire was developed to gather data on seven
health components and health related variables: functional limitations, commom complaints, emotional balance, social integration,
global ratings of actual health status and chronic impairments, utilization behaviour, disease conditions in the past 12 months, and
additional information on demographic and socioeconomic characteristics of the respondents.

The questionnaire was sent by mail. Two reminders followed. In cases
of non-response interviewers contacted the persons in their homes
and presented the questionnaire personally, but respondents filled
them out by themselves. Previous investigations on survey methodology comparing varying interview strategies did not show any superior quality of personal to mail interviewing(6,7).

2.3 Scales of Functional Limitations (FLS) and Common Complaints
(CCS)
The functional limitations component of the health status measure
should indicate disturbances of elementary functions in daily life
which might be consequences of disease conditions. Most investigators who constructed survey measures for functional limitations explored six categories: physical, self-care, mobility, role, household, and leisure activities (8). For the sake of brevity we concentrated upon mobility (3 items), physical activity (4 items), role
and self-care (3 items), and one item concerning unspecified limitations. Items read e.g.:"Do you spend most of your time indoors because of your health ?" or "Are you unable to perform certain activities regarding your job or household because of your health ?".
Categories for answering were:"never/sometimes/ever".

To measure the amount of complaints we used a list of 24 somatic or
emotional complaints, dysfunctions and misfeelings. Part of the
items is concerned with the general level of vitality, e.g. tired-
ness, boredom, whereas others deal with more specific complaints,
e.g. headaches, or pain in the stomach. The items were selected from
the so-called "Beschwerdenliste"(9), a well-known German check-list
for complaints. As selection device from the original 48 items we
used the ratings of a group of physicians, patients, and blue-collar
workers about the importance of the items for the description of a
person's health status(11). The opening question reads:"How much do
you suffer from the following complaints ?" Answers might be:" Not
at all/scarcely/moderately/strongly".

Computation of scale values for the Functional Limitation Scale
(FLS) and for the Common Complaints Scale (CCS) followed an additive
linear scoring model. We scored the answer categories "0/1/2" in the
case of the functional limitation items and "0/1/2/3" in the case of
the complaints and summed up to the respective scale scores.
Theoretically FLS-scores may vary from zero to 22 and CCS-scores
from zero to 72.

3. RESULTS

3.1 Reliabilities and Distributions of FLS and CCS

To estimate the reliability and homogeneity of the scales we computed internal consistency coefficients (11) for both scales and coefficients of reproducability and scalability of the GUTTMAN-scal-
ing-model (12) for the FLS. Table I gives an overview of the coefficients for the two scaling models.

Table I
RELIABILITY COEFFICIENTS FOR FLS AND CCS

Scale	Index of reproducability	Index of scalability	Internal consistency
Functional limitations	.94	.59	.86
Common complaints	---	---	.93

The GUTTMAN-coefficients for FLS indicate a sufficient degree of
scalability. Internal consistencies of the FLS and CCS are very
high, especially for the CCS. This allows the reduction of the
number of items without substantial loss of reliability for survey
purposes.

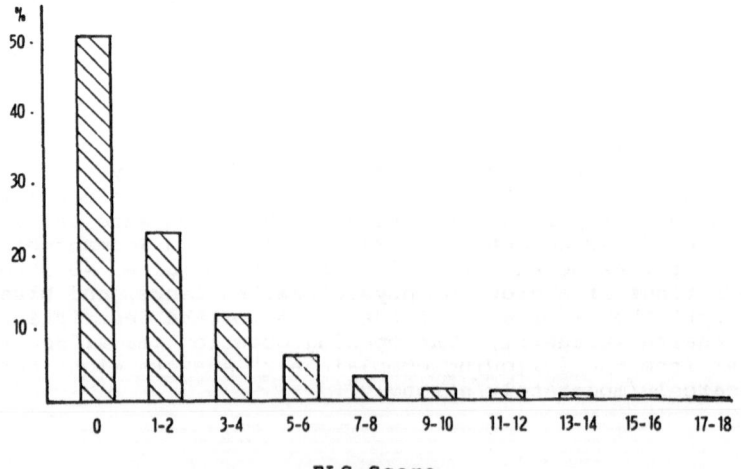

FLS-Score

Figure 1: Functional Limitations in the Munich Population, N=1384

The distributions of scores (see Figures I and II) are highly skewed
to the left, towards the "healthy" ends of the scales. 50% of the
sample report no functional limitations at all. The frequency of
scores declines monotonically and extreme scores occur almost never.
This may be due to the age restriction in the sample and the exclusion of all persons living in hospitals or nursing homes. Special
studies on the prevalence of functional limitations in groups thus
not represented in the sample will be conducted in the
near future. In contrast to the prevalence of functional limitations
only 4% of the sample report no complaints. The distribution is
nevertheless markedly skewed to the left and fades out to the right.
This means that a small amount of complaints with little intensity
is natural in a general population but prevalence of high scores is
low.

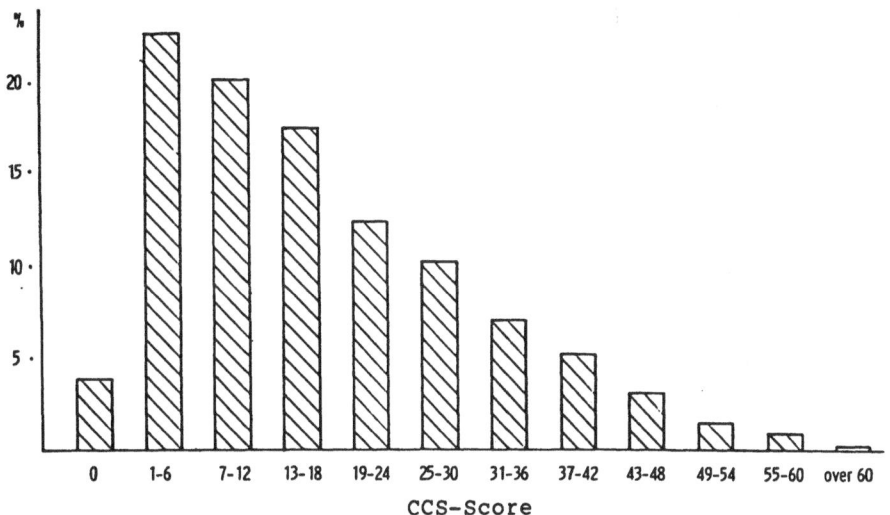

Figure 2: Common Complaints in the Munich Population, N=1384

3.2 Validation of Health Status Components

Preliminary evidence whether the health component scales elict meaningful and representative information about the health status of a
person can be gained by an inspection of the verbal content of the
scale-items themselves. This approach, called content or face validation, should by all means be complemented by an empirical investigation whether the measured constructs fit into a network of health
related variables and whether associations between them follow those
that can be postulated from theory and previous empirical studies.
This procedure of construct validation (3) plays an important role
in demonstrating the explanatory and predictive power of the health
status concepts.

From previous research the following propositions can be made:
a) FLS and CCS shall be strongly and positively related to each other;
b) the amount of functional limitations and complaints shall increase monotonically with age;
c) women shall report more complaints than men;
d) FLS and CCS shall have substantial associations with the number of diseases a person has experienced and with general self-ratings of health status and chronic impairments;
e) FLS and CCS shall be positively related to utilization behavior, namely the number of contacts with physicians and the amount of drug consumption.

An overview of the product-moment-correlations between FLS/CCS and the above variables is presented in Table II. Eta-statistics (with FLS and CCS dependent) allow the evaluation of the linearity of the association.

Table II
ASSOCIATIONS BETWEEN FLS, CCS, AND RELATED VARIABLES

Variables	Functional limitations		Complaints	
	r[1]	eta[2]	r[1]	eta[2]
Age	.36	.38	.25	.27
Sex	.02	.03	.20	.21
Contact to physicians in the past two weeks	.30	.30	.25	.26
Drug consumption in the past two weeks	.41	.42	.46	.45
Number of chronic conditions in the past year	.46	.47	.59	.60
Global rating of actual health status	.40	.48	.46	.57
Global rating of chronic impairments and complaints	.58	.59	.51	.54

[1] Product-moment-correlations
[2] Eta-statistics, functional limitations and complaints dependent

Association between FLS and CCS. The product-moment-correlation between functional limitations and complaints is .58. Eta is .60. The similarity between the two association measures indicates that the relationship is essentially linear.

Age. The associations between functional limitations and complaints are significant but weak (see Table II). Both scores increase monotonically and nearly linearly with age. Functional limitations are more directly related to age. This agrees with the theoretical idea that ageing is accompanied by a loss of functioning and an increase in dependency on other people.

Sex. In agreement with previous research we found that women report more complaints than men. The difference in mean CCS-scores for women (x=20.1) and men (x=14.6) is substantial. It amounts to approximately 9% of the whole range of observed scores. Women suffer especially more from headaches, dizziness, sensitivity to changes in the weather, and anxiety.

Utilization behaviour. Contacts to physicians two weeks prior to the interview (none/one or two/three or more) and amount of drug consumption (regular/occasional/seldom/never) were used to estimate the utilization of medical services. Correlations between FLS/CCS and contacts to physicians are positive but rather weak (see Table II). This may be due to several reasons: a considerable part of contacts to physicians may be motivated by other factors than states of existing diseases, e.g. preventive diagnostic screening for cancer or vaccination. Besides this the recall-period of two weeks is rather short, failing to include longterm periodic visits of chronically ill persons to the doctor. Perceived barriers like long ways to the doctors office or waiting times may hinder the decision to see a doctor in states of minor complaints. Consumption of drugs shows - as predicted - a stronger positive relationship to both health status measures.

Reports of experienced disease and general self-ratings of health. As hypothesized we found strong positive associations between the scores for FLS and CCS and other direct self-ratings of health status. Product-moment-correlations between the health status components and the number of disease conditions in the last 12 month (e.g. rheuma, hypertension), global ratings of chronic impairments (strong/moderate/weak/none), and global assessment of health status in the past two weeks (excellent/good/satisfactory/bad/was ill for shorter or longer period) range between $r=.46$ and $r=.59$ (see Table II). The pattern of correlations reflects that functional limitations are more likely associated with chronic impairements whereas the complaints score may be viewed as an indicator of the actual health status.

4. DISCUSSION

The construction and evaluation of valid, feasible, and acceptable health status indicators has to take several goals and criteria into account. In this paper we reported results on the FLS and the CCS that demonstrated that both health status components can be reliably measured and that their associations with biological variables and other health related constructs demonstrate that they are meaningful and valid operational definitions of health. In addition our health status measures have several practical and theoretical advantages and shortcomings. To start with the advantages:
- The FLS and the CCS provide sensitive descriptive tools for health statuses on various aggregation levels: e.g. individuals, patients of local medical facilities, regional or social population groups, general population. This allows the formulation and testing of very specific hypotheses concerning the distribution and determination of levels of health.
- FLS and the CCS are not restricted to measure specific effects of single diseases on health. So comparisons of the impacts of diverse disease conditions on the quality of life are possible.

On the other hand there are some shortcomings and areas of further development:
- The measurement of health based on the FLS and the CCS does not take into account the case of mortality. Besides the apparent conceptual deficiency this creates the paradox that the longer persons live or the higher the life-expectancy in a population is the more "unhealthy" they will be because of the increase of functional limitations and complaints with age.
- The relevance of our health status concept to the measurement of the effectiveness of medical services on health has yet to be demonstrated empirically.

- In this paper we treated FLS and CCS as seperate health measures.
  To combine them to a unitary index of health requires a model to
  unify both scales. This implies the explicit weighting of the relative importance of both components by relevant actors in the
  health field, e.g. physicians, patients, and health administrators.

To solve these problems further research is necessary. Up to now
first applications of the FLS and the CCS in a community survey on
the prevalence and impacts of hypertension and in an evaluation effort of the effectiveness of German rehabilitation clinics are conducted. We expect that the results of these studies strengthen the
medical validity of our health status measures and support their
usefullness as effectiveness measures for health service purposes.

4. REFERENCES

(1)   SULLIVAN D.F., Conceptual Problems in Developing an Index of
      Health. National Center Statistics, Series 2 No. 17,
      Washington,1966
(2)   MOONEY A., NORFLEET W.R., Measures of Community Health Status
      for Health Planning. Hlth Serv Res. 1978; 13: 129-145
(3)   KAPLAN R.M., BUSH J.W., BERRY C.C., Health Status Indexes:
      Types of Validity and the Index of Well-Being. Hlth Serv Res
      1976; 4: 478-507
(4)   BERGNER M., BOBBITT R., KRESSEL S., et al., The Sickness Impact
      Profile: Conceptual Formulation and Methodology for the
      Development of a Health Status Measure. Int J Hlth Serv 1976;
      6: 393-415
(5)   Statistisches Landesamt der Stadt München, Die Verteilung der
      Nettoeinkommen der Münchener Haushalte. Münchener Statistik
      1980; Heft 4: 86-94
(6)   HOCHSTIM J.R., A Critical Comparison of Three Strategies of
      Collecting Data from Households. J Amer Stat Ass 1967; 62:
      976-989
(7)   SIEMATYCKI J., A Comparison of Mail, Telephone, and Home
      Interviewing Strategies for Household Health Surveys. Amer J
      Publ Hlth 1979; 69: 238-245
(8)   STEWART A.L., WARE J.E., BROOK R.H., et al., Conceptualization
      and Measurement for Adults in the Health Insurance Study: Vol.
      II, Physical Health in Terms of Functioning. Santa Monica. The
      RAND-Corporation 1978
(9)   ZERSSEN D.v., Die Beschwerdenliste. Weinheim. Beltz Verlag 1976
(10) Internationales Institut für wissenschaftliche Zusammenarbeit
      e.V., Entwicklung eines Fragebogens zur Beurteilung des
      Gesundheitszustandes und zur Einschätzung des Erfolgs von
      stationären Heilbehandlungen (1978/79).Schloß Reisensburg.
      Forschungsbericht 1981
(11) LORD F.M., NOVICK M.R., Statistical Theory of Mental Test
      Scores. Reading. Addison-Wesley 1968
(12) SIXTL F., Meßmethoden der Psychologie. Beltz Verlag. Weinheim
      1967

STATISTICAL COMPARISON OF TWO RADIOGRAPHIC METHODS FOR SCREENING FOR CANCER OF THE BREAST [x]

by

H. Prestele [1] and E.M. Paterok [2]

[1] Institute of Medical Statistics and Documentation
(Director: Prof. Dr. L. Horbach)

[2] Department of Obstetrics and Gynecology
(Director: Prof. Dr. K.G. Ober)
University of Erlangen-Nuremberg, Erlangen, Germany

1. Introduction

Mammography permits detection of cancer of the breast before the malignancy becomes clinically apparent. This widely used and indispensable method involves some radiation hazard for the patient however. A few years ago, the so-called "low-dose" film-screen combination was developed for mammography (1, 2). By the use of that film-foil combination, the radiation exposure for the patient can be lowered significantly, approximately by a factor of 10, as compared with the use of an industrial non-screen film, e.g. "KODAK Definix Medical".

This paper deals with the question, whether this new technique is valid and appropriate for screening for cancer of the breast. If low-dose pictures would basically result in the same findings for all types of breasts, the method would even allow for repeated x-ray investigations in an individual patient while keeping the total accumulated dose of radiation below the level received by the patient during a single shot using the conventional method. As a result, the efficiency of the screening procedure might be improved with simultaneous reduction of the radiation hazard for the patient.

---

[x] Supported by the Deutsche Forschungsgemeinschaft, Sonderforschungsbereich 118: Methods of Early Detection and Evaluation of Processing of Cancer.

2. Planning of the Study

Figure 1 shows the principal standard views used in mammography. We determined that radiographic views should be taken in the oblique direction both by the conventional and the low-dose technique.

Figure 1:
Standard views, mammography

1. cran.-caud. view
2. oblique projection
3. med.-lat. view

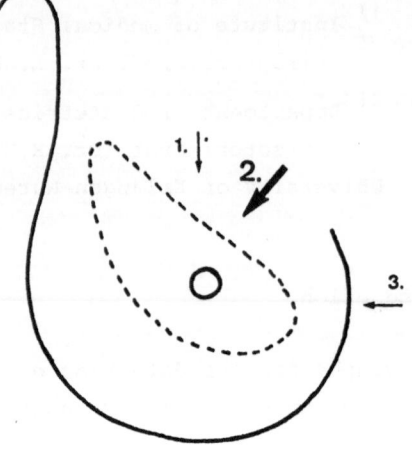

Accurate interpretation depends upon detection of significant micro- and macro-calcifications and evaluation of the low-contrast soft-tissue structures of the mammary gland. But, remarkable findings may only be possible indicators of a malignant status of the breast, since cancer cannot be diagnosed directly by mammography. To get objective results, these criteria should be reviewed independently for the two pictures, but by only one radiologist to avoid a possible bias due to different examinators. In order to satisfy this condition, the radiologist should not be able to "search" in one picture the characteristics of the other. Therefore, the two pictures are to be diagnosed in a randomized sequence and the second picture at least two months after the first one. Because of the large number of pictures to be reviewed, remembering the corresponding findings by the first diagnostic method can almost be ruled out.

3. The Statistical Model

Just as the technical conditions, the statistical model and the analysis of the study was planned before the patients had been investigated. First, some notations shall be explained:

When a population is screened, one may consider the following numbers (table I):

M = number of individuals attending the screening
N = number of cases of disease at the screening
s = number of cases of disease detected during the screening
a = number of false positives at the screening
c = number of false negatives at the screening

Result of Screening	True disease status		total
	present (D_+)	absent (D_-)	
positive (S_+)	N - c	a	s
negative (S_-)	c	M - N - a	M - s
total	N	M - N	M

Table I: Subjects classified by true disease status (D) and result of screening (S).

Let Se be the probability that the screening detects a diseased patient. Clearly, Se is the sensitivity of the screening method. Equivalently, the specificity Sp is the probability of screening negatively if the individual is truly negative. If all the numbers of table I are known, Se and Sp are estimated as

$$\widehat{Se} = (N - c) / N \qquad\qquad (3.1)$$

$$\widehat{Sp} = (M - N - a) / (M - N) \qquad\qquad (3.2)$$

In our study, we consider a screening program in which patients are screened by two different methods. The following notations are used in accordance with table II:

s_i = number of cases of disease detected at the i-th screening (i=1,2)
b = number of cases of disease detected at both screenings
S_{i+} = i-th screening method positive (i=1,2)
S_{i-} = i-th screening method negative (i=1,2).

Table II represents the situation of our study in such a way that, in accordance with radiological possibility, D_+ means the existence of macro- or micro-calcification or irregular mass density respectively. These symptoms may occur alone or in combination and are possible

Result of Screening		True disease status present (D_+) absent (D_-)		total
positive	$(S_{1+}S_{2+})$ $(S_{1+}S_{2-})$	b $s_1 - b$ $s_2 - b$	a	s
negative	$(S_{1-}S_{2+})$ $(S_{1-}S_{2-})$	c	$M - N - a$	$M - s$
total		N	$M - N$	M

Table II: Subjects classified by true disease status (D) and result of two screening methods (S_1 and S_2).

indicators for cancer. The use of the conventional radiographic method, say S_1, may yield a positive (S_{1+}) or a negative (S_{1-}) result of the screening, i.e. it may detect the one item D examined. In both cases, cancer may be present or absent. Analogous notations hold for the low-dose technique S_2.

The aim of this study is to examine whether the two screening methods result in the same radiologic diagnosis, especially for patients with cancer of the breast. Thus, estimating the sensitivities of the two methods and comparing them with respect to the clinical importance of the findings was preferred to statistical tests, e.g. McNemar's test for dependent frequencies.

Usually, the numbers of true positives and negatives are not observed. The number of true positive cases of disease in the population is the number of observed positive cases during the screening who are truly diseased plus the unidentified false negatives. Therefore, a binomial capture-recapture model according to the paper of GOLDBERG and WITTES (3) was taken into consideration to estimate the unknown value N of diseased patients and the sensitivity of each screening method.

The classical capture-recapture problem estimates the number N of fish in a lake: s_1 fish are caught, marked, and returned to the lake. When the marked animals have freely mingled with the unmarked, a random sample of size s_2 is caught, of which b are found to be marked. The biased maximum likelihood estimator of the total number of fish in the lake is

$$\hat{N} = s_1 s_2 / b \qquad (3.3).$$

As shown in (3) or (4), a nearly unbiased estimator of N is

$$\hat{N} = (s_1 + 1) (s_2 + 1) / (b + 1) - 1 \qquad (3.4).$$

The use of the same letters is intended to explain the correspondence between the capture-recapture model and the underlying screening program. Thus, the numbers of fish of the first respectively of the second capture correspond to the numbers of patients screened positively by the low-dose (s_1) respectively by the conventional (s_2) technique. The number b of marked fish out of the second sample corresponds to the number of patients detected by both screening methods.

As outlined in the paper of GOLDBERG and WITTES (3), it is assumed that a = 0 (cf. table II). In practice, this is equivalent to assuming that all false positives are identified by subsequent clinical evaluation. The sensitivities of the two methods are then estimated as

$$\widehat{Se}_1 = b / s_2 \quad (\text{if } s_2 \neq 0) \tag{3.5}$$

$$\widehat{Se}_2 = b / s_1 \quad (\text{if } s_1 \neq 0) \tag{3.6}.$$

4. Results

During a period of 18 months, all 3.987 patients of our outpatients' department entered the study. 7.375 breasts were x-rayed in the oblique direction both by the standard technique (S_1) and by the low-dose film-foil combination (S_2). Table III gives a survey of the radiological findings.

	Macro-calcification	Micro-calcification	Tumour, mass density
S_1+S_2+	1.221	1.662	1.714
S_1+S_2-	3	10	4
S_1-S_2+	8	4	7
S_1-S_2-	6.143	5.699	5.650
total	7.375	7.375	7.375

Table III: Radiological findings of 7.375 breasts of 3.987 patients, simultaneously screened by conventional (S_1) and low-dose (S_2) mammography.

More detailed informations mainly of clinical importance are reported in (2), for instance the fact that some micro-calcifications detected only by the conventional mammography were small calcific deposits in breasts of very dense tissue, or that skin, nipple and subcutaneous areas were demonstrated best by the low-dose radiograms.

The correspondence of the two methods was surprisingly high, for
instance only in 4 + 7 = 11 cases the reports differed with respect
to detection of tumours. Clearly, for many breasts there was no indication for further investigation despite of radiological findings.
Thus, in only 461 breasts invasive clarification was needed in accordance with the total medical evidence (palpation, sonography a.s.
o.). In 154 out of these cases, a carcinoma was diagnosed by histological examination. Table IV shows the results of this group.

	Macro-calcification	Micro-calcification	Tumour, mass density
$S_{1+}S_{2+}$	55	75	146
$S_{1+}S_{2-}$	1	0	0
$S_{1-}S_{2+}$	1	1	0
$S_{1-}S_{2-}$	97	78	8
total	154	154	154
$\hat{N}$	58	76	146
$\hat{Se}_1$	0.98	0.99	1.0
$\hat{Se}_2$	0.98	1.0	1.0

Table IV: Radiological findings of 154 malignant mammary
glands; $\hat{N}$: estimated totals: (3.4), $\hat{Se}_i$: estimated sensitivity (i=1,2): (3.5), (3.6).

Cancer was associated with detectable macro- and micro-calcifications in about 37% respectively 50% of the cases. In about 95%, con-
spicuous tumours were found, if at all, by both screening methods.
Applying formula (3.4) separately to the three diagnostic items, it
is seen in table IV that $\hat{N}$ underestimates the number of malignant
breasts. Furthermore, we are interested in the sensitivity of each
screening method, i.e. the probability of detecting a cancer if it
truly exists. The estimated values according to formula (3.5) and
(3.6) are all equal to or close to 1.0. Since they are related to the
number of cases detected by mammography only, they cannot signify the
essential sensitivities of the two methods and therefore the merit of
the mere values is rather poor. These results are based on the fact
that principally a cancer may be undetectable when one restricts the
investigation to a single characteristic and even when using mammography only. Also in our study, a cancer was found by other medical
investigations in 3 cases where mammography did not give a hint for

the existence of a malignant lesion.

Despite of these facts, the low number of cases in which the two screening methods differed and the close correlation of the corresponding sensitivities favour the low-dose technique. It was demonstrated that the low-dose mammography results in the same radiologic diagnosis in nearly all breasts. Because of lower radiation exposure for the patient, the low-dose technique should be preferred as compared with conventional mammography.

Summary

7.375 breasts were x-rayed both by conventional mammography and by a new technique with lower radiation exposure for the patient. Independent evaluation of the two pictures was related to detection of calcifications and irregular mass densities which are possible indicators for cancer. The correspondence of radiological findings was surprisingly high. Therefore, the application of a capture-recapture model resulted in almost equal but overestimated sensitivities for the two methods. Despite of this, the close correlation of the two methods favours the low-dose technique because of lower radiation exposure for the patient.

References

(1) Friedrich M. Neue technische Entwicklungen der Röntgen- und Ultraschalluntersuchungen der Mamma. Röntgenpraxis 1981; 34: 181-195.
(2) Paterok EM, Säbel M, Weishaar J, Prestele H. Klinische Erprobung der Mammographie mit Film-Folien-Kombinationen. Röntgenpraxis (in press).
(3) Goldberg JD, Wittes JT. The Estimation of False Negatives in Medical Screening. Biometrics 1978; 34: 77-86.
(4) Darroch JN. The Multiple-Recapture Census; I. Estimation of a Closed Population. Biometrika 1958; 45: 343-359.

Correspondence should be addressed to:

Dr. Hans Prestele
Institut für Medizinische Statistik und Dokumentation
Waldstr. 6
D 8520 Erlangen
Fed. Rep. of Germany

COST-BENEFIT ANALYSIS IN INTENSIVE CARE MEDICINE.

Lis Dragsted, Qvist J, Janstrup F, Johansen SH.
Department of anesthesia, Herlev Hospital, 2730 Herlev, Denmark and
Danish Institute for Clinical Epidemiology, Svanemøllevej 25,
2100 Copenhagen, Denmark.

SUMMARY.

By using many resources the intensive care units have been much critic-
sed.   The use of cost-benefit analysis on intensive therapy can show
what is cost-effective and what is cost-ineffective.   It is emphasized
that cost-benefit analysis concern the treatment of patient or disease
categories, not the single patient.   To avoid the most cost-ineffective
it is important to avoid patients in the end-stage of a disease and
this stresses the importance of the early recognition of the end-stage
patient.   The cost-benefit analysis can be of use when establishing
criterias for selection of patients for intensive therapy.

The number of intensive care units (ICU) has increased considerably during the last twenty years and such units are now found in
almost all acute hospitals.

Despite the improved survival rates from diseases that formerly
were considered mortal, the ICU have been viewed with criticism
especially because of the resources used in ICU for the benefit of a
"few" patients.   The ICU's require qualified personnel, advanced
technology, expensive drugs and space in order to provide optimal care.
By many it is considered as waste of money.

The problem is if it is such a bad investment to have ICU's, this
question is almost impossible to answer.   A possible solution to the
problem is to make a cost-benefit analysis on the intensive therapy.

The benefit must be the patients survival, preferably totally
restored to normal health status.   Here is made the assumption that
the patients would have died if not treated in the ICU.   The next
assumption is that the longer lifetime after discharge the better
benefit for the patients.   The costs can be calculated as the financial
expenditures; it is a useful, but not a perfect reflection of the costs.

It is necessary here to emphasize that cost-benefit analysés are
concerning patient or disease categories, not the single patient, determining what are cost-effective and what are cost-ineffective.   To use
the cost-benefit in determining the treatment of the single patient is
impossible.

H.Bendixen (1977) (1,2) did propose this model for estimating the cost-benefit of intensive therapy, which we have found very useful.

$$\frac{cost}{benefit} = \frac{cost\ per\ day\ \times\ length\ of\ stay}{survival\ fraction\ \times\ expected\ lifetime}$$

This gives the cost per year of survival for one survivor. This is
based on the former mentioned assumptions, that the survival is due to
intensive therapy and that the alternative to intensive care is demise.

The cost per day varies with the therapeutic intervention needed
and can roughly be divided into 3 groups, one for critically ill patients who need maximal therapeutic efforts, in our unit it amounts to
approximately 2500 $ per day; the next group of patients demand a
lesser therapeutic effort and the cost per day is approximately 1200 $,
and the last group consists of patients who do not require many therapeutic interventions, but still cannot be treated in the ordinary ward;
these cost about 700 $ per day.

The survival fraction gives the fraction of the number of patients
in the disease group who survived the hospitalization, a high survival
fraction is found, i.e. patients with a diabetic ketoacidosis, whereas
a low survival fraction is found i.e. patients with a cirrhotic liver
and upper gastrointestinal bleeding.

The expected lifetime is the number of years that the average
survivor may be expected to live after discharge from the hospital.
This is the determinant factor in the equation. The best cost-benefit
ratio is found in the young patient with a high survival fraction and
a long expected lifetime, whereas the worst cost-benefit ratio is found
in patients with a poor survival and a short expected lifetime. The
cost-benefit in treating the young patient who can be restored to normal
or near normal lifespan is better than in treating an elderly patient
with the same disease.

It is easy to find predictions of remaining lifespan for any given
age group of the normal population, but for patients who have been
critically ill there does not yet exist any reliable data concerning
their remaining lifespan. Furthermore only very few data are available
concerning the quality of life after discharge. In our studies we
have found that one year after discharge about 50% of the surviving
patients are back in normal activity, about 50% are in limited activity,
a few percent are still hospitalized, while approximately 45% of the
admitted patients have died. This distribution has also been found
by LeGall et al. (3) and Cullen et al. (4). More specified data on
the quality of life does not exist presently and a prospective study
would be very cumbersome and time consuming, besides being very expensive.

This model for cost-benefit analysis shall not be used in the decision whether a patient shall be treated in the ICU or not, but it can be used in the evaluation of which disease categories that can be admitted to the ICU.

As shown the worst cost-benefit is found in treating end-stage diseases. It would be very valuable to find out what characterizes the patient with end-stage disease that is not considered for admission to the ICU. Often such a patient has been followed and evaluated for a long time and the decision on therapy in the end-stage has often been taken. ICU has no role to play when the patient has reached the end-stage, and intensive therapy can only prolong the end, only making it more painful and even more costly than necessary.

REFERENCES.

1. Bendixen HH (1977) In: Costs, Risks and Benefits of Surgery, p.372. Editors: J.P.Bunker, B.A.Barnes and F.Mosteller. Oxford University Press, New York, N.Y.
2. Bendixen HH (1981) In: Anaesthesiology. Proceedings of the 7th World Congress of Anaesthesiologist Hamburg, September 14-21 1980. Editors: E.Rügheimer, M.Zwidler. Excerpta Medica. Amsterdam-Oxford-Princeton.
3. Le Gall JR, Latournerie J, Plevin D, Trunet P, Candau P. Evaluation de l'etat de santé avant et apres hospitalisation en reanimation (1981) In: Medical Informatics Europe 81. Editors: F.Gremy, P. Degoulet, B.Barber and R.Solamon. Springer Verlag, Berlin-Heidelberg-New York.
4. Cullen DJ, Ferrara LC, Briggs BA, Walker PF, Gilbert I. Survival, hospitalization charges and follow-up results in critically ill patients. N.Eng.J.Med. 1976; 294:982.

ARE COMPUTERS USED APPROPRIATELY IN PREVENTIVE CHILD HEALTH?

C. Hopton[1], J. Davison[2], H. Fearn[3], J.A. Beal[3] and A.J. Hedley[2]

1 Nottinghamshire Area Health Authority. 2 Department of Community Health, University of Nottingham. 3 Derbyshire Area Health Authority.

SUMMARY

Standard computerised systems have been developed to facilitate the delivery of preventive child health care. Technical details of these systems have been described elsewhere[1,2], but there have been no evaluation studies which have examined the impact of computerised systems on the overall process of preventive child health. This paper describes some results of such a project in a health authority using a computerised child health system. The introduction of computers imposed some degree of structure and uniformity on records and the collection of clinical information, and improved access to records. However the reliability and quality of recorded information was variable. Links between computer and manual records were poor and files did not hold information which would allow screening procedures to be evaluated. Computer-based scheduling procedures were subject to delays because of batch processing methods. The conclusion is drawn that the further development of computer-assisted child health records requires radical rethinking.

1. INTRODUCTION

1.1 The computerised systems which have been developed for use in community child health services have two basic functions:

i)   the scheduling of appointments for vaccination and immunisation, and screening examinations.

ii) the recording of information which is potentially of use for planning, monitoring and evaluation purposes.

1.2 In the course of this study it was possible to gain some insight into the efficiency of the scheduling and information storage functions and the overall contribution of these to community child health services.

2. METHODS

2.1 The principal aim of the study was to examine the quality of
information in child health records which document the activities
which together comprise preventive child health care. Both computer
and manual based methods of record keeping were investigated.

Two sampling frames for children were derived from the 1976 birth
register of the Derbyshire Area Health Authority:
> One sampling frame comprised children born and still living at
> the time of the study in small urban towns along the eastern
> Derbyshire border.
> The other sampling frame comprised children born and still living
> at the time of the study in Derby City.

For historical reasons, relating to the administration of health
services before the 1974 National Health Service reorganisation, the
Derby City children were not included in a computerised developmental
screening programme, although they were eligible for immunisation and
hearing test programmes which were computer assisted. The children
from the east Derbyshire towns were eligible for the full computer
assisted programme of developmental screening. A study of these two
groups provided an opportunity to compare the completeness, consistency
and utility of information on manual and computer held records, and the
uptake of immunisation and screening procedures. The final samples were
derived by a multi-stage sampling technique which for the east Derbyshire
sample yielded 154 children in the care of 17 health visitors in 5
different urban centres (Sample 1). The Derby City group comprised 147
children in the care of 14 health visitors in 5 areas in Derby (Sample 2).

2.2 Access was provided to all manual records relating to the preventive
health care of these children from 0 to 2 years of age. Additionally all
corresponding computer records for children in both samples were examined.
A number of variables including birth weight, maternal age and parity
were compared for the two samples, but no evidence of unequal distribution
of bias was found.

3. RESULTS

3.1 Number of records in use and the quality of information documented

For both samples the main repository of information on each child was a semi-structured child health record book. This is designed to hold the structured forms completed for birth notification, neonatal discharge, immunisation consent and the first health visitor report, which are initially used as computer input documents. The record books also contain a variable amount of hand written unstructured data on immunisations, screening examinations, clinic attendances and home visits.

Additional manual record sources of information were clinic cards held at the 'well baby' clinic attended, and for the Derby City children there were further manual records, developmental progress charts, completed by health visitors. Computer-held records for both samples of children included the initial birth data, results of immunisation and hearing test procedures and for the east Derbyshire group details of developmental screening examinations.

The main findings from examination of these records are summarised below:

Completeness of information

Information relating to statutory documents, ie birth notification and initial health visit, was relatively complete, whereas information derived from non-statutory documents was variable and frequently incomplete. For example, in Sample 1 15% of discharge forms and related data were missing. Computer output and/or written entries detailing the results of immunisation and hearing test procedures were missing from many manual records (Table I).

	1st	2nd	3rd	Measles
Sample 1	2.7 (4)	5.1 (7)	1.6 (2)	4.8 (5)
Sample 2	59.7 (83)	37.6 (50)	9.8 (12)	8.4 (8)

TABLE I

Proportion of completed immunisations (Diphtheria/Tetanus/Pertussis/Polio/Measles) with no entry in the manual child health record.

For the Derby City children (Sample 2) who had not been part of the computerised screening programme, references to screening examinations carried out by health visitors were recorded on a number of different unstructured documents which were not linked (Table II).

	Record type	Total no. of entries	Cases where entry appears exclusively in this record type
1	Child health record	339	65
2	Clinic notes	43	5
3	Developmental progress chart	407	116
4	Form 10M	24	8

TABLE II

Use of clinical records by health visitors and medical officers for recording developmental assessments in Sample 1; distribution of entries in different record types.

For the east Derbyshire children in the computerised programme references to examinations in the child health record were more systematic but were confined to manually recorded unstructured notes and did not necessarily include information archived in the computer.

Consistency of information

For the data captured on the birth notification and other structured forms there was a high level of consistency between computer and manual records in both samples, but inconsistencies on computer and manual records were found with the information relating to immunisations and screening tests. For example, stated dates for the procedures in computer and manual records were most frequently at variance, which for development examinations occurred in 1 in 5 records.

Utility of information

Extraction of information from manual records was laborious, time-consuming and inefficient, lack of structure and missing information being the main problems. Computer records provided readily

accessible data, but the value of much of the information was
questionable. For example, the diagnoses recorded at developmental
examinations and archived on computer comprised a wide range of
conditions from 'napkin rash' to congenital dislocation of the hip.
It was apparent that some of the conditions recorded were 'inactive'
problems while others were current conditions perhaps revealed by
the examination or already known and reported by the parent.
For both samples there was no information in the routine records,
for example from general practice or hospital record sources, which
would have allowed further investigation of the validity of
diagnoses.

3.2 Uptake of immunisation and screening procedures

Both samples of children were eligible for the computer assisted immunisation and hearing test programmes. The uptake of immunisation was
similar in the two groups and was higher than the national average.
However 1 in 20 children received no doses of vaccine and of the remainder
1 in 12 received only partial courses. Eight children out of the total of
301 received more than the recommended three doses of primary Triple or
Diphtheria/Tetanus vaccine. For hearing tests information from the
computer file indicated that 90% of the east Derbyshire sample were
screened compared with 80% of the Derby City children (approximate 95%
confidence limits being 94 - 84% and 87 - 73% respectively).

Records of developmental screening showed that in the Derby City group
screened by health visitors, the proportion of children seen at any of the
prescribed examinations was lower than in the computer scheduled group.
Eighty percent of children in the computer programme group received three
assessments, whereas 74% of children in the non-computer group received
three or more assessments. In the groups of children for whom developmental examinations were eventually completed, long delays occurred
beyond the recommended examination date for up to 20% of the population.
These delays tended to be longer in the computer group.

4. DISCUSSION

4.1 The results raise a number of important issues. First, where

computer assisted methods are introduced there are likely to be potential
benefits in terms of the efficiency of specific surveillance activities.
Reasonably high uptake rates for immunisation and for developmental
screening in the computer group demonstrate this. The question must be
asked whether this was the direct result of a computer system or due to
the introduction of a system where none previously existed. Second,
there were problems in fitting batch processing to the practical working
of health visitors, with consequent inefficiency of the scheduling system
producing delays and sometimes confusion. Many of these problems might
be alleviated with closer monitoring of the overall function of the
system, but equally they are likely to be inherent features of scheduling
procedures which are entirely dependent on very large scale batch
processing systems. Third, the impact of computer-assisted records on
the continuity of care may not necessarily be the positive one that has
been claimed[3]. Unless routine feedback of information on screening and
immunisation and the correct handling of this output is assured then
coordination of the different components of preventive child health will
not be promoted. The system studied did not generate a 'hard copy' report
on examinations or provide periodic routine feedback of results. If
health visitors and others are not provided with such information then
they can have no clear basis for planning the allocation of their time and
skills to the different children and families on their caseload. In both
systems the use of multiple records stored in different locations
increased the difficulty of extracting information. Although the
computer system led to some reduction in the number of records in use
there was no attempt to link those used by different personnel.

4.2 The contribution of computerised systems to the collection of data
for research and management purposes needs reassessment. Computer-
assisted records can greatly facilitate access to data, however in this
study the information which was complete and accurate was usually already
available from existing information systems, eg OPCS returns. The uptake
of screening procedures may be enhanced and can be monitored more easily
with computerised systems, but in this study appropriate information
necessary for their evaluation was not archived.

5. CONCLUSIONS

It is necessary to consider how far the findings of this study can be
generalised and in particular how they relate to the potential effects
of the new National Child Health Computing System. The main conclusion
of this paper is that there are fundamental problems in creating,
maintaining and linking health records in preventive child health.
There are still important gaps between the setting of objectives for
collecting this type of health information and its use either for care
of individuals, predicting risk in subgroups of the population under
surveillance or for measuring the efficiency and effectiveness of
services. There are likely to be many difficulties in the use of a
large scale centralised register with batch processing methods to meet
the needs of health personnel and clients in this type of clinical
activity. With better links between records, personnel and tasks and
the use of interactive systems, for example based on dedicated microcomputers, computer assisted records may be able to make a much more
valuable contribution than is the case at present.

REFERENCES

1. Department of Health and Social Security (1979). The Standard Child
   Health System - Pre-School Health. An Outline.
2. Parkinson J.S. (1979). A Review of the National Standard Child
   Health Computer System and its Potential Benefits. Proceedings of
   MIE 78. Cambridge.
3. Walker C. (1980). 'Batch' or 'On-line' for Child Health - a Review.
   Brit Med J 2 : 90 - 92.

ACKNOWLEDGEMENTS

This study was supported in part by a grant from the Trent Regional
Health Authority.

ON THE EVALUATION OF SOME CORONARY CARE UNITS

C.L.Tuinstra (1), K.I.Lie (2), A v.d.Laarse (3)

(1) Dept Medical Information Processing
Medical Faculty, PB 9500
LEIDEN,the Netherlands
(2) Dept Cardiology, Amsterdam
(3) Dept Cardiobiochemistry, Leiden

1.0 SUMMARY.

The evaluation of treatment of patients with heart diseases in
six coronary care units (CCU) in the Netherlands is described.
According to the preliminary diagnosis, about 32% of the admitted
patients have suspected, acute or recent infarction. Results are
presented which show differences and similarities between CCU's.
Relations of clinical entities with infarction size as determined by
biochemical methods are shown.

2.0 INTRODUCTION.

The Interuniversity Cardiological Institute embraces a
cooperation of the cardiological departments of six Dutch university
hospitals. The Institute stimulates and coordinates research in
cardiological fields.   One of the current projects evaluates the
treatment in the CCU, the prognostic value of certain variables and
the effect of interventions in patients with coronary heart disease.

The problem in evaluation of treatment is quite often the lack
of a firm reference and the fact that not all types of treatment can
be evaluated in double blind studies. To be able to compare the
treatment results in the different CCU's this project establishes a
common clinical database for all patients in the participating
CCU's.

While the hospitals are located throughout the country and
while the CCU's developed completely autonomously their own specific
routines in the patient care, very strict rules for the
datacollection were necessary to avoid that variables would have
different meaning in the different CCU's. It needed a strong effort
to have all participants agree on the layout and content of the
necessary forms, and to have the forms completed regularly (1).

3.0 DATACOLLECTION.

Data on patient history,previous treatment on CCU and discharge
information are collected on forms. In the present stage of the
project these forms are mailed to the data-coordination centre

(Leiden) where they are screened and entered into a common database. Integration of the datacollection in the Hospital Information System ZIS (2) is under developement. This will offer the possibility of on-line, on-site data quality control.

One of the most important variables to be registrated is the quantitative measurement of the infarction size. It is determined by means of the enzyme method described by Rosalki (3) and Witteveen (4) using alpha hydroxy butyraat dehydrogenase (HBDH). This enzyme has the advantage that the release is rather slow, so that infarction size can also be estimated in patients who came in with 24 hours delay, and that blood sampling can be limited to once a day. Moreover , the biochemical test is relatively easy to standardize and is available in all centres. Reference samples are sent to the participants at regular intervals to maintain quality control on the quantitative measurements.

The participating CCU's send their completed forms to Leiden where the database is updated on a daily base and review reports are sent to the participants every week.

4.0   RESULTS.

Up to october 1981, more than 4000 cases were registrated in the database. They come from the six CCU's over a period of about one year.The preliminary diagnosis of the patients is 22% angina pectoris, 32% suspect, acute or recent infarction, 20% rhythm disturbances, 10% pumpfunction problems, 10% atypical angina and 6% other diagnoses.

4.1 Differences between CCU's.

From the many variables we choose a small number to be presented in this paper to show differences and similarities in the CCU's. Figure 1 shows the distribution of sexes in the populations. Each bar represents a participating CCU, except for the leftmost, which represents the sum of all CCU's. There is very little difference between the populations. In all places 70% of the patients are male and 30% are female. This figure has been constant since the start of the study. Figure 2 shows the age distribution, which is typical for each CCU. The patients in hospital 1 are significantly older than in hospital 4.

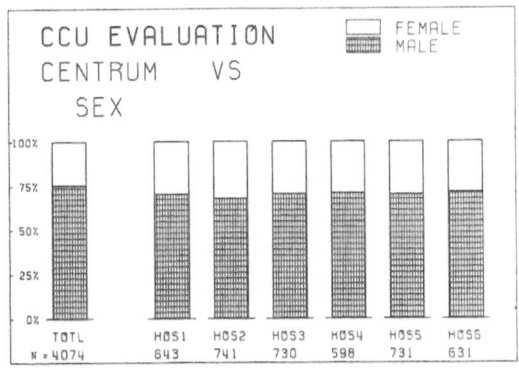

figure 1. Sex distribution in the different hospitals.

Table I shows that the social circumstances of the population in hospital 1 may be different from hospital 2 where less 'non-workers' are admitted. Table II shows mortality in the CCU. There are two hospitals in which the mortality is high (>10%) with respect to the other hospitals. Although the age distribution might have a some influence, we have as yet no explanation.

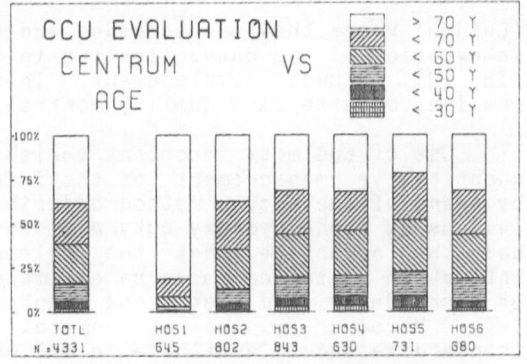

figure 2. Age distribution in the different hospitals.

TABLE I   CENTRUM vs SOCIAL ACTIVITY

	Worked 100%	partially	not working	not applic.	unknown
HOSPITAL 1	91	49	127	23	24
HOSPITAL 2	317	117	152	153	17
HOSPITAL 3	238	107	266	161	24
HOSPITAL 4	227	132	194	13	52
HOSPITAL 5	284	96	203	34	114
HOSPITAL 6	279	95	192	100	10
TOTAL	1436	596	1134	484	241

TABLE II   CENTRUM vs MORTALITY on CCU

	Dead on CCU	Survival
HOSPITAL 1	77	568
HOSPITAL 2	24	738
HOSPITAL 3	90	708
HOSPITAL 4	23	598
HOSPITAL 5	32	699
HOSPITAL 6	39	641
TOTAL	285	3952

4.2 Relation of observations with infarction size.

Table III shows the relation of some clinical entities with infarction size as estimated 96 hours after the onset of complaints. This infarction size can be computed in about 10% of all admitted patients, and in 25% of all patients with a preliminary diagnosis "infarction". The size cannot be calculated if the infarction is too old or if the patient leaves the CCU within 48 hours. No blood samples are taken if the patient has a prelimanary diagnosis of 'rhythm disturbances'.

TABLE III.

INFARCTION SIZE DEPENDENCE.

Infarction size in U/l	Mortality on CCU Dead on CCU	Surv.	Preliminary Diagnosis Angina Pecto.	Recent Infarct	ECG at admission Normal Q	Pathol Q	AV conduction delay Normal	2 + 3 cond del
< 300	0	48	7	6	25	7	40	1
301-450	0	45	2	5	20	20	38	0
- 600	2	39	2	6	16	17	28	1
- 750	1	33	2	3	14	17	26	1
- 900	1	26	0	4	8	15	23	0
- 1050	3	26	0	3	7	20	22	0
- 1200	1	30	3	3	12	17	20	0
- 1350	1	26	0	7	8	16	23	0
- 1500	1	17	0	6	5	13	12	0
- 1650	1	18	1	4	5	14	13	2
- 1800	1	13	0	4	2	10	12	0
- 1950	2	13	0	5	4	11	8	2
- 2100	4	9	0	3	0	12	10	1
- 2250	2	13	1	6	1	13	10	2
- 2400	0	5	0	0	1	4	5	0
- 2550	0	2	0	0	1	1	0	1
- 2700	0	6	0	1	1	5	5	0
- 2850	0	4	0	1	0	4	2	0
- 3000	0	2	0	0	0	2	1	0
> 3000	1	6	0	2	0	6	6	0
P =	0.01		< 0.001		< 0.001		0.02	

Table III. Infarction size dependence of mortality,preliminary diagnosis and ECG. Absolute frequency is tabulated in classes of 150 U/l. P-values according to Kolmogorov-Smirnov non-parametric tests.

The infarction size distributions have a non-Gaussian shape, there is a long 'tail' towards the higher size values. Therefore we used the Kolmogorov-Smirnov non-parametric test to judge the significance level of observered differences. Figure 3 and figure 4 illustrate the numbers given in table III.

Significant size differences (p < 0.01) occur between those who died on CCU and the survivors.

The preliminary diagnosis seems to estimate the infarct size rather well. Sizes are significantly larger (p < 0.001) in 'Acute infarction' than in 'Stable angina pectoris'.

Highly significant differences are found between patients with pathological Q-waves in their ECG at admission (p <0.001), and those without abnormal Q-waves. Second and third degree AV-block occur more frequently with larger infarctions. (p=0.02)

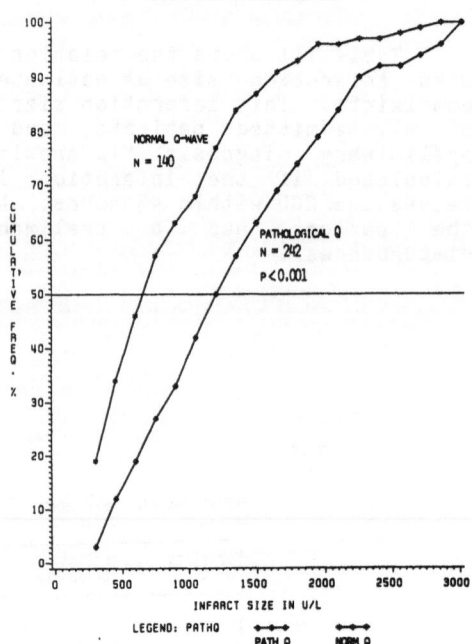

CUMULATIVE FREQUENCY FOR (NON) TRANSMURAL INFARCTS

figure 3

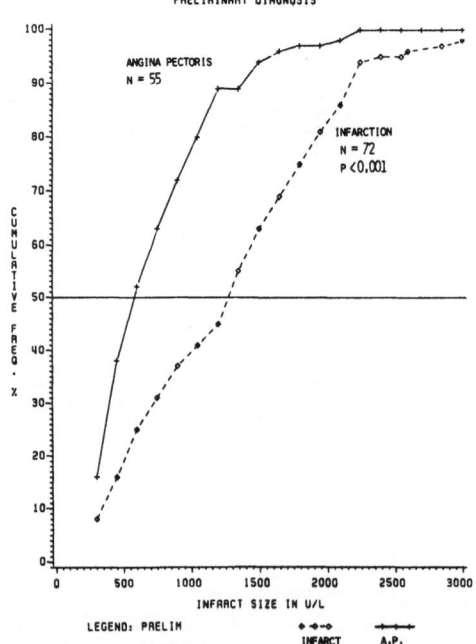

CUMULATIVE DISTRIBUTION FOR A.P. VS INFARCTION

figure 4.

5.0 DISCUSSION.

While the project is in full progress, not many conclusions can be drawn. It has turned out that organisation of datacollection at different places in a strictly uniform way is difficult, but possible.

The feasibility of the calculation of infarction size from HBDH enzyme on a routine base has been shown.

6.0 REFERENCES.

(1) Tuinstra CL, e.a. : A dataprocessing structure to registrate data from geograffically dispersed CCU's. in : Medical Informatics Europe 81', Springer Verlag, Berlin, 1981, 253-257.
(2) Bakker AR, : Scope and limitations of a mini-based centralized hospital information system. in : Medinfo 80', eds Lindberg DAB and Kaihara S, North Holland Publ., Amsterdam, 1980, 505-9.
(3) Rosalki SB and Wilkinson JH : 'Reduction of alphaketo butyrate by human serum. in Nature (London) 1960 ; 188; pp 1110-1111.
(4) Witteveen SAGJ,e.a. :"Quantitation of infarct size in man,

by means of plasma enzyme levels.' Brt Heart J. ; 1975;37;

pp 795-803.

Northwest-German Hemophilia Study
An Example of Descriptive Epidemiology and Evaluation of Health Care

W.D. Hoffmann, O. Rienhoff

Medical School Hannover, Institute of Medical Informatics
(Director: Prof. Dr. P.L.Reichertz)
D-3000 Hannover, W.Germany

1. INTRODUCTION

In 1976, hemophiliacs in Northwest-Germany (Figure 1) asked for an intensivation of contacts between their attending physicians and themselves. This led to the formation of a study group of hemophilia centers aiming at an improved information exchange. Since then this group has met regularly two or three times a year in working sessions. In 1977, a pilot study for the documentation of hemophilia treatment was initiated. Data of 148 patients were collected at that time in 12 centers and were evaluated with descriptive statistics.

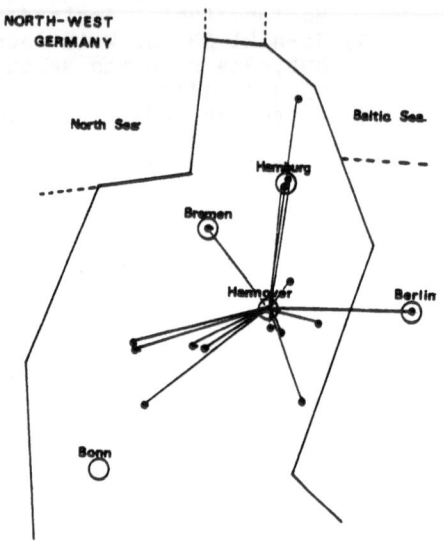

Figure 1: Map of the participating centers in Northwest Germany

The results served as a basis for intensive discussions between patients and physicians on one hand and between the members of the study group on the other. In 1979, the participating centers decided to use a data base system (IMS) to handle the patient files and to improve the possibilities for data evaluation (1). The number of patients increased from 180 in 15 centers in 1979 to 208 in 15 centers in 1980 and since then has still been rising.

2. RESULTS

Quarterly reports are printed of the data collected. These reports contain important information about the frequency and localization of bleeding episodes per patient, and the date and amount of units of factor-concentrates applied. On the basis of these data the physician has the control of the treatment of individual patients as well as of his patient collective as a whole. Thus he can see whether the therapy or prophylaxis had been successful or should be altered. This is especially important for all cases of home therapy and can be considered as a model for quality assurance in the therapy of hemophiliacs.

At the end of each year the data are evaluated with descriptive statistics for the stimulation of discussions and activities during medical working sessions. Further the results serve as basis for epidemiologic research (2,3).

As no valid dosage recommendations for the treatment with factor-concentrates exist up to now, the applied amounts of factor-concentrates are influenced in most cases of substitution therapy or prophylaxis by the subjective, intuitive impression of the therapist. In this context the Northwest German Hemophiliac Study is not able to substitute a controlled clinical trial comparing alternative treatments, but it helps doctors to be more conscious about the course of the individual therapies and to discuss documented results with colleagues from other cities. In addition, the annual statistics have a 'hypothesis generation-function', thus inaugurating special trials. This explorative function is of great value, as ethical limits are rather close within research of hemophilia treatment.

As the patients know that the sensitive information about their disease are protected against unauthorized access and supports their treatment most of them actively cooperate and the data captured are becoming more and more complete.

3. DISCUSSION

The growing number of participating centers, the improved cooperation with the patients, and the response of the physicians involved show that the documentation is accepted by patients and physicians.

During the regular working sessions of this work study group the physicians ask more and more for additional evaluations of the collected data, resp. for subsequent investigations of the patient collective.

4. PARTICIPATING CENTERS

Dr.Beck, Universitaetskinderklinik, Berlin; Dr.Bock, Staedt. Krankenanstalten, Bielefeld; Dr.Fenne, Kinderklinik, Braunschweig; Dr.Holzhueter, Bremen; Dr.Leithaeuser, Allgemeines Krankenhaus, Celle; Dr.Moesseler, Universitaetskinderklinik, Goettingen; Prof.Tilsner, Chir. Universitaetsklinik, Hamburg; Dr.Kurme, Hamburg; Dr.Skrandies, Dr.Kramarz, Krankenhaus St. Georg, Hamburg; Dr.Barthels, Medizinische Hochschule, Hannover; Dr.Schulz, Kinderklinik St. Bernward, Hildesheim; Dr.Lasson, Universitaetskinderklinik, Kiel; Prof.Asbeck, Medizinische Universitaetsklinik, Muenster; Dr.Mertner, Muenster; Dr.Bartsch, Sarstedt; Prof.Barthelmai, Rehabilitationsanstalten, Volmarstein.

5. REFERENCES

(1) Klonk J, Hoffmann WD. A Data Base for the Study of Therapeutical Strategies for Hemophiliacs. to be published in Abstracts of MIE'82, Dublin 21.-25.3.1982, Springer-Verlag, Berlin Heidelberg New York.

(2) Hoffmann WD, Rienhoff O. Multi Center Study for Monitoring Ambulatory Therapy of Hemophiliacs in Northwestern Germany. Abstracts of the 1st International Hemophilia Conference, Bonn, F.R.Germany, 3.-7.10.1980.

(3) Hoffmann WD, Klonk J, Rienhoff O. Organization Scheme and Data Flow Chart of the Multi Center Study of Hemophiliacs in Northwestern Germany. Abstracts of the XIV Congress of the World Federation of Hemophilia, San Jose, Costa Rica, 3.-7.7.1981.

Acknowledgement: This study is supported by:

Behringwerke AG, Frankfurt/Main; Immuno GmbH, Heidelberg; Travenol GmbH, Muenchen

STUDY OF SUDDEN CARDIAC DEATH

An Example for the Use of a Hospital Departmental System
for a Follow-up-study

by P. Wenzlaff and O. Rienhoff

Medical School Hannover, Instiute of Medical Informatics
(Director: Prof. Dr. P.L.Reichertz)

In 1978/9 the Division of Clinical Cardiology (Director: Prof.Dr. P.R. Lichtlen) at the Medical School Hannover (MHH.) started defining a study of the socalled Sudden Cardiac Death. By this study the correlation between the incidence of chronic life threatening arrhythmias and morphological and physiological changes of the left ventricle of patients with advanced sclerosis should be analyzed and algorithms for the prognosis of the Sudden Cardiac Death should be derived. For this purpose data of 300 patients with coronary heart disease, a heart-catherization and a 24-hours-ECG are analyzed.

In a first step the 24-hours-ECG tracings are analyzed (ventricular premature beats) and compared to the angiographic data (coronary sclerosis resp. ventricular wall akinesis) (1). In a period of at least 3 years for each patient a half-yearly (or yearly) follow-up examination is performed. For the determination of the influence of risk-factors (social/familiar/individual) also the patient's history, the clinical status, and different labtests are considered.

With little modifications or supplementations existing EDP-systems are used for data collecting. Most of these belong to the Data Interpretation and Evaluation System (DIES) (2). DIES allows the input and storage of data from different input mediums (optical mark reader form (OMR), optical character reader form (OCR), On-line, cards, tape, etc.), some elementary plausibility-checks, the creation of standardized medical reports by an own macro-language and some simple descriptive statistics. The DIES-system is not storing the collected data in a central organized data base, but for each application separated in single files on magnetic tapes.

The following (DIES-)application-systems, which serve routine functions in the Division of Clinical Cardiology, are used for this study:

(I) Heart-catherization:
The input of data obtained from two heart-catherization-labs is done by a documentation-clerk by an on-line-application of DIES. Also a standardized medical report is generated.
Contents of this data set:
Technical data of heart-catherization (approx. 20 different parameters), haemodynamics (90), angiocardiography (90), coronarography (450), coronarography of bypass-grafts (130).

(II) Quantitative angiocardiography:
Additional data are determinated by the GRAFOMED-computer, which respectively computes the $\pm$ variation (in %) of the 36 semi-axes and of the longitudinal axis for the RAO- and LAO-projection of the left ventricle. Together with the patient-identification the parameters are punched on cards (2 cards/case) and stored in a separate tape-file by a PL/1-program-system, that also creates a simple medical report.

(III) 24-hours-ECG tracings (complete finding):
Analog ECG tapes are analyzed automatically by a special purpose computer (PATHFINDER). The data obtained are merged with additional data of this 24-hours-ECG to the following data set:
technical data for 24-hours-ECG (approx. 20 different parameters), medication data (15), ECG-findings (values for the whole duration of this ECG) (50).
The handling and execution of these data is done analogous (I).

(IV) 24-hours-ECG tracings (condensed raw data):
Further the PATHFINDER produces a punch-tape containing data of some important types of supra-ventricular and ventricular primature beats for each hour respectively. These data are translated, transferred on a separate tape-file (with some elementary checks of the record format) and a data-listing is created by a program-system (COBOL/PL1), that is already used within the European Infarct Study (EIS).

These four EDP-systems yield data for answering the most important questions of the study. The medical reports created by the computer-systems allow a first reliability-check by being controlled by the cardiologists.

Besides these 'main' data sets for the study the following existing EDP-systems can be used:

(V) ECG-data gathered on an OMR form in the ECG-lab:
ECG physician readings are stored by a DIES-application in a separate tape-file and a standardized medical ECG-report is created too.

For the collection of the data of exercise (ECG), which will be analyzed at each follow-up examination of the study, no EDP-sytem exists up to now. These data shall be gathered by a new EDP-system.

In case of death of patients included into the study the last hours of the patient are analyzed (e.g. sudden death, time, weather, activity, medication, etc.). Therefore a cardiologist will interview the closest relatives of the deceased. This data noticed on a standardized sheet will be punched on cards (1 card/case) and stored by a PL/1-program in an extra file. By this file it is also possible to support the organization of patient's flow by computer (excluding of these patients out of the further run of the study).

In August 1981 nearly 150 patients are included into the study. (i.e. the data of the first examination of (I),(II),(III), and of the first follow-up-examination of (III) are almost completely stored).

Literature:

(1) Bethge KP, Graf A, Bethge HC, Lichtlen P. Regionale linksventrikulaere Wandveraenderung und Haeufigkeit von Kammerextrasystolen bei Koronarpatienten. Zeitschrift fuer Kardio- logie (Suppl.) 1976, III: 101-109.
(2) Pocklington PR. The Necessity for Requirements of and Basic Design of a General Data Interpretation and Evaluation System (DIES). In: Anderson J, Forsythe JM (Edit.). MEDINFO 74. (Amsterdam, Oxford, New York: North-Holland 1974) 411-418.

Acknowledgement

This study is supported by the Fritz Thyssen Stiftung and the Federal Ministry of Research and Technology.

STRATEGIC PLANNING OF A CARDIOVASCULAR REGISTRY
FOR THE PROVINCE OF ALBERTA

Denis H.J. Caro
Cardiac Care Evaluation
Department of Medicine
The University of Alberta

#910, 10711 Saskatchewan Drive
Edmonton, Alberta, CANADA T6E 4S4

The Province of Alberta is presently examining the possibility of establishing a Provincial Cardiovascular Registry. This is being done as an Alberta Heritage Savings Trust Fund Project under the aegis of the University of Alberta in Edmonton, Canada. The overall purpose of this Registry is to integrate and expand upon present cardiac care information systems in such a way as to facilitate an increased understanding of current morbidity and mortality patterns of cardiac disease in the Province. This understanding will hopefully lead to the development of effective preventive strategies and rehabilitative and restorative programs in cardiac care for the population.

The Cardiovascular Registry will be cardiac disease - specific and will consist of an integrated set of records of patients, who have coronary heart disease in the Province, regardless of the hospital to which the patient was admitted and regardless of the services provided that patient. This will include patients both for an adult population of 30 years of age or over (ICD-9-CM diagnostic codes 400-448) and for a pediatric and adolescent population of 19 years of age or under (ICD-9-CM codes 390-398, 746, and 747). Clinic users and researchers primarily in Edmonton and Calgary will have access to this database using distributed processing technology.

Through the mechanism and controls of the Cardiovascular Registry, patient information would, for the first time, be highly integrated, complete, reliable, valid, tailored to user needs, readily available, and finally, provided in a format meaningful and relevant to the users. The Cardiovascular Registry will provide integrated and valid information on patients with cardiac disease in a format and in a time frame appropriate to the clinical and research users. In particular, it could

- facilitate patient care continuity,
- readily identify patients at high risk for heart disease,
- readily identify families with a potential high risk of cardiovascular disease,
- assist and promote effective epidemiological surveys and studies,

- assist and facilitate health services research studies of the cardiac
  care system,
- provide critical information to cardiologists and cardiovascular
  surgeons who wish to improve the quality of their practice, and
- provide information on the incidence and prevalence of all types of
  heart disease.

Hence, once implemented over the course of the next four to five years,
clinic users and researchers will have access to a centralized database of
patients with cardiac disease in the Province of Alberta through distributed
processing technology. Through the application of a rigorous and carefully
designed approach to the evolution of this database, it is planned that the
goals of the Registry could be fully realized and that preventive and
rehabilitative programs for cardiac disease be effectively designed and
implemented.

SIMPLE MEASURES IN A COMPLEX REALITY
Indices on the frequency distribution
of diagnoses in Dutch hospitals.

Chrit van Ewijk
Dept. of Statistics
Stichting Medische Registratie
Postbus 14074 3508 SC UTRECHT
The Netherlands

'The identification of dimensionality in disease is only a first step in the development of case mix measures. Further conceptual and methodological development is required before proper applications and interpretations of measures can be carried out'
(Roice D.Luke 1979 (1)).

The hospital information system of the SMR (Medical Records Foundation) has discharge data of approximately 90% of all general in-patients in the Netherlands. Annually standard hospital utilization statistics are presented to the 194 participating general and teaching hospitals and their medical staffs.

Subsystems generate additional information, e.g. on expected length of stay and service populations. At present the SMR is developing other indices on hospital and medical specialist performance. These should facilitate the analysis of admission and reference policy, specialization and role differentiation, both at the hospital level and the specialist level.

1. Diagnostic proportions

The Infrequent Diagnoses Index (IDI) is based on case mix information, as represented in table I.

Table I: Hospital diagnostic case mix information

main diagnosis (three digit ICD-9-CM codes)	1	2	3	.	.	.	N
hospital proportions (percentages)	P_{1j}	P_{2j}	.	.	.	.	P_{Nj}
national pool proportions	P_1	.	.	.	.	.	P_N
weights per diagnostic category	w_1	w_2	w_3	.	.	.	w_N

An univariate index was constructed for each hospital H_j: $IDI_j = \sum_{i=1}^{N} w_i P_{ij}$.
The choice of weights is directed by the expected or required use of the index (2) (3) (4). We wished to distinguish between <u>exceptional</u>, i.e. infrequently occurring diseases and frequently occurring <u>common</u> diseases (cf. Lave and Lave (5)).

Therefore the weights were related to the pool frequencies of the diagnostic categories: $w_i \sim P_i^{-\frac{1}{2}}$ (inversely proportional).
The 'exceptionality' weights ranged from 0.3 t 99.6. The average case weight was set
at 1.0.

2. Structure of Classification of Diseases

The index uses available diagnostic information coded on three digit level. Unfortunately the underlying Classification shows irregularities: some parts of it are
clearly more elaborated than others. The ICD-system offers a comprehensive range of
coding possiblities for infective diseases, whereas the number of codes available for
heart diseases is limited. This certainly reflects the historical growth of clinical
medicine and the fact that morbidity statistics stem from mortality statistics.
As a consequence most measures are more sensitive to case mix variations in the 'older' rather than in the 'newer' branches!
Also in our case the degree of exceptionality depends on the national frequencies of
diagnostic categories. These in turn depend on the coding system: the number of sub-
divisions(codes) within groups of diseases. If no correction is made, the average exceptionality in several departments will inevitably be low (table II).

Table II

group of diseases	dept.generally respon- sible for admission	number of codes	average case exceptionality
heart diseases	cardiology	24	0.6
injuries	general surgery	149	2.2
infective diseases	general medicine/pediatrics	121	1.9
musculoskeletal diseases	orthopedic surgery/rheumatology	40	0.8

We adjusted the weights w_i to equalize the department average case exceptionalities.
Now the contribution of each department to the hospital index is roughly proportional
to its number of admissions.

The corrections also diminished another problem, equally seldom mentioned in literature. Diagnostic proportions usually are presented as relative frequencies (percentages). Consequently certain large categories may to a large degree characterize the
case mix. Admission policies for e.g. tonsillectomies or deliveries may strongly influence the average hospital case load. This actually disturbed Souteyrand, who used
the Evans/Walker information theory measure to characterize French hospitals (6)(7).

3. Hospital and specialist profile analysis

To facilitate the interpretation of the hospital index value, we created a 'table of weighed differences'. It ranks the numerical values of $(p_{ij} - P_i) w_i$. Summation leads to $\Sigma p_{ij} w_i$ (hospital index) $- \Sigma P_i w_i$ (poolindex = 100), in order to make the hospital distribution comparable with the pool distribution.

Furthermore decomposition of the hospital index was made possible by constructing specialist - indices ($IDIS_k$). The national patient census was divided in 30 specialism subpools according to the specialism responsible for admission. Again specialism diagnostic proportions, subpool proportions and exceptionality weights were defined and combined to form an index.
These indices may also serve to analyze the role differentiation among specialists working in different hospitals (university teaching hospital, general hospital et cetera).

4. Dissections of reality

Measures based on weighing resource utilization of diagnostic categories (8) (9) are useful, but their feasibility depends on the functional homogeneity of hospitals. Treatment patterns may be very dissimilar (3). Measures based on frequency distributions seem to be very rewarding, provided that a coherent regional or national admission/reference pattern exists. This holds true for the Netherlands and probably for other countries as well (10). This is what makes measures of the Evans/Walker type (complexity) and the SMR type (exceptionality) very interesting. Although in a complex, living reality adequate measures can be no more than clever 'dissections'.

5. References

(1) Luke RD. Dimensions in hospital case mix measurement. Inquiry 1979; 16: 38-49.
(2) Rafferty J. Hospital Output indices. Econ Businesss Bulletin 1972; 24: 21-27.
(3) Klastorin TD, Watts CA. On the measurement of hospital case mix. Med Care 1980; 18: 675-685.
(4) Griffith JR. Measuring hospital performance. Chicago, Inquiry Books, 1978.
(5) Lave JR, Lave LB. The extent of role differentiation among hospitals. Health Serv Res 1971; 6: 15-39.
(6) Evans RG, Walker H D. Information theory and the analysis of hospital cost structure. Can J Econ 1972; 5: 398-418.
(7) Souteyrand Y. Caracteristiques de la clientèle et dispersion des coûts entre hôpitaux publics français en 1976. Aix-en-Provence, Université d'Aix-Marseille II, 1979.
(8) Goodisman LD, Trompeter T. Hospital case mix and average charge per case: an initial study. Health Serv Res 1979; 14: 44-55.
(9) Fetter RB et al. Case mix definition by diagnosis-related groups. Med Care 1980; 18 No. 2 Supplement: 1-53.
(10) Horn SD, Schumacher DN. An analysis of case mix complexity using information theory and diagnosis related grouping. Med Care 1979; 17: 382-389.

SPANISH MEDICAL LITERATURE DATA BASES: IME AND BILIME

M.L. Terrada, E. Casaban
Centro de Documentación e
Informática Biomédica
Avda. V. Blasco Ibáñez, 17
Valencia-10, Spain

The data base of the Indice Médico Español (IME) and the data base of the Bibliometrics of Spanish Medical Literature (BILIME) are presented.

IME: The area of coverage, indexing characteristics, information retrieval language utilized and the informatic schema of the IME data base with the characteristics of automatic retrieval tools are described.

BILIME: The material analyzed in the bibliometric study, the information furnished by BILIME and the characteristics of the automatic data processing are described.

1. INTRODUCTION.

The IME and BILIME data bases are two products of the Centro de Documentación e Informática Biomédica (CEDIB) at the University of Valencia. The fundamental aim of IME is to provide information, both in retrospective and up to date, about article published in Spanish journals. The aim of the BILIME data base (Bibliometrics, etc.) is to provide a series of indicators on the scientific activity of Spanish physicians and medical institutions.

2. IME DATA BASE.

The IME data base is the automated version of the Indice Médico Español, bibliographic index which has been published four times yearly since 1965. At present it is the only data bank of Spanish medical information.

2.1. Coverage and general characteristics.

The IME analyzes 180 Spanish medical journal which represents about 100.000 bibliographic references, with an annual increase of 5.000 new articles.

Since 1978, the indexing by subject matter has been accomplished as much from title as from summary or text. The number of key-words selected follows a mean of five per article, which enter to form part of a master file for information retrieval.

All journals are analyzed from cover to cover, with the exception of articles with out references. Conferences, symposia, meetings, etc., are also analyzed when they are published in spanish journals.

The analysis of each document is accomplished by CEDIB's Staff (physicians specialized in Medical Documentation), who establish a network of other professional physicians in diverse areas of medicine.

At present, the articles indexed may be retrieved by subject-matter, by author, by the journals in which they were published, and by the year of publication.

2.2. The IME thesaurus.

At present the IME data base utilizes the thesaurus IME as a descriptors language both for its elaboration of the subject file and for information retrieval. It is structured in nineteen categories and is brought up to date quaterly through nearly 1.500 analysed articles which entails a new contribution of terms; approximately 18.000 per year.

Semantic problems of synonymity, eponymity, and related terms, as well as the proper places in the tree of classification, are presented and solved for each preferred term or descriptor.

The IME thesaurus also aspires to confront the complex problem of the equivalences between the different nomenclatures and classifications in medical terminology, towards the end of contributing to an authentic international cooperation between the various data bases.

2.3. The informatic support of the IME.

The automatic processing of the Indice Médico Español resolves the following points:

1) Automatic creation and management of the master file. This file contains records of distinct natures, but of identical structure.

2) Quaterly listing of a subject matter index and an index of authors for the corresponding volume of the Indice Médico Español. Each of the index's terms is accompanied by a numerical code that facilitates its localization in the printed repertory.

3) Automatic retrieval of works in the commulative represented by the master file. Works may be retrieved (off-line or on-line) by author, subject matter, journal, or year of publication or of incorporation in the Indice Médico Español.

These processes were accomplished by an IBM 4331/1 computer of 1024 KB, with IBM 3370 disk units and IBM 3279 polychromatic screens.

The software is composed of the IBM DMS/CICS/VS panels as well as the COBOL ANS and FORTRAN programs.

The new system permits the use of software for STAIRS searches. This has improved considerably the power of the search and the response time.

The system has a master file and, besides, there are sequential alphabetical files of authors and subjects, and of journals sorted by year and code.

The master file is of the type KSDS/VSAM and its records, although of identical structure, contain distinct information. The conceptual unit of information is "article-published-in-journal". Each one of these units is composed by the following records on the master file:

1) Names of the authors (a registry for each author).

2) Title of the work (in the published language: castilian, catalán, etc.).

3) Abbreviation of the journal of publication.

4) Key-words (a record for each key word).

5) Institutions, cities, and professional status of each author.

The key to the master file's records is a structuring key composed of seventeen digits.

Table 1.

Digits	Items
1-2	Volume number of Indice Médico Español.
3-5	Journal's code.
6-8	Page of Indice Médico Español.
9-12	First page of the article.
13-15	Type of paragraph. (author, title, etc.).
16-17	Sub-paragraph's number. various authors, various records to contain the title, etc.).

The creation and management of the master file has been accomplished on the basis of the design of the DMS/CICS panels and their corresponding programming. In this way the visualization of whichever record, the addition of new records and the modification or deleting of existing records is resolved in real time.

The automatic retrieval of works is accomplished with an alphabetic profile (whether by author or by subject) or with a numerical profile (in the case of a search by journal or year). The keys of the articles are in the sequential files, and with these access in gained to the totality of information in the master file KSDS/VSAM. The references of the retrieved works are printed from there.

Besides the programs mentioned, five COBOL ANS programs have also been designed for the trimonthly edition of the Indice Médico Español.

3. BILIME DATA BASE.

This is a data base of the bibliometric type whose aim is to provide the results of an analysis of Spanish medical literature. The resulting files permit us to construct bibliographic indexes, scientometric analysis of the production and use of information and the posibility to inform individually the persons and institutions which are effected the contribution.

3.1. Coverage and general characteristics.

The material analyzed in medical publications by Spanish authors from 1973 to 1977. 2.864 books, 21.292 articles from Spanish journals, 1662 Spanish papers published abroad, and 2.233 institutions were studied.

At present the results of the 1978-1980 period are being added.

This data base furnishes information about:

1) The productivity of Spanish medical authors (observed and theoretical, distribution, Lotka's law, signature/work index, etc.).

2) Analysis of the journals where Spanish medical works are published (incidence, Bradfor's law, country of publication, language in which said works were published, etc.).

3) The work's originating institutions (collaboration between institutions, distribution by cities and countries, etc.).

4) Analysis of Spanish use of medical information (distribution by languages and country of origen, years of publication of th cited references, obsolescence of medical literature, etc.).

5) Institutions of origen, cities and professional status of the authors of the analysed works.

3.2. Informatic support.

The informatic support permits the retrieval and operation of these files, and the number of programs elaborated toward this end are 25 COBOL ANS programs and 10 FORTRAN programs.

4. DEGREE OF UTILIZATION OF IME AND BILIME.

Since 1965 3.000 copies of the Indice Médico Español are publisheed quaterly and distributed to the medical professionals and institutions (such as hospitals, schools of medicine, information centers, etc.). Information retrieval is currently performed under request from spanish and foreign users (about 500 searches/year).

Advances of the BILIME results are cited in the references (2, 3 and 4).

5. REFERENCES.

(1) Indice Médico Español (1965-1981). Vols. 1-66. Valencia. Centro de Documentación e Informática Biomédica.

(2) Terrada ML. La literatura médica española contemporánea. Estudio estadístico y sociométrico. Valencia. Centro de Documentación e Informática Biomédica. 1973.

(3) Terrada ML, et al. Bibliometría de la literatura científica española publicada en revistas extanjeras 1973-1977. Valencia. Centro de Documentación e Informática Biomédica. 1980.

(4) Terrada ML, et al. Bibliometría de la producción y el consumo de literatura médica en España, 1973-1977. Valencia. Centro de Documentación e Informática Biomédica. 1981.

SEMANTIC REPRESENTATION: A MODEL FOR INFORMATION RETRIEVAL FROM MEDICAL LITERATURE

B.J. KOSTREWSKI, Centre for Information Science, The City University,
Northampton Square, London EC1V 0HB

J. ANDERSON, King's College Hospital Medical School, Denmark Hill, London SE5

Abstract

The work is concerned with the definition of data structures. It delineates a model for medical semantics. The outcome is the condensation of information in a formatted manner to allow rapid and accurate retrieval of medical data for decision support.

Introduction

Published information has been increasing rapidly yet the systematic representation of document content has not matched this progress mainly because of our lack of understanding of the nature of semantic mechanisms.

It is now recognized that the integration of linguistic devices into the representation of document content has not significantly increased the performance of bibliographic storage and retrieval systems (1). Indeed the integration of such parameters is now deemed redundant. Instead there is an emphasis on the user interface and the representation of a user's state of knowledge (2) and the definition of conceptual networks at the user/database interface underlines this approach. This is the philosophy underlying the ASK approach (2,3) which allows for the interpretation of individual networks and the incorporation of changing patterns both as a result of bibliographic output from the system and because of knowledge acquired otherwise over time. The above approaches are aimed at a research audience and aim to find a balance between the expression of the users knowledge structure and a broad definition needed for the support of creative effort.

Information Retrieval from Medical Documents

Medicine is heavily dependent on published information. Abstracts, e.g. in the MEDLINE system, can be a direct source of information; however, they are not formatted and retrieval is not direct. Unpublished data has been used to derive a structured reference base of experience. To this class belongs the processing of pathology and radiology reports (4,5) and the hypertension database founded on records of patients attending a hypertension clinic at Duke University, North Carolina (6). Both approaches make available the wealth of experience which is not normally available for reference. Clearly there is a need for the integration of clinical experience based on the literature presented in a manner which will approximate closely to the clinical reasoning process and thus allow for rapid retrieval of data.

The MYCIN approach (7), while being implicitly organized towards decision support, represents a knowledge structure and attempts to represent the reasoning process associated with the domain of bacterial therapy. The explicit definition of the reasoning process demands the delineation of entities and the definition of interrelationships and interaction in order to represent the structure.

Published documents represent a different type of structure. The reasoning process is within the context of that which is known, and in this case, captured by the direct-ional and definitive semantemes. This approach allows for the expression of a wider range of interrelationships, characteristic of the development of new ideas. It also allows for the expression of interdisciplinary relations (8).

The Representation of Medical Concepts for Data Retrieval

Medicine is dependent upon language based data. To this end attempts have been made to derive nomenclatures and standardize terminologies (8,9,10,11). Moreover, these formalized reference languages show some adaptation of structure commensurate with their applications (12). These approaches fulfil an encoding function and have inte-grated into their organization an element of semantic power.

While the structure of reference languages is an important element in their capacity to capture the message contained in a document, mapping on to a template which repre-sents the cognitive dimensions of a domain is a novel approach. Implicit in this approach is the idea that there are levels of information which are units in themselves and yet they have some relational association to the whole, which, as items of inform-ation can stand alone. In the unfolding of information, each stage has an element of dependence upon the preceeding and successive stage and implications for association throughout the entire schema.

The schema is based on the interdependence of information elements as depicted by the aims of medical activity, and drawn from the medical record as the primary document of medical experience (8,13). Its principle explicit use is the encoding of patient data. Implicitly it is also a physical record of cognitive activity showing patterns of associations which in the formulation of a schema should be made explicit. The rules define the positions of words according to the type of document and the subject nature of the data.

The Schema comprises of two major elements:
(1) Rules for the representation of document content.
(2) The "Medical template" upon which the rules are based and to which the appropriate data is subsequently mapped.

The schema itself provides a set of rules for the analysis of specific types of docu-ments, since these differ in aim and organization.

A range of types of medical publications has been identified as follows (13,14): Reviews; Case Studies; Experimental Work; Notes and Letters; Reports of case studies in Letters.

The common aim of publication is to show some element of novelty, to report new observ-ations and to synthesize, thus the structure is different in terms of semantic organ-ization, and varies according to document type with important implications for content representation. The organization of semantic flow dependent upon the interplay of macro and microsyntax, has been defined according to the following semantemes (14):

Directional   -   Relates the work to the domain within the confines of the Semantic class.

Definitive   -   Defines the aims of the present work in relation to the Directional Semanteme.

Operative   -   Defines methods and results.

Conclusive   -   Defines results in relation to the domain and defines their place in the overall reference framework.

This information framework defines the sequence of information flow. The approach is based on three further assumptions viz:

(1)   That the work under examination bears some relation to the overall domain under consideration.

(2)   That there is a message contained within the document which fits into the overall framework.

(3)   That the transmission of the message in a structured form allows for a more accurate representation of meaning.

Thus to have total meaning we are aiming to represent all levels of information contained in the document and to capture the essence of the message. Hutchins (15) has made the theoretical distinction between 'aboutness' and 'meaning' and postulated the integration of structure for the transfer of meaning through indexing (16). Message analysis overcomes this dilemma but demands a rigorous approach to document analysis.

The subject related model

The definition of the aim is the bridge between the semantic representation and the medical framework. The four principal classification parameter which reflect the goals of medicine have been identified (17); these are Diagnosis, Therapy, Management and Prognosis. Moreover certain types of medical communication tend to be associated with specific aims.

Diagnosis   -   (1) Reviews; (2) Case reports; (3) multiple patient studies, (4) letters and notes, (5) epidemicological studies, (6) statistical studies.

Therapy   -   (1) Experimental studies on animals, (2) clinical trial data, (3) case reports, (4) studies on interactions, contra-indications and adverse effects.

Management   -   (1) Reviews, (2) Case studies.

Prognosis   -   (1) Reviews, (2) Case studies.

A semantic model for Therapy

The semantic class THERAPY presents the most complex structure and captures some elements which appear in the other classes. The wide range of data elements contributing to this class are showed in Figure 1; qualitative data and its semanteme distribution is shown in Figure 2 and quantitative data is shown in Figure 3. These examples represent the most complex information both in terms of number of information elements

FIGURE 1: Data Elements contributing to Therapeutic Information

Patient Details	Treatment	Trial Design	Adverse Effects
Numbers	Dose	No details given	None found
Age	Route	Single blind	Identity those found
Sex	Frequency	Double blind	Frequency
Weight	Concurrent medication	Open	No details
Height	Previous medication	Multicentric	
Criteria inclusion		Comparison a)Drug	
Criteria exclusion		b)Placebo	
Withdrawals		Crossover technique	
		Randomised	
		Duration	
Drug Monitoring	**Statistical Analysis**		
Parameters measured	Sample size		
Frequency	Statistical methods		
Methods			

FIGURE 2: Classes of concepts represented in documents about Therapy:Distribution

Concepts	Semanteme	Concepts	Semanteme
Administration of drug/dose	OPERATIVE	In vitro	OPERATIVE
Control	OPERATIVE	In vivo	OPERATIVE
Diagnosis/Disease	DIRECTIONAL/ DEFINITIVE	Medical history (in case reports)	DEFINITIVE
Drug	DIRECTIONAL/ DEFINITIVE	Patient data	DEFINITIVE
Efficacy	CONCLUSIVE	Placebo	OPERATIVE
Prophylactic action	OPERATIVE	Symptoms	DEFINITIVE
Time Period	OPERATIVE/ DEFINITIVE	Therapy	AIM
		Types of clinical trial	DEFINITIVE
Further research required/recommended	CONCLUSIVE	Significance	CONCLUSIVE

FIGURE 3: Quantitative information in documents relating to Therapy: Distribution

Information	Semanteme	Information	Semanteme
Number of patients	DEFINITIVE	Cell concentrations	OPERATIVE
Duration of treatment	DEFINITIVE	Plasma osmolality	OPERATIVE
Drug doses	OPERATIVE/ DEFINITIVE	Renal clearance	OPERATIVE
		Radioactive quantities	OPERATIVE
Age Distribution	DEFINITIVE	Concentrations	OPERATIVE
Percentages	CONCLUSIVE	Indices and Scales	OPERATIVE
Serum drug concentrations	OPERATIVE	Increases/decrease	CONCLUSIVE
Serum hormone levels	DEFINITIVE/ OPERATIVE		

and the complexity of interrelationships.

Semantic Parameters in the transfer of meaning

True representation can only be effected through the interplay of the subject related model and semantic mechanisms. These have been defined as follows:

(1) **Aims**: These are linked with the four principal semantic classes. Psychological theory provides an explanation in McDougall's theory of purposive behaviour (18) which identifies the step-by-step process to achieve a goal.

(2) **Context**: The definition of context is paramount for efficient understanding and hence needs to be integrated into information retrieval systems which are dependent on language based data. The formatting of language based data has been contextually restricted because meaning was evident and character strings had well defined meanings. Thus, when the body of medical knowledge is considered, an element of partitioning must be introduced. Within the schema of this model this is effected both by the aims as defined by the semantic classes of Diagnosis, Therapy, Management and Prognosis coupled to conventional classifications of entities such as components of body systems, diseases and drugs made explicit in the Directional Semanteme.

(3) **Inference**: Represents the dynamic concept of semantics, restricting the kinds of information elements that are likely to be associated. The integration of inference into computerized information retrieval systems demands sequential partitioning of data such that blocks of information can be identified and inference formalized between the blocks. This approach represents semantic flow (13). In practice this is demonstrated by the semanteme structure designed for the transfer of meaning.

Inference embodies a wider concept than that conveyed by classificatory systems. The types of inference incorporated into knowledge base systems are dependent upon the nature of the information. Thus "tight" and "loose" inference frameworks may be described. A "tight" inference framework details the network of associations defining all associations and operates in well defined contexts and within explicit schema (Fig.1). A "loose" inference framework allows for flexibility in interpretation, as in keyword based systems. The tolerance allowed by 'tight' and 'loose' inference structures depends on the level of application. The role of inference in the unfolding of meaning was emphasized by Parker-Rhodes (19).

The following levels of inference are therefore in operation:
(1) word level - anticipatory character sequencing, linked with morphemes.
(2) sentence level - grammatical unfolding based on word sequences.
(3) semanteme level - distribution of vocabulary and discrete types of information which result in the unfolding of meaning.

A synthesis: Semantic parameters and medical framework

In this context the decision support system is taken to mean a direct question answering system; this requires well structured inference frameworks. The network of interrelationships is restricted but all inference must be made explicit. For example in a file of therapeutic compounds, (Figure 2), the question "What is the dosage of

Propanolol?" would require additional patient information to be truly meaningful; e.g. the patient's condition (diagnosis), age, current malfunction, and associated therapy. At this level a meaningful network of relationships emerges with a definite inference structure. The integration of the network of associations in structure is important in the encoding of knowledge. Hendrix (20) presents a case for the partitioning of a domain. Van Djik (21) has rightly pointed out that semantic representation involves reduction and abstraction. For data retrieval systems this means both semantic and syntactic reduction with the transference of the macrosyntax.

The novel element contained in the document is set within the context of that which is already known and from the information point of view the latter constitutes the redundant element. This was realized by Schwarzlander (22) who proposed the Information Item File (IIF); the aim of the IIF was to encode each unique information element once only.

In medicine this approach has limited applications since, in the reporting of patient data, the "context" is essential and unique for each item of patient information.

The Integration of Semantic Devices

The development of the information structure can be viewed in terms of:

1. The interdependence of units of information.
2. The dynamic element of the semantic framework is inference which in turn allows for modification and explanation of the argument.

Thus the unfolding of the message in structured terms can be viewed along the vertical axis and links well both with semantemes and with the framework within the medical record. The organization effected by punctuation can only be integrated by analyzing what it is that punctuation actually does while the condensation effected through semantic analysis concentrates the information and indeed produces a different organization.

This organization is reflected in the rules for condensation and in the organization of the structured terminology. This schema represents the interdependence of medical concepts.

References

(1) SPARK-JONES, K. and KAY, M.(1976) Linguistics and Information Science in Natural Science, edited by Walker, Kalgren and Kay. (Skriptor, Stockholm)

(2) BELKIN, N.J. (1977) The problem of "matching" in information retrieval. in Theory and Application of Information Research. Proceedings of the 2nd International Research.

(3) ODDY, R.N. (1974) Reference Retrieval based on induced dynamic clustering. (PhD Thesis. University of Newcastle upon Tyne, UK).

(4) DUNHAM, G.S., PACAK, M.G. and PRATT, A.W. Automatic Indexing of Pathology Data. J.AM. Soc.Inf.Sci. 1978; 29; 81-90.

(5) GRISHMAN, R. and HISCHMAN, L. Question Answering from Natural Language Databases. Artificial Intelligence. 1978; 11; 25-43.

(6) ROSATI, R.A. and McNeer, J.F. (1975) A new information System for Medical Practice: Archives of Internal Medicine, Vol.135, pp 1017-24.

(7) SHORTLIFFE, E.H. (1977) A rule and approach to the generation of advice and explanations in clinical medicine. In:Computational Linguistics in Medicine, edited by W. Schneider and A.L. Sagvall Hein.

(8) ANDERSON, J. The Computer: Medical Vocabulary and Information, Brit.Med.Bull. 1968; 24; 3; 194-198.

(9) International Anatomical Nomenclature Committee (ed). Nomina Anatomica, 4th.Edn. Amsterdam. 1977.

(10) CÔTE, R.A. Systematized Nomenclature of Medicine (SNOMED). College of American Pathologists, Skokie, Illinois. 1976-1979.

(11) International Classification of Diseases WHO, Geneva. 1978.

(12) MAJOR, P., KOSTREWSKI, B. and ANDERSON, J. (1978). Analysis of Semantic Structures of medical languages: Part II. Analysis of the semantic power of MESH, ICD, and SNOMED. Medical Informatics 3(4), p. 269-281.

(13) KOSTREWSKI, B. and ANDERSON, J. (1980). Document Content: The transfer of meaning in Proceedings of AWAMI, May 1980.

(14) ORMISTON, T. (1980) Structural analysis of medical documentation. M.Sc. Dissertation, The City University.

(15) HUTCHINS, W.J. (1978) The Concept of "aboutness" in subject indexing. Aslib Proc. 30 (5), p. 172-181.

(16) HUTCHINS, W.J. (1975) Language of Indexing and Classification: a linguistic study of structure and function. (Peter Perigrums, Stevenage)

(17) KOSTREWSKI, B. and ANDERSON, J. (1979) Structural Consideration for the encoding of Medical Data: a formalism for Medicine, in Barber, B., Gremy, F., Uberla, K. and Wagner, G. Proceedings MIB79 International Conference on Medical Computing, Berlin, September 17-20, p. 269-281.

(18) McDOUGALL, W. (1923) Purposive or Mechanical Psychology? Psychological Review 30, 273-288.

(19) PARKER-RHODES, A.F. (1978) Inferential Semantics. (Harvester Press, Sussex)

(20) HENDRIX, G. (1979) Encoding knowledge in Partitioned Networks. p 51-92 in Associated Networks, Representation and Use of Knowledge by Computers,edited by N.V. Findler. (Academic Press, New York)

(21) VAN DIJK, T.V. (1977) Perspective Paper: Complex Scientific Information Processing, in Walker, D.E., Kalgren, H. and Kay, H. ed, Natural Language and Information Science, p 127-163. (Skriptor, Stockholm)

(22) SCHWARZLANDER, H. (1970) Encyclopeadic storage of scientific and technical knowledge. IEEE Transactions of writing and speech. vol.13; 2; 48-57.

Literature and Research Data-Bases in the Field of Medicine and
Health-Care
- an International Review with Enduser's Aspects

Rüdiger Schneemann
Head of the Department
Technische Universität Berlin
Universitätsbibliothek
Straße des 17. Juni 135

D-1000 Berlin 12

Abstract

The most important database systems, the used retrieval languages and the communication networks are described. The databases, which are relevant to medical
sciences in the broadest sense, are given with their producers and sizes. The
essential aspects of valuation are named and the growing influence of the information industry is mentioned.

Zusammenfassung

Literatur- und Forschungsdatenbanken in Medizin und Gesundheitswesen -
ein internationaler Überblick mit Bewertung für den Endbenutzer.

Nach einer allgemeinen Erklärung von Literatur- und Forschungsdatenbasen wird
auf die wachsende Bedeutung, insbesondere für den Bereich Medizin und Gesundheitswesen eingegangen. Die wichtigsten Datenbanksysteme, Retrievalsprachen und
Kommunikationsnetze werden erklärt. Die Datenbasen, die im weitesten Sinne mit
der Medizin zu tun haben, werden mit Hersteller und Umfang genannt. Nach einer
Aufzählung von Bewertungskriterien wird auf die wachsende Bedeutung des Infor-
mationssektors hingewiesen.

1. Topics

1.1. Literature and Research Data-Bases

Traditionally libraries list their monographies, series and journals in card indexes. The authors or titles are set up in alphabetical order. Mostly, a subject catalogue exist also which gives the user a general view of special field required. By covering articles from journals, newspapers and books, the usual aim of the library – the cataloguing – is surpassed and one step in the direction of documentation is taken. The function of documentation means the gathering of all kinds of references which can be retrieved in various special fields. For many decades, bibliographies with qualified abstracts and comprehensive registers (printed card indexes) belong to the tools of the scientist. In the late fifties the dataprocessing technology has made it possible to have the indexed literature online, to search with simple strategies in databases and obtain bibliographies with individual profiles.

Each year, the mass of publications grows exponentially. The international complexity in the fields of economics, politics and sciences has increased the demand for literature databases. An information market has come into existence. Besides the bibliographic databases, so-called " numerical databases ", which are built up by evaluated bibliographies or have arisen by special research work { e.g. databank of products, databank of conferences).The information systems do not only inform about publications but answer questions directly. Here they are called research databanks because of their task to support the researchers.

1.2. Medicine and Health Care

Abstract services in medicine are as old as those in the traditional sciences physics, chemistry and mathematics. In the same measure as the plain natural science aspects lost their significance because more and more economical, political and technical conditions are essential to the application of medicine health care, hospital care, preventive medicine etc. obtain greater importance. At the same time the demand for interdisciplinary literature grows, e.g. Health Economics, nuclear medicine. The mentioned shift of the main point caused the foundation of relevant databases.

Particularly in respect of the research work in medicine the technical or natural science based databanks in chemistry, biology, food sciences and pharmacy continue to be very important.

1.3. End - user

Interested in literature and research databases could be anyone who works in the field of medicine or parts of it. Not only the medical staff, nursing staff, or scientists, are users but also an increasing member of administrators, planners, economists and architects ask for literature.

In principal the training or the specialization of the interested persons is not a relevant factor to formulate the search; each inquires receives the identical literature. For the evaluation of the references the training standard is of course important.

2. Importance of the Literature Data-Base

The groups mentioned above, know the value of the databases, which is based on one simple regulation: ayone who works scientifically publishes. By means of a literature retrieval one can find out who has dealt with what, where and when. The successful principle of the Science Citations Index is based on a further generalization: only persons who have written " good articles " will be cited. The SCI registers anyone, who has been cited and receives all essential and important results of the sciences in this way.

The tendency towards a complete coverage of the essential sciences by online databases has been arrived at within the last five years. The reason being: the equipment of both university and industry with a better computer capacity, which inturn is supported by the trend to " computerize " all knowledge. The importance of the databases has also grown due to the following facts: Economical obligations, which require a rapid utilization of scientific results, (in relation to practice), and double research with can be excluded as far as possible. On the other hand the big research institutes - it is through their work that science is developed further - use the databases because of their obligation to be informed quickly, reliably and rationally.

But also for the so-called practice, the use of the existing information systems is obvious. Consulting offices use the information services of the databases for the qualified handling of problems. Without noticing, customers seeking advice often pay a certain amount for the literature retrieval, which included in the fee. The databases are used by an even increasing number of people, who are interested in obtaining information about every day problems at a moment's notice. Certainly they have neither the money nor the time to use a consulting office. They try for themselves or ask the information-transfer for help.

3. International Review

3.1 Retrieval Systems, Producer

The present development of the International Information Industry has become
more confusing. The growing number of acronyms, logograms, and names of communication networks are more bewildering than helpful.[1] The aim of the following
diagram (Fig. 1) is to support the explanation of the information sector as a
whole:

Host and Retrieval language	Database Producer					Communication network		
	Eng.Index (Compendex)	NTIS	Predi-casts	NLM (Med-lars)	DOMA	Telenet/ Tymnet	EURONET	Others
Dialog – Dialog (Lockheed)	x	x		x		x		
SDC – ORBIT	x	x		x		x		
BRS – BRS		x	x	x		x	x	
Data Star – BRS (Radio Suisse)		x	x				x	
IRS – Quest (ESA) (CCL)		x		x			x	ESANET
DIMDI – DIRS (CCL)				x			x	DIMDI-NET
INKA – DIRS (CCL)	x	x			x		x	

Fig. 1
Examples for the information market

Explanation of Fig. 1 :

Host:

Dialog (Lockheed), SDC and BRS are only database administrators. They provide
systems effective user services by adequate software and hardware retrieval
languages and database structures which are advantegeous to the user and
sufficient store capacity.

It is easy to learn the retrieval language which enables the searcher to effect
a retrieval in several databases, sometimes with the same descriptors and logic.
The Information Retrieval Services (IRS) of the "European Space Agency" (ESA)
and INKA started as database producers.They have a continuous interest in
completing their offer through a take over of other databases and to obtain a
host.
The following service items belong to the quality standard of a host:

- A telephone that is free of charge
- An online-Keyword index for all existing databases of the host
- Online-ordering of the literature that has been found
- Keyword-in-context
- Save search

Retrieval languages:

A simple and time saving dialogue language, which considers the specific interests
of the own database, is expected to be a market advantage.[2] For that reason
each host tries to develop " its" own language. Retrieval languages drawn up
for general purposes e.g. GOLEM (Siemens) or STAIRS (IBM), are accepted with
reservations (but BRS is similar to STAIRS).
The EURONET-Language CCL (Common Command Language), which has to be adopted by
each connected host, will be similarly used.[3]

Data Base Producer:

The first are database producers. They offer no own equipment for retrieval by
externals. They give their magnetic tapes to the hosts. But, the National
Library of Medicine (NLM) offers within their own net (MEDLINE) MEDLARS and all
the other databases produced in their institution (meanwhile MEDLARS is also
offered by Dialog, BRS and SDC).

Communication Networks:

Genuine data-transport-nets (package-transfer-technology) are Telenet and
Tymnet in the USA. By using them, DIALOG and SDC are within reach in Europe by
satellite. EURONET/DIANE as a system of European postal-administrations (also
package-transfer-technology) fulfil additional cooperation and coordination tasks.
ESANET and DIMDINET are small direct-call-systems, with knots-processors and
continuous connections knot exist in addition to EURONET.
The normal communication with the database is done by telephone, which is
connected to a modem or acoustic-coupler with a continous or dial line, or with
Datex. Also Telex-connections are used (separated networks). Telefax and
video-text are further possibilities.

3.2. Databases

The most intersting Databases are listed in the figure 2 below; additionally in
the bibliography is given a list of some of the most well known online-directories.

Database	Producer	Host	Entry-date	Doc. Units (ths.)	Printed Versions
MEDICINE					
MEDLARS	NLM,USA	BRS DIALOG SDC EU:BLAISE DIMDI	1964	4.100	Index Medicus Int. Nursing Index Index to Dental Lit.
EMBASE	Excerpta Medica,NL	DIALOG SDC EU:DIMDI	1974	1.700	Exerpta Medica Sect.1-51
ISI/ BIOMED	ISI,USA	BRS DIALOG SDC EU:DIMDI	1979	660	Science Citation Index
SOCIAL SCISEARCH	ISI,USA	BRS DIALOG SDC EU:DIMDI	1973	950	Science Citation Index
PREMED	BRS,USA	BRS EU:Data-Star	1981	7	-
CATLINE	NLM,USA	BRS DIALOG SDC	1965	210	-
BIOSIS PREV	BIOSIS, USA	BRS DIALOG SDC EU:DIMDI ESA-IRS INFOLINE	1969	2.950	Biolog. Abstracts Biosearch Index
PASCAL- MEDICINE	CNRS,F CDST,F	EU:Questel ESA-IRS	1973	3.000	Bulletin Signal- etique
SPECIAL MED.					
BIOETHICS	NLM,USA George- town,USA	MEDLINE	1973	7	(Fact-Base)
PTF (Pat. Treat.File)	Veterans Adm.,USA	-	-	30	(Fact-Base)
NAT. KIDNEY REC.Pool	UCLA, USA	-	-	8	(Fact-Base)
DZF (Biomed. Technik)	DZF,D	EU:INKA	1979	43	Referatedienst
BLDIS	Blood Inf. Serv.,USA	-	1968	108	-

Database	Producer	Host	Entry-date	Doc. Units (ths.)	Printed Versions
CANCER- -LIT -PROJ -PROT	NCI,USA	MEDLINE EU:BLAISE DIMDI ESA-IRS	1963 1974 1977	250 20 2	Cancer Theory Abstracts Carciogenisis Ab.
CANCER-NET	DKFZ, D Gustave-Roussy,F	EU:Questel	1979	140	Bulletin Signal-etique
INKA NUCLEAR	INKA,D FU	EU:INKA	1970	696	Literaturdienste Nuklearmedizin INIS-Atomindex
MEDLIST	INKA,D	EU:INKA	1981	2	-
ARAMIS	Am.Rheum. Ass.,USA	-	1977	6	(Fact-Base)
BEHAVIOUR. SCIENCE					
PSYCINFO	PASAR,USA	BRS DIALOG SDC EU:DIMDI	1967	360	Psychological Abstracts
SOC.AB.	Sociolog. Abstr.,USA	DIALOG	1963	120	Sociological Abstracts
HEALTH CARE					
HECLINET	IFK,D DKI,D	EU:IFK	1969	50	Informationsdienst Krankenhauswesen
HEALTH	NLM,USA AHA,USA	BRS DIALOG SDC EU:BLAISE DIMDI	1975	180	Int. Nursing Index Hosp.Lit.Index
idis	idis,D	EU:idis	1969	300	Dokumentation So-zialmedizin
ILO	Int.Labour Org.,CH	EU:ILO SPIDEL	1974	-	CIS-Abstracts
NTIS	NTIS,USA	BRS DIALOG SDC EU:ESA-IRS INKA	1964	418	Gov. Rep. Announcements
TOX./PHARM.					
RTECS	NIOSH,USA	MEDLINE EU:BLAISE DIMDI	1978	49	(Fact-Base) Toxic Substances List
TOXLINE	NLM,USA	MEDLINE EU:BLAISE DIMDI	1940	1.175	-
TDB(Toxic Data Base)	US Dep.En., USA	-	-	5	(Fact-Base)
RINGDOC	Derwent,GB	SDC EU:INFO-LINE	1964	500	-
PESTDOC	Derwent,GB	SDC	1968	100	-

Database	Producer	Host	Entry-date	Doc. Units (ths.)	Printed Versions
DRUGINFO	Univ.of Minn.,USA	BRS	-	-	-
GIFTPOOL	BGA,D	EU:DIMDI	1974	85	(Fact-Base)
INTDIS	Uppsala,S	EU:INTDIS	-	-	Int.Drug Info.Serv.
IPA	Am.Soc.Hosp. Plan.,USA	DIALOG	1970	70	Int.Pharma Abstr.
PNI	Data Courier USA	BRS DIALOG	1975	50	Pharm. Newsl.Index
CRDS (Chem.Re-act.Doc. Service)	Derwent,GB	SDC	1944	40	(Fact-Base)
CAS (CHEMABS, CHEMLINE)	Am.Chem. Soc.,USA	BRS DIALOG SDC EU:ESA-IRS BLAISE DIMDI	1976	490	CA-Condensates Chem. Abstracts (Fact-Base)
VET.MED. CAB-ANIMAL	Common-wealth Agric. Bureau,GB	DIALOG EU:DIMDI	1972	616	Abstracts
LADB (Lab.An. Data B.)	Battelle, USA	-	-	-	(Fact-Base)
FOOD SCI. FSTA	IFIS,GB	DIALOG SDC EU:ESA-IRS DIMDI GID	1969	210	-

Fig. 2

Databases in the Field of Medicine

4. Assessment

4.1 Technical and logical accessibility

In general, the user requests the library of his university, factory, or research institution etc., to help him search in databases. For this task of information-transfer, the library has at its disposal a typewriter-terminal with acousticcoupler (300 baud) or a display with modem (1200 or more baud).

The actual distribution of EDB-equipment and the possibility to use the many existing bureaus of information-broker or technology adviser reduce the problem of technical accessibility.

Important for the logical accessibility and the choice of the suitable databases are the following points:

> software   - rapid searching = low charges
>
> user help   - toll free phone with trained staff
>
> online
> order   - order of the found literature as e.g. DIAL-
>   Order (Dialog) or Electronic Maildrop (SDC)

At present, it is very difficult to estimate the importance of the price. If the user knows that he has to pay, he or his transmitter decides the choice of a host by such criterias as comfort, fastness of printouts, and completeness than by fees. A calculation in advance is very difficult. It depends on the following factors: phone-charge, net-charges, connecting time, number of printouts, licence charge, postal charges. Therefore, information offices calculate with standard charges. The price is very important indeed, if the literature search is part of a general consulting task. In this way, the information officer supplies a refined product by reading, evaluating, and combining the searched literature.

4.2 Completeness and Hit-Rate

Instruments of the hosts, a correct search, and points of evaluation for use are:

> Pre-search   - search, which database should be the
>   bastion for the users's question,
>   e.g. DIALINDEX

| Online-thesaurus | – defined, specialized vocabulary to find the correct Keyword, in context with broader or narrower terms or refer-to-connections, e.g. Mesh (Medical Subject Headings) |
| Keyword in Context | – comfort by numerous databases and by the possibility to save or transmit the search-descriptors besides different thesauri |

A point for the user is the hit-rate, i.e. to find the literature as accurately as possible. Supposed is, that all possible databases are involved and, on the other hand, that every requested database is searched as intensively and extensively as possible. Every relevant article should be found, and not a single one should be disregarded. However, no partial or non-relevant literature should be printed. In addition the whole number should be in a reasonable frame, e.g. below 100.

By these means it is recommendable to select a well-trained information-officer, not only in respect of the EDB-equipment but also of the search quality.

4.3 Possibilities for Comparison

In general, it is very difficult, or nearly impossible, to say to a physician or pharmacist: this is your correct database. The enourmous economical interests that exist in the information market do not allow such general phrases. (Here only the millions of Dollars paid to buy SDC by Burroughs or BRS by Thyssen-Bornemisza in 1980 have been mentioned.)[4]

But apart from that, it is though only by defining the conditions and the knowledge of the gaps that one is able to search for the correct things. In general, one has to consider that a good search depends on a search in several databases.[5] The user should start in the base with the highest hit-likelyhood.

> Example: The task is to look into job-sharing of physicians. Recommendable databases are: Medlars, Embase, Health, HECLINET and ILO.
>
> It is necessary to know that Medlars is an American based system which includes only some foreign literature, but especially non-English

literature;

Health is a subsystem of Medlars, which combined with
datas of different American hospital institutions and
is subject to the same restrictions;

Chiefly, Embase is medically and clinically orientated;
e.g. literature about nursing is not included;

HECLINCET is a German and Scandinavian based system[6]
(about 60 %);

the ILO database content rates literature from the
viewpoint of ergonomics.

A European user should start with HECLINET and complete
with Health. An American user should proceed vice versa
but actually theydo not like to read European or German
literature.

Apart from the knowledge about the contents the user has to be aware
that the same database in different hosts has different conditions.
It is possible that in one case the base is stored with abstracts,
and in another case without. Some categories could be implemented
in one host contrary to another one. They could be searchable or
not; a free text-search depends on the software and the retrieval
language of the different hosts.

The amount of literature that compares the substantial or formal
aspects for the user, is reasonable but highly specialized and it
does not allow general statements. More helpful could be an quantitative analysis of libraries; the background and the cause for copy-
orders or loan-outs based on online-searches gives a (even if very
vague) feedback of the user behaviour and user-satisfaction.[7]

5.   Tendencies

The user has an increasing possibility to effect a pinpointed search
for the desired literature with the help of capable systems.

As before, he will carry out short-searches (quick and dirty) in
printed versions. Intensive searches with a certain claim to
quality and quantity will be done increasingly online. The direct
operating of EDB-equipment by the ultimate user will be increased
but only relating to their profession.

The development of the information market will concentrate the available databases in very few hosts. The quality of software, hardware and research systems will be more similar. On this background, the price and quality of the offered databases are more relevant to the user. Numerical databases will obtain more importance than literature databases.

References

1) Penke, K.; Schneemann, R.
   Besuch bei SDC and Dialog in Kalifornien. Bericht von einer Studienreise.
   Bibliothek, Forschung und Praxis; (1982) No. 1

2) Krichmar, A.
   Command language ease of use: a comparison of DIALOG and ORBIT.
   Online Review; 3(1981) No. 3, S. 227 ff.

3) Common Command Language: Ironing out the differences.
   Diane News; (1981) No. 24, September, p. 10

4) See e.g. Online; 5 (1981) No. 1, S. 9

5) Bechtel, H.
   Eine Datenbasis ist nicht genug.
   Nachrichten für Dokumentation; 32 (1981) No. 2, S. 78-84

6) Schneemann, R.; Swertz, P.
   HECLINET - Advanced European Cooperation for Literature Documentation in the field of Hospital Care
   Proceedings of the 3rd Annual WAMI Meeting. May 1980
   Paris 1980, S. 70-82

7) Bake, H.; Kühnen, F.J.
   Information und Literaturanforderung. Eine Untersuchung bei einer zentralen Fachbibliothek.
   Nachrichten für Dokumentation; 31(1980) No. 6, S. 232-241

Online-Directories

Am. Soc. Inf. Science
Computer Readable Data Bases - a Directory and Source book
Washington 1979

Codlin, E.M. (Ed.)
Aslib Directory - volume 2
Information Sources in Social Sciences, Medicine and Humanties
London: Aslib 1980, 871 pp.

Commission of the European Community
EURONET - DIANE Directory 1981
Brüssel-Luxemburg: EEC 1981, 72 pp.

Cuadro Ass. (Hrsg.)
Directory of Online Databases
Santa Monica; 1(1979) ff.

GID (Hrsg.)
ODIN-Datenbankführer
Heidelberg: GID 1981, 377 pp

GID (Hrsg.)
Verzeichnis Deutscher Informations- und Dokumentationsquellen
Ausgabe 3, 1978/1979
München: Saur 1979, 463 pp.

Hall, J.L.; Brown, M.J.
Online Bibliographic Databases
2nd. ed. 1981
London: Aslib 1981; 213 pp.

Information Trade Directory, 1981
Oxford: Learned Information 1981, 217 pp.

Kruzas, A.T. (Ed.)
Medical and Health Information Directory
2nd ed.
Detroit: Gale 1980, 855 pp.

Kruzas, A.T.; Schmittroth Jr., J. (Ed.s)
Encyclopedia of Information Systems and Services
4th ed.
Detroit: Gale 1981, 930 pp.

Morton, L.T.
Use of Medical Literature
2nd ed.
London, Boston 1977

Tomberg, H. (Ed.)
EUSIDIC Database Guide 1981
Oxford, New York: Learned Information 1981

CLEARING-HOUSE FOR ON-GOING RESEARCH IN CANCER EPIDEMIOLOGY

C.S. Muir   K. Schlaefer   G. Wagner

Div. of Epidemiology & Biostat.   Institute for Documentation,
    International Agency for   Information und Statistics
      Research on Cancer   German Cancer Research Center
    150, cours Albert Thomas   Im Neuenheimer Feld 280
      69372 Lyon, France   6900 Heidelberg, F.R.G.

The ever increasing volume of research projects and the continuously growing costs of research make it imperative that overlap and reduplication of investigations be avoided as much as possible. In fast moving fields of science (e.g. molecular biology or virology), information about on-going research gets relatively rapidly out of date. In other fields (e.g. cancer epidemiology), however, it takes anywhere from 3 to 5 years to complete scientific studies. During this time, it frequently happens that very similar projects are initiated at different places, not knowing that work in the same field is already being carried out elsewhere. In order to facilitate the exchange of information on current projects, the International Agency for Research on Cancer (IARC) in Lyon and the German Cancer Research Center (DKFZ) in Heidelberg with the support of the National Cancer Institute (NCI) of the USA have set up a Clearing-House for On-Going Research in Cancer Epidemiology on which we want to report in the following.

1. AIM AND STATUS OF THE CLEARING-HOUSE

The purpose is to maintain a central data bank from which epidemiologists and other interested scientists can obtain information about on-going studies in cancer epidemiology and to facilitate direct contact and communication between researchers in the field.

Information about on-going research projects is procured by a circular letter with which a questionnaire developed for the Clearing-House is sent to about 12,000 scientists who are known or supposed to work in this field.

The information received is essentially reproduced in the annual Directories. In addition to the project descriptions, different indices with key-words facilitate the searching special projects.

The key-word indices arranged according to the different subject groups afford a purposeful access to the projects in the main part. In a list of scientists and countries the key-words and the corresponding project numbers are arranged in alphabetic order.

Special Permuterm indices are used as a connection between the key-words (e.g. the key-words of the TERM group and the sites investigated and vice versa). This leads to the following indices: (1) Investigators, (2) so-called "Term"-key-words, (3) tumour localisations, (4) chemicals investigated, (5) occupations, (6) type of study and (7) countries, where the data are collected.

Numerous suggestions for improvement with regard to contents and formal matters have been submitted by the users of the directories which have appeared since 1976 of which a considerable part could be taken into consideration in the course of the years whereby the layout and the information content of the directories was steadily improved.

The list of "formal" suggestions for improvement reached from the hint that "Nedlands" was but a suburb of Perth via typographical requests ("Titles should stand more out"), other wishes with regard to the form of presentation (countries as titles of columns) up to the form of the indices (introduction of special forms of Permuterm indices).

The most important proposals with regard to contents that could be realized in the meantime referred to the creation of a new section with bibliographic data on already published studies, the possibility for authors to suggest descriptors and the introduction of new indices for chemicals and occupations.

This interest on the part of the users, also expressed by numerous positive letters, shows clearly that there exists a great demand for information on current research projects and that the user of such information is prepared to cooperate so that "his" information system may be optimally to his requirements.

2. BIBLIOMETRIC RESULTS

A further problem is the detection of scientists working in the field of cancer epidemiology who are prepared to place at the disposal of the Clearing-House information on their research projects in time, i.e. at the beginning of the project or even in the planning stage.

The searching for investigators in this field is based on the assumption that scientists who once published in cancer epidemiolgy will continue to work in this domain. Therefore, the addresses of those scientists were ascertained who had published epidemiological papers on cancer in the past or who had participated in such publications. In this way, of course, many researchers were approached who had merely acted as consultants for a certain project.

In order to attain a separation between possible participants and casual co-workers, all scientists approached were classified according to their reply or non-reply and stored in two different databases. In the case of the researchers addressed for the first annual Directory 1976 - but not yet classified - we reached a reply rate of roughly one fifth: out of 5,619 scientists 980 replied; 242 of them informed us that they were not working in the field of cancer epidemiology; a further 187 informed us that they had no project running at the time; 91 projects reported did not fall into the framework of the Clearing-House. In all, 460 researchers reported 622 projects - a success rate of 8.2 percent.

After the first mailing cycle the address database was divided into possible participants and non-participants. In the meantime, a total file of 11,458 addresses has been attained. After the number of newly approached researchers had increased at the beginning, it went down to about 2,500 in the last cycle; the rate of answers seems to find its level at about 10 %. The number of new projects thus shows furthermore a dependency on the number of newly addressed researchers (Figure 1). It must, therefore, be assumed that it has not yet been possible to make out all epidemiologists ready to cooperate.

When the project was started in 1974, we assumed that the running time of a typical epidemiological project would be three to five years. An analysis of the duration of the projects from 1976 to 1981 about confirms this. However, the share of projects with a duration of only

one to two years is surprisingly high (24.4 %); projects with a longer
duration (more than 10 years) also form a considerable part with
20.1 %, among them projects of 20 years and more running time with
3.8 %. With many projects their duration is not yet fixed at the
beginning; with one fifth to one third (1976 and 1977) of the projects
nothing was said about their termination. The fact that the so-called
"smooth" figures (5, 10, 15, 20, ...) are mentioned so frequently shows
that some of the statements concerning duration are rather vague. In
some cases, the end of a project is sure to be determined by external
factors which cannot always be considered, such as the discontinuance
of project financing causing a premature end or difficulties arising in
procuring the necessary data which may delay the planned termination.

In all, a minor shift in the mean duration of projects can be seen:
from 1976 to 1978 the peak lay at two years, in the years 1979 to 1981
at three years. For example the year 1978 is represented in Figure 2.
In the years 1976 to 1980 the median had the value 4, in the year 1981
it reaches the value 5. The arithmetic mean developed from 5.3 years
in 1976 to 6.6 years in 1981.

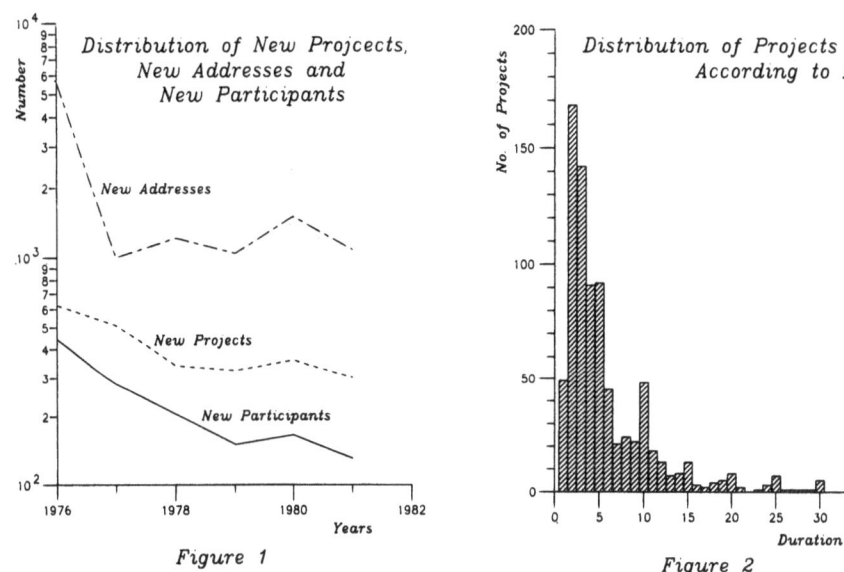

Figure 1

Figure 2

The mean project duration of 6.6 years means that 15.0 % of all
projects are eliminated from the database every year due to their
termination. The real development tends to the following value: of the
622 projects in the 1976 Directory 27 were eliminated after the first
year, i.e. 4.3 %. Of the 1,261 projects of the 1980 Directory 171
projects, i.e. 13.6 %, have been eliminated.

Contrary to literature information systems, project descriptions do not
remain unchanged: the progress of the projects is to be documented in
the new Directories by annual update actions. The share of replies
thereby doubled from 22.35 % (139 projects) in 1976 to 45.5 % (574
projects) in 1980. The share of investigators who replied demanding no
change in the descriptions increased from 9.0 % (1976) to 12.8 %

(1980). Since the epidemiologist have recognized the value of the Clearing-House, the non-response-rate decreased from 64.3 % in 1976 to 28.2 % in 1980. All the same, this share of more than a quarter is still high. The development of these percentages is illustrated in Figure 3.

The essential cooperation of researchers consists in their participation by reporting projects. Here, too, some noteworthy changes have taken place during the years 1976 - 1981 as the following schema shows:

DISTRIBUTION OF PROJECTS TO PARTICIPATING COUNTRIES

COUNTRIES	1976	1977	1978	1979	1980	1981
USA	239	324	370	374	438	463
United Kingdom	85	139	143	142	158	160
Japan	12	37	45	61	67	73
Canada	33	45	42	58	72	61
France	16	27	34	34	45	50
Italy	15	19	18	24	36	44
India	21	21	26	24	31	33
Sweden	11	16	21	29	30	33
Australia	16	27	32	31	33	31
Federal Rep. of Germany	25	28	31	29	30	28
Israel	14	18	22	20	21	23
Denmark	10	12	13	14	17	23

All other countries in all years less than ten projects

TOTAL OF PROJECTS	622	906	1025	1092	1261	1313
NUMBER OF COUNTRIES	55	61	63	66	69	70

While the "large" countries (USA, United Kingdom) show an absolute increase, their relative share decreased by several percent which in all probability is due to an increase in the number of participating countries on one hand and to initial difficulties with some countries (Japan, France, Italy) underrepresented at the beginning on the other hand. A further group (Canada, Australia) shows a continuous increase of reported projects, its relative share stagnating. In some countries (e.g Germany) the number of reported projects remained about equal. India is the only developing country represented among the first ten countries.

Although there has been a 20 % increase in the total number of studies since 1978, a slight fall in the number and proportion of projects from Africa and South America occurred, while a concomitant minor increase in the proportion of studies from Western Europe, Japan and the United States is noted. However, the geographical pattern of study source has in general remained remarkably constant.

Reffering to the number of projects per one million inhabitants (Figures from the year 1980), this rank order has somehow changed: while the Anglosaxon countries remain in the first half, the "smaller" countries advance from the back places to the peak; Japan and India show a marked decrease (Figure 4). For the purpose of comparing the development the proportion to the projects of the year 1976 is also shown.

3. NATURE AND GEOGRAPHICAL DISTRIBUTION OF STUDIES REPORTED

One of the functions of the Clearing-House for On-going Research in Cancer Epidemiology is to monitor changes in the sites of cancer being studied, the hypotheses being tested, and the epidemiological methods used, with a view to suggesting where further effort is required, as well as assessing the level of epidemiological effort on a national and regional basis.

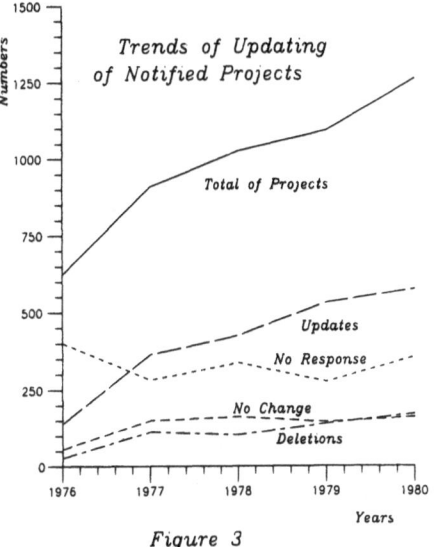

Figure 3

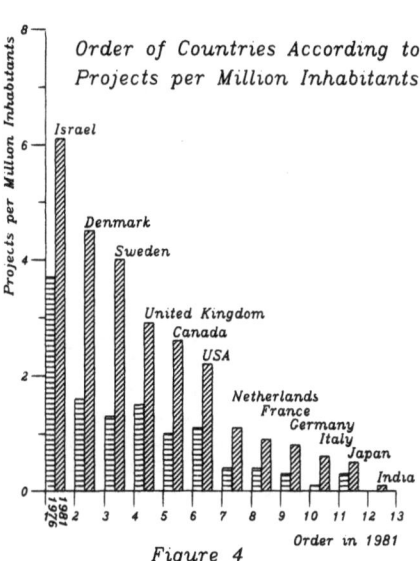

Figure 4

Such analyses have been carried trough for the materials for the years 1978, 1979 and 1981 and a comparison will be tried. Each study was assigned to one, or rarely two, broad categories in alphabetical order:

- case characteristics: studies in which the characteristics of cancer patients are examined with a view to hypothesis formulation;
- case-control: studies in which hypotheses are tested by comparing the replies of cancer patients and their controls to questions about their habits and exposures;
- cohort: studies in which groups with specific exposures are followed to determine whether they are associated with an increased cancer risk (see also high risk groups and occupational exposure);
- correlation: studies to determine whether there is a parallelism at the population level between an exposure and the risk of cancer;
- morphology: studies relating the microscopic appearances of cancer to epidemiological features;
- occupational exposure: studies to assess the risk of cancer, usually by the cohort method, in groups with defined occupational exposures;
- radiation: examines risk in persons exposed to ionizing radiation;
- screening: relates to studies in which the effect of screening programmes is being evaluated;
- statistics: covers those investigations - incidence, mortality or relative frequency - assessing the magnitude of the cancer problem in a county or region. This heading also includes studies dealing

with statistical methods;
- virus: studies in which a viral hypothesis of aetiology is being tested irrespective of the epidemiological method used;
- other: a residual category for those studies which could not be assigned to one of the above.

Where the same investigation dealt with more than one anatomical site, these were considered separately, particularly when involving different systems of the body. For many studies, notably those of a statistical nature and cohort studies, cancer developing in any organ is of interest and hence "All Sites" is the largest category in the tables.

Clearly, this approach is simplistic and, while an attempt was made to allocate study type and the site under study in as uniform a manner as possible, it is likely that there would be differences of opinion between classifiers concerning the assignments.

Since 1978 there has been a substantial increase in the proportion (and number) of case-control studies with a more or less equivalent fall in the studies of case characteristics. There has been little change in the proportion of cohort studies relating to occupation or other exposures.

The case-control study was almost twice as frequent in the US as in UK, cohort follow-ups, including those of industrial exposure, being about equally frequent in both countries (Table 1). Increasingly frequent are cohort studies in which a case-control investigation is also undertaken in relation to those cohort members who develop cancer. This technique is useful when it is desired to examine the effects of confounding variables, such as smoking, withouth going to the expense of collecting such data for all cohort members. As would be expected, statistical studies tended to be proportionately more frequent in those areas where analytical studies were uncommon (Table 1). Although analysis of the total database implies that it may be some time before a change of pattern is evident, there has been remarkably little change in the sites studied between 1978 and 1981. The lung is still by far the most frequent one, and over half of these investigations related to occupational exposures (Table 3). Studies of lung cancer were rather more common in Western Europe (excluding UK) than elsewhere (Table 3). Only 8 of the 23 projects dealing with pleural or peritoneal mesothelioma were directly associated with occupation (Table 2). There were a few more studies of urinary tract cancer than in 1978 and somewhat fewer dealing with male genital cancer, malignant lymphoma and leukaemia.

Not only does the Clearing-House indicate where epidemiological work is being done, the sites studied and the techniques being used, it also permits assessment of those areas which are currently not being adequately covered. Thus there is still little work on cancer of the pancreas, which is increasing rapidly in both sexes on a worldwide basis, and on cancer of the prostate, one of the most common forms of malignancies in occidental males.

Finally the 1981 Directory shows that although diet and life style, probably responsible for over half of the cancers in females, are being increasingly studied, emphasis still tends to be on the identification on discrete chemical carcinogens.

Thus, the directory also reflects the most important focal points of research of the present time in the field of cancer epidemiology.

Table 1. Geographical distribution of on-going epidemiological studies in 1981 by study type

	Case Characteristics n	Case Characteristics %	Case-Control n	Case-Control %	Cohort n	Cohort %	Correlation n	Correlation %	Genetic, Familial n	Genetic, Familial %	High Risk Groups n	High Risk Groups %	Morphology n	Morphology %	Occupational Exposure n	Occupational Exposure %	Radiation n	Radiation %	Screening n	Screening %	Statistics n	Statistics %	Virus n	Virus %	Other n	Other %	Total	% of Total
Africa	10	23	4	9	2	5	5	11	2	5	1	2	3	2	3	2	–	–	–	–	6	14	7	16	1	2	44	3.2
Canada	1	2	20	32	9	15	4	6	–	–	–	–	–	–	12	19	3	5	2	3	11	18	–	–	–	–	62	4.5
Europe, East (incl. USSR)	3	4	16	22	5	7	6	8	–	–	4	6	2	3	11	15	2	3	4	6	19	26	–	–	–	–	72	5.2
Europe, West (excl. UK)	13	5	47	17	17	6	23	8	5	2	11	4	11	4	42	15	13	5	21	8	56	21	10	4	3	1	272	19.8
Far East (excl. Japan)	9	15	11	18	6	10	2	3	3	5	1	2	1	2	–	–	–	–	1	2	19	31	7	11	2	3	62	4.5
Japan	3	4	17	23	7	9	9	12	2	3	2	3	2	3	4	5	5	7	4	5	18	24	2	3	–	–	75	5.5
Middle East	5	11	10	22	1	2	7	16	–	–	1	2	1	2	4	9	1	2	–	–	7	16	6	13	2	4	45	3.3
Oceania	4	9	9	20	2	4	2	4	1	2	1	2	–	–	5	11	3	7	1	2	18	39	–	–	–	–	46	3.3
South America	4	4	7	26	1	4	–	–	–	–	3	11	1	4	–	–	–	–	1	4	12	44	1	4	–	–	27	2.0
UK	4	2	23	14	23	14	22	13	2	1	4	2	1	1	40	24	9	5	8	5	25	15	3	2	1	1	165	12.0
USA	12	2	118	23	60	12	38	7	19	4	18	4	12	2	101	20	32	6	14	3	57	11	20	4	4	1	505	36.7
All countries	65		282		133		118		34		46		34		222		68		56		248		56		13		1375	
% of Total	4.7		20.5		9.7		8.6		2.5		3.3		2.5		16.1		4.9		4.1		18.0		4.1		0.9			

Table 2 Type of on-going epidemiological studies in 1981 by primary site of cancer

Case	All Sites	Oral Cavity 140-146	Nasopharynx 147	Oesophagus 150	Stomach[*] 151	Intestine 152-154	Liver, Gallbladder 155-156	Pancreas 157	Nasal Sinus, Larynx 160-161	Lung[*] 162	Mesothelioma[*] 163.0	Bone, Soft Tissue 170-171	Melanoma of Skin 172	Other Skin	Breast 174	Cervix 180	Other Female Genital 181-184	Male Genital 185-187	Bladder, Kidney, Urinary Tract 188-189	Eye, Brain, etc. 190-192	Endocrine 193-194	Malignant Lymphoma 200-203 incl. BL	Leukaemias 204-207	Childhood Neoplasms	Other	Total	% of Total
Case Characteristics	8	4	–	2	2	–	1	1	–	6	2	1	5	1	5	3	10	1	3	–	–	3	2	4	1	65	4.7
Case-Control	21	3	1	5	16	11	9	7	6	28	1	3	11	3	42	10	22	8	24	10	2	15	10	9	5	282	20.5
Cohort	43	8	–	1	6	9	2	–	–	12	3	–	–	1	15	5	6	2	3	1	2	2	4	5	4	133	9.7
Correlation	36	1	–	4	14	5	7	–	1	15	4	–	–	4	7	2	3	2	–	–	3	5	2	2	–	118	8.6
Genetic, Familial	11	1	–	–	1	2	2	–	–	–	–	–	3	–	3	1	1	–	–	1	–	3	1	3	1	34	2.5
High Risk Groups	8	4	–	2	3	6	–	–	–	2	1	–	–	1	9	3	–	–	2	1	–	3	–	1	1	46	3.3
Morphology	6	1	–	2	5	6	2	2	–	3	1	–	1	–	1	1	–	–	1	–	2	1	–	–	–	34	2.5
Occupational Exposure	100	–	3	–	2	1	5	–	4	64	8	3	–	–	–	–	1	5	5	3	–	8	8	–	2	222	16.1
Radiation	24	1	–	–	1	–	–	–	–	12	–	2	–	1	3	–	–	1	–	1	5	2	11	2	2	68	4.9
Screening	1	–	–	–	2	5	1	–	–	8	–	–	–	–	18	18	3	–	–	–	–	–	–	–	–	56	4.1
Statistics	124	2	2	1	14	4	5	1	1	14	3	4	5	6	8	3	3	4	2	4	4	10	2	16	6	248	18.0
Virus	1	–	6	–	1	–	21	–	–	–	–	1	–	–	1	10	1	4	–	–	–	6	–	–	–	56	4.1
Other	2	–	2	–	–	–	1	–	–	2	–	–	–	–	–	3	1	–	–	–	–	1	1	–	–	13	0.9
Total	385	26	14	17	67	49	56	11	12	166	23	14	25	17	112	60	51	27	40	21	18	59	41	43	21	1375	
% of Total excl. All Sites		2.6	1.4	1.7	6.8	4.9	5.7	1.1	1.2	16.8	2.3	1.4	2.5	1.7	11.3	6.1	5.2	2.7	4.0	2.1	1.8	6.0	4.1	4.3	2.1		
% of Total	28.0	1.9	1.0	1.2	4.9	3.6	4.1	0.8	0.9	12.1	1.7	1.0	1.8	1.2	8.1	4.4	3.7	2.0	2.9	1.5	1.3	4.3	3.0	3.1	1.5		

[*]Stomach includes gastrointestinal tract
Lung includes respiratory tract
Mesothelioma includes pleural and peritoneal mesothelioma

Table 3. Geographical distribution of on-going epidemiological studies in 1981 by primary site of cancer

	All Sites	Oral Cavity 140-146	Nasopharynx 147	Oesophagus 150	Stomach* 151	Intestine 152-154	Liver, Gallbladder 155-156	Pancreas 157	Nasal Sinus, Larynx 160-161	Lung* 162	Mesothelioma* 163.0	Bone, Soft Tissue 170-171	Melanoma of Skin 172	Other Skin 173	Breast 174	Cervix 180	Other Female Genital 181-184	Male Genital 185-187	Bladder, Kidney, etc. 188-189	Eye, Brain, etc. 190-192	Endocrine 193-194	Malignant Lymphoma 200-203 incl. BL	Leukaemias 204-207	Childhood Neoplasms	Other	Total	% of Total
Africa	8	3	—	3	2	—	11	—	—	3	1	—	—	—	3	—	1	—	—	—	—	6	3	—	—	44	3.2
Canada	16	1	—	—	2	1	1	—	—	13	—	—	2	—	10	2	2	2	3	2	—	1	2	1	1	62	4.5
Europe. East (incl. USSR)	22	1	—	—	8	2	—	—	1	10	—	1	2	2	10	2	4	—	—	—	—	2	1	2	2	72	5.2
Europe. West (excl. UK)	78	5	3	7	15	14	7	2	4	37	7	6	—	2	22	13	8	4	8	5	4	7	4	7	3	272	19.8
Far East (excl. Japan)	13	7	1	1	1	—	10	—	—	7	—	—	1	—	1	8	1	1	1	1	1	3	—	3	1	62	4.5
Japan	22	—	1	1	9	3	6	—	1	8	—	—	1	—	4	5	4	—	1	3	1	—	3	3	—	75	5.5
Middle East	12	1	1	3	1	1	—	—	—	5	4	—	—	1	3	1	3	—	1	—	—	4	2	1	—	45	3.3
Oceania	13	—	—	—	2	3	1	1	—	4	1	1	4	1	2	1	1	—	2	—	—	7	1	1	—	46	3.3
South America	8	—	1	—	1	—	1	—	—	1	—	—	2	—	2	6	—	1	1	—	—	3	1	—	—	27	2.0
UK	39	2	1	1	12	7	1	—	3	25	6	—	3	2	13	7	5	5	8	1	—	5	4	9	6	165	12.0
USA	154	6	6	1	14	18	19	8	2	53	4	6	11	9	42	15	22	14	15	9	12	21	20	16	8	505	36.7
All countries	385	26	14	17	67	49	56	11	12	166	23	14	25	17	112	60	51	27	40	21	18	59	41	43	21	1375	
% of Total excl. All Sites		2.6	1.4	1.7	6.8	4.9	5.7	1.1	1.2	16.8	2.3	1.4	2.5	1.7	11.3	6.1	5.2	2.7	4.0	2.1	1.8	6.0	4.1	4.3	2.1		

*Stomach includes gastrointestinal tract
Lung includes respiratory tract
Mesothelioma includes pleural and peritoneal mesothelioma

INFORMATION MEDIATION FROM THE VIEWPOINT OF INFORMATION SPECIALISTS. A DELPHI STUDY CONCERNING THE BIOMEDICAL COMMUNICATION NETWORK DIMDINET.

Birgit SCHWARZ and Peter L. REICHERTZ
Institute for Medical Informatics
Medical School Hannover, D-3000 Hannover 61, FRG

Information mediation and the functions of intermediaries from the subjective viewpoint of information specialists were subject of an inquiry concerning biomedical information services and its communication network DIMDINET. This paper primarily focusses on a few major aspects: profile of requirements of qualification and education of information specialists, organization structure and problems of centralization and decentralization of information centers, the role of commercial information brokers, the end-user as searcher. The inquiry was based on the Delphi technique.

1. PROBLEM DESCRIPTION

The development of information technology and the growing need for information, access to information, information transfer including the need for a mutual co-operation in this field has led in the USA and Europe to both an 'information industry' and several telecommunication networks, e.g. EURONET. These networks are established for access to computerized factual and bibliographic data bases covering a wide spectrum of subject fields of science and technology. Information services are provided by different types of persons or institutions which are service companies or public bodies: data base producers, information providers ('spinners'), intermediaries, information brokers. Recipients of information services are heterogeneous groups of end-users (e.g. experts or laymen interested in various subject fields; familiar or non-familiar with EDP etc.) needing to use information for their specific purposes and interests (e.g. technical or biomedical informations etc.). Intermediaries are established to act as a link between the system (data bases, data banks, information systems) and end-users. Information mediation and the role and functions of intermediaries from the subjective viewpoint of information specialists were subject of an investigation concerning biomedical information services and its communication network DIMDINET (3). DIMDINET was established on the national level with connection to EURONET for access to data bases covering the subject fields of biosciences, in particular, bibliographic data bases, e.g. MEDLARS etc.(1). Primary

589

concern of this investigation was dedicated to the problem that little is known about the chain of information origin - information bases - information transfer - end-users. In this context, information mediation respectively the functions of the intermediary (i.e. information center /institution or information specialist /person) play an important role on both a) as an essential connecting link between system and end-user and b) for an adequate and efficient supply of information.

2. MATERIAL AND METHOD

An inquiry, using the Delphi technique (2), was conducted to gain insight into opinions, ideas, experiences, motivations and assessments of information specialists according to the following topics resulting in a list of criteria:

1) Which are the requirements on education, professional qualification and activities of information specialists working in the field of information mediation and counseling ? 2) How should information centers - functioning as intermediaries - be organized (structure, functions, personnel) and located (centralized vs. decentralized; in private companies vs. public bodies) ? 3) Which are the requirements and outcomes of information centers respectively information specialists in regard to end-users ? 4) Which are the future trends concerning information brokerage on the private, commercial sector ?

The main goal of the Delphi technique is to obtain in a structured, multiphased group communication process knowledge, experiences and subjective assessment of a group of individuals - or experts - in order to deal with a complex problem. The main assumption of this method is that the view of a group of individuals (i.e. group judgement) has a better chance to be correct than the view of one individual (i.e. individual judgement). The inquiry, using questionnaires, comprised 3 Delphi rounds. A sample of 64 institutions with information centers respectively 147 'experts' participated in this inquiry. These institutions are or were DIMDINET-users, mainly working in the field of biosciences. Participant and return ratio of the inquiry are illustrated in table 2. In order to contrast opinions, the sample was divided into 2 main panels with sub-panels:

1. panel of institutions: (a) libraries of universities (human and veterinary medicine, bioscience, science and technology), (b) industry (pharmacy, chemistry, cigarettes), (c) institutional information and documentation centers (I+D) (energy/physics/mathematics, nutrition, health care, cancer research, psychology, sports), (d) research and authorities (health care, ecology, agriculture /forestry, pharmacy).
2. panel of 'experts': (a) information specialists, (b) ·heads of

information centers, documentation centers, libraries.

3. RESULTS

3.1 Information specialist

3.1.1 Education and professional qualification

The inquiry in the 3 Delphi rounds showed that much concern was
expressed by the participants on the subject field of education and
training. Which type of education is necessary for the information
specialist working in the wide and interdisciplinary field of biosciences: university vs. non-university education? Which type of non-university education ? Did the different panelists (library, industry,
I+D center, research and authorities) prefer specific profiles of
requirements in education ? Did the opinion of information specialists
contrast with the opinion of heads of information centers, documentation centers and libraries ?

The results showed a consensus of opinions (80% of panelists) that the
information specialist should be highly skilled and should have an
education on an university level rather than on non-university level.
The group judgement concerning efficiency of education of information
specialists showed:

very efficient: university (graduated)
efficient: doctor's degree, advanced specialized colleges
less efficient: university (not graduated)
not efficient: (exclusive) training on the job, special colleges,
                 apprenticeship.

Preferences for a doctor's degree were expressed by the panels libraries, research and authorities as well as by the information specialist
himself and the heads of I+D centers and libraries. Naturally, the
expressed opinion of the information specialists is effected by their
own education level and their environment. About 90% of the information specialists are graduates of universities (about 40% have a doctor's degree) and about 10% are educated on a non-university level,
e.g. special colleges etc.

Reasons for an university education were specified as follows:
The information specialist should have a wide, detailed, well-founded
knowledge of specialties and good knowledge of the specific terminology and terminology of the data base(s). He should be an adequate
partner in communicating with experts and scientists in the subject
field. He must be able to clearly understand the background, content
of (scientific) search requests of the user and must be able to analyze and solve the problems in an optimal manner in order to transpose
them in an optimal data base search respectively use the data base(s)

efficiently. This includes qualifications in analytical and methodological thinking.

Different opinions and profiles of requirements in education could be
obtained according to the different panelists. Libraries of universities prefer an university education (83%), desirable is a doctor's
degree. Less suitable is an education on a level of an advanced specialized college. Research and authorities: All panelists prefer an
university education. 84% expressed that a non-university education
is conceivable. Preferable is a doctor's degree; suitable an advanced
specialized college education and less suitable an university education without graduating. I+D centers: 88% of the panelists felt that
an university education is necessary. Less necessary is a doctor's
degree. Suitable is the education on the advanced specialized college
level; less suitable an university education without graduating.
Industry: The panel industry differs from the other panels in regard
to requirements in education. 54% expressed that an university education is necessary; 39% less necessary and 7% not necessary. University education is as well preferred as education on advanced specialized colleges respectively university education without graduating.
Here, the application orientation corresponds to the pragmatic view of
science in industry.

Concerning the education in biosciences on the level of advanced specialized colleges, the results showed that the model curriculum for
documentalists in bioscience established in Hannover, Germany (4)
could be suitable in future for education of information specialists.
The group judgement showed that - based on present opinion and without
corresponding experiences with graduates of this type of curriculum -
the bioscientific documentalist could become a professionally acceptable alternative to the university graduates (58%). However, the panelists felt that the bioscientific documentalist is at present and in
future time neither preferable nor equal to a graduate from university
(specialist).

3.1.2 Information specialist and auxiliary personnel

80% of the panelists stated that it is (very) desirable to relieve the
information specialist from non-specific tasks in information mediation, especially main and auxiliary administrative tasks. These tasks
should be delegated to specially skilled and auxiliary personnel.
Specially skilled personnel, i.e. assistants of the information specialist, should mainly perform search requests, e.g. manual searches,
simple computer searches - perhaps under supervision of the information specialist - as well as main administration tasks, e.g. sorting

search requests, pre- and postselection of printouts etc. (90% of the panelists). Auxiliary personnel should mainly perform administrative (auxiliary) tasks, e.g. typing addresses, filing papers, sorting results, some parts of search statistics etc.

96% of the panelists would prefer an organizational structure of an information center of the type of a team compared to a one-man position. This team should - in the opinion of the panelists - have a team-leader, educated on university level (specialist). He should be chief of the information specialist(s), assistant(s) and auxiliary personnel. Such a construction could facilitate the employment of differently skilled persons on different educational levels (table 1).

3.1.3 Information specialist and end-user as searcher:

Another main question was related to the information specialist as a link to end-users. Although the panelists characterize the end-user as interested, active co-operating and useful, 76% of the panelists would accept the end-user as recipient of information services only, but not as searcher. Based on experiences and probably self-assessment, the panelists expressed apprehensions if the end-user would perform search requests in different data bases himself. The results showed a divergency of opinions: on the one hand, pro user as searcher and on the other hand, contra user as searcher. Reasons pro user searches were specified with: provided, information systems will become more user acceptable (easier in handling the system etc.) the user could be accepted as searcher. On the other hand, apprehensions were stated by the panelists based on the insufficient professional competence, insufficient knowledge of specialties and data bases (terminology, retrieval etc.). However, a general conclusion should not be drawn from these opinions because, in this context, the heterogenity of end-users and user's behavior as well as the location of information centers (library of an university, industry etc.) must be kept in mind.

3.2 Information center

3.2.1 Centralized vs. decentralized information centers

72% of the panelists prognosticated an increasing number of institutions with information centers in the next years, occupying highly skilled specialists and information specialists, as intermediaries for external data bases (defined as decentralized information centers). 54% prognosticated this trend also for institutions providing own data bases (defined as centralized information centers).

3.2.2 Location of centralized and decentralized information centers

According to the following priority scale, centralized information centers with own data bases should be located in:

1. information centers of a specific subject field (e.g. the German
   Institute of Medical Documentation DIMDI, covering the subject
   fields of biosciences etc.),
2. commercial data base producers and or data base providers (e.g.
   Lockheed, Excerpta Medica etc.),
3. in large institutes,
4. in industrial enterprises.

Decentralized information centers not providing own data bases should
be located in libraries, e.g. close to or in connection with universities (87%). As an alternative to libraries, locations were considered
desirable by the panelists:

1. demand-intensive research institutes,
2. large institutes with a sufficient volume of requests,
3. universities,
4. institute or faculty,
5. national specialized information centers with additional facilities, e.g. information analysis, contact with experts,
6. libraries of faculties (with different subject fields of data
   bases),
7. industrial enterprises.

less desirable:

8. close to the library,
9. commercial information brokers and or information consultants.

3.3 Information brokers

78% of the panelists prognosticated a growing trend in the field of
commercial information brokers. This trend was expected to start
rather in 1980-85 (71%) than in 1986-90 (27%) or 1991-95 (2%). 85%
supposed, that commercial information brokerage will become a new
market providing e.g. small and medium-sized enterprises with information services. 64% from 85% of the panelists agreed with this trend,
21% supposed that it is indispensable respectively the only possibility to provide the small and medium-sized enterprises with scientific
and technological information.

4. CONCLUSION

From the results of the investigations suggestions and recommendations
in regard to curricula aspects and research planning were expected.
According to 'information industry' much concern should be dedicated
to the commercial information brokerage and counseling, especially
under the aspect to offer the end-user information services from factual data bases.

REFERENCES

1. Fritz R, George R, Kurzwelly HE, Plate G. DIMDINET. Bedarfsgerechte und benutzernahe Informationsversorgung durch Errichtung und Betrieb eines Informationsnetzes: Modellvorhaben im Bereich der Biomedizin. Bundesministerium fuer Forschung und Technologie (ed.), Forschungsbericht ID 81, Bonn, 1981 (in press).
2. Linestone HA, Turoff M (eds.). The Delphi Method. Techniques and Applications. Addison-Wesley, London, 1975.
3. Reichertz PL, Schwarz B. Informationsvermittlung aus der Sicht des Informationsvermittlers. Eine Delphi-Studie als Begleituntersuchung zum Projekt DIMDINET. Bundesministerium fuer Forschung und Technologie (ed.), Forschungsbericht ID 81-004, Bonn, 1981.
4. Rienhoff O. From medicine to bioscience. A modified concept for the education of documentation clerks. In: Lindberg DAB, Kaihara S (eds.): MEDINFO 80, North-Holland Publ., Amsterdam, 1980, 349-352.

Table 1:

Table 1: organizational structure of an information center
(according to different panels)

libraries of universities:
1. leader: specialist (university)
2. information
   specialist: specialist (university)
   bioscientific documentalist (advanced spec. college)
3. assistants: bioscientific documentalist (advanced spec. college)
   documentation clerk (special college)
   librarian (special college)
4. auxiliary
   personnel: administrative employee

industry:
1. leader: specialist (university)
2. information
   specialist: bioscientific documentalist (advanced spec. college)
   specialist (university)
3. assistants: documentation assistant in medicine (special college)
   documentation clerk (special college)
   laboratory assistant (special college)
4. auxiliary
   personnel: administrative employee

I+D centers:
1. leader: specialist (university)
2. information
   specialist: bioscientific documentalist (advanced spec. college)
   specialist (university)
   librarian (advanced specialized college)
   documentalist (advanced specialized college)
3. assistants: librarian (special college)
   documentation assistant (special college)
   documentation assistant in medicine (special college)
4. auxiliary administrative employee
   personnel: secretary

research and authorities:
1. leader: specialist (university)
2. information
   specialist: specialist (university)
   bioscientific documentalist (advanced spec. college)
   scientific employee without a special education in
   information mediation
3. assistants: bioscientific documentalists (advanced spec. college)
   documentation clerk (special college)
   documentation assistant in medicine (special college)
   documentalist (advanced specialized college)
   librarian (advanced specialized college)
   librarian (special college)
   scientific employee without a special education in
   information mediation
4. auxiliary secretary
   personnel: administrative employee

Table 2:

Participant and return ratio of 3 Delphi rounds
(institutions, information specialists and heads of
information and documentation centers, libraries)

institutions n=64		return	
	round 1	round 2	round 3
	51 (80%)	37 (58%)	41 (64%)
panels:			
library (27)	24 (89%)	18 (67%)	2o (74%)
industry (19)	14 (73%)	9 (47%)	11 (58%)
I+D centers (1o)	6 (60%)	4 (40%)	5 (5o%)
research and authorities (8)	7 (88%)	6 (75%)	5 (63%)
participants:	n=147	n=142	n=139
return:	95 (65%)	56 (39%)	63 (45%)
information specialists	59 (62%)	33 (59%)	36 (57%)
heads of I+D centers,libr.	36 (38%)	23 (41%)	27 (43%)

INFORMATRICS:

THE CLINICAL TRIAL SYSTEM OF CIBA-GEIGY

R. Bieri, N. Palmer, L. Penin, M. Turri

CIBA-GEIGY AG
CH-4002 BASEL SWITZERLAND

1. Summary

The main objectives of INFORMATRICS, the clinical trial system of Ciba-Geigy, are to improve the quality of the data and to speed up the completion of trials and the registration process. The system consists of a worldwide network of intelligent terminals connected with central interrelated data bases using an english-like query language. Its main benefits and drawbacks are discussed.

2. Introduction

One of the most time-consuming parts of drug development is the period of clinical trials, when the preparation is administered according to a pre-specified plan to selected populations in order to assess its efficacy and tolerability. In its nature this has to be a deliberative process, but a further delay is imposed by the frequency of errors and deviations from plan in the execution of the trials. We frequently found that data foreseen in our trials was not in fact usable, for several reasons:
- The trial plan was misunderstood.
- Restrictions on patient recruitment were overlooked and a non-homogenous sample collected.
- Omissions were not noticed until the data was analysed, by which time they could not be remedied.
- Initial estimates of patient intake were higher than the patient numbers actually collected.

We felt, then, that it would be worth investing a good deal of effort in the construction of a system which would allow us to process clinical trial data during the trial while it is still possible to correct mistakes.

Coupled with this, we wanted to create an integrated information system bringing together in easily-retrievable form all the information available on clinical trials from all the branches of the company.

3. Objectives

We decided that the new system should aim at the following objectives:
- Early data validation
- Control of trial progress from the planning stage right through to the archieving stage
- Centralization of information allowing general searching (by cross-referencing all aspects of trials)
- Improvement of the design of new trials
- Decentralization of data entry and correction
- Access to data for local branches
- Possibility of interim analysis during a trial
- Improved information exchange between branches via Headquarters
- Early data entry and storage to help monitor progress
- Standardised classification of medical terminology.

4. Structure of the system

Each Ciba-Geigy branch has an intelligent terminal (a Data General Micronova or Nova) which they use for input, corrections and requests for output. This communicates with our central (IBM 3033) computer via a further Nova acting as a "front-end" for the central machine. The front-end is available 24 hours a day and exclusively used by Informatrics (unlike the central computer), so that branches can be confident of having the machine available to pass on their data and requests.

Data are centrally stored in the IBM 3033 using a relational data base management system (INQUIRE, © INFODATA). This enables us to group together similar data from all our international trials and get the overview of progress and the broader picture of trial results which are needed to meet the objectives listed above. Separated but interrelated data bases are used to describe:
- the trial plan
- the validation criteria checking that the data collected are plausible, consistent and complete
- the drugs used in the trial
- the planned and actual timing and patient numbers
- the classification of medical terminology encountered in textual data (e.g. side-effects)

This data bank is used for a variety of functions described below. In particular, it automatically generates the data entry/correction programs for the terminals on the basis of the plan description and the validation criteria, thereby avoiding the need for special programming after each trial. These programs are written using standard data entry and communications software from the London consultants LOGICA Ltd. (who adapted the software for us to the clinical trial context). It was the availability of this software on the Data General family of machines which most influenced us to opt for the Micronova and Nova. The system works in practice as follows:

Before a trial starts, the following specifications are entered in the central system, making use wherever possible of data from similar trials already in the bank:
- Administrative trial data
- Drug regimens
- Treatment groups using these regimens
- Patient numbers randomly allocated to these treatment groups
- Trial plan and content/format of case record forms
- Validation criteria
- Format and content of lists and tables for reporting during trials (automatic or on request)

The central system now generates automatically from these specifications:
- Packing instructions and labels for the trial drugs
- Data entry and correction programs for the terminal
- A data base to record patient results
- A set of validation programs on the central computer
- A set of programs which will on request convert the current data into SAS, the Statistical Analysis System (© SAS Inc.) with flags marking doubtful data which have been confirmed in consultation with the investigator.
- Full documentation on the above tools for this trial.

If the trial starts on time, we move to the next stage. If it does not,then individual warnings are sent to the local and Headquarters staff for appropriate action, e.g. amendment of the expected starting date. The system therefore provides a constantly updated picture of trials in preparation, ongoing or concluded.

<u>During the trial</u>, the following steps are taken:
- During the patient's visits, the investigator records all required data on the case record form (patient's condition, laboratory results, any adverse effects, etc.).
- After completion, this form is sent to the local Ciba-Geigy branch as soon as possible.
- On receipt, <u>all data</u> on the form including texts are entered in the terminal <u>in their original form</u>.
- During data entry, checks are made for each line for format and plausibility, and the data are packaged by the terminal for transmission and processing on the central computer.
- The data are transmitted (via normal dial-up telephone) to Headquarters central computer via the front-end. They are then distributed to the relevant data bases, texts being automatically coded and stored in directories for later classification.
- The central computer runs its validation programs for all trials with fresh data. Error messages and lists required for each trial are automatically generated and sent to the appropriate local and Headquarters staff via the front-end.
- Local staff discuss error messages with the investigator and enter corrections, which are dealt with as in the 2 previous steps.

This process continues until the trial is completed. At any time, anyone using the system can ascertain the current state of progress, but detailed patient results are disclosed only to the staff directly involved, even then concealing the allocation of patient data to treatment groups, so that the staff are not biased by premature conclusions. At the end of the trial this security restriction is lifted. Patients are identified, of course, by number only, so the company is unaware of the patient's name.

<u>After trial completion</u>, the following steps are taken:
- The data is converted into SAS format for analysis
- After analysis, the data and programs used are "frozen" in long-term storage to facilitate re-analysis if questions should arise at a later date.
- Results regarding efficacy/tolerability are summarized in tables and short comments for later overviews.
- References to all internal and external documents on the trial are stored for future retrieval.

5. Present status

The system has been fully productive since March 1981, with data transfers so far between 20 Ciba-Geigy branches in Europe, Canada, South Africa and Australia and a routine turnaround time between data entry and output reports of 1 day. It has enough capacity to run all clinical trials monitored by Headquarters.

6.Shortcomings

During several months of intensive use, we have found the following shortcomings:
- A good deal of preparatory specification is required before a trial starts, and at present this can only be done at Headquarters. This limits the independence of the local branches in using the system and to some extent inhibits its acceptance. In the long run, this problem may be mitigated by further developments allowing some decentralization.
- The new tools place greater demands on paramedical personnel at Headquarters compared with earlier systems, making recruitment more difficult and necessitating more in-house training.

7. Benefits

The main benefits experienced so far have been:
- The processing costs have been reduced by 40%.
- Information on trial progress is available in time for appropriate action.
- The general retrieval capabilities of INQUIRE (©) and its convenient English-like query language give all users worldwide access to any clinical research-related data, subject to the security restrictions noted above.
- Few data processing-related constraints are imposed on case record form design.
- The interface with SAS (©) allows us to produce easy-to-read outputs in the form of tables, histograms and multidimensional graphs.

- The system is able to process all medical texts: all previously used terms are automatically coded, while all new terms receive new codes automatically. A central classification unit is able to use the system to refer all new terms (which may be in various languages) to preferred English terminology, creating new preferred terms as necessary. The preferred terminology is in turn classified by (for medications) composition and therapeutic and pharmacological classes using WHO principles, and (for symptoms and diseases) by systems and organs, function, etiology, morphology, and other categories following a microglossary based on SNOMED and ICD. The original texts are therefore retained in the system, but the statistician has the classification ready-made before starting the analysis.

8. Conclusion

The main effort went into the automatic parts of the system, and it is evident that a manually-controlled system would have been possible much more quickly. However, this would have required special programming for each trial, and the basic goal of speeding up drug testing to make the preparation available sooner would have been lost. We consider that the consequent benefits, both to the company and in social value, justify the effort, and hope that this abbreviated summary of our experiences may be useful to others in similar situations.

9. Acknowledgement

Before designing the system described here, experience was gained by developing a conceptually different one with more emphasis on the proper design of clinical trials, in cooperation with Professor Joyce of Ciba-Geigy Project Innovation, Medical Department, and with K. Hammond Associates of Boulder, Colorado, USA.

10. Members of Project Team

Medical Data Analysis (MDA), Medical Department:
    R. Bieri, G. Cameron, T. Mitterhofer, N. Palmer (Project Leader), M. Rainisio, M. Turri (Head of MDA), P. Weis
Scientific Computing Centre (WRZ):
    B. Bodmer, R. Bucher, P. Hadorn, S. Hamdy, K.H. Kuny, I. Moshfegh, L. Penin (technical Project Leader), D. Pole, F. Sandor, H. Schmitt.

CARDIOCOD DATABASE - CLINICAL USABILITY AND RESPONSIVENESS EVALUATION (1979-1981)

Henryk KRUG, Franciszek ZERBE, Tamara CIESLICKA,
Institute of Cardiology, Medical Academy, Poznań, Poland

Piotr J. JASIŃSKI
Technical University of Poznań, Poznań, Poland

Clinical usability and responsiveness of research-oriented CARDIOCOD database system [1] have been evaluated in this study.

The term <u>usability</u> is referred to ease of use of the database system by casual, non-programming clinical users, namely physician who uses the CARDIOCOD database as a tool supporting his research activity. The relational, algebra-based query language has been taken as a subject of a study. Two groups of voluntarily selected physicians (three physicians aged over 40 and three physicians aged over 30, all previously not engaded in a design of CARDIOCOD system) were given equal training in query language. After training consisted of 2-hours lectures and a selflearning from 16-pages user's manual they were examined with questions concerning CARDIOCOD database contents. All exams results were precisely evaluated for accuracy of formulated queries and time it took to complete a set of questions. The evaluation shows that:

- the relational query language proposed is relatively easy to learn,
- simplification and/or modification of certain language constructs (join, complex selection conditions) may reduce the amount of syntax errors in queries formulation,
- understanding of logical principles of data structure could be improved by more informative design of source clinical documents and would therefore simplify and shorten the necessary training for clinical users.

The term <u>responsiveness</u> is referred to the question how well the system responds to clinical user requirements and of what clinical research value are the data received. Therefore, apart from individual and not preplanned accesses to the database, we recognized a need of more generalized, retrospective evaluation of CARDIOCOD database contents. On the basis of clinically heterogenous population stored within CARDIOCOD system (October 1978 - September 1981, approx. 2500 patients) the evaluation of acute myocardial infarction (AMI) patients has been designed. The outline of analyses is given in Figure 1.

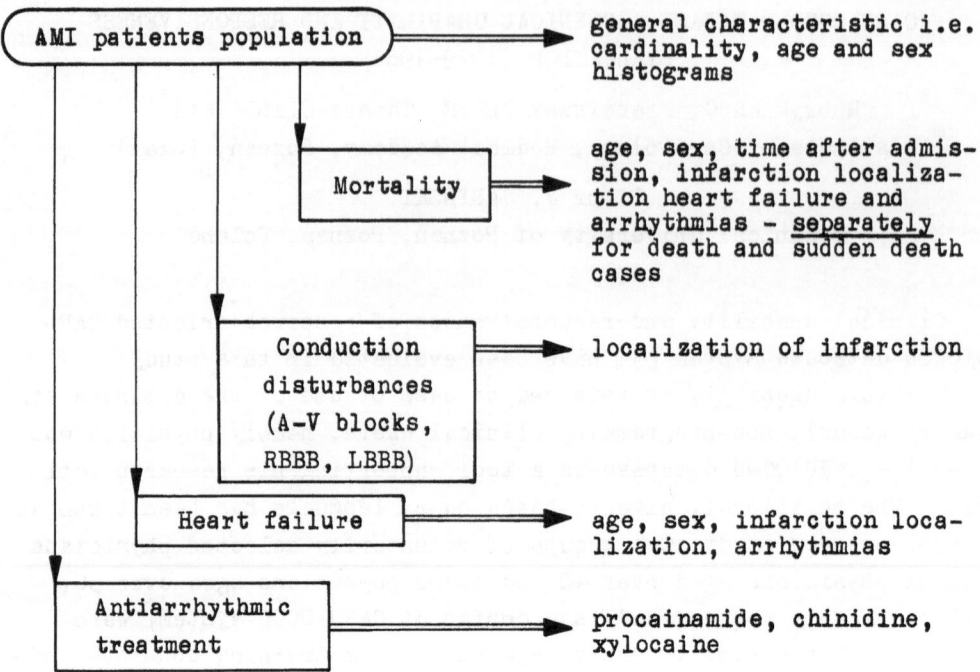

note: vertical lines (───►) represent selection of subgroups from
      AMI patients population; horizontal lines (═══►) lead to more
      detailed description of analyses performed.

Figure   1

   The analyses of cumulative data received from CARDIOCOD database
system show some intelligible discrepencies, as compared to the
literature data. However, the overall results of responsiveness
evaluation are an evidence that the availability of computer database storing our patients data could be of considerable practical
value in the statictical assessment of clinical events.

[1] Jasiński P.J., Krug H., Talkowska B.: Relational database CAR-
    DIOCOD: a tool for clinical research in cardiology. Medical
    Informatics Europe 81, Lecture Notes in Medical Informatics 11,
    Springer-Verlag 1981, 512-519.

A COMPARATIVE EVALUATION OF SOURCES OF INFORMATION ON OCCUPATIONAL DISEASES

Dr R A Burley   and   Miss A M C Kahn

Research Librarian   Chief Librarian

Industrial Injuries Advisory Council   Department of Health

Friars House   and Social Security

157-168 Blackfriars Road   Alexander Fleming House

LONDON   Elephant and Castle

SE1 8EU   LONDON

                                                                    SE1 6BY

This evaluative study of sources of information on occupational diseases was
carried out as part of a research project, in co-operation with the DHSS library,
investigating methods of setting up a current awareness information system for the
Industrial Injuries Advisory Council. The work of the Industrial Injuries Advisory
Council requires the provision of current information pertinent to the causation,
incidence and occupational links of occupational diseases. A considerable problem
in monitoring published information on occupational diseases arises from the fact
that the literature of the subject is widely dispersed. A number of potentially
useful abstracting and indexing publications and databases cover this subject area,
and an evaluative study was undertaken to identify material which is both relevant
and timely to the work of the Industrial Injuries Advisory Council. Over a one-year
study period, a selected group of primary journals, abstracting and indexing
publications were regularly scanned and a number of databases searched for relevant
articles, and retrieved items were systematically recorded using a card index
system. Analysis of the results of the study has revealed differences in the
coverage and timeliness of the various sources dealing with occupational diseases,
and has enabled the recommendation of an effective method of monitoring published
information for the Industrial Injuries Advisory Council.

ETAT DE SANTE

de la population française masculine à 20 ans

Alain GUILLOREAU *   Nathalie BOULARD *   Philippe GRANDHAYE **   Thierry LAMBERT ***

For 130 years, and still now, a law prescribes that morbidity's statistics concerning Military Staff must be published every year.

Five years ago the Army Health Service set a number of automated applications which help not only to obtain precise epidemiological data on the sources of the Staff's attrition but also to evaluate the general sanitory state of 400 000 young people, and eventually to get an idea of the general epidemiology of the country, at least for the male population with a very short notice to obtain the information.

Depuis 130 ans une loi impose la publication annuelle de statistiques de morbidité concernant les personnels militaires.

Depuis cinq ans le Service de Santé des Armées a mis en place un certain nombre d'applications automatisées qui lui permettent non seulement d'obtenir des données épidémiologiques précises sur les causes de l'attrition des effectifs mais aussi de situer l'état sanitaire général d'une population jeune de 400 000 individus et accessoirement d'approcher l'épidémiologie générale du pays tout au moins pour sa population masculine, avec un très court délai d'obtention des informations.

The military administration has always wanted to know about the morbidity and mortality of its staff :

- for the purposes of prevention,

- with the aim of casting the possible use of the armed forces,

- finally in order to prepare and plan necessary sanitary means.

Since January 1851 law prescribes usual annual publication of this compulsory information.

The health service has progressively set a system of information derived from the previous intention to evaluate the technical activity of medical staff. This system presently allows with an average three monthes notice to get :

- activity date;

- the main diseases in the armed forces in the mother country and overseas;

- the reasons for exemption or elimination of national service;

- detailed supervision of some particular diseases.

Most of these epidemiological data can be reduced to a precise referential.

- homogeneous and known population,

- specified geographical surroundings,

- I.C.D. 75 from the W.H.O.as semantical reference.

*   Centre de Traitement de l'Information Médicale des Armées - 69, Avenue de Paris - 94160 St-MANDE
    Téléphone 374.12.40 - Poste 45.40

** Université de Nancy I. Faculté de Médecine - 54500 VANDOEUVRE

*** Service de Pharmacologie Pr. TILLEMENT - Faculté de Médecine - 94000 CRETEIL

They can be used by :

Military administration :

to set medical means aimed at preventing or reducing the risks;

to establish possible consequences of the use of the aimed forces in a given place from operational research studies.

Public health

to estimate sanatory state of all French twenty years old males and to draw the consequences concerning health care at school and at work.

Medical research

to focus at national level some diseases for which little information is quickly available.

Eventually, an overall survey of the male population pathology can be given by the system. However all these potentialities can be maintained only if the system gives reliable information.

All the efforts made by the health service aim at bettering the quality of the data by :

- organisational procedures;

- complete integration of different sub-systems;

- motivation of the providers and users of the information.

the followings will be successively studied;

- the elements of the reference set;

- the different aspects of the set of sub-systems.

- motivation of the providers and users of the information.

the followings will be successively studied;

- the elements of the reference set;

- the different aspects of the set of sub-systems;

- the obtained results and products,

- the problems encountered and further developments.

I - THE ELEMENTS OF THE SET OF REFERENCES.

1.1. - Population

The system provides an overview of all military population morbidity (600 000 people). But the rules of medical practice only allow us to take into account the "contingent" part of this group.

This includes all French young males aged 18-27 (average 20 yeard old). That is 400 000 people.

These people receive medical supervision according to two methods :

- one static questionnaire which they receive at 18, when they go through medical examination for aptitude to national service, 25 % are exempted;

- the other, one, dynamic during the national service (12 to 16 monthes) which concern 300 000 people. For them any pathological manifestation is known.

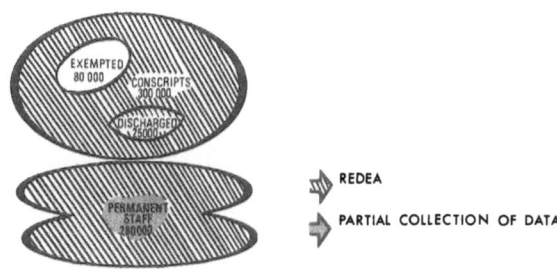

1.2. - Geographical surrounding

The information given allows us to attribute pathology to a definite geographical surrounding where the patients' units are located.

This geographical definition corresponds to epidemiological countries integrating 1 to 5 metropolitan departments or overseas sectors. However, under certain circumstances it is possible to situate events to a department or even a city which can be those where the patient lives or is born

1.3. - Semantical reference

Since the beginning of 1979, the use of I.C.D. (1975) has been extended to all statements of disease in the Army.

II - SET OF SUBSYSTEMS

2.1. - Hardware and Software.

For the described system, a computer CII HB IRIS 55 is used.

The software has been developed by "Centre de Traitement de l'Information Médicale des Armées".

The others can be analysed according to three groups :

- those corresponding to the first stage of selection,

- those corresponding to the normal active National Service,

- those corresponding at least to the studies of particular diseases.

2.2. - The selection

This medical examination is always done in ten specialized centers spread in the whole country, in order to determine physical and professional aptitude of all French young men for army jobs. An automated system's allows to obtain in one month's time :

- statistical data on activity;

- non confidential general information on medical classification (1 to 7) of the young people examined;

- precise biometric data (height, weight);

- all exemption's reasons in reference with 75 I.C.D. (80 000 annual cases).

Table I : Reasons for exemption from Military Service : Mental disturbances

TABLEAU RECAPITULATIF DU 1 SEMESTRE 1981 - TOTAL GENERAL DES CENTRES

EXAMINES 214795
EXEMPTES GLOBAL 48567

	NOMBRE EXEMPTES PAR			POURCENTAGE PAR RAPPORT AUX			
CHAPITRE 05	CHAP.	SOUS-CHAP.	MALA-DIES	EXAMINES	EXEMPTES CENTRE	EXEMPTES DU CHAP	EXEMPTES DU S/CHAP
TROUBLES MENTAUX	15329			7,13	31,56		
SOUS-CHAPITRE							
. ETATS PSYCHOTIQUES ORGANIQUES		98		0,04	0,20	0,63	
. AUTRES PSYCHOSES		956		0,44	1,96	6,23	
PSYCHOSES SCHIZOPHRENIQUES			627	0,29	1,29	4,09	65,58
ETATS DELIRANTS			28	0,01	0,05	0,18	2,92
TROUBLES NEVROTIQUES, DE LA PERSON-NALITE ET AUTRES NON PSYCHOTIQUES		10549		4,91	21,72	68,81	
DEVIATIONS ET TROUBLES SEXUELS			356	0,16	0,73	2,32	3,37
PHARMACODEPENDANCE			41	0,15	0,70	2,22	3,23
ABUS DE DROGUES CHEZ UNE PERSONNE NON DEPENDANTE			398	0,18	0,81	2,59	3,77
TROUBLES DE L'ADAPTATION			44	0,34	1,53	4,85	7,05
RETARD MENTAL		3726		1,73	7,67	24,30	

2.3. - The active service

Two complementary applications give elements in one month :

- on the real reasons for elimination from active service (Reformes),

- on all pathologic phenomena observed in a reference population (REDEA).

They are both founded on organisational procedures which transmit to the data store pieces of information derived from the normal administrative work part of the hospital trained service, or of a medical Doctor's office.

"Reformes" involve the epidemiological problem in its relation to the selection of use (subevaluation of a pathologic disease, omission, or intercurrent affection) trying to determine medical reasons of staff illness, and their direct or indirect relations with the quality of medical care (2oo ooo cases are observed every year).

REDEA application collects all the pathological symptoms of the concerned population :

- in hospital environment and in sanitary units of health service,

- in force unit's nurseries,

- or in civilian care centers by the means of unit physicians.

Its conceptual basis is founded on the patient physician. It allows to get 16 variables for any declared cases according to a certain level of gravity:

- activity suspension,

- para-clinical confirmation

All the data are dated, geographically situated, but do not refer to individual identity.

200 000 cases where collected for the concerned population in 1980, which was the first year this system was put into effect, and 80 000 other cases for the rest of active military population.

2.4. - Study of particular pathologic cases

Many computerized subsystems were set to observe more accurately some pathologic facts which interested the Head staff on medical research.

These works help to control the reliability of REDEA data. Two of them function already.

- one concerning the TOXICOMANIA,

- the other self agression conducts.

Table II : Number of cases observed per month in 1980, some examples :

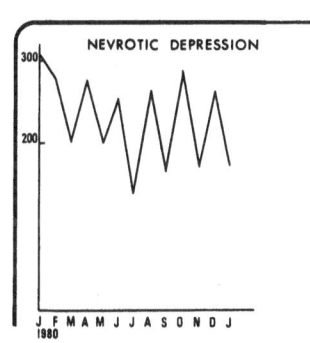
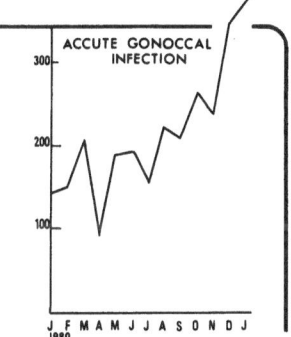

III - RESULTS AND PRODUCTS OBTAINED

Evaluation of the medical staff's activity :

- the system can give in a short time (about two months) the awareness of recent diseases spread on a wide territory and concerning a homogeneous and young population (REDEA);

- it can also give an instantaneous idea about the health of all French 18 years old males.

TOUTES ARMEES CHAPITRES CIM-75		TOTAL GENERAL	RECAPITULATION ANNUELLE REDEA														ANNEE 1980			
		JANV	FEV	MARS	AVRIL	MAI	JUIN	JUIL	AOUT	SEPT	OCT	NOV	DEC	TOTAL	DECES	CAA	AP.T	COLL.	AC.S
1 MAL INFECTIEUSE & PARASITAIRE	TOT	2270	2462	2328	1715	2133	2180	1760	1759	1840	2109	1914	2234	24704	15		1	646	5
	CTG	1588	1709	1558	1236	1361	1471	1104	1179	1157	1248	1063	1173	15827	11		1	293	3
2 TUMEURS	TOT	151	121	108	94	87	120	76	80	92	117	92	84	1222	59				
	CTG	112	77	69	59	48	66	38	51	49	53	34	37	693	4				
3 MAL ENDOC. NUTRI	TOT	163	213	154	178	131	171	69	139	104	192	104	156	1774	2	2			1
	CTG	78	136	76	115	64	109	40	92	47	107	39	92	995	1	2			
4 MAL SANG ET ORG HEMATOPOIET	TOT	54	54	40	58	47	56	28	33	38	44	40	48	540	4				
	CTG	41	44	32	45	33	43	21	29	26	30	23	28	395	2				
5 TROUBLES MEN-TAUX	TOT	1733	1906	1386	1763	1328	1748	1141	1777	1293	1977	1104	1899	19055	5	233	521		7
	CTG	1558	1689	1127	1573	1114	1528	963	1605	1088	1744	891	1589	16469	5	206	489		7
6 MAL SYST NERV. ORG. DES SENS	TOT	1149	1124	1089	1020	888	992	683	775	766	1015	751	852	11104	9	4	1	88	12
	CTG	853	833	768	780	625	720	473	575	528	713	471	586	7925	5	2	1	3	7
7 MAL APPAREIL CIRCULATOIRE	TOT	601	639	507	537	430	571	335	465	436	629	436	529	6115	55	1	1	6	3
	CTG	396	458	278	376	236	358	197	342	223	394	189	317	3764	10	1	1	6	2
8 MAL APPAREIL RESPIRATOIRE	TOT	7012	8293	14111	7708	5073	4389	3070	2504	3293	5809	4105	5084	70451	8	3	1	422	10
	CTG	5030	6622	11019	6118	3630	3134	2271	1932	2230	3850	2599	3600	52035	3	2	1	53	10
9 MAL DIGESTIF	TOT	1733	1478	1364	1184	1221	1365	1044	1053	1189	1376	1199	1139	15345	6		2	41	4
	CTG	1262	1110	981	890	881	946	795	826	878	975	709	726	10979	1		2		2
10 MAL ORG. GENITO URINAIRES	TOT	607	600	534	552	469	532	392	538	479	612	455	487	6257	3	1			2
	CTG	485	479	378	430	347	384	275	425	322	434	250	321	4530	1	1			1
11 COMPLIC. GROSSESSE. ACCOUCH	TOT	12	16	21	21	20	14	7	9	14	16	6	10	166					
	CTG	6	4	8	14	7	4	5	2	2	3			55					
12 MAL PEAU.TISSU CELLUL S/CUTANE	TOT	1489	1449	1331	1066	1174	1387	1117	1118	1256	1447	1073	1174	15081		5		67	8
	CTG	1121	1070	937	834	857	997	789	846	896	1041	723	795	10906		4		26	8
13 MAL OS-ARTICUL. MUSCLES-T CONJ	TOT	2097	2030	1932	1580	1562	1884	1316	1470	1635	2070	1550	1517	20643	1				22
	CTG	1398	1373	1112	1079	928	1259	856	1063	1037	1319	870	927	13221	1				15
14 ANOMALIES CONGENITALES	TOT	112	128	136	125	102	131	75	106	108	119	79	118	1359		1	1		1
	CTG	99	103	97	106	89	108	64	93	102	53	92	1100				1		1
16 ETATS MORBIDES MAL DEFINIS	TOT	1921	2104	2404	2041	1560	1834	1170	1549	1474	1864	1313	1702	20936	28	18	2	49	12
	CTG	1427	1670	1590	1599	1043	1366	867	1256	1046	1374	869	1230	15337	7	10	1	5	7
17 TRAUMATISMES EMPOISONNEMENTS	TOT	6076	5853	6064	5187	5640	6068	4679	5027	5456	5973	5200	4807	66030	431	413	2	88	32286
	CTG	4470	4271	4055	3942	4016	4397	3435	3852	4018	4058	3317	3115	46946	200	328	2	66	21255
TOTAL	TOT	27180	28470	33509	24829	21865	23442	16962	18402	19473	25369	19421	21840	280762	626	680	531	1407	32373
	CTG	19924	21648	24065	19196	15279	16890	12193	14169	13640	17445	12100	14628	201177	248	556	498	452	21318
DONT DECES	TOT	35	25	45	80	64	67	38	65	48	70	50	39	626	626	72	1		118
	CTG	17	11	19	29	31	25	14	27	12	31	15	17	248	24	25			38

The analysis of those results hasn't yet produced; practical applications since the medical supervision of people before they are 18 yeard old does not concern the military health service. Nevertheless the results given by REDEA after one year have already allowed to approach or recognize some problems concerning :

- recollection of elementary rules of hygiene,

- discovery of rare diseases in the army environment,

- more suited medical means used according to the morbidity rate.

Moreover, one of the aims of the system was to motivate the physicians, the purveyors and the people responsible for the information, placing them in an epidemiological environment. This aim has not been reached because the system took to much time to answer.

Nevertheless, thanks to the fast publication of the collected data, the almost immediate availability and easy access to the information stored on magnetic devices.It tend to be increasingly used for clinical research concerning the awareness of the epidemiological fact.

IV - THE PROBLEMS MET AND FUTURAL DEVELOPMENTS

A long survey of information implies :

- the purveyors' interest in feedback of their action,

- the limitation of the required work,

- the perfect understanding of it.

The setting up of these informatical treatments, based on an epidemiological aim, in a wide geographical surrounding concerning more than 1 000 physicians; encountered difficulties due to lack of knowledge of epidemiological problems, of their consequences and of their use in a prevention perspective. According to the result already obtained, and thanks to the spreading of the informations, the state of mind is progressively changing, but an active and permanent participation will be long to obtain.

On the technical side the practical use of I.C.D. 75 without previous experience was not easy and elaborate control programs had to be set up, in order to allow detection and correction of anomalies by specialised physician staff. Moreover the detection of repeated cases without individual identification created many problems. Now the global reliability of data is estimated to 90 %, in spite of subdeclaration true or pathological cases implying legal medical consequences.

As for results the employment of useful information giving precisions on an epidemiological environment, is difficult to obtain rapidly. Studies presently run, try to define indicators whose variations would be significant of an extensive or even future pathology. On the other hand, self-formation of users for a better definition of the products to be obtained is just beginning and the possible consequences of the system are not yet entirely forseen.

CONCLUSION

The automated system set by the Health Service already allows to obtain, by different ways, precise epidemiological data which were not available until now, for a certain part of the french male population. An extrapolation allows to get an overall idea on the whole population, with the data collected from active staff. The studies run to test the reliability of informations, allow to think that their quality is satisfactory after one year of exploitation. However, the present deficiency of experience, and the important problems due to the availability of this information have not yet allowed to define all of the possibilites of use.

BIBLIOGRAPHIE

- "REDEA" ARMEES D'AUJOURD'HUI n° 63 Septembre 1981.
  Médecin en Chef Jean DUTERTRE

- Les statistiques épidémiologiques des Armées - CRESSA/DOC Rapport n° I Décelbre 1975
  D. BEZSONOFF - G. VINCENT - D. COUTURIER - J. DENJEAN

- "L'HOPITAL DES ARMEES ET L'INFORMATIQUE"
  A. GUILLOREAU - MEDECINE ET ARMEES 1969/3/211/221

- "GESTION DE L'INFORMATIQUE MEDICALE"
  B. PHILIP - A. GUILLOREAU - INFORMATIQUE ET GESTION 1972/1/34/93/96.

COMPUTERIZED EPIDEMIOMETRIC MODEL OF SHIGELLOSIS AND ITS USE IN ASSESSING POTENTIAL USEFULNESS OF NEW TOOLS FOR DISEASE CONTROL

Jadranka Božikov, Gjuro Deželić and Branko Cvjetanović

Andrija Štampar School of Public Health, Medical School, University of Zagreb and University Computing Centre, Zagreb, Yugoslavia

SUMMARY

A computerized prototype of the epidemiometric model of bacillary dysentery was developed in order to study its potential usefulness in public health. The multistate model was built on the basis of the natural history of shigellosis by formulating an appropriate set of difference equations relevant to the flow of population between epidemiological classes. Necessary software was developed for performing interactive simulation games. Simulations included studying the natural course of the disease in a stable endemic situation, the results of the application of different types of vaccines, both real and hypothetical. The epidemiometric model of shigellosis also appears to be useful in the evaluation of the projects aimed at the development of new control measures, such as new vaccines against this disease. Further investigation of shigellosis modelling is needed in order to design realistic models of this disease with complex etiology.

1. INTRODUCTION

Multistate epidemiological models have multiple uses. Among the most important of them are: planning and evaluation of the disease control programmes, their cost-effectiveness and cost-benefit analyses. Such models, formulated mathematically and simulated by use of computers were developed so far for diseases such as typhoid fever, tetanus, cholera, cerebrospinal meningitis, dyphteria and whooping cough /1/, poliomyelitis, measles /2/ and some other diseases.

The modelling of bacillary disentery encounters difficulties inherent in model formulation of the disease entities caused by several etiologic agents /1/. However, in view of the public health importance of bacillary disentery and its control it was considered useful to attempt the construction of a model of this disease. The term "epidemiometric" is used in connection with the present model in order to emphasize its quantitative character.

In the attempt to develop a model for bacillary dysentery well established techniques in building of the models of acute bacterial disease /1/ were used. The model was explored for the assessment of the potential usefulness of new tools for disease control, namely of new vaccines, still to be developed.

The advances in bacterial genetics and immunology open almost unlimited opportunities to develop new anti-dysentery vaccines using genetic engineering and other techniques, and preparing the so-called tailor-made vaccines with desired characteristics has real prospects. Thus an attempt was made to explore potential usefulness of new hypothetical vaccines with different biologic activity which are reflected accordingly in the model.

2. FORMULATION OF THE MODEL

In view of the fact that the etiology of bacillary dysentery is far from being homogeneous, we limited our model to shigellosis, considering it as a group of similar but not identical disease entities.

For the construction of the prototype of the natural history of the dynamics of shigellosis we took the parameters which meet consensus /3/, as shown in the flow-chart /Figure 1/. In order to study the effect of immunization a class of immunized was added.

Mathematical relationships between the ten epidemiological classes shown in the flow-chart are expressed in the system of difference equations shown in Figure 2. The symbols used are those applied in earlier models /1/. The force of infection /RI/ which governs the transfer from the class of susceptible /X_1/ to those infected /X_3/ is determining the incidence level and represents the totality of external factors which affect the transmission of the infection.

The symbols X_i denote the number of persons in class i at a given moment. $R_{i,j}$ denote the coefficients of exit from the given classes. The definitions of $R_{i,j}$ and the daily rates of exit /P's/ are given elsewhere /1/.

A computer program according to the adopted model was written in FORTRAN and included interactive data input for performing simulation games and graphical output. The simulations were performed on a UNIVAC 1100/42 computing system with TEKTRONIX 4051 Graphics and CALCOMP Plotter.

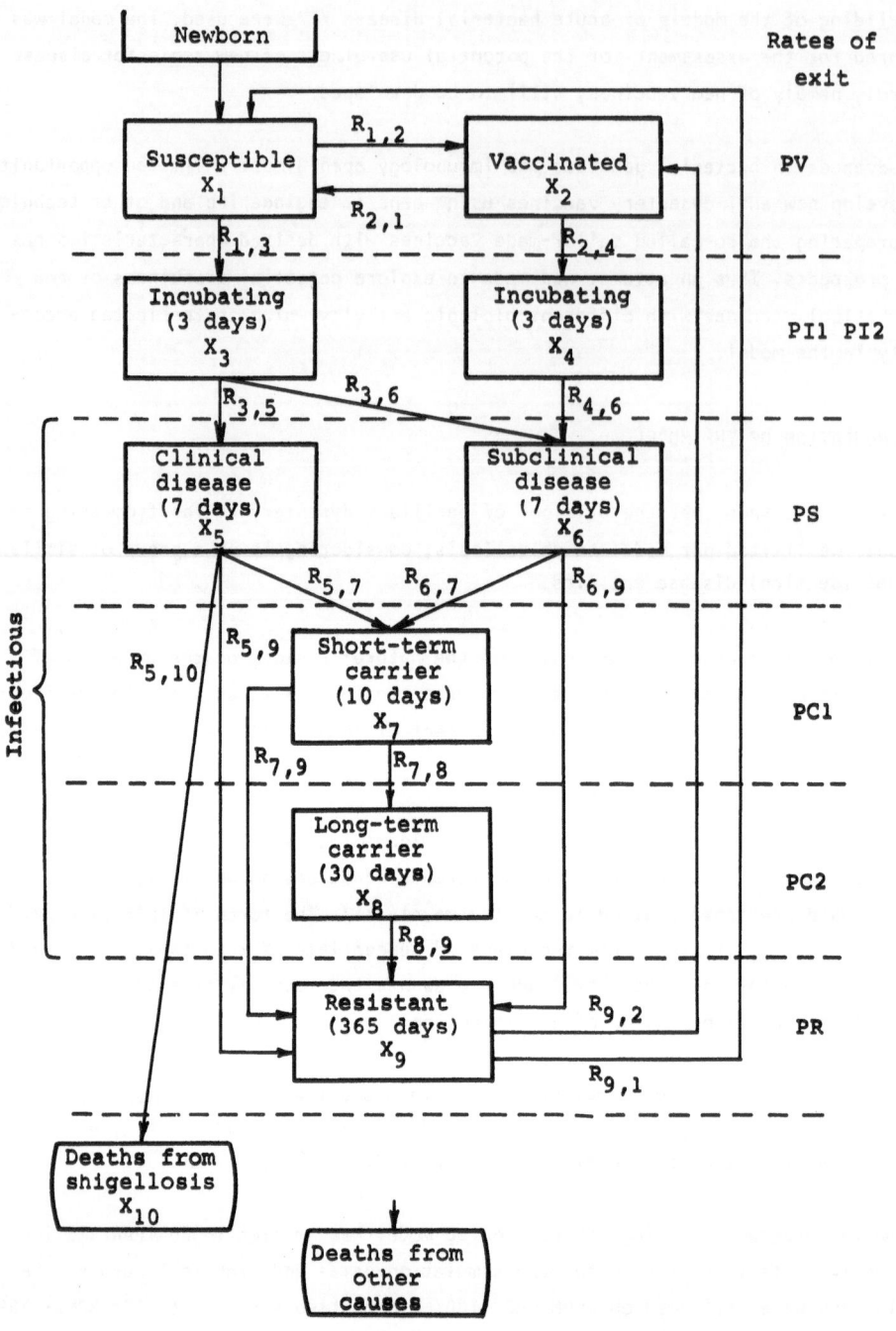

Figure 1. Flowchart of the dynamics of shigellosis

$$\Delta X_1 = -X_1 \frac{X_5 + X_6 + X_7 + X_8}{X_T} R_{1,3} \, RI - X_1 R_{1,2} + X_2 R_{2,1} \, PV +$$

$$+ X_9 R_{9,1} \, PR + X_T PB - X_1 \, (PD - \Delta X_{10} / X_T)$$

$$\Delta X_2 = -X_2 \frac{X_5 + X_6 + X_7 + X_8}{X_T} R_{2,4} \, RI + X_1 R_{1,2} - X_2 R_{2,1} \, PV +$$

$$+ X_9 R_{9,2} \, PR - X_2 \, (PD - \Delta X_{10} / X_T)$$

$$\Delta X_3 = X_1 \frac{X_5 + X_6 + X_7 + X_8}{X_T} R_{1,3} \, RI - X_3 R_{3,5} \, PI1 - X_3 R_{3,6} \, PI1 -$$

$$- X_3 \, (PD - \Delta X_{10} / X_T)$$

$$\Delta X_4 = X_2 \frac{X_5 + X_6 + X_7 + X_8}{X_T} R_{2,4} \, RI - X_4 R_{4,6} \, PI2 - X_4 \, (PD - \Delta X_{10} / X_T)$$

$$\Delta X_5 = X_3 R_{3,5} \, PI1 - X_5 R_{5,7} \, PS - X_5 R_{5,9} \, PS - X_5 R_{5,10} \, PS -$$

$$- X_5 \, (PD - \Delta X_{10} / X_T)$$

$$\Delta X_6 = X_3 R_{3,6} \, PI1 + X_4 R_{4,6} \, PI2 - X_6 R_{6,7} \, PS - X_6 R_{6,9} \, PS -$$

$$- X_6 \, (PD - \Delta X_{10} / X_T)$$

$$\Delta X_7 = X_5 R_{5,7} \, PS + X_6 R_{6,7} \, PS - X_7 R_{7,8} \, PC1 - X_7 R_{7,9} \, PC1 -$$

$$- X_7 \, (PD - \Delta X_{10} / X_T)$$

$$\Delta X_8 = X_7 R_{7,8} \, PC1 - X_8 R_{8,9} \, PV2 - X_8 \, (PD - \Delta X_{10} / X_T)$$

$$\Delta X_9 = X_5 R_{5,9} \, PS + X_7 R_{7,9} \, PC1 + X_8 R_{8,9} \, PC2 + X_6 R_{6,9} \, PS -$$

$$- X_9 R_{9,1} \, PR - X_9 R_{9,2} \, PR - X_9 \, (PD - \Delta X_{10} / X_T)$$

$$\Delta X_{10} = X_5 R_{5,10} \, PS$$

Figure 2. Differential   equations of the model of shigellosis shown in
Figure 1

3. SIMULATIONS

Simulations were first made to establish validity of the model /1/. The basis for simulations was: /i/ the natural course of the disease in a stable endemic situation, and /ii/ its course during an epidemic. Various endemic and epidemic patterns were obtained by suitable changes of the daily force of infection /RI/. To these well defined states of stable endemicity the impact of different types of vaccines and of various immunization schedules and schemes /with varied programmes/ were simulated. Figure 3 shows some of the typical examples of simulations performed. Output results may be plotted with all classes shown in the flowchart, but for the present discussion the monthly incidence of clinically ill persons /class X_5/ per 1000 inhabitants was choosen.

The effect of the presently available vaccine, the live Streptomycin dependent /SmD/ vaccine /4/, on disease dynamics over longer periods is shown in examples /a/ and /b/, whereas the potential effect of a hypothetical vaccine is shown in /c/ and /d/. The SmD vaccine protects one year and only against the clinical disease, whereas the hypothetical vaccine was thought to be able to protect against both the clinical and subclinical form three years. Different immunization schedules with one to three mass immunizations at different time intervals /shown by arrows/ were applied covering 60 % of the population with the vaccine effectiveness of 90 %.

As an interesting phenomenon a rather sharp rise in the number of cases is observed /with the hypothetical vaccine having longer protection/. This vaccine protects the population quite well during the protection period, but after that the number of susceptible persons becomes high enough to provoke temporarily higher incidence until its stabilization at the endemicity level. As the result of the simulation it is suggested that much care has to be taken when one starts with a mass immunization programme, because it is possible to predict potential unwanted outbreaks of the disease if the immunization schedule and scheme has to be broken.

Potential vaccines having longer and more complete protection could undoubtedly be more effective. However, their relative cost-effectiveness and cost-benefit depend on other factors, namely on vaccine costs and other costs of immunization and treatment /1/. It has to be noted that the described prototype of the model of shigellosis is not reflecting the actual epidemic process which consist of several paralel infections with different serotypes of Shigella. A set of parallel models would better reflect the real situation.

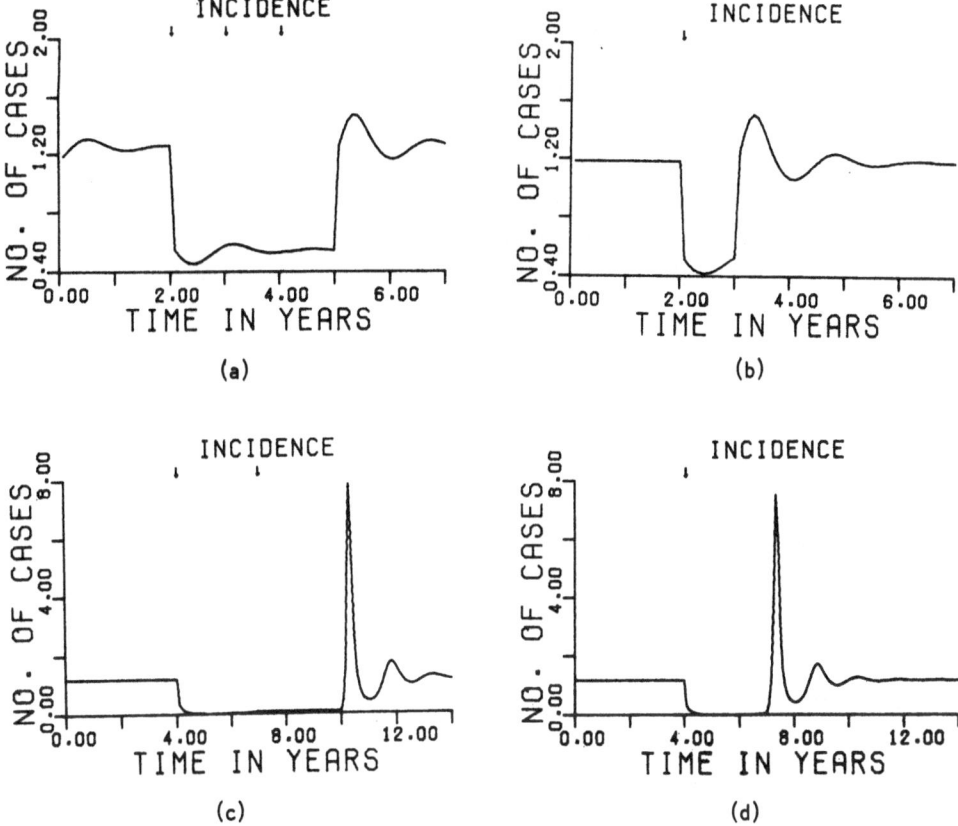

Figure 3. Incidences (per 1000 inhabitants, monthly) in dependence of time at a immunization coverage of 60 %, on effectiveness of 90 % and a force of
infection RI = 0.12; arrows denote mass immunizations;

(a) Immunization by the SmD vaccine in three consecutive years;
(b) Immunization by the SmD vaccine once only;
(c) Immunization by the hypothetical vaccine twice in a three-years span;
(d) Immunization by the hypothetical vaccine once only.

4. DISCUSSION

Besides other uses it seems that the epidemiological models can be used also in evaluating possible health and economic benefits of research projects aimed at the development of new control tools. The models thus could be used as an additional method for helping make decisions on allocating the priorities in public health programmes. However, in decision-making various complex biological, social and other factors should be also considered besides the simulations of epidemiometric models, such as the one presented. There is a need for further studies in this direction before potential usefulness of the models in this particular field could be determined.

Much further work is also needed to simulate more realistically multiple types of shigellosis possible by parallel running of several slightly different models in the same population. Further, besides the above deterministic approach for the study of outbreaks, stochastic elements should be introduced in the model.

5. CONCLUSIONS

The attempted epidemiometric model of shigellosis could be used in epidemiological studies and planning of control measures. There is the potential value of such a model in assessing possible benefits of contemplated research projects aimed at the development of new vaccines against this disease.

REFERENCES

1. Cvjetanović B, Grab B, Uemura, K. Dynamics of Acute Bacterial Diseases, Supplement No. 1 to Vol. 56 of the Bull. WHO, Geneva, 1978.

2. Cvjetanović B, Grab B, Dixon H. Epidemiological Model of Poliomyelitis and Measles and their Uses in the Planning and Evaluating of Immunization Programmes, Bull. WHO /In print/.

3. Benenson A /editor/. Control of Communicable Diseases in Man, 11th Edition, American Public Health Association, New York, 1970.

4. Mel DM, Arsić BL, Nikolić BD, Radovanović ML. Studies on Vaccination Against Bacillary Dysentery. 4. Oral Immunization with Live Monotypic and Combined Vaccines. Bull. WHO 1968; 39:375-380.

   Mel DM, Gangarosa EJ, Radovanović ML, Arsić BL, Litvinjenko S. Studies on Vaccination Against Bacillary Dysentery. G. Protection of Children by Oral Immunization with Streptomycin-Dependent Shigella Strains. Bull. WHO 1971; 45:457-464.

MONITOR
A System for the Evaluation of Mortality Data

N. Becker, R. Frentzel-Beyme, G. Wagner
Institute of Documentation, Information and Statistics
Director: Prof. Dr. G. Wagner
German Cancer Research Center
Im Neuenheimer Feld 280
6900 Heidelberg 1

Summary

The system MONITOR permits the descriptive epidemiological evaluation of
incidence and mortality data respectively in dialog. Apart from tables,
graphic presentations as well as regional distributions in the form of
maps can be generated on graphic terminals or plotters.

Introduction

In many countries of the world, among them the Federal Republic of Germany, mortality data is being collected, coded by causes of death and
stored. These ever growing data collections permit the observation of
temporal trends in diseases as well as the investigation of regional
differences in the frequency of certain causes of death. As a means for
the formulation of new hypotheses they supply a valuable basis of epidemiological research.

Rather uniform modes of presentation are used in epidemiology for the
analysis of mortality data (1,2). In order to establish whether a tumor
form is gaining or losing importance, temporal trends are recorded, the
increase or decrease compared to a reference year calculated in percentages, individual age groups followed in their movement over time, etc.
Furthermore, birth cohorts analysis has provided its value for a more
sophisticated investigation of the problem. The forms of presentation
mentioned can be purposeful for the absolute numbers of death as well as
for crude or age-standardized rates. The cartographic presentation seems
to be suitable for demonstration of the regional distribution of causes
of death.

For the descriptive analysis of mortality the data are processed mainly
by fixed patterns. The extent of the available data as well as the number of possible problems suggest that these preprogrammable steps of

epidemiological research be transferred to a DP system. For this purpose, the system MONITOR was developed at the German Cancer Research Center (3) permitting the speedy setting up of tables, graphs and cartographic presentations of mortality data.

The Data

The data collected by WHO are available in uniform format so that each set begins with a code consisting of the year in question, the international country code and a sex code. Subsequently, the deaths of the respective ICD number and sex which occurred in the year and the country mentioned are detailed in 22 age groups. This data is used by us directly as the data base for MONITOR with a population data base of equal structure (except for the code for causes of death) as reference values. The described identification of the sets is used as a key for direct access to the data. In dialog mode the user is asked for the information required for a complete code and the respective sets in the mortality and population data base are immediately accessed with the thus defined code. Since the databases are continuously kept on disc, the system attains a high working speed with answering times in the range of seconds, even with extensive queries.

The Interpreter

MONITOR is an interpreter with a command language whose scope is specially tailored to the need of descriptive epidemiology. For the user this language is divided into three sub-languages for

- the production of tables,
- the production of graphs,
- the production of maps.

In these the desired evaluations are defined and the result is immediately shown (on terminals) in the form of tables or (on graphic terminals) in the form of graphs. Demographic maps are also defined in a short dialog and then put out via a raster plotter.

For example, the sequence of commands

```
GRAPHICS
TIME TRENDS
COUNTRY      4100
CAUSE        A 046, A 047, A 048, A 049, 157
SEX          1
TITLE        FRG/MALES
LEGEND       OESOPHAGUS, STOMACH, COLON,
             RECTUM, PANCREAS

PLOT
```

supplies the presentation of the secular trends of malignant tumors of the digestive organs for men in the Federal Republic of Germany (Figure 1).

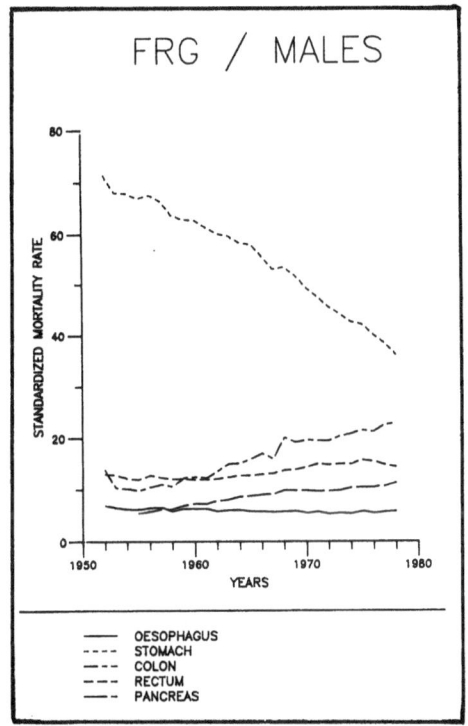

Figure 1

With the three commands

          SEX   *2*

          TITLE   *FRG/FEMALE*

          PLOT

one obtains the same presentation for women (Figure 2).

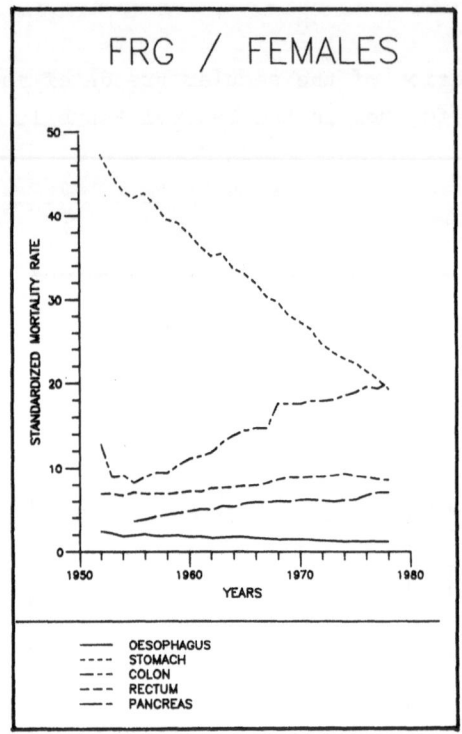

Figure 2

Correspondingly, other causes of death for several countries etc. could be plotted by changing the parameters of the commands CAUSE or COUNTRY.

In the background of the interpreter a syntax analyzer is at work inter-
cepting syntax errors as well as offering language aids if the user makes
a mistake, does not know how to continue or is not informed about the
scope of the language. In this connection it is worthwhile dealing with
the technology of the generation of the interpreter.

MONITOR was developed with a program generator (4). The basis is a definition of the command language in the form of a grammar and a semantics
program containing the substance of operation pertaining to every syntactic rule in a programming language (here SNOBOL). From the grammatical
rules the generator generates the syntax analyzer and from the semantics
part the actual executive program of the system.

Through the high modularity attained by this method of development the
programming and testing times are considerably reduced for one thing and,
moreover, system extention are rendered much easier. An additional command merely requires the introduction of the grammatical rule in question
and the syntactic operation related to it; the rest is done by the generators.

Calculation of Cumulative Rates

Apart from the above mentioned usual methods for the evaluation or presentation of mortality data, the user in MONITOR may also avail himself
of the "cumulative rate" which during the last few years, has been used
to an increasing extent (5,6) and offers some advantages as compared to
other standardized procedures. It can be derived by describing the mortality in a population as a stochastic process with integer-valued jumps,
i. e. describing it as a Poisson process. With it the risk of an individuum is indicated of dying from the respective cause of death in the
course of his life of an average length of 75 years. This risk is mostly
stated in per cent.

$$CMR_{0,75} = 1 - e^{-\int_{0}^{75} \lambda(u)\, du}$$

The hazard function λ (u) can be approximated by the mortality rates MRi, i = 1,..,22 given in the 22 age groups $\triangle t_i$ so that the formula is simplified to read

$$CMR_{0,75} = 1 - e^{-\sum\limits_{1}^{22} MR_i \cdot \triangle t_i}$$

Since CMR estimates the risk of an individuum and since only the rates are required to approximate the hazard function, CMR does not depend on a standard population; in spite of this or rather just because of this it is generally comparable. This is what renders its application so attractive. Moreover, confidence intervals may easily be given for it so that statistically significant differences in the spatial or temporal distribution of the risk can be directly established.

$$CMR_{0,75} = 1 - e^{-\left(\sum\limits_{1}^{22} MR_i \triangle t_i \pm X_\alpha \cdot \sqrt{v}\right)}$$

On account of these advantages CMR is applied in the German Cancer Research Center as a basis of that part of MONITOR used for setting up cancer maps where the significant deviation of regional mortality rates from the mean value is of particular importance.

REFERENCES

(1) Lilienfeld AM, Levin ML, Kessler II. Cancer in the United States. Harvard University Press Cambridge 1972.

(2) Muir CS, Choi NW, Schifflers E. Time Trends in Cancer Morality in some Countries. Skandia International Symposia Medical Aspects of Mortality Statistics Stockholm 1981.

(3) Becker N. MONITOR Ein Programmpaket zur epidemiologischen Auswertung der Mortalitätsdaten der BRD. Deutsches Krebsforschungszentrum, Abt. Epidemiologie, Technical Report Nr. 1 Heidelberg 1979.

(4) Becker N, Osterburg G, Schadewald K. PAULA - Generator für LL (k)-Parser und lexikalische Analyseprogramme. Deutsches Krebsforschungszentrum/ZDV, Technical Report Nr. 10 Heidelberg 1977.

(5) Miettinen OS. Principles of Epidemiologic Research. Department of Epidemiology and Biostatistics, Harvard School of Public Health, Unpublished Course Text Boston 1978.

(6) Day NE. A New Measure of Age-Standardized Incidence, the Cumulative Rate. In: Waterhouse J, Muir C, Corvea P, Powell J. Cancer Incidence in Five Continents Vol. III. IARC, Lyon 1976.

DEMOGRAPHIC MODELS AND THE FINNISH MENTAL HOSPITAL POPULATION

A. Hakkarainen
The National Board of Health
P.B. 223, 00531 Helsinki 53
Finland

SUMMARY

A Lexis diagram is applied to the mental hospital population which is divided into two subpopulations according to the length of stay. These are the short-stay and the long-stay populations. Their characteristics are described. It is found that the Finnish long-stay mental hospital population resembles the stationary population model while the short-stay one does not. The connections between the Lexis diagram and hospital data systems are discussed. The mental hospital population processes are compared with other population phenomena and the explanation of the processes is discussed.

1. INTRODUCTION

Projections of mental hospital populations have been done since the beginning of the 60'ies. They started the application of demographic methods in psychiatry. Von Korff (1) has referred to seven English and American studies from the years 1961-77. He states that these studies do not usually refer to a clearly specified model and as such they do not greatly contribute to understanding of the population dynamics of the mental hospital. He has himself applied the life table methodology and the theory of stable populations. There are some studies where stationary population model has been used (2, 3), although the use of a demographic model can be concluded only from the mathematics used. In Finland the projections of mental hospital population have been compared with the stable population theory (4).

The motive of this study was to find the causes of the regional differences in the accumulation of long-stay mental patients in Finland. The first task was to define the concept of the explanandum which is the incidence of long-term hospitalization. This is a study of the population processes to be explained.

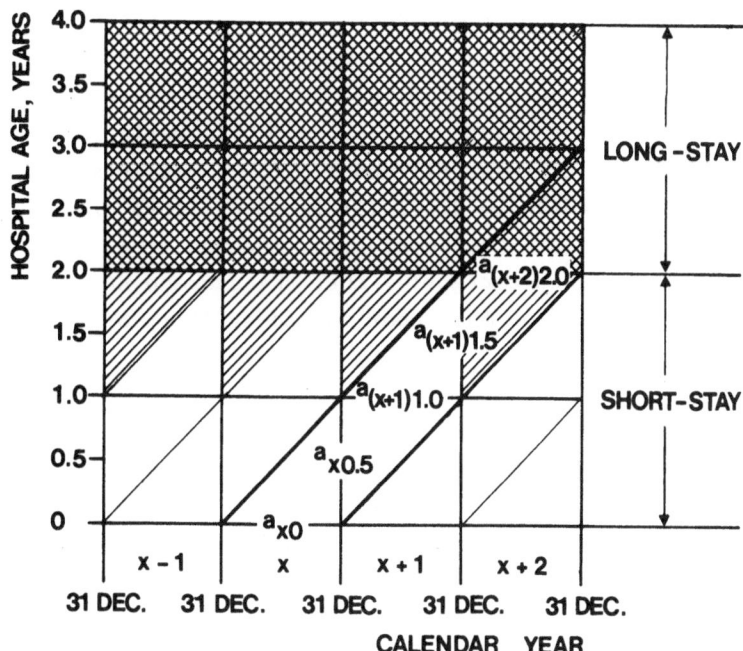

Figure 1.   The attrition of a cohort of patients admitted to mental
             hospitals in year x by calendar year and hospital age and
             the limit of long-term hospitalization.

2.   THE LEXIS DIAGRAM

The term long-stay patient has been used in several studies. It has
been found that the patient's probability of separation decreases
greatly when he/she starts the third year in mental hospital. Brown
(5) has shown this tendency in 16 studies of schizophrenic patients
during the period 1900-1951. These studies were based on separation
data.   If census data are used the operational definition of long-
stay patient is different. Figure 1 illustrates these definitions in a
so-called Lexis-diagram (6). In it the term hospital age (HA) refers
to the amount of time an inpatient has been continuously hospitalized
at any point in time prior to separation (1). It is measured at census
and in calculations the admission day is usually excluded. The length
of stay (LOS) is the hospital age of an inpatient on the day of
separation.

Figure 1 shows the decline of a cohort admitted in year x. At admission its size is a_{x0}, at census on 31 Dec. year x there are $a_{x0.5}$ patients left. When the cohort is followed further there are $a_{(x+1)1.0}$ patients whose LOS is at least one year, $a_{(x+1)1.5}$ patients are present at census on 31 Dec. year x+1 and $a_{(x+2)2.0}$ patients' LOS is at least two years. According to Brown (5) these patients are long-stay and $a_{x0}-a_{(x+2)2.0}$ patients are short-stay. The notation used in the figure assumes (not quite correctly) that the average HA of the cohort is at census the average of the upper and lower limit of the HA-category of that cohort.

If Brown's definition of long-stay patient is used the researcher needs data on admissions and separations. Very often the separation data are not available, but there are patient censuses at certain intervals. If the interval is one year as in figure 1, the census data can be used in the evaluation of LOS. The number of patients $a_{(x+1)1.5}$ on 31 Dec. in year x+1 can be called the new long-stay patients. Their HA is 365-729 days, if the admission day is excluded. Then there are $a_{x0}-a_{(x+1)1.5}$ short-stay patients in the cohort and their LOS varies from 1 day to 729 days. These two patient groups are partly overlapping but it does not bias the calculations markedly. This method has been used by several researchers. It can be shown that the results of the census method are very similar to those based on separation data.

The processes of admission and separation define the size and the composition of hospital population. This study applies the census method. The admission process according to it is described above. The separations can be defined as follows: According to the notation used in figure 1 the number of separated short-stay patients is $a_{x0}-a_{x0.5}+a_{(x-1)0.5}-a_{x1.5}$ in year x. The number of separated long-stay patients in year x is $a_{(x-1)1.5}-a_{x2.5}+a_{(x-1)2.5}-a_{x3.5}+, \ldots, + a_{(x-1)(m-0.5)}$. It is assumed that the highest possible LOS is m.

The total population at census on 31 Dec. year x is accordingly $a_{x0.5}+a_{x1.5}+a_{x2.5}+, \ldots, +a_{x(m-0.5)}$. The population of short-stay patients at census is the accumulation of patients whose HA is under one year and who will be separated before the next census. On 31 Dec. year x it is $a_{x0.5}-a_{(x+1)1.5}$. At census there also is a group of patients waiting for entrance to the long-stay population. On 31 Dec. year x its size is $a_{(x+1)1.5}$. The population of long-stay patients on 31 Dec. year x is accordingly $a_{x1.5}+a_{x2.5}+, \ldots, +a_{x(m-0.5)}$.

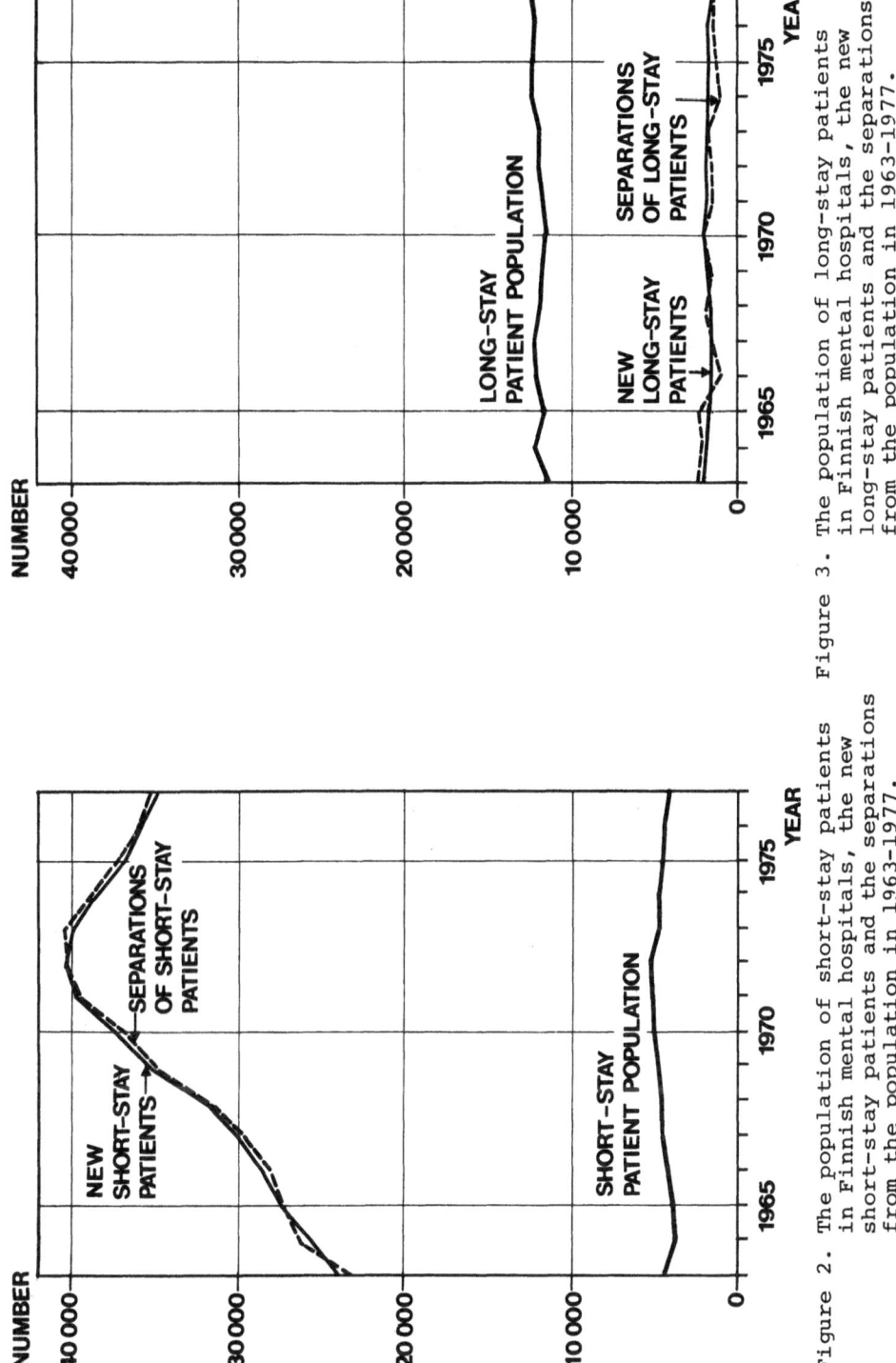

Figure 2. The population of short-stay patients in Finnish mental hospitals, the new short-stay patients and the separations from the population in 1963-1977.

Figure 3. The population of long-stay patients in Finnish mental hospitals, the new long-stay patients and the separations from the population in 1963-1977.

3. THE FINNISH MENTAL HOSPITAL POPULATION

Figures 2 and 3 illustrate the short-stay and the long-stay mental hospital populations in Finland in 1963-1977 using the census method based on the Official Statistics of Finland. It can be seen that the long-stay population resembles the stationary population model, although there is some growth, abt 1 percent per year. The average size of the population has been abt 12 000 patients at census. The number of admissions equals to separations, on the average 1 800 patients per year. In a stationary human population the birth and death rates are equal and they are equal to the reciprocal of the life expectation at birth (6). Applied to this hospital population the LOS expectation of the patients would be abt 7 years. Yoshitake (2) and Weeke and others (3) have also found stationary long-stay mental hospital populations.

When the figures 2 and 3 are compared it can be seen that the two populations have behaved in quite different ways. The long-stay population is large, abt 70 % of the resident population. The trends of long-stay admissions and separations have not changed markedly during the follow-up period of 14 years. The size of the short-stay population has slightly changed, but the change of the admission and separation trends is very marked indeed. This population is not stationary. It is assumed that some of these short-stay patients have multiple readmissions which result in a long aggregate stay in hospital.

4. DISCUSSION

The strategies of different hospital data systems can be seen in a Lexis diagram. If only census data are used we can measure HA; if separation data are available we can measure LOS. Together these data provide the number of admissions during an observation period, usually one year. Analogous to the general population statistics, the census is the first and the least expensive method which provides useful approximations in case of long-term care. Additional information is provided by separation data but the expenses are higher. In case of short-term hospitals (LOS< 30 days) separation data are preferable. It can be assumed that the population processes in long-term institutions resemble those found in this study of mental hospitals.

629

The information concerning the general population phenomena may be useful if the researcher wants to find the causes of the variation in hospital populations. The upper limit for the growth of a human or an animal population is set by the available space and food. The space has not yet become critical, but food has been. There have been transitions of the human population, when the supply of food has changed.

In hospitals the space is both the upper and the lower limit for the growth of population. The number of beds and the size of population are regulated by political decision. The other aspect of hospitals comparable with food in other populations is the available treatment. Food is a necessary condition for life, medical treatment may decrease LOS.

These ideas seem to find some support in mental hospital data. Since the birth of the asylum there has been "moral treatment" based on the interaction between the patient and the personnel (7). The new psychotropic drugs which have been used since the 50'ies cure the psychotic symptoms. In some countries this has started a transition of the mental hospital population. In New York it declined by a third in 1964-70 (1), in Ireland by 16 percent in 1963-71 (8). In Finland the mental hospital population has remained unchanged. It is now abt 4.1 per 1 000 of population.

The transitions of the general population suggest that the factors which explain the regional and the temporal variation of the mental hospital population are the resources. They are the available beds and the forms of treatment. The variation of drug utilization and various forms of psychotherapy are of interest. However, that is not enough. They may be the necessary conditions, but not the sufficient ones. It is the moral of the society, its values and norms, that determine the need for "moral treatment". Its best indicator may be the incidence of formal admissions. It varies in different regions.

BIBLIOGRAPHY

(1) Von Korff M. The dynamics of the public mental hospital population of Duchess County, New York 1964-1970. Thesis submitted to
the School of Hygiene and Public Health of the Johns Hopkins
University. Baltimore 1977.

(2) Yoshitake Y. The length of stay in planning hospitals. Translation
by Kusaka A. Transaction of Architectural Institute of Japan
1960.

(3) Weeke A, Kastrup M, Dupont A. Long-stay patients in Danish
psychiatric hospitals. Psychol. Med. 1979; 9: 551-566.

(4) Hakkarainen A. Pitkäaikaissairaat psykiatrisissa sairaaloissa,
havaintoja ja ennusteita. Lääkintöhallituksen tutkimuksia 21.
Helsinki 1980.

(5) Brown GW. Length of hospital stay and schizophrenia: a review
of statistical studies. Acta Psychiat. Scand. 1960; 35: 414-430.

(6) Pressat R. Demographic analysis. Chicago, Edward Arnold 1972.

(7) Foucault M. Madness and civilization. A history of insanity in
the age of reason. USA, Tavistock Publications 1979.

(8) O'Hare A, Walsh D. The Irish psychiatric hospital census 1971.
The Medico-Social Research Board.

RELIABILITY OF THE AID ANALYSIS IN SAMPLES FROM FIXED POPULATIONS

Vesa Kuusela

The Rehabilitation Research Centre
of the Social Insurance Institution
20720 Turku 72, Finland

Merja Kronström

Institute of statistics
University of Turku
20500 Turku 50, Finland

1.   SUMMARY

Monte Carlo study was conducted to achieve a rough description of the small sample
properties of AID. The study shows that when the distribution on the dependent variable is normal (symmetric), and the distances between terminals and groups are considerable then the sampling properties of the AID are adequate. The more the generated
population differed from the first one the more there was variability in the results.
A study was also made on an epidemiological material. The variation of the results
of the samples was considerable.

2.   INTRODUCTION

Since Sonquist, Baker and Morgan (1) published the Automatic Interaction Detector
within the OSIRIS statistical package it has been used widely in epidemiological surveys. The program is based on the principle invented by Morgan and Sonquist (2) and
its algorithmic version published a year later (3). The program has been developed in
several phases ever since and the one meant in this context is called AID3.

When the first version was published (and ever since) the method has been criticized
sharply although its popularity in application has grown. Einhorn (4) and Cramer (5,6)
were the first to focus attention on the drawbacks of the method. Severe criticism is
found also in Doyle (7) and Feinberg (8) . One of the points criticized was the lack of
information concerning statistical significance.[†]

Kass (10) was the first to try to develop a stopping criterion of statistical nature for
AID. The result was a statistic for rather simple situations, which was developed further
by Scott and Knott (11) and Ecob (12). None of these authors, however, focused attention to the fact that the whole structure is stochastic. In addition to the stopping
criterion also the selection one of the competing variables in the model and its point
of division (into two subgroups) is liable to sampling error. The permutation of the
structure variables lead to a different partition of sample, which actually is the
main result of the method.

The present study was focused on the stability of the tree structure in random sampling
from fixed populations i.e. the robustness of the AID model.

[†]Sonquist (9) did not take the possibility of sampling error very seriously: ",but
seeing a number of crows of varying sizes, shapes, and ages who are, in fact, black
lends credence to the proposition that all crows are black."

3.   METHOD OF STUDY

AID does not actually use a mathematical model and this makes an analytical study very difficult. Therefore, a Monte Carlo study was conducted. The aim was to get a rough description of the stability in order to decide the need for further investigations.

A population of 18 210 cases with a predetermined tree structure was generated by a random number generator (Figure 1). The distribution of the dependent variable in each terminal group was either normal or log-normal with fixed means. Various research situations were generated by varying the variances of the distributions. Several random samples were drawn from each generated population and the effect of different sampling schemes was described by varying the sampling fraction.

The first structure generated was normally distributed in each terminal group with a constant variance ($\sigma^2 = 10.0$). The means of the distributions were chosen in order to keep distances between groups considerable.[†] To validate the generated model an AID analysis was made of the whole population. The model discovered by the program matches almost completely with the theoretical model (Figure 1).

The AID3 program was used with the free option. Other options which have an effect on the model had default values in order to imitate a standard user.

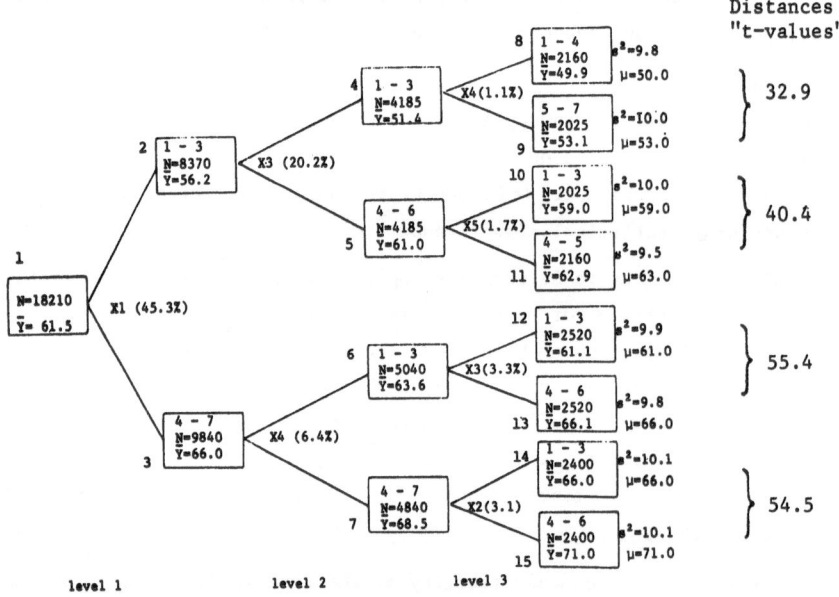

Figure 1. Theoretical and observed AID-structure. The means on which the generation of the structure is based are indicated by μ, and s^2 indicates the observed variance. Distributions in terminal groups are normal.

[†] Students t-statistics was taken as distance measure.

4.   RESULTS

4.1.   Normal distributions in terminal groups

When the AID tree structure is as regular as described above and the distances between terminal groups are considerable $(t > 30.0)$, the algorithm performs its function as

Sampling fraction Sample size	20 % 3642	10 % 1821	5 % 911	2 % 364
level group				
1 1	3(3)/3	3(3)/3	3(3)/3	3(3)/3
2 2	2(3)/3	3(3)/3	3(3)/3	3(3)/3
3	3(3)/3	3(3)/3	3(3)/3	3(3)/3
3 4	3(3)/3	3(3)/3	2(2)/2	2(2)/2
5	3(3)/3	3(3)/3	3(3)/3	3(3)/3
6	3(3)/3	3(3)/3	3(3)/3	3(3)/3
7	3(3)/3	3(3)/3	3(3)/3	3(3)/3
Number of samples	3	3	3	3

Table I. Results of samples from normal populations. Levels and groups refer to figure 1. Each entry in the table means: no. of correct divisions (no. of correct points of division)/no of divisions.

expected. The results of the 12 different samples are shown in table I. The population structure was detected in the correct form in every sample expect one with 5 % and one with 2 % sampling fractions. In these cases the division of the fourth group was not done at all. Results were identical in respect to the points of divisions.

When distances were changed by varying the variances of the terminal groups none of the populations structures were discovered by the algorithm. Different structures were found from samples not only as to the variables but also as to the point of division. Only in the two smallest samples attempts of division in the third level were made but most of them happened according to wrong predictor (Table II). Not in one case the correct structure was found.

4.2.   Log-normal distributions in terminal groups

The distribution of the independent variable should not be "too skew". When the distribution is "too skew", it is not explained in any way and hence the common practice is ignore the danger. The effect of the shape of the distribution was analyzed by changing the terminal distributions into log-normal ones.

In the first population generated the distances between terminal groups were considerable in respect to the measure of distance. The results of 16 samples from this population are shown in table III. We notice that the beginning of the model building has been unsuccessful in regard to both variables and the points of division.

Sampling fraction	20 %	10 %	5 %	2 %
Sample size	3642	1821	911	364
level group				
1 1	7(6)/7	7(5)/7	6(3)/8	4(1)/8
2 2	–	1(0)/1	0(0)/4	0(0)/7
3	–	3(1)/3	2(0)/5	0(0)/7
3 4	–	–	–	0(0)/3
5	–	–	0(0)/1	1(0)/4
6	–	–	0(0)/1	2(0)/3
7	–	–	0(0)/2	0(0)/2
Number of samples	8	8	8	8

Table II. Results of successive divisions when the distance between groups varied between 6.0 and 0.17. In addition there were some divisions in levels 4 and 5.

Sampling fraction	20 %	10 %	5 %	1 %
Sample size	3642	1821	911	364
level group				
1 1	4(4)/4	4(4)/4	4(4)/4	4(4)/4
2 2	4(4)/4	4(4)/4	3(3)/3	4(3)/4
3	4(4)/4	3(2)/4	3(1)/4	4(1)/4
3 4	–	–	–	–
5	–	–	–	1(0)/1
6	2(1)/2	4(1)/4	2(0)/3	2(0)/2
7	4(4)/4	3(1)/3	2(0)/4	2(0)/4
Number of samples	4	4	4	4

Table III. Results of AID tree construction when the terminal distributions were lognormal and distances between groups were considerable (t > 6.0). In addition there were diverse divisions in the levels 4 and 5 in all sizes of samples except the biggest one.

The AID algorithm also discovered some points of divisions of diverse variables in levels 4 and 5 which are not included in the model of the generated population.

When the population structure was changed by changing the variances of the distributions the results did not change much (Table IV).

Sampling fraction	20 %	10 %	5 %	1 %
Sample size	3642	1821	911	364
level group				
1 1	4(4)/4	4(4)/4	3(3)/4	4(2)/4
2 2	4(4)/4	4(4)/4	4(4)/4	3(2)/3
3	4(4)/4	4(4)/4	3(3)/4	3(2)/4
3 4	–	–	0(0)/2	0(0)/1
5	–	–	–	0(0)/1
6	–	–	0(0)/1	0(0)/2
7	1(0)/1	0(0)/1	1(0)/2	0(0)/3
Number of samples	4	4	4	4

Table IV. Results of AID tree construction when the terminal distributions were lognormal and distances between groups varied between 4.3 and 0.4. In addition there were diverse divisions in levels 4 and 5 in two smallest samples.

4.3. Epidemiological population

In order to get some highlight to the behaviour of AID with ordinary epidemiological data, a material of 4597 cases concerning an angina pectoris symptom was chosen as the population. Predictors were place of living (1), sex (2), age (3), nature of work (4), body mass index (5), systolic blood pressure (6), diastolic blood pressure (7), haematocrit (8), cholesterol (9), glucose (10) and smoking (11). The only predictor discovered from the whole material was age, which explained 1.8 % of the variance.

Four samples with 40 % and 20 % sampling fractions were drawn. The results are presented in table V. It is quite easily observed that different structures were achieved from distinct samples. Age was most common predictor in the first level but not in every sample. On other levels the predictors are more diverse. As a matter of fact, two similar structures were not detected. Even the point of divisions of the predictor age at first level varied between samples.

Predictor level	group	1	2	3	4	5	6	7	8	9	10	11	No. of divisions
1	1			3(2)			1(2)						4(4)
2	2			(1)		(1)							-(2)
	3	1				1(1)					2(1)		4(2)
3	4					(1)							-(1)
	5		(1)										-(1)
	6				1					1	(1)		2(1)
	7			1									1(-)
4	.												.
	6						1						1(-)
	.												.

Table V. Divisions of the epidemiological material with 40 % and 20 % sampling fractions. The results of the smallest samples are in parenthesis.

The detailed results of the study will be presented in the Publications of the Social Insurance Institution, Finland (Series M) by the authors.

5.   DISCUSSION

A criterium in judging statistical models is their stability in random sampling from fixed populations. Absolute stability is seldom reached and therefore information concerning the sampling error of the model should be attached to the results. The AID model, however, does not provide any information of it. That is the motivation of the study, to elucidate the behaviour of the AID in random sampling from fixed populations.

The results show that only in unrealistically regular cases the algorithm discovers the population structure correctly from samples. Although the terminal distributions are symmetric and the distances between groups are "significant" but not "considerable, the algorithm could not discover the AID structure of the population. Skew distribution of the dependent variable made the performance of the program more unstable. The results are probably too optimistic because the distance measure is sensitive to skewnes.

The results also show that when the sampling fraction decreases the algorithm is inclined to discover; predictors of even two levels more than exists in the population in some cases. Presumably the explanation is rather the decreasing sample size than the decreasing sampling fraction.

The results of an ordinary epidemiological material revealed serious unstability of the AID model within epidemiological surveys. On the other hand the material did not fulfill all the assumptions of AID but this kind of data is common in surveys.

According to the present study the results of AID should be verified by cross validation procedures. Easiest way to do this is to split the sample into two groups and analyze both parts with AID. The model is approved if both parts are similar. It should be noticed that the parts must not be of equal sizes because sample size may have an effect on the model.

Before AID can be regarded as a reliable survey method, information concerning its sampling error should be attached to the results. The method of Stone and Geisser (12, 13) would probably be suitable for this purpose.

6.   REFERENCES

(1)   Sonquist JA, Baker EL, Morgan JN. Searching for structure. Michigan: The University of Michigan, 1971.

(2)   Morgan JN, Sonquist JA. Problems in the analysis of survey data, and a proposal. JASA 1963; 58: 415-35.

(3)   Sonquist JA, Morgan JN. The detection of interaction affects. Monograph n:o 35. Survey Research Centre, Institute for Social Research. Michigan: University of Michgan, 1964.

(4)   Einhorn HJ. Alchemy in the behavioral sciences. Public Opinion Q 1972; 36: 367-378.

(5)   Cramer EM. Review of multivariate model building by Sonquist J.N. Psychometrika 1971; 36: 440-442.

(6)   Cramer EM. Review of searching for structure (Alias-AID-III) by Sonquist, Baker and Morgan. Psychometrika 1975; 40: 263-265.

(7)   Doyle P. The use of automatic interaction detector and similar search procedures. Operat Res Q 1973; 24: 3: 465-67.

(8)   Feinberg S. Soc Indication Res 1975; 2: 119-126.

(9)   Sonquist JA. Multivariate Model building. Michigan: Institute for Social Research, University of Michigan, 1970.

(10) Kass GV. Significance testing in automatic interaction detection (A.I.D.). Appl Statist 1975; 24: 178-189.

(11) Scott AJ, Knott M. An approximate test for use with AID. Appl Statist 1976; 25: 103-106.

(12) Ecob R. The distribution and power properties of the AID criterion. In: Corsten LCA, Hermans J, eds. Compstat 1978. Proceedings in Computational Statistics. 3rd Symposium held in Leiden 1978. Wien: Physica-Verlag, 1978: 253-58.

(13) Stone M. Cross-validatory choice and assesment of statistical predictions. J R Stat Soc Series B; 1974: 36: 111-133.

(14) Geisser S. The predictive sample reuse method with applications. JASA 1975; 70: 320-328.

NATURAL HISTORY OF ALCOHOL DEPENDENCE AND
ALCOHOL RELATED DISABILITIES

M.L. Fleming

A.R. Unwin
Department of Statistics
Trinity College, Dublin

J.P. Meehan
St. Patrick's Hospital
Dublin

Summary

This study investigates the sequencing of symptoms of alcohol dependence
and alcohol related disabilities for a sample of problem drinkers. Our
findings are that the dependence symptoms studied can be grouped as
early, middle-stage or late experiences in the dependence process. Disabilities related to alcohol do not appear to occur at any particular
stage in this process.

1.   Introduction

Recurrent themes in alcoholism research include (a) does it have a
biological basis? and (b) what are the diagnostic criteria? Jellinek (1)
proposed that certain types of alcoholism included cellular pathology
and could be looked upon as disease entities. Edwards and Gross (2)
delineated the clinical syndrome of alcohol dependence. Both these
formulations, the former at the cellular level and the latter at the
clinical level, constitute elements of the disease concept of alcoholism.
Another important element of any disease concept is its evolution or
natural history. Orford and Hawker (3) demonstrated a natural ordering
in symptoms of alcohol dependence but not in items related to social
damage. Chick and Duffy (4) demonstrated that the sequence of
symptoms in alcohol dependence was not random .

The purposes of this study were firstly to replicate Chick and Duffy's (4)
work in a different environment and secondly to investigate the combined
sequencing of both symptoms of alcohol dependence and alcohol related
disabilities.

2.   Population Studied

The sample consisted of forty six consecutive admissions to a
psychiatric hospital in Dublin who were diagnosed as having an alcohol

problem. Nine of the sample (ie less than 20%) were females. Their ages ranged from 22 to 65 years with a mean age of 42.6 years. Thirty two (70%) claimed that they would describe themselves as alcoholics; eleven (24%), in their view, were not alcoholics but did recognise that they had a drinking problem; the remaining three (6%) did not see their drinking behaviour as constituting a problem.

To study relevance of ordering of symptoms in another population with alcohol related problems 109 outpatients from a Gastro-Intestinal-Tract (GIT) clinic were interviewed.

3.   Methodology

Chick and Duffy's Alcohol Dependence Schedule (4) along with our own questionnaire on alcohol related disabilities were administered during a structured interview. The questions on these forms referred to twenty three dependence symptoms and twelve disabilities related to alcohol. Each time an item was acknowledged by the patient, the interviewer put aside a card naming that item. At the conclusion of the interview the patient was asked to place these cards, each naming an item he had acknowledged, in order of first occurence of each item. The order of the cards was then recorded by the interviewer. A Severity of Alcohol Dependence (SADQ) score was obtained for each patient using Stockwell et al.'s questionnaire (5).

In analyzing the data a test of randomness based on analysis of variance by ranks was used (6). A modal ordering was obtained for the dependence symptoms and the alcohol related disabilities. The modal sequence obtained by Chick and Duffy (4) was compared with our data using a trend test also based on unified analysis of variance by ranks (6). Patients' SADQ scores were correlated with numbers of disabilities experienced and with other variables. Cluster analysis of the items and of the patients were carried out using Ward's method and a relocate procedure (7).

4.   Results

A sequence of symptoms of alcohol dependence was elicited from each of the forty six patients in this study. The frequency with which each of the twenty three symptoms was experienced is given in Table 1 along with the frequencies obtained in an earlier study (4). The test of randomness yielded an H statistic H = 89.98. This result is extremely

significant (p < .001) and supports Chick and Duffy's conclusion that
the ordering of symptoms of alcohol dependence by patients with an
alcohol problem is not random.

An analysis of rank sums yielded a modal sequence which in many ways
resembled classical descriptions of alcoholism. The modal ordering
obtained in Chick and Duffy's study was compared with our data and
resulted in a Z value of 7.52 (p < .001) This large positive value of
Z indicates that the overall sequencing of symptoms by patients in each
of the two studies follows similar trends. The modal sequences from
this study and that of Chick and Duffy are given in Table 1. Symptom
descriptions are listed in the appendix.

TABLE I - *Modal Ordering of 23 Symptoms as Found in this Study (A), and
in a Previous Study by Chick and Duffy (B).*

	(A)			(B)	
Symptom	% Frequency of Occurrence	Criterion	Symptom	% Frequency of Occurrence	Criterion
9	69	-3.49	10	47	-3.34
5	61	-2.63	9	58	-3.17
12	41	-2.56	11	45	-2.24
6	54	-2.50	5	39	-1.76
4	56	-2.38	4	68	-1.72
3	59	-2.14	23	92	-1.53
8	24	-0.82	12	31	-1.35
10	43	-0.68	3	45	-0.87
13	9	-0.53	6	37	-0.82
1	13	-0.15	1	21	-0.21
2	4	0.29	8	55	0.19
11	37	0.33	2	8	0.24
23	74	0.51	19	66	0.37
15	67	0.55	13	26	0.53
7	59	0.65	14	84	1.03
16	54	1.12	7	66	1.03
19	56	1.19	16	74	1.44
14	65	1.34	18	55	1.45
20	4	1.69	20	3	1.60
17	24	2.08	15	79	2.07
18	56	3.14	22	29	2.50
21	19	3.61	17	24	2.87
22	59	3.82	21	21	3.91

Care must be taken when interpreting the modal ordering of the items.
This ordering does not represent the sequence of symptoms that an alcohol
dependent person would necessarily follow. Not all persons with alcohol
problems will experience all of the twenty three symptoms listed in this
study. In fact, one patient in the present sample, who claimed his
drinking behaviour was a problem, said he experienced none of these
symptoms. The modal ordering does not imply that persons who experience

some of the 'early symptoms' will inevitably experience later symptoms sometime in the future. The modal sequence states only that, if a person experiences some of the symptoms listed, they will tend to occur in the order suggested by the sequence.

Patients in this study were assessed for presence or absence of twelve disabilities related to alcohol consumption. Patients ranked, in order of first occurrence, those disabilities which they had acknowledged. There is only weak evidence for an ordering of alcohol related disabilities (H = 21.09; p = 0.032).

There is no relation between the number of disabilities and the severity of alcohol dependence as measured using the SADQ. Figure 1 is a plot of SADQ score against the number of disabilities experienced. The correlation coefficient r is r = 0.31.

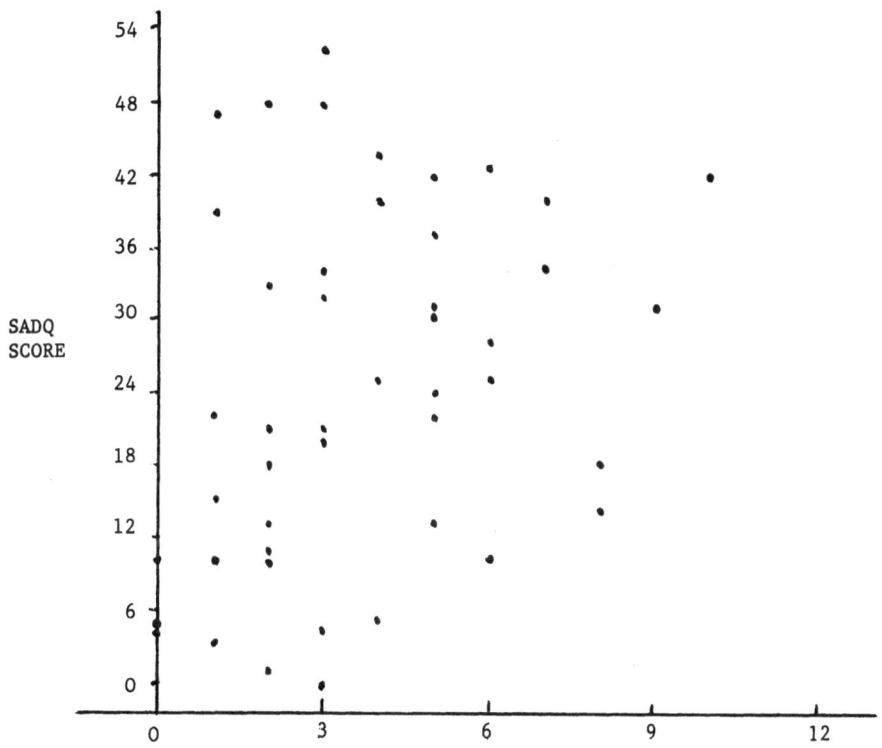

No. of Disabilities Experienced

Figure 1

Clustering patients on the basis of dependence symptoms resulted in two very different clusters. These two groups differed in terms of the number of symptoms experienced and SADQ score. There is no evidence that symptoms of alcohol dependence or alcohol related disabilities tend to occur in clusters either when examined separately or both together.

Nineteen patients from a GIT clinic who were detected as suffering from alcoholism on the basis of the Michigan Alcoholism Screening Test (MAST) (8) did not acknowledge the dependence items experienced by the hospitalised sample.

5. Discussion

The results of our study demonstrate a definite sequence of the symptoms of alcohol dependence. Behavioural and subjective symptoms occur early in the sequence and physiological symptoms occur at a later stage. This adds further confirmation to Jellinek's hypothesis of discrete developmental stages. The later appearance of the symptoms of physiological dependence again emphasises the increasingly predominant role that alcohol itself plays in the perpetuation of the pathological process. The origins of alcohol dependence are probably multifactorial but as the condition evolves the pattern of drinking at the clinical level becomes increasingly stereotyped.

Cluster analysis was used to investigate whether different groups of patients experienced different sets of symptoms. The findings support the overall unity of the concept of alcohol dependence as the only clustering obtained split the patients into two groups, those who experienced many symptoms and those who experienced few.

Alcohol plays such a predominant role when physical dependence is initiated because the motivation for drinking is to avoid the unpleasant effects of alcohol withdrawal. Previous studies have tended to ignore the drug effect of alcohol itself in the process of dependence. Thus physiological alcohol dependence is the final common pathway for a multiplicity of aetiological factors.

Previous diagnoses of alcoholism have often been influenced by cultural norms. The second significant result of this study has been the cross cultural replication of Chick and Duffy's findings. The dimension of alcohol dependence whilst being influenced in its

expression by the individual's environment nevertheless remains a
concept that has wide application.

Alcohol related disabilities are often single events rather than on-
going pathology. Whilst there was weak evidence that the ordering of
disabilities was not random the sequence evolved did not have clinical
meaning. The incidence of disabilities did not affect the ordering of
the symptoms. There was no correlation between the severity of alcohol
dependence and the number of disabilities recognised (Figure 1). A
related conclusion may be drawn from the results of screening out-
patients at the GIT clinic . The manifestations of alcoholism in this
population appear to be physical damage and not the syndrome of alcohol
dependence. It is possible that this group is a different species of
alcoholic and could be categorised as Jellinek's Beta species whereas
the sample from the psychiatric hospital would be more similar to
Jellinek's Gamma and Delta species. This again illustrates the need
at the clinical level to spearate the syndrome of alcohol dependence
from other alcohol related disabilities.

Acknowledgements

We thank the staff and patients of St. Patrick's and Sir Patrick Dun's
hospitals, Dublin, for their cooperation, and the Statistics and
Operations Research Laboratory, Trinity College for assistance.

References

1. Jellinek, E.M., The Disease Concept of Alcoholism, Millhouse
    Press, Connecticut, U.S.A., 1960.

2. Edwards, G. and Gross, M.M., Alcohol Dependence: Provisional
    Description of a Clinical Syndrome, British Medical Journal, 1,
    1058-1061, 1976.

3. Orford, J. and Hawker, A., Note on the Ordering of Onset of
    Symptoms in Alcohol Dependence, Psychological Medicine, 4,
    281-288, 1974.

4. Chick, J. and Duffy, J.C., Application to the Alcohol Dependence
    Syndrome of a Method of Determining the Sequential Development of
    Symptoms, Psychological Medicine, 9, 313-319, 1979.

5. Stockwell, T., Hodgson, R., Edwards, G., Taylor, C. and Rankin, H.,
    The Development of a Questionnaire to Measure Severity of Alcohol
    Dependence, British Journal of Alcoholism, 74, 79-87, 1979.

6. Meddis, R., Unified Analysis of Variance by Ranks, British Journal
    of Mathematical and Statistical Psychology, 33, 84-98, 1980.

7. Wishart, D., Clustan - User Manual, 3rd Edition, Inter-University/
    Research Councils Services, Report No. 47, 1978.

8. Selzer, M.L., The Michigan Alcoholism Screening Test: The Quest for
    a New Diagnostic Instrument, American Journal of Psychology, 157,
    86-94, 1971.

Appendix - Symptoms of Alcohol Dependence

1. Change to drinking same on work day as day off
2. Change from drinking according to mood to not drinking according
    to mood
3. Giving up interests because drinking interferes
4. Missing main meals regularly because of drinking
5. Spending more time drinking
6. Restless without a drink
7. Times when can't think of any thing else but getting a drink
8. Organising day to ensure supply
9. Needing more than companions
10. Completely unable to keep to a limit
11. Difficulty preventing getting drunk
12. Difficulty cutting down
13. Passing out while drinking in public
14. Trembling after drinking the day before
15. Morning drink
16. Morning retching or vomiting
17. Wakening up panicking or frightened
18. Sweating excessively at night
19. Tense on waking
20. Withdrawal fit
21. Hallucinations
22. Decrease tolerance
23. Amnesia

APPLICATION OF TIME SERIES ANALYSIS TO RETROSPECTIVE DATA
OF A CENTRAL LONDON CLINIC FOR THE TREATMENT OF
SEXUALLY TRANSMITTED DISEASES

PETER A WIGODSKY

Department of Genital Medicine
St Bartholomew's Hospital
West Smithfield
LONDON   EC4
England

The Polytechnic of North London
Eden Grove Building
Holloway Road
LONDON   N7 8DB
England

SUMMARY

This paper identifies the situation where retrospective data, when employed in Time Series Analysis for the purpose of forecasting future trends, may not necessarily be used in the traditional form. Where both seasonal and cyclical variations occur for such data it may be necessary to initially replicate the data in a seasonal blocking, before attempting to produce acceptable forecasting models.

INTRODUCTION

The need for such Time Series Analysis and model fitting for patients of Sexually Transmitted Diseases (STD) is obviously necessary for provision of services in the future.[1,2,3,4] The retrospective data available on BARTS I and the DHSS Quarterly Return form SBH60 were used for this purpose. Unknown at the time, the information respective to the year of episode entered on BARTS I was incorrect and it was necessary to use only copies of SBH from 1963 to 1979 (inclusive).

Due to the fact that the volume of patients diagnosed with syphilis or gonorrhoea were very limited indeed, the following results and discussions are for all diagnoses together.

The only published work on any form of model fitting was found to be by Drs. P Balasubromian and A Ravindran on Syphilis patients in Chicago, Illinois.[5] The model proposed by these authors is relatively straight forward for suitable application by databases containing data for both clinics and private Physician. Unfortunately, the model will not function without both these sources and is thus invalid for the data available.

Again in the USA Drs F N Judson and R A Wright have discussed seasonal patterns of STD's in Denver Colorado.[6] Their volume of patients would be suitable for application to the above 'Chicago Model' but as yet no such work has been tried.

The most productive works concerning Time Series Analysis in the UK come from Dr C B S Schofield and concerns work he has done in Scotland during 1972-76.[7]

METHOD

The data available was then employed in two investigations:

(1) A typical seasonal Quarterly Time Series Analysis and fitting a line of Best Fit from which a linear model was obtained and tested. This was prepared so as to make comparisons with the previously published works.

(2) A Quarterly Replicated Time Series Analysis looking at patterns of initially the first quarters throughout the time period, then the second quarters and so on. A line of best fit was completed and again, a linear model was obtained and tested. The impetus for this type of Time Series Analysis comes from the fact that the graphical presentation of the data from the first method led to erratic lines of best fit, and subsequently to debatable logistic models. In this second method, the data was more in order to application of a line of best fit.

In both methods the data was trichotomised for male patients, female patients and an aggregated total population.

RESULTS

(1) Seasonal Quarterly Time Series Analysis.

The following give the results for male patients (9009), female patients (5045), and the aggregated total population (14054). Calculations using the eight point moving averages led to the opportunity of Seasonal Differences and Seasonal Adjustments. In all three sets of the data there is overall high patient visits during the third quarter (i e the months of July, August and September). For both male and total populations, the least quarter of patient visits was the first quarter (i e January, February and March) and for the female patients the minimal quarter was the second quarter.

Once the moving average points were plotted, an attempt was made to fit a suitable line of best fit. As mentioned previously, this was somewhat difficult and infact several suitable slopes were possible and it was at this stage that I felt that suitable analysis should take a different avenue. Nevertheless, suitable linear models were fitted and tested and it is possible to have a certain degree of confidence in the models obtained for each of the data sets.

(2) Quarterly Replicated Time Series Analysis.

As above, the results are for each of the three named data sets. A replication has been employed in each set, there were a total of twelve tables produced (four quarterly replicates). Naturally, it was impossible to calculate the seasonal differences as occurred above. The plotted moving averages led to drawing a line of best fit and in the majority of cases this was an extremely straightforward process without similar difficulties as obtained in the previous method. Linear models were fitted and tested and one has more confidence in these twelve models as being more functional

EXAMPLE 1

Quarterly Time Trend: Female Patients

First Quarters : 1963 - 1979

YEAR	OBSERVATION	4PT	8PT	MOVING AVERAGE
1963	65			
1964	88			
1965	86	321	662	82.75
1966	82	341	696	87
1967	85	355	750	93.75
1968	102	395	854	106.75
1969	126	459	1022	127.75
1970	146	563	1259	157.375
1971	189	696	1545	193.125
1972	235	849	1853	229.375
1973	279	986	2054	256.75
1974	283	1068	2187	273.375
1975	271	1119	2295	286.875
1976	286	1176	2370	269.25
1977	336	1194	2545	318.125
1978	301	1351		
1979	420			

Fit model from the Line of Best Fit.

Taking two points from the graph : 1963 and 1977

$y = mx + c$ where y = frequency, x = year, c = constant

$315 = 15m + c$ (1)

$25 = 1m + c$ (2)

$290 = 14m$ $\therefore$ m = 20.71

Subst   (1)   .315 = 310.71 + c .$\therefore$. c = 4.29

Check   (2) =   20.71 + 4.29 = 25

$\therefore$ $\underline{y = 20.71x + 4.29}$

EXAMPLE 1 : FEMALE PATIENTS : FIRST QUARTERS   PEARSON'S   r = 0.986

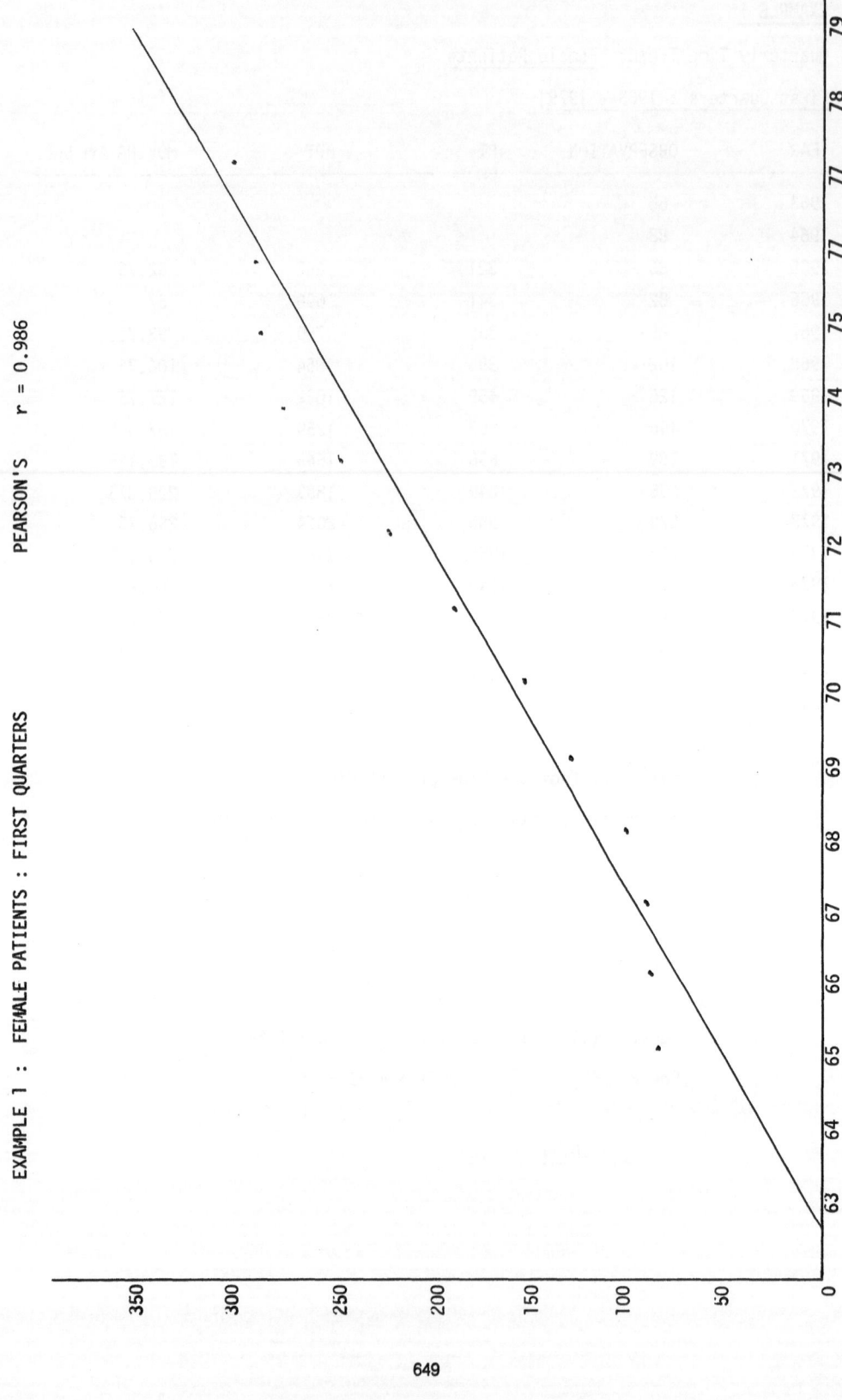

than those obtained from the more orthodox method of time series analysis.

DISCUSSION

The aforegoing results show clearly that there exists a seasonal variation in the number of patient visits; seasonal variation in human behaviour has a major effect on diseases incidence. The data sets show a pronounced increase in late summer and early autumn in total patient visits, in normal findings on clinical examination and in total episodes. These occurrences are similarly bourne out by the Denver Study and the Scottish Study.

The factors leading to this seasonal pattern are many but may in part depend on some variables which directly affect sexual behaviour and clinic attendance. For example, weather conditions may make winter transportation difficult in some areas, and thus cause difficulty for patients in finding sexual partners and in using clinic facilities. Substantial seasonal variation in degree of sexual exposure could also determine the observed patterns, in that summertime could be a favourable catalyst for sexual activity.

The problem of illness behaviour with respect to S T D's has to be considered. The most recent work is by R M Harrison[8] at the Middlesex Hospital. It is suggested from an examination of records, that 75% of women consulted a doctor within six weeks of noticing a symptom, and men, within two weeks. If this is true say, throughout the London population then their inclusion in one quarter or another will vary. However, as is indicated in the results of the prospective study at St Barthomew's shows quite a different pattern indeed.

Further work on illness behaviour has been done in the USA, producing the Kalimo Study[9] and the Rosenstock Study[9]. The two reports both put forward a formal list of criteria covering medical, social and available resources elements and as Harrison rightly suggests, "it is true that these (demographic) variables do discriminate to some extent, but within any particular cultural or socio-economic group variation exists, which as yet, students of illness behaviour have largely been unable to explain".

BIBLIOGRAPHY

1   Bacon P M   Social Distribution of Sexually Transmitted Diseases: A Survey of Female Clinic Registrations. British Journal of Venereal Diseases, 1979 55, 295-299.

2   Heywood C P Bacon P M   Social Background and Diagnosis - Survey of Male Registrations. British Journal of Venereal Diseases, December 1975.

3   Kampmeir R   The Special Clinics for Venereal Disease in the United Kingdom. Journal of the American Venereal Disease Association, September 1975.

4   Woodcock K   How useful are our present statistics on S T D?   British Journal of Venereal Diseases, June 1975.

5   Balasubramanian R and Kavindran A   A Time Series Aggregation Model for Predicting the Incidence of Syphilis. Journal of the American Venereal Disease Association, 1979 January - March, 14-18.

6   Wright R A Judson F N   Relative and Seasonal Incidences of the Sexually Transmitted Diseases.   British Journal of Venereal Diseases, 1978, 54, 433-440.

7   Schofield C B S   Seasonal Variations in the Reported Incidence of Sexually Transmitted Diseases in Scotland, 1972, 96.   British Journal of Venereal Diseases, 1979, 55, 218-222.

8   Harrison R M   Illness Behaviour and Sexually Transmitted Diseases. British Journal of Venereal Diseases 1979, 55, 125-126.

9   Health Education Council - Medical Research Department. Report 32. Motivation and Behaviour in Seeking Treatment for Venereal Diseases.

EDUCATION IN MEDICAL INFORMATICS

- THE ROLE OF THE APPLICATION AREA IN A

CURRICULUM OF APPLIED INFORMATICS -

by

F.J. Leven*, J.R. Möhr**

* Fachbereich Medizinische Informatik, Fachhochschule Heilbronn
Max-Planck-Str. 39, D-7100 Heilbronn

** Fakultät für Theoretische Medizin, Universität Heidelberg,
Im Neuenheimer Feld 325, D-6900 Heidelberg

SUMMARY

Two classes of application areas of informatics are distinguished:
   (1) areas with formalized problems, like mathematics,
       and
   (2) areas with problems of limited formalizability, like medicine.
With respect to curricula in case (1) application-specific education does not
differ significantly from that in core informatics, whereas in case (2) the application area exerts a considerable impact on the respective curriculum. This leads -
as exemplified in the case of medicine - even to curricula specialized to the
application field and to concepts of corresponding postgraduate curricula.

1. INTRODUCTION

Informatics as a science does not fit into the conventional classification of
sciences: It neither belongs to the natural sciences - its objects are no phenomena
of nature - nor is it a part of mathematics - contrary to mathematics it deals with
the dynamic behaviour of complex variable objects - nor is it a human science or
one of the classical engineering sciences. (2)

As a self-contained science it deals with investigating the fundamental procedures
of information processing and the general methods of the application of such
procedures in the various application areas.

For the following discussion of curricula in informatics the application areas are grouped into two classes

1. theoretical sciences with great affinity to informatics as to methodology and reasoning, like mathematics
2. practical sciences with problems of limited degree of formalization and empirical deductive reasoning, like medicine.

According to this classification the impact of the application area on the corresponding curriculum of applied informatics will be outlined and exemplified for medicine as a practical science.

2. CURRICULUM MODELS IN INFORMATICS

Various curriculum models have evolved in several countries during the last ten years in connection with the development of the "new" science of informatics.

One curriculum model with more than ten years of practical application at about 20 universities in the FRG follows the "recommendations of the GAMM/NTG" (the Association for Applied Mathematics and Mechanics and the Association for Telecommunication Technology) (2,4).

In this model core informatics - comprising theoretical, practical and technical informatics - is emphasized with about 80% of the lectures and courses. Roughly 20% are reserved for electives and an application area such as mathematics, economics or medicine.

The aim of offering an application area is not to provide application specific competence. It is assumed that job-specific knowledge and capabilities may grow obsolete after a short while. Students are supposed to get a broad, theoretically based primary education and become familiar with the methods of scientific research in order to be able to keep pace with the rapid development in the area. The introduction into an application field has a mere exemplary function. Application areas are considered interchangeable.

3. THEORETICAL AND PRACTICAL SCIENCES AS APPLICATION AREAS OF INFORMATICS

3.1 Mathematics - a theoretical science

The theoretical concepts are the dominant principles of a theoretical science. All efforts are directed at refining the systems of axioms and theorems which make up the theory underlying the science. In this way the realm of discourse is highly formalized. The practical relevance of the system of theories is unimportant. The validity of the concepts is limited in time. They are replaced as soon as better concepts emerge. Internal inconsistencies are not tolerated. If the theoretical science is also a natural science, the experiment which is characterized by highly standardized conditions, repeatability and the modelling of complex structures is the characteristic tool of investigation.

Mathematics is considered as a representative for a theoretical application area. Its relation to informatics may be examined from two different points of view:

> "First, informatics education was often developed in connection with an existing mathematics education system.
> Secondly, the use of informatics and its methods needs appropriate mathematical skills and determines the part mathematics is taking in the development of informatics." (12)

The development of informatics thus is characterized by its strong theoretical foundations with the most important notions defined clearly and generally. "The more progress is made in building theoretical foundations of informatics the more complicated and advanced mathematical methods are involved in that process". (12).

Though the relation between mathematics and informatics is certainly unique compared with other sciences, one can state that there is a strong relationship between theoretical application areas and informatics with respect to methodology, terminology and the way of reasoning. This means that a theoretical application area can be represented in a curriculum of applied informatics rather simply, because application-specific courses do not differ significantly from those in core informatics: Much of the methodology of the application subject is already contained in that of core informatics.

3.2 Medicine - a practical science

Medicine is a practical science. In practical sciences the underlying theoretical systems play a different role than in theoretical sciences.

The requirement to take action and to influence an object system entails that practical success becomes the dominant criterion. The necessity to take action even if no theoretical basis for this action is available, may demotivate from the research necessary to define such a theoretical basis, as long as the chosen action is successful. On the other hand failure of practical action and the failure of a theory to result in practical success may lead to a continuous search for alternative theories and hence to a proliferation of alternative theoretical systems.

Finally theories - even if wrong - may persit undisturbed if they do not disturb practical success.

Typically the advent of a new instrument such as the computer stirs new interest in the theoretical foundations of a practical science. Introduction of computers in medicine has renewed the interest in such fundamental concepts as diagnosis and efficacy of medical action. It is characteristic for a practical science like medicine that it cannot be completely defined by the theoretical tools it employs - be it mathematics or pathophysiology. The theoretical sciences underlying medicine have ancillary functions.

This situation is responsible for a deep conceptual gap between practical and theoretical sciences. Even if applied informatics is essentially a practical science, its concepts have been formulated as concepts of theoretical sciences. And this conflict also exists between informatics and its application subjects. This conflict is characterized by differences in goals, language, way of reasoning, and the pragmatic environment created around the two sciences that try to meet in order to solve a given problem.

4. EDUCATION IN MEDICAL INFORMATICS - APPLIED INFORMATICS IN MEDICINE

Perhaps it is not by accident that the concept of "medical informatics" has evolved as a special term for applied informatics in medicine. Investigating some curricula in medical informatics offered in the Federal Republic of Germany for almost ten years will show how they try to bridge the conceptual gap between medicine and informatics.

4.1 Concepts of Medical Informatics

Some conceptual difference is already discernible if one compares the following characterizations of medical informatics which we owe to a representative of core informatics (SEEGMÜLLER) and a physician (REICHERTZ). (Figure 1):

Whereas the informatician emphasizes the application of algorithms - supposing the formalizability of the application problems - the physician stresses the support of information processes - a sort of operational characteristics - considering the problems of describing such complex systems as human beings: "Human beings belong to the most complex systems we know and each schematizing and simplification for the purpose of algorithmization claims sacrifices as to the precision of the mapping of reality" (ÜBERLA, from (11) translation by the author). Besides the interface problems between medicine and informatics as well as between informatics and medical informatics there is also - according to MOEHR - a significant difference between medicine and medical informatics: For the physician the patient is

655

```
┌─────────────────┐
│    MEDICAL      │
│ ┌─────────────┐ │
│ │ INFORMATICS │ │
│ └─────────────┘ │
└─────────────────┘
```

characterized

by

```
┌──────────────────────┐        ┌──────────────────────┐
│ an Informatician     │        │ a Physician          │
│ (SEEGMÜLLER)         │        │ (REICHERTZ)          │
├──────────────────────┤        ├──────────────────────┤
│ MEDICAL INFORMATICS  │        │ TASKS OF             │
│ IS THE SCIENCE OF    │        │ MEDICAL INFORMATICS  │
│ FEATURES;            │        │ ARE                  │
│ REPRESENTATION;      │        │ DOCUMENTATION        │
│ CONSTRUCTION AN      │        │ ANALYSIS             │
│ REALIZATION OF       │        │ CONTROL              │
│ ┌──────────┐         │        │ SYNTHESIS            │
│ │ALGORITHMS│         │        │ OF                   │
│ └──────────┘         │        │ ┌──────────┐         │
│ FOR THE AREA OF      │        │ │INFORMATION│        │
│ MEDICAL SCIENCES     │        │ │PROCESSES │         │
│ AND                  │        │ └──────────┘         │
│ MEDICAL PRACTICE     │        │ IN MEDICINE          │
└──────────────────────┘        └──────────────────────┘
```

Fig.1: Aspects of medical informatics

the dominant object of interest, for the medical informatician however, the patient is only a part of the system of medicine: Medical informatics deals in a more comprehensive way with medicine as a whole comprising patients and institutions that form our health care system.

Whereas a curriculum of medicine ranges from anatomy, pharmacology etc. to psychology the scope of medical informatics includes in addition - in a highly interdisciplinary way - eg economics, medical sociology and structure and organisation of the health care system and its components.

4.2 Curricula in Medical Informatics in the FRG

To meet the special requirements of education in medical informatics a joint commission of the GMDS and GI (The German Association for Medical Documentation, Informatics and Statistics and the Association for Informatics) has worked out a frame of contents for formation in medical informatics in 1973 (1). These concepts together with the GAMM/NTG recommendations form the basis of the following two types of curricula in medical informatics in the FRG:

(i) Curricula in core informatics with medicine as an application subject

The first curriculum type corresponds exactly to the GAMM/NTG recommendations as outlined. It is offered at 7 universities: Hannover/Braunschweig (Hannover Medical School and Braunschweig Technical University), Dortmund, Erlangen, Frankfurt, Hamburg, Kiel and Munich (Technical University). Though there are differences as to the content of the lectures between the various universities one common problem for some of them is that medical subjects are a mere selection from lectures prepared for medical students, nurses or technicians. For students of informatics, however, such lectures are often overloaded with medical details for which bases are sometimes lacking, and which are therefore hard to comprehend. Also they tend to lack specific subjects such as organization of health care institutions which are relevant for students of medical informatics.

(ii) A spezialized curriculum for medical informatics

A methods-oriented curriculum specialized in medical informatics is jointly offered since 1972 by the University of Heidelberg and the Heilbronn School of Technology (3,6,7). The main feature of this curriculum is an allocation of more than 30% of its time for lectures and courses to the application area. (Figure 2). The total amount of lectures exeeds the GAMM/NTG recommendations also by approximately 30%.

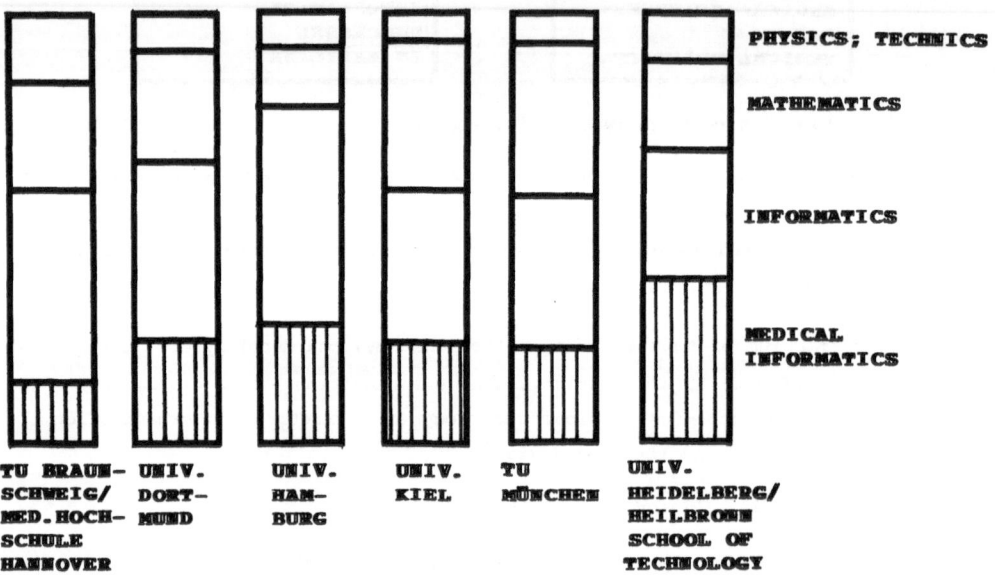

Fig. 2: Relative weight of subjects in curricula for medical informatics.

Structure and features of the entire curriculum are summarized in Figure 3. The first study section comprizes the foundations in informatics, mathematics, natural sciences, medicine and economics. The second section contains number of electives in addition to the core of mandatory lectures. The possibility exists to choose among three major subjects for graduation

    1 computer aided organization of health care systems

    2 information systems

    3 technical medical informatics

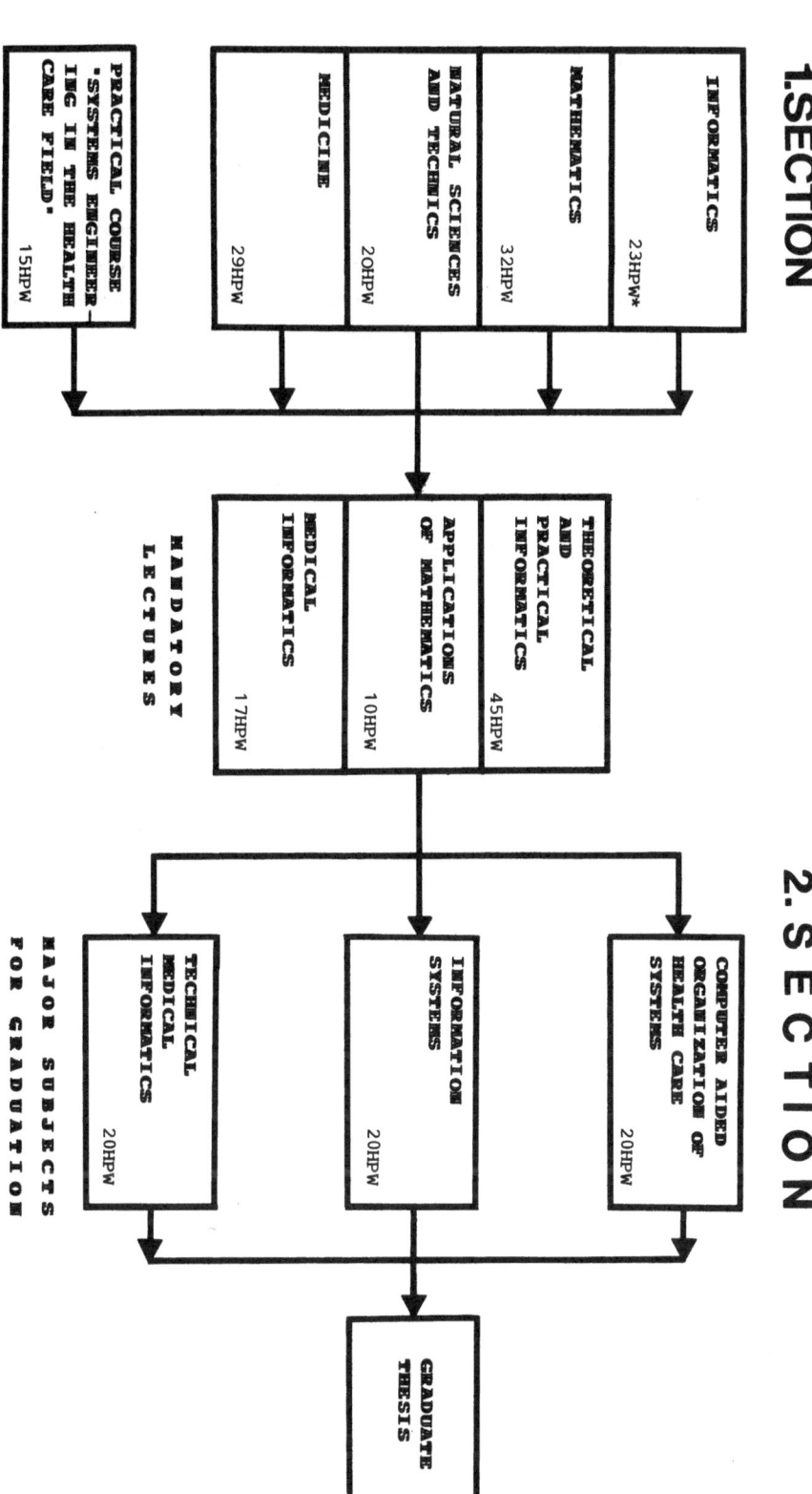

Fig.3. Structure of the HEIDELBERG/HEILBRONN curriculum for medical informatics

* Hours per week

The first major subject includes computer center management as well as health care facility management; the second is concerned with scientific medical applications, and the third covers computer networks as well as process control and biosignal processing.

An essential feature of the curriculum is that basic medical subjects - presented in a way tailored to students of this curriculum - form an integrated part of the curriculum from the beginning. An introduction to medical informatics during the first semester provides for a link between seemingly unrelated subjects such as mathematics, anatomy, and technical informatics. Another important subject is a practical course on "systems engineering in the health care field" (9) which is offered in the 4th semester. It aims at confronting the students with practical problems of the health care field and at practicing systems engineering techniques. Fifteen hours per week are allocated to this course which takes place in the actual work environment of the health care field:

Practical problems existing in health care institutions such as hospitals, doctor's offices, insurance companies and the like are analyzed by the students. The changing subjects include eg aspects of textprocessing, reorganization of a medical records department in a hospital and the conception of an information system for an insurance company. The general problem is broken up into subtasks which are solved by students in groups of 1 to 6. The results are reported orally and in writing, and assembled into a report. In this way the students get an introduction in project management, team work and practical application of systems engineering techniques. The course is supplemented by demonstrations of selected health care institutions mostly connected with local hospitals.

An essential difference between the two curriculum types may become evident if one tries to answer the question of STIEGE (10): "How many subjects are there mandatory in the field of medical informatics that can not at all or not in sufficiently short time be learned postgraduatly?" Independent of the answer to this question the need for postgraduate education in the area of medical informatics is generally considered relevant.

(iii) Post-graduate education in medical informatics

A common concept of postgraduate education has been proposed on the basis of the already mentioned recommendations of the GMDS/GI joint commission.

The prerequisites for obtaining a certificate as 'medical informatician' which is issued jointly by the GMDS and GI (8) include recommendations for postgraduate training for medical doctors, informaticians and graduates of other curricula.

Primary prerequisites are:

1   a university degree in either computer science or medicine
2   at least five years of pertinent and successful professional
    performance - an operational qualification
3   a "complementary" postgraduate education, which means education
    in those subjects that are not part of the applicant's pregraduate
    education.

This approach of postgraduate education thus can be characterized as a hybrid concept of university education and on-the-job-training for medical informatics. It accounts for the need for profound familiarization with the application field which is not conveyed by classical university education in informatics. However the process of offering courses etc. which convey the knowledge postulated as a prerequisite is relatively slow. Initiatives have been taken by the responsible societies. The difficulties encountered in meeting the demand may be taken as an additional indication of the justification of a specialized curriculum.

5. Conclusions

We propose that the role of the application area in a curriculum of applied informatics should depend on the type of the application area. The conceptual affinity between informatics and a theoretical application subject can be accounted for in curricula in which no great differences between lectures in core informatics and the application field exist.

Practical application areas, however, like medicine, may exert a remarkable impact on the corresponding curricula. As is exemplified for medicine this is due to a great conceptual difference in terminology, methodology and way of reasoning between informatics and the application area. To bridge this distance curricula are needed that take care of these interface problems. This may even lead to curricula specialized to the application area. Furthermore education in this case has to consider ways of postgraduate curricula in order to combine university education with on-the-job-training.

REFERENCES

(1) Anonym: Reisensburger Protokolle. Red: Reichertz, P.L.,
Medizinische Hochschule Hannover, Dept. für Biometrie und Medizinische Informatik
(German).

(2) Brauer, W., Haacke, W., Münch, S., Studien- und Forschungsführer Informatik, Gesellschaft für Mathematik und Datenverarbeitung, Bonn, and Deutscher Akademischer Austauschdienst, Bonn-Bad Godesberg 1980, (German).

(3) Hofmann, J., Leven, F.J., Diplom-Informatiker der Medizin - ein neues Berufsbild im Gesundheitswesen, Medizinische Technik 96,6 (1976), 112-115, (German).

(4) Koeppe, P., Überlegungen zur Gesataltung einer Vorlesung "Medizinische Informatik", in: Köhler, C.O., Wagner, G. (Eds.), Interaktive Datenverarbeitung in der Medizin, Schattauer, Stuttgart, New York, 1976, 345-367, (German).

(5) Koeppe, P., Reichertz, P.L., Übersicht über den Stand der Ausbildung in der Medizinischen Informatik, in: Möhr, J.R., Köhler, C.O. (Eds.), Datenpräsentation, 6. Frühjahrstagung der GMDS, Heidelberg 1979, Springer, Berlin, Heidelberg, New York, 1979, 220-231, (German).

(6) Leven, F.J., Studium des Diplom-Informatikers Fachrichtung Medizin, in Gaus, W. (Ed .), Ausbildung in Medizinischer Dokumentation, Statistik und Datenverarbeitung, Springer, Berlin, Heidelberg, New York, 1980, 11-32, (German).

(7) Möhr, J.R., Hofmann, J., Leven, F.J., A specialized curriculum for medical informatics, review after 6 years of experience, in: Barber, B., Grémy, F., Überla, K., Wagner, G. (Eds.), Medical Informatics Berlin 1979, Springer, Berlin, Heidelberg, New York, 1979, 61-72.

(8) Möhr, J.R., Zertifikat Medizinischer Informatiker, Schriftenreihe der Deutschen Gesellschaft für Medizinische Informatik und Statistik, Heft 2, Schattauer, Stuttgart, New York, 1978, (German).

(9) Möhr, J.R., Rothemund, M., Boese, J., On introducing professional practice into a curriculum of applied informatics, publication in preparation.

(10) Stiege, G., Ausbildungsfragen Medizinische Informatik: Aspekte aus der Sicht des Informatikers, in: Möhr, J.R., Köhler, C.O. (Eds.), Datenpräsentation, 6. Frühjahrstagung der GMDS, Heidelberg 1979, Springer, Berlin, Heidelberg, New York, 1979, (German).

(11) Überla, K., Probleme zwischen Informatik und Medizin - die Sicht des Anwenders, Informatik-Spektrum 1 (1979), 4-11, (German).

(12) Waligorski, S., Mathematics and informatics, in: Lecarme, O., Lewis, R. (Eds.), Computers in education, IFIP 2nd world conference on computers in education Marseille 1975, North Holland, Amsterdam, Oxford 1975, 659-660.

INFORMATION SYSTEMS AND COMPUTER SCIENCE MODULE IN THE TRAINING OF COMMUNITY PHYSICIANS IN DEVELOPING COUNTRIES: THE EXPERIENCE IN LAGOS, NIGERIA.

O.O. Hunponu-Wusu, A.P.Curran and N.R.Rao, Department of Community Health, College of Medicine, University of Lagos, Lagos, Nigeria.

ABSTRACT.

   Training in information systems and computer science was introduced as part of the course in the post graduate degree programme in public health (M.P.H.) of the University of Lagos.   The academic staff of the department of Community Health with the cooperation of specialists in the allied fields reviewed the module of the information systems and computer science in conjunction with the module of medical statistics for the M.P.H. course.   The need for the knowledge, the syllabus of the module and the examination aspects are discussed.   The University of Lagos Faculty concludes that it is reasonable to continue to allocate 10% of the academic teaching time to these topics.

   Since they are often consulted to advise on the applications of these topics, trainee community physicians should be encouraged to master this area of knowledge.

COMPUTERS AND CONTINUING EDUCATION IN THE HEALTH SCIENCES

Phil R. Manning,
Barbara Silva,
Development & Demonstration Center in
Continuing Education for Health Professionals
University of Southern California
School of Medicine
Los Angeles, California 90033
USA

Methods of continuing medical education have centered around reading, attending courses and conferences, and informal conversations with colleagues. Computer technology now makes it possible to link education to real events in practice. Current efforts to develop physician profiles, provide information at the time and place it is needed, and provide guidance in difficult cases should be extended.

0. INTRODUCTION

There is no doubt that lifelong learning in the health sciences is necessary, but there is considerable disappointment among academicians in traditional continuing medical education, that deals with the transfer of information rather than ways in which that information can be utilized. Formal continuing medical education, as well as undergraduate education, usually fails to teach students how to determine their own educational needs, nor does it offer techniques for organizing medical practices in order to facilitate continuing education by relating learning to events in actual practice. The transfer of information in continuing medical education is possible through a variety of avenues, both in a formal setting and in the physician's own office. In studying the techniques physicians use to keep up with new developments in their field, studies continue to show that the professional journal continues to be most frequently cited as the main learning source. (1,2) For example, in a survey of physicians it was determined that physicians learned about cimetidine primarily from medical journals and meetings, as well as conversations with peers. (3)

1. NON COMPUTER TECHNOLOGY

To keep up with the rapid expansion of knowledge, new technologies are being developed which allow the physician to update his knowledge on a subject by way of television, radio, telephone, audio and video tapes, and this transfer of information can be taken out of the classroom and delivered to the physician in his office, home, or automobile. (4) Developments in audiovisual media show promise of excellent potential for simulated problem solving as well as information transfer. But these technologies must be coordinated to prevent the physician from being so inundated that most of the material will go unused. We personally believe that the approaches using the classroom paradigm are helpful, but will not produce a major change in CME. While a physician's knowledge may be adequate, this fact is not always reflected in the physician's actual performance with patients. (5) To best serve the physician, continuing education should be available at the time and place needed, when the physician is developing his diagnostic and therapeutic plans, thereby improving the quality of care. Thus, we agree with Eisele's views on CME: that it be (1) continuous; (2) community-hospital based (we would add office-based); and (3) directly related to the physician's daily activities regarding patient care. (6) While this concept has been agreed to for decades, manual techniques to implement the concept are time consuming and cumbersome.

2. SUCCESSFUL STUDIES

Let's examine four studies cited by Sanazaro that relate improvement in the quality of care to educational activities. (7) The deDombal study of computer-assisted diagnosis, required that a group of surgeons in England provide clinical data to a team of investigators. (8) In providing this data, the diagnostic skills of the surgeons was improved. Another study that involved the development of a protocol to aid physician's assistants and nurse practitioners in diagnosis and treatment of sore throat, was also found to improve the performance of physicians. Protocols were also used in the McDonald study in order to identify insufficient, excessive or dangerous treatment. (9) A computer warning system was utilized to alert one group of physicians if such a situation arose, along with suggestions for remedy, while the control group received no such warning. For the group receiving the computer printouts, there was significant change in treatment behavior. The Stapleton study concerned itself with a comparison of the quality of care in teaching

and nonteaching hospitals. While the certification or noncertification
of physicians showed little or no effect on the quality of care, the
teaching environment produced superior care when compared to the care
given in hospitals not associated with a medical school. (10) In all
of these studies, the attention of the physicians is focused on specific
problems through the act of compiling data or by receiving reminders on '
their practice from a computer or residents, and the learning experience
is applied to the physician's day-to-day routine. This, no doubt, accounts for the improvement in the physician's behavior.

3. LINKING CME TO REAL EVENTS IN PRACTICE

Thus, in spite of the ever increasing technologies available to deliver
knowledge; in order for continuing education to be most effective, it
should be linked to the actual events in practice. Sir William Osler
expressed this concept when he said, "In what may be called the natural
method of teaching, the student begins with the patient, continues with
the patient, and ends his studies with the patient, using books and lectures as tools, as means to an end." (11) Promoting such a linkage
will probably be the computer's most significant contribution to continuing medical education. It is here that research and development should
be strengthened, since every physician's office will probably soon be
equipped with a computer terminal.

4. HOW THE COMPUTER MAY HELP LINK EDUCATION TO PRACTICE

The computer may help the physician continue education based on real
events in practice in at least three ways: (1) indexing office records
for educational needs assessment; (2) providing information when needed;
and (3) providing guidance in decision-making.

4.1. Indexing Office Records for Educational Needs Assessment

Most American physicians file charts by patient name only. Manually
cross-filing by patient problems is more difficult, but it does allow
the physician to study his practice and profit from his experience when
he can pull the files of all patients who have presented with the same
condition to compare his experience with others'. Computer technology
can facilitate the organization of data with use of a multiple cross-

filing system. Braunstein from South Carolina and Green of Denver have
described a system that readily permits the cross-filing of patient data
according to (1) the problems that a physician is seeing in his practice;
(2) social and demographic characteristics of patients; (3) medications;
(4) laboratory studies; and (5) vital signs. (12,13) This method allows
physicians to analyze many aspects of their practice and to direct their
study accordingly. For example, it would be possible to assemble the
charts of the last twenty patients with hypertension and review the diagnostic and therapeutic plans with an expert. This would be very indi-
vidualized instruction.

4.2. Providing Information When and Where Needed

Computer technology permits rapid, direct access to information when the
physician is developing his diagnostic and therapeutic plans. An example
of this is the hepatitis data base developed at the Lister Hill National
Center. (14) This system does not directly guide the decision-making,
since the physician must still apply the computer information appropriately in the management of the patient's problem.

4.3. Providing Guidance

Computer technology can also provide the physician with guidance in
decision-making. The system "Caduceus" formally "Internist" being developed at the University of Pittsburgh, offers guidance by mimicking
the diagnostic behavior of the "excellent clinician." (15) The system
developed by Dr. Lawrence Weed and co-workers at the University of Vermont is organized around the problem-oriented record, which consists of
four major parts: the data base (patient history, physical examination,
and laboratory studies); a list of the patient's problems as they are
understood; diagnostic and therapeutic plans; and progress notes organized around individual problems. (16) Information related to a problem is contained on more than 45,000 frames or displays. Appropriate
medical knowledge relating to a specific problem may be displayed within
milliseconds. In addition, when a physician is puzzled about a diagnosis, he may obtain a list of diagnostic possibilities as well as information about procedures to confirm or exclude certain options. Possible
side effects, dosages, and cost of drugs can be displayed, as can normal
values, indications, contra-indications, and costs of laboratory tests.

5. CONCLUSIONS

Lifelong learning is recognized as necessary in the health sciences, but time constraints make it difficult for many professionals to pursue. To date, most CME has consisted of information transfer by the printed page, classroom activities, or audiovisual media. These methods may not relate to problems confronting the physician at a given moment, nor do they aid the physician in applying his knowledge to actual treatment of patients. Current computer technology makes it possible to relate education to actual events in practice when the physician must devise his diagnostic and therapeutic plans. Continuing education must place less reliance on strict memory and enhance the possibilities for professional growth from experience. Efforts to further develop, perfect, and field-test the linking of computerized continuing medical education to real events in practice should take precedence over simulation techniques and simple transfer of information.

REFERENCES

(1) Manning PR, Denson TA. How cardiologists learn about echocardiography: a reminder for medical educators and legislators. Ann Int Med. 1979; 91:469-471.

(2) Stross JK, Harlan WR. The dissemination of new medical information. JAMA. 1979; 241:2622-2624.

(3) Manning PR, Denson TA. How internists learned about cimetidine. Ann Int Med. 1980; 92:690-692.

(4) Manning PR, Millard WL. Technology for continuing medical education. HSRC/HCPC Health Care Technology Compendium Series, University of Missouri, Columbia, Missouri, September 1979.

(5) Pinkerton RE, Tinanoff N, Willms JL, Tapp JT. Resident physician performance in a continuing education format: does newly acquired knowledge improve patient care? JAMA. 1980; 244:2183-2185.

(6) Eisele CW. The medical audit in continuing education. J Med Educ. 1969; 44:263-265.

(7) Sanzaro PJ. Medical audit, continuing medical education and quality assurance. West J Med. 1979; 125:241-252.

(8) deDombal FT, Leaper DJ, Horrochs JC. Human and computer-aided diagnosis of abdominal pain: further report with emphasis on performance of clinicians. Brit Med J. 1974; 1:376-380.

(9) McDonald CJ. Use of a computer to detect and respond to clinical events: its effect on clinician behavior. Ann Int Med. 1976; 84:162-167.

(10)   Stapleton JF, Zwerneman JA.   The influence of an intern-resident
staff on the quality of private patient care.   JAMA.   1965; 194:135-140.

(11)   Cushing H.   The Life of Sir William Osler.   Oxford University
Press, New York.   1940; p. 328.

(12)   Braunstein M.   The computer-based medical record in family practice.   In Medalie JH.   Family Medicine.   Baltimore.   The Williams &
Wilkins Company, 1978.

(13)   Green LA, Simmons RL, Reed FM, Warren PS, Morrison JD.   A family
medicine information system: the beginning of a network for practicing
and resident family physicians.   J Fam Prac.   1978; 7:567-576.

(14)   Schoolman HM, Bernstein LM.   Computer use in diagnosis, prognosis
and therapy.   Science.   1978; 22:926-931.

(15)   Pople HE, Meyers JD, Miller RA.   In proceedings of the Fourth
International Joint Conference on Artificial Intelligence, USSR, Tablishi,
1975.

(16)   Weed LL.   Your health care and how to manage it.   Vermont: Essex
Publishing Co., Inc., 1978.

INTEREST OF A MICROCOMPUTER PILOTING SLIDES AND VIDEOTAPE
IN MEDICAL PROGRAMMED TEACHING

L. PERLEMUTER M.D., F. VASSE M.A., F. LEGRAND ING E.C.P., AND A. COGET
UNIVERSITÉ PARIS XII-HOPITAL HENRI MONDOR - 94000 CRETEIL

SUMMARY

Un micro-ordinateur a été utilisé pour piloter un projecteur de diapositives
et un magnetoscope. Cet équipement a permis de réaliser des programmes d'ensei
gnements pour des étudiants et des malades. Les avantages de la méthode
(mémorisation rapide des données et acquisition des comportements) sont discutés
ainsi que les inconvénients (coût en matériel et temps .

INTRODUCTION :

Pedagogy in medicine has two main aims : acquisition of knowledge which is memorized and organized in specific structures and acquisition of behaviour allowing
the physician to make a decision when facing different situations.

The tremendous amount of facts and data which have to be learnt by medical students
clearly shows that new methods should be used for teaching.

Experiments in programmed teaching have been carried out in Iowa and Missouri
Universities (1) New York (2) Newcastle U/Tyne (3).

A survey has been made by Brigham and Kemp (5) to point out the status of computed
assisted methods of instruction.

Our purpose was to develop a method of programmed medical teaching using an
individual computer and audo-visual possibilities of a slide projector and video
cassette recorder to enhrance both the efficiency of teaching and assessment.

MATERIAL

We chose a micro-computer manufactured by SHARP the MZ 80 K Model because of the
following advantages :

- compacity : the screen, the keyboard and the tape recorder are in on piece
- 48 K of RAM and removable BASIC language of 12 K
- large possibilities of interfacing which enabled us to connect a projector of
  slides and a portable videotape recorder
- relatively low cost : 8200 FF for the computer and the interfacing cards
- reliability of the system

The slide projector is a Caramate (manufactured by SINGER) whose carrousel is
controlled by the computer.

The videotape is a portable V H S from J.V.C. : model HS 2200 allowing forward
and backward quick searching as well as pause and image by image functions. It is
also piloted by the MZ 80 K. Films are done with a portable J V C color camera.
We would also develop our programs on the microcomputer GOUPIL 2 manufactured
in France by S M T.

METHODS

1) Programs for students

Before doing a program we had to determine the precis pedagogic objectives we
wanted the students to reach.

For example, if an intermediate objective was : "describe the symptoms and signs of
Graves disease" it was also necessary to define specific objectives such as :
"describe the symptoms which are present in more than 70 % of cases of Graves
disease" : " describe the ophtalmologic signs, significant of severe ophtalmopathy
in Graves disease" etc...

This first step is a rather difficult one for the medical teacher because he has
to wonder why he should teach this item and for what purpose.

The second step consists of making a flowchart of the pedagogic program. Cutting
the whole program in smaller and well defined parts corresponding to the specific
objectives is the most important job.

We chose a ramified type of program. In this conception each objective may be
considered as a unit of knowledge. The main line of the program progresses when
the student has correctly answered the questions assessing the acquisition of
each unit of knowledge.

Assessment of knowledge may be performed by multiple choice questions using the
ON GOTO possibilities of the computer. In other cases it is better to ask the
student to print a short answer on the keyboard.

At each step, if a wrong answer is given, explanations and new information are
brought. The program may then loop the unit of knowledge that has still to be
acquired or leads previously to a parrallel line of program.

The third step consists of the choice of appropriate illustration for the different
units of knowledge.

These may be :
- texts
- animated drawings on the screen of the computer
- slides
- movies

Each one of these possibilities may be the best for a particular item

2) Programs for patients

We developped a program of self assessing choice of food for diabetics.
The aim was to compare the choice made by patients and the ideal calculations done
by the computer.

DISCUSSION

Programmed teaching has many advantages. On the one hand the medical teacher has
to determine his precise objectives. Then he must choose the best way of teaching
the items. When this choice has been made the same program may he presented to
many students avoidingrepetitions and waste of time.
On the other hand for the student :
- success in learning is obligatory
- retroaction is immediate
- the rhythm of learning is individual
- attention is permanently stimulated
- interest in the method is almost constant, partly because this way of learning
seems like a game. Our conclusions are the same than in (4)
In an experience in a program teaching how to prescribe insulin in diabetics all
the items were quickly learnt by fifty five students after having performed one
to three times the programs. A control was done after one month without a single
error.
For the patients they learnt quickly how to avoid serious errors in selecting
their diet.
After one month a control has shown a good memorization as concerning the quantity
and the sharing out of carbohydrates in the diet. With the videotape the patients
learnt self control of blood glucose.
Nevertheless certain problems should not be overlooked : this method does not
suit every purpose. Other ways are often more economic especially when only simple
memorization is required. In our opinion the best application of programmed medical
teaching with a computer is the study of clinical cases and more generaly all kinds
of situations where the student must learn how to make a decision or how to
behave in precise circumstances.
The second problem is the realization of the program itself. The ratio between
the cost of the "hard" (computer, slides, videotape, camera) and the number of
students that can be taught is not bad at the present time and will be even better
in the next few years. But the "soft" is costly , especially in time. Even if the
medical teacher is interested in pedagogy and computers he could hardly do all the
work himself. A team consisting of physicians, medical students and computer specialists together would give the best and quickest results.
The third problem is that the standardization of the programs is uneasy because of
the different curricula existing in many universities : thus exportation of programs and, by the way, their profitability are not obvious.
Despite these obstacles we think that programmed teaching will expand in the near
future because it opens upnew methods in pedagogy.

1 - KENT Th. and all
   Field test of programmed tests for teaching general pathology.
   Journ. of Medical Educ. 1972, 47, 873-878

2 - PORTNOV A.L., GLASSER N.A.
   Four years experience with a programmed test in clinical pathology
   Journ of Medical Educ. 1974, 49, 457-459

3 - OWEN S.G.
   Comparison between programmed learning and reading in teaching electro-
   cardiography.
   Journ. of the Association for programmed learning Vol. 1, 1964

4 - D'IVERNOIS J.F., MARQUIS Y., BIASPEYRE J.
   Enseignement de la cardiologie par ordinateur : bilan d'une expérience.
   Union Med. Canada, 1975, 544-546

5 - BRIGHAM C., KAMP M.
   The current status of compared assisted instructions in the health sciences.
   Journ. of Medical Educ., 1974, 49, 278-279

Training Anaesthetists to cope with an Emergency in the Operating Theatre: the Use of the Microcomputer

BY

B. Richards#, M.E. Dodson∅, B.R.H. Doran∅, C. Jeffery#, R. Longbottom∅,
A. Poyser# and P. Stellar∅.
≠ University of Manchester Institute of Science and Technology
∅ Department of Anaesthetics, University of Manchester

SUMMARY

A program has been written which indicates the best courses of action to
be taken during a crisis in a real or simulated operation. In the early hours
of the morning, it is often the lot of less experienced anaesthetists to take
charge of the patient about to undergo an emergency operation. Usually everything
will go well but, on sufficient occasions for it not to be a rarity, the unexpected will happen and an emergency will occur whilst the patient is undergoing the
operation. The patient may have a cardiac arrest and then a life threatening situation
presents itself. Less dramatic, but nevertheless, still of great importance, the
patient may become cyanosed (turn blue) and be in danger of oxygen starvation to the
brain. Likewise, the dangers to the patient from high or low Blood Pressure, high
or low Central Venous Pressure, high or low Heart Rate, or abnormal heart rhythms
(heart block or ectopics) must not be diminished. In situations like these the
anaesthetist would like to have his consultant at his side but, alas, the latter
may be many miles away. The authors have put the expertise of several consultants
in a desk-top micro and the computer can now cope with almost every type of patient
emergency. The usefulness of such a program from the training point of view is
enormous. Junior staff can now simulate crisis situations in the computer and test
their own reactions to such situations. They can decide on what they would do
at each critical point and then press the button and see what the team of consultants
would have done in those same circumstances.

INTRODUCTION

Computer models of physiological processes have been in existence for some time,
one of the best known being the 'MacPuf' model of human respiratory structures and
functions [1],[2]. However, apart from these two projects cited, very little has
been published. At present these models are used particularly in the field of
education and this is one of the major uses of the program described here for coping
with an emergency in the operating theatre.

It is possible for many potentially dangerous conditions to arise during an
operation, such as abnormal heart rhythms, hypotension or hypovolaemia and action
needs to be taken quickly to stabilise the patient. In an emergency situation like

this, the Anaesthetist, who is the person responsible for maintaining the physiological condition of the patient, will sometimes require experienced help, especially if still only a junior member of staff.

The program can run interactively on a microcomputer sited in the operating theatre. The program indicates the best course of action to be taken, according to the conditions prevailing, to stabilise the patient. The courses of action suggested are based on the experience of a group of consultants. Conversely, the program can be used in a teaching environment by the lecturer or even by an individual who would wish to test his own responses to a crisis situation in theatre.

The program runs on a Commodore Pet Microcomputer equipped with a floppy disk drive and a printer. This computer is easily available at many hospitals, takes up little space, and is relatively simple to use. The program is stored on a diskette and so is readily portable.

METHOD

The program is loaded into the computer at the beginning of the operation, either simulated or real, and basic details concerning the patient are requested. These include the name, sex, age, weight, height and clinical condition present on admission to theatre, allergies, temperature, blood pressure and blood sugar level of the patient. The blood pressure is checked to see if it is within the range of normality for the patient's age. The values for weight and height are used in the calculation of blood volume and body surface area if necessary. A clock is integrated into the program and the date and time on the twenty four hour clock are indicated at the start. The program then waits for help to be requested, if an emergency occurs.

Once the computer has been asked for help, an instruction is immediately given to increase the inspired oxygen, then a 'master' or 'control' program asks questions to assess the nature of the emergency. On the basis of the answers given, one of three subprograms is brought into operation, which asks further questions and indicates actions to be taken.

In addition to controlling the routes in and out of the subprograms, the master program also sets up a database containing current values of variables and details of drugs that can be administered. Some of the variable values will have been set pre-operatively, but others will not be assigned a value until the appropriate subprogram requests it. Any unknown variable is set to the value -1 in the database. Hence a subprogram that requires a value will check back to the database to see if -1 is present and if it is it will ask for a value to be entered. Every variable entry is paired with the time at which it was recorded.

Only certain values will change due to a change in status of the patient; a subprogram assesses which ones might have changed and asks for new values. Those values which will not have been altered by the change in status, are extracted from the database, if available.

With regard to the drugs recorded in the database, the number of times any one drug is given is counted. This is used in assessing whether or not a drug has been administered previously, with whatever that might imply, as, for example, in the case of atropine. A marker is placed against any drug that the patient is allergic to and that drug will not be used by the program.

The first question asked by the master program is whether or not the patient has suffered a cardiac arrest. If this is the case, then the cardiac arrest team are called and the cardiac arrest program is activated. Assuming no arrest has taken place, the next question to be asked is whether or not cyanosis is present. If it is, then control is passed to the cyanosis program. There are two main branches in this program; the first deals with peripheral cyanosis and the second with central cyanosis. The latter is by far the larger program.

Depending on the responses given, various courses of action will be suggested. With an intubated patient in deep cyanosis, action starts with checking the apparatus. When checking and adjusting has been carried out and the patient is still not stable, then treatment regimes are indicated. These include discontinuing anaesthetics, hyperventilating,or administering an intravenous infusion of dextrose and saline.

Activation of alternative subprograms is always via the master program, i.e. control is transferred back to the master program on leaving a subprogram.

When cyanosis is not present then any changes in heart rate, blood pressure central venous pressure and heart rhythms are investigated. In other words, help can be provided by the program when the patient is suffering from bradycardia, tachycardia or hypotension, Blood pressure, heart rate,and central venous pressure are all divided into low, normal,or high and heart rate as being in sinus rhythm, heart block state, or having ventricular ectopics more frequently than one ectopic every five beats. When the above values are entered for the patient, the program classifies them accordingly. There are 3^4 (i.e. 81) different combinations of categories of blood pressure, heart rate, central venous pressure and state of the heart, and, depending on the responses given, 1 out of the 81 subroutines is activated to provide advice. As with the cyanosis and cardiac arrest programs, control is switched back to the master program on leaving one of the 81 subroutines that make up this program. An example of the conditions prevailing and the actions indicated for nine of the subroutines is shown in Figure 1.

		HEART RATE		
		<60	60-120	>120
BLOOD PRESSURE	>110	**1** If H.R > 50 then observe If H.R. ≤ 50: Atropine Isoprenaline Pace	**4** Normal	**7** Go to Tachycardia subroutine
	70-110	**2** As 1 plus Dextrose 5% then Colloids	**5** Dextrose 5%) Colloids) slowly	**8** As 5 but fast
	<70	**3** As 1 plus Dextrose 5%) Colloids) fast	**6** Dextrose 5%) Colloids) quickly	**9** As 5 but very fast

FIGURE 1: ACTIONS INDICATED BY THE SUBROUTINE FOR VARYING BLOOD PRESSURE AND HEART RATE AT LOW CENTRAL VENOUS PRESSURE (<+5) WITH THE HEART IN SINUS RHYTHM

A record is kept of the events occuring during the operation and at the end of the operation this can be output onto printer paper.

```
DATE: 20/06/81
TIME: 02.20

PLEASE ENTER THE FOLLOWING DETAILS PREOPERATIVELY:-

NAME OF PATIENT? [A.N. OTHER]
HOSPITAL NUMBER? [81/96231]
SEX? [MALE]
AGE(YRS)? [46]
WEIGHT (KG)? [75]
HEIGHT (CM)? [173]
CLINICAL CONDITION? [PERITONITIS]
PLANNED OPERATION? [REPAIR OF PERFORATED DUODENAL ULCER]
ARE THERE ANY KNOWN ALLERGIES E.G. HALOTHANE (Y/N)? [N]
TEMPERATURE? [37.5]
BLOOD PRESSURE (S/D)? [140/100]
SODIUM (MMOL/L)? [132]
POTASSIUM (MMOL/L)? [3.9]
BLOOD SUGAR (MMOL/L)? [10.2]

HAVE YOU DONE THE ONE HOSE TEST (Y/N)? [N]
I WILL WAIT WHILE YOU DO IT

WHEN YOU HAVE DONE IT PRESS ANY KEY

    [PRESS]

IF AND WHEN HELP IS REQUIRED PRESS ANY KEY

    [PRESS]

INCREASE INSPIRED OXYGEN THEN PROCEED AS DIRECTED
```

FIGURE 2: PRE-OPERATIVE BASIC INFORMATION

RESULTS

Computer output from the log-in and from two main sections of the program are shown in figures 2, 3 and 4. The patient parameters are those which send the computer to that particular routine. The dialogue itself is easily understood.

```
CARDIAC ARREST PROCEDURE
 ABSENT MAJOR PULSE (CAROTID OR FEMORAL)

 DISCONTINUE ANAESTHETIC AND SURGERY
 CLEAR AIRWAY
 HAND VENTILATE WITH 100% OXYGEN

 INITIAL SHARP BLOW TO STERNUM MAY RESTART HEART

 START EXTERNAL CARDIAC MASSAGE:-
     HEELS OF HAND OVER LOWER PART OF STERNUM
     DEPRESS 4-5 CM AT RATE 1/SEC, 4 TO EACH BREATH
     AVOID FRACTURING RIBS

 INTUBATE TRACHEA IF NOT ALREADY DONE

 WHEN YOU ARE READY FOR FURTHER INSTRUCTIONS PRESS ANY KEY

     [ PRESS ]

 ASSESS ADEQUACY OF CIRCULATION BY:-
     1)COLOUR OF LIPS/TONGUE
     2)PREVIOUSLY DILATING PUPILS NOW CONSTRICTING
     3)PALPATION OF MAJOR PULSE (CAROTID OR FEMORAL)

 WHEN CIRCULATION HAS BEEN ASSESSED PRESS ANY KEY

     [ PRESS ]

 CONNECT ECG MACHINE

 CANNULATE VEIN-PREFERABLY CENTRAL VEIN,EXTERNAL
 OR INTERNAL JUGULAR IS USUALLY VISIBLE

 START INFUSION OF 100 MLS SODIUM BICARBONATE 8.4%
     TO RUN OVER 10-15 MINS UNLESS PERIOD
     OF ARREST LESS THAN 5 MINS

 SEND FOR MOST EXPERIENCED IMMEDIATELY AVAILABLE HELP
 ==================================================

 TO CONTINUE PRESS ANY KEY

     [ PRESS ]

 WHICH OF THE FOLLOWING APPLY:-
     1)ANAPHYLACTOID REACTION
             -FLUSHED SKIN BECOMING CYANOSED
             -BRONCHOSPASM
             -ECG SHOWS TACHYCARDIA
     2)ASYSTOLE
     3)VENTRICULAR FIBRILLATION
     4)PROBABLE HYPOXAEMIA

 ANSWER 1,2,3,OR 4? [2]
 ASYSTOLE
 GIVE 1)0.5 TO 10 MLS OF 1 IN 10,000 ADRENALIN
         SLOWLY I.V.
      2)10 MLS OF CACL2 10% I.V.
         (NOT WITH BICARBONATE)

 RESPONSE:-1)ASYSTOLE CONTINUES
           2)VENTRICULAR FIBRILLATION
           3)CARDIAC RHYTHM WITH PALPABLE PULSE
           4)CARDIAC RHYTHM WITH NO PALPABLE PULSE
```

677

YOU WILL NOW RECEIVE INSTRUCTIONS ON HOW TO DEAL WITH CYANOSIS

IS THE CYANOSIS CENTRAL (Y/N)? `Y`

  1)CHECK LEVEL OF INSPIRED OXYGEN
  2)CHECK MECHANICS OF VENTILATOR

IS THE PATIENT INTUBATED (Y/N)? `Y`

CHECK THAT THE ET TUBE IS IN THE TRACHEA

  I WILL GIVE YOU A MOMENT TO DO THAT

IS THE CYANOSIS DEEP (Y/N)? `Y`

HAND VENTILATE WITH 100% OXYGEN

  I WILL GIVE YOU A MOMENT TO DO THAT

IS THE VENTILATION PRESSURE HIGH, NORMAL OR LOW (H,N,L)? `N`

WHAT IS THE PATIENT'S PULSE RATE? `120`

WHAT IS THE BLOOD PRESSURE(SYS)? `100`

WHAT IS THE PATIENT'S TEMPERATURE? `37.5`

POSSIBLE DIAGNOSES:-
    A)POSSIBLE PULMONARY EMBOLUS
    B)LOBAR COLLAPSE POSSIBLY DUE TO FOREIGN BODY OR MUCUS
    C)LEFT VENTRICULAR FAILURE
    D)RIGHT TO LEFT SHUNT

SEND ARTERIAL BLOOD SAMPLE FOR PO2

TAKE CHEST X-RAY

IF PO2 IS NORMAL DIAGNOSIS:-METHAEMOGLOBINAEMIA

DO YOU REQUIRE TREATMENT FOR A,B,C OR D ABOVE?
ANSWER A,B,C,D OR N? B

ENSURE ADEQUATE OXYGENATION
BRONCHOSCOPY, IF ANY OBSTRUCTION IN MAIN BRONCHI
BAGGING AND SUCKING AND POST-OPERATIVE PHYSIOTHERAPY

                    FIGURE 4: CYANOSIS PROGRAM

```
ANSWER 1,2,3,OR 4? [1]

REPEAT 10 MLS 1 IN 10,000 ADRENALIN INTRACARDIAC INJECTION
       INTO THE 4TH INTERCOSTAL SPACE CLOSE TO THE STERNUM
       10 MLS OF CACL2 10% I.V. (NOT WITH BICARBONATE)

RESPONSE:- 1)ASYSTOLE CONTINUES
           2)VENTRICULAR FIBRILLATION
           3)CARDIAC RHYTHM WITH PALPABLE PULSE
           4)CARDIAC RHYTHM WITH NO PALPABLE PULSE

ANSWER 1,2,3,OR 4? [3]

WHAT IS THE BLOOD PRESSURE? [80]

WHAT IS THE QRS RATE? [88]

SEND BLOOD FOR-ARTERIAL BLOOD GAS ESTIMATION
              -SERUM K
              -HAEMATOCRIT

GIVE METHYLPREDNISOLONE 2GM I.V.

WHEN READY FOR FURTHER INSTRUCTIONS PRESS ANY KEY
```

FIGURE 3: CARDIAC ARREST PROGRAM

DISCUSSION

The fact that the program is written for use on a microcomputer and can be easily stored on a floppy diskette makes it suitable for use in many other teaching institutions and hospitals.

The program is ideally suited to use as an educational tool in the teaching of anaesthetists and indeed others in the medical field. It is possible to simulate a very wide variety of emergency situations and responses to treatment, the scope of which would not generally be encountered during operations until after many years as an anaesthetist. The student is able to learn without the pressure of a real life and death situation on their hands. The program can also be used in the operating theatre and experience has shown that the use of the computer in the theatre enables a more accurate and systematic approach to the treatment of the patient than does the reliance on the unaided human [3].

REFERENCES

1.   Dickinson, C.J. "A Computer Model of Human Respiration", Medical and
     Technical Press, Lancaster, 1977

2.   Kelman, G.R. "A new lung model: An investigation with the aid of a digital
     computer". Comput. Biomed. Res. $\underline{3}$, 241 - 248. (1970)

3.   Richards, B. et al. "Control of open heart surgery with a stand-alone
     microcomputer" Medinfo 80, North-Holland Publishing Co. Amsterdam (1980)

THE EDUCATION OF DOCUMENTALISTS AT THE ADVANCED
SPECIALIZED COLLEGE LEVEL

An Example of New Educational Concepts in Medical Informatics

by O.Rienhoff, W.-D.Hoffmann, K.-W.Hartmann and J.Klonk

Medical School Hannover, Institute of Medical Informatics
(Director: Prof. Dr. P.L.Reichertz)

1. INTRODUCTION

A model curriculum for documentalists in the biosciences has been established at the advanced specialized college level in Hannover, Germany (1). Being the result of a three years' federal research investigation teaching objectives, methods and equipment have been directed
towards a methodologically oriented approach. For occupational flexibility the scope has been broadened from medicine to bioscience.

The concept has been discussed at MEDINFO '80 in Tokyo on an international basis and was found to be in accordance with e.g. the extensive
work of the van Bemmel Group in Belgium (2,3).

The duration of the education was set to 7 semesters or 3.5 years. As
the college education is supposed to be close to the actual work, 9
months of training courses have been integrated into the approach as
well as the design and evaluation of a project during the last three
semesters. Altogether more than 2000 hours of theoretical education
will be given for eventually 240 students.

2. SPECIAL DETAILS OF THE CURRICULUM

2.1 Special Courses

During the first two semesters all basic knowledge is taught to the
students. They share most of their courses with student-librarians.
Main themes of education are literature-documentation, bibliography,
data-documentation, and informatics.

After one year the students leave college to work for six months in
three different institutions to get a first impression of the everyday

life within their profession. After one further semester of more specialized training the students leave their college for another three
months for practical training, this time in a library.

The last two semesters are devoted to rather complicated themes within
medical documentation and the students are systematically trained how
to run documentation projects - and, how to 'handle' scientists (4).
A final report written about their 'personal' project and a final examination are the last steps in their education.

Through all these semesters special courses are given to the documentalists to basically educate them in biology and medicine (Fig.1).

```
--------------------------------------------------------------------

 Number   Titel                                          Teaching Hours

  6.3     Analytical Statistics                               51

  8.3     Institutions in the field of Biology-Documentation  17

 16.1     Medical Terminology, Basic Biology                  51

 16.2     Aims, Methods and Institutions in Medicine          34

 16.3     Cytology, Histology, Morphology, Embryology         85

 16.4     Physiology                                          68

 16.5     Biochemistry                                        51

 16.6     Human Pathology                                     51

 16.7     Data Bases in Biology                               34

 17.0     Specialized Documentations in Biology and Medicine  85

--------------------------------------------------------------------
```

Fig.1: List of all special courses in which basic biological and medi-
       cal themes are taught.

2.2 The 'Bio-Lab'

A laboratory has been installed (besides several other workshops for practical training), where the students have the possibility to perform several basic physiological experiments and use microscopes within the courses of morphology. This lab was introduced into the media-concept of the curriculum to enable the students during their training to get a personal touch of practical difficulties within everyday work in biology and thus make them better understand the problems of the later users of their information systems.

Literature:

(1) Bock G, Hoffman WD, Hueper R, Klonk J, Raters E, Reichertz PL, Rienhoff O (ed.). Studienrichtung 'Biowissenschaftliche Dokumentation' an der Fachhochschule Hannover. Schriftenreihe der GMDS 3. Stuttgart-New York, Schattauer Verlag, 1980.

(2) Rienhoff O. From Medicine to Bioscience - A Modified Concept for the Education of Documentation Clerks. in: Lindberg DAB, Kaihara S (eds.). MEDINFO '80. North Holland, Amsterdam, New York, Oxford, 1980; 349-352.

(3) Rienhoff O. A Curriculum for Short-term-training in Medical Documentation for Developing Countries. (in print) presented at the Symp. International de Informatica Medica, Mexico City, 20.8.81.

(4) Rienhoff O, Reichertz PL. The Communicational Structure of Medical Information Systems and its Educational Consequences. in: Andersson J. Medical Informatics Europe 78. Berlin-Heidelberg-New York, Springer-Verlag, 1978; 315-327.

Acknowledgement:

This study is supported by the Federal Ministry of Education and Science.
The Curriculum is implemented at the Fachhochschule Hannover, Fachbereich Bibliothekswesen, Information und Dokumentation, Hanomagstrasse, 3000 Hannover, West Germany.

POSTGRADUATE EDUCATION OF 'NON-PHYSICIANS' TO SPECIALISTS IN MEDICINE IN THE FIELD OF MEDICAL INFORMATICS - A NOVEL SYSTEMIC APPROACH TO AN OLDER PROBLEM -

Joachim Elsner and Dieter Schreiter
Medizinische Akademie "Carl Gustav Carus" Dresden,
Organisations - und Rechenzentrum
GDR - 8019 Dresden, Fetscherstr. 74.

Modern medicine as an applied science cannot do without the utilization of the methods and results of the natural sciences, technical sciences, psychology, sociology and last but not least of mathematics and informatics. Bearing this in mind, every opportunity should be taken to highlight the role which specialists in these areas play in the joint effort with the physicians and medical scientists in patient care and medical research and also in training and education. An increasing number of these paramedical scientists are occupied in medical facilities. Together with the essential continuing education in their own original discipline there is an additional requirement for them to gain a deeper insight into the nature of medical science, its features, methodology, structure, etc., and to obtain a better and more comprehensive understanding of the manyfold activities in the health service and health care delivery. Moreover, comprehensive specialized knowledge and experience have to be acquired in the very field of their daily work which is often on the medical 'borderlines'. Some efforts have been made and some solutions have been found in several countries as how best to tackle these problems. These efforts were concerned mostly with one of the abovementioned paramedical specialities. More-over, they were uncoordinated in respect to duration, mode, contents, etc. of the postgraduate education.

Recently, by the Ministry of Health, GDR, a novel systemic solution for this actual problem was proposed and a relevant law enacted. For eighteen medical/paramedical fields a postgraduate specialist education is now possible. These fields cover nearly all potential modes of engagement of 'non-physicians' in medicine, for example, biochemistry, clinical chemistry, biophysics, biomedical engineering, physiology, genetics, immunology, clinical psychology, cytology/histology, toxic-ologic chemistry, radiation physics, physiology, microbiology, hygiene, medical sociology and some other ones and last not least biomathematics and medical informatics. The good experiences gathered from the obligatory five years' postgraduate training necessary for all medical graduates in the GDR to become a specialist in medicine, formed the model for the training in these fields. Thus, the final goal and underlying philosophy of this novel systemic approach is to achieve an optimum increase in quality of patient care and research work by an advanced training, excellent cooperation with physicians and, in certain respects, equality of the status within the medical community. But it must be emphasized that these paramedical scientists never become any kind of a physician, of course have no right to treat patients a. s. o. A general prerequisite for the admission to the postgraduate education is a one year's full-time occupation in a discipline of the health science. The specialist's training then takes no less than four, but no longer than five years with an examination. A diploma will be obtained by which the student is certified as a specialist in medicine for his original discipline, for example, "specialized chemist of medicine". The postgraduate education comprises self-instruction modules, on-the-job training, lectures, supervised practicals. The curriculum in medical informatics is generally designed for medical informatics and biomathematics, but with a subspecializing for either field owing to the typical characteristics and diverse applications of each of them. Common for both specialities are the basic education in the health sciences and some other basic items of mathematics-biostatistics and informatics. The curriculum has been worked out by a board set up by the Ministry of Health comprising biomathematicians, medical informaticians, physicians.

Provisional regulations are provided for those graduates in the abovementioned fields who have been successfully occupied in a health care facility or an institute for more than ten years.

The curriculum for the education in medical informatics a. o. covers nearly all known fields of computer application to medicine. During the postgraduate education a project and dissertation is carried out. The computer centre of the Medical School of Dresden, existing for about thirteen years, is designated as the GDR centre for post-graduate education in medical informatics. It is assumed that through this state-run coordination a rapid and considerable progress will be achieved in medical care, research, and, finally, in the further development of our discipline 'medical informatics'.

FINDING SOURCES FOR RESOURCES.

Genevieve M. Hibbs,
West London Institute of Higher Education,
300 St. Margarets Road, TWICKENHAM TW1 1PT.

ABSTRACT.

The need for sources of information for management, administration and occupational health practice is demonstrated along with users requirements.

Manual methods used included a pamphlet file and thesaurus, rotary address and equipment files, a register of articles and a bibliography. Microfilming had limited value. The need for automation by inability to maintain the information using typing service available and using the Twinlock strip system is mentioned.

The process of automation is described using Wordstar, Datastar, Mailmerge and Supersort software packages.

The way books, journals and other sources are found, used and checked is indicated. Information, thesaurus, microfilming, autoation, bibliography software packages.

PRIVACY, DATA DECAY AND THE LONG TERM MEDICAL RECORD

A. L. Rector and M. G. Sheldon
Department of Community Health
University of Nottingham Medical School
Nottingham   NG7 2UH
England

SUMMARY

The medical significance of certain information in the medical record declines
much more rapidly than does its potential to do harm. The protocols for
accessing to and transfer of information in an automated information system
should therefore be governed in part by the time since it was collected. In
setting up these protocols, the potential value of the information should always
be weighed against the harm it might do.

INTRODUCTION

The arrival of practical computer-based medical record systems means that the time
is approaching when the life-time medical record can become a reality rather than
a pious hope. Do we really want it? What are the implications to patients'
privacy of a dossier covering most of their lives? What safeguards need to be
built into such a system?

The time is long since past when the medical profession can claim that its records
are purely private; the medical care system has simply grown too large. Many
people have a legitimate need for access to clinical notes, especially to
hospital records, and there is therefore a limit to the degree of security which
can be provided practically. The degree of protection which can be afforded
varies with the institution, and we must therefore establish standards for the
transfer of information both between institutions within the health service and
between the health service and outside institutions. It is important that old,
possibly inaccurate, potentially damaging information not be allowed to circulate
even within the health service itself.

In manual systems information is transferred primarily via **referral** and **discharge** summaries. Information is only transferred if explicitly included by the doctor. The default condition is that information is <u>omitted</u>.

The default condition is quite different if medical information is to be transferred between institutions automatically as has been widely advocated[1]. Much information will be transferred unless explicitly deleted by the doctor or subject to special conditions. The default condition will be <u>included</u>. This is equally true whether the transfer is by computer printed summaries used as part of referral letters or by totally electronic means.

It must be seriously questioned whether it is reasonable to expect the hard pressed and busy doctor to expend much effort on the vigilance required to ensure that no potentially sensitive or out-dated information is transferred. Maintaining the confidentiality of computer held medical records therefore requires a more formal approach than in the case of manual records[2]. Besides overall security precautions, this should take several forms:

a)   Discipline in what data is entered on the system;

b)   Controls on who has access to information on the system;

c)   Controls on the transfer of information;

d)   Special provisions for the protection or deletion of information held for long periods of time.

Data protection legislation and practices are now being formulated in most western countries. The next few years are crucial for setting standards for how data will be handled in an electronic age[3]. Current medical practice is based on experience with manual records whose very shortcomings of illegibility and liability to loss provided some protection. The problem of engineering the decay of data has not arisen because it has occurred naturally. These practices must be carefully examined in the light of a society in which information is much more likely to be harmful than previously and in which the medical record could be made permanently available and retrievable.

DATA DECAY AND PRIVACY

In the UK a person convicted of a minor criminal offence may be 'rehabilitated' after three years and the record virtually expunged. Psychiatric patients and others with potentially damaging information on their medical record enjoy no such right. The information in most manual record systems is protected to some extent by their sheer bulk and illegibility. Computer based records designed specifically to make information more accessible have no such 'safeguards'.

The medical significance of much information wanes with time, but its sensitivity does not[4]. Details of most past episodes of illness are of little consequence once that episode is past. Even the occurrence of isolated self-limiting illnesses are of little significance once the episode is past. Rarely are the details of such importance that the essential information can not be gained from the patient.

Furthermore, determining the meaning of 'soft' medical data many years after the event may be virtually impossible. How is a doctor to evaluate a diagnosis of 'personality disorder' or 'anxiety neurosis' written by an unknown general practitioner fifteen years previously? Even a diagnosis such as 'borderline hypertension' may be difficult to evaluate without specific knowledge concerning the events in the patient's life and the criteria in force at the time.

These statements may have been important at the time they were made, but their value many years later is dubious. Their potential to harm the patient however, decreases more slowly.

Although it is always possible to construct a hypothetical case to argue for the retention or transfer of any item of data, the potential value of having the data on record must be weighed against the potential harm which it might do. An unconfirmed (and perhaps erroneous) diagnosis of hypertension made at some time in the past might well cost a patient the opportunity of a job if it were accepted as 'fact' because it was entered on a computer system. Psychiatric diagnoses can be particularly harmful and are particularly difficult to verify. (See for example, the case of the 'man from the Pru', Times, 17th March, 1978).

The harm may also be medical. Research has shown that doctors tend to form hypotheses early in their interviews and to seek information which would tend to confirm them[5]. Diagnostic errors are often made because only one line of attack was followed up thoroughly. Information concerning a previous 'diagnosis' may serve only to obscure the current illness. This problem is confirmed by much anecdotal information - consultants who want to approach the case afresh without prior information. Is a patient who presents with a bowel complaint more or less likely to have a correct diagnosis of cancer of the colon made if there is a diagnosis of 'functional bowel disease' appears on the record from many years previously?

Outdated information can also lead to more subtle medical problems. One patient has written to the author to describe how her dealings with the hospital out-patient department are affected by the record of a brief period of psychiatric care. Informal discussions with both patients and staff suggest that this is not an isolated instance. It is one of the curious side effects of more and more psychiatric in-patient stays being in general hospitals, that the existence of a psychiatric admission is often more evident than was formerly the case.

IMPLICATIONS FOR THE DESIGN OF SYSTEMS

The sensitivity of certain medical data decays much more slowly than its significance. If the access controls built into systems do not reflect this fact, then systems will either release too little information to be useful, or too much to be acceptable.

The details of the methods used will vary from system to system to system, but certain basic requirements can be identified:

The information must be coded so that it can be interpreted by the system. Free text data which is not closely linked to coded information is extremely difficult to control adequately;

The system must contain a strong model of time;

It must be possible to specify the accessibility of information according to complex criteria including time based primitives.

Although these requirements impose some overheads, the first two are generally desirable for other reasons in complex medical information systems. The third implies a more elaborate system of access controls than are generally used. However, if the access controls are integrated into the general information display system, the overheads need not be unacceptable.

The authors have proposed a data model for their work (Rector, 1981) which allows such criteria to be included in the data dictionary scheme. Rules may set up to alter the accessibility of information according to the time since it was collected, the use to which it is to be put, or other information currently available in the data base. Such a system has the potential to improve current practice significantly since information can be made available highly selectively - for instance, an old obstetric history made available if the problem were gynaecological rather than surgical. Furthermore, it has the advantage of allowing the system to present a well edited, pertinent record which does not inundate the doctor in irrelevant detail.

Although the details of this scheme are not appropriate in all environments, some such mechanism is essential if we are to be able to satisfy the public and the medical profession that our systems are safe and valuable.

REFERENCES

1. CLARKE, D.J., FISHER, R.H., AND LING, G. (1979) Computer held patient records: the Exeter Project. Inf. Privacy, 1. (4) March.

2. ZIMMERMAN, J. & RECTOR, A.L. (1978) Computers for the physician's office. J. Wiley and Sons, New York.

3. LINDOP, SIR N. (1978) Report of the Committee on Data Protection HMSO.

4. RECTOR, A.L. Data Decay, Significance and Confidentiality: a time orientated data model for comprehensive care. Medical Informatics. 6 : 3 pp 187-193.

5. ELSTEIN, A.S., SCHCELMAN, L.S., SPRATKA, S.A. (1978) Medical Problem Solving: An Analysis of Medical Reasoning. Cambridge Moss. Harvard University Press.

MEDICAL COMPUTING AND INDUSTRIAL RELATIONS.

D. White, Department of Health and Social Security, London, S.E.I.

Summary

This paper considers the growing dependence on computing of the delivery of health care, assesses the likely effects of industrial action by computing staff and discusses ways of arresting that action and minimising its effects.

Background 1. Unionisation

1. The National Health Service (NHS) of the UK is a highly monolithic organisation. Although divided into regions, each with considerable autonomy, its health care policies and priorities are centrally directed, resources centrally allocated and its health care delivery systems are highly standardised. Similar tendencies to standardisation can be found in many countries' health services, particularly (in Europe) in the Scandinavian countries.

2. The larger the scale of any organisation, whether state, industrial or commercial, the more it is obliged to develop formalised systems of categorising, grading and rewarding staff. And in the latter half of this century health services have experienced a rapid growth in the unionisation of staff. In the NHS all staff (even hospital doctors) are organised into an elaborate system of occupational classes, each with its internal hierarchy of job titles and grades and its own scales of pay and conditions of service including systems of annual incremental salary progression, rules for promotion, annual holidays increasing with length of service and systems of financial allowances reflecting the demands of particular occupations. An estimated 70% of more than 1 million NHS employees are members of trade unions or staff/professional associations of some kind. Unsurprisingly the primary aim of these organisations is constantly to maximise these rewards. And the greater the number and variety of the rewards, the larger are the number of pressure-points at which unions can seek to compel management to make improvements. The ability of these staff associations and unions to exert pressure on management by impeding or halting patient care, whether directly (eg by halting ambulance services) or indirectly (eg by preventing the payment of commercial suppliers of goods), is great.

Background - 2. Computing

3. A very wide variety of computing equipment is used in the NHS, from large multi-access to microcomputers, and of systems, from administrative to clinical. A special effort has been put into attempts to standardise equipment and systems. The regional headquarters (14 in England and 1 in Wales) have roughly the same configuration of computer, supplied by the same manufacturer. The main systems are standardised. Consequently the NHS now has standard pay roll and accounting systems and many other standard computer-based procedures, including a child health registration and immunisation system, and a manpower planning and personnel information system.

"Model" or "transferable" medical and patient-orientated systems are less common, but similar systems exist for pathology, radio-therapy planning, patient administration and nursing.

4.   Computer-based procedures can be divided into those with direct consequences for patient care (eg radiotherapy treatment, ECG analysis, clinical decision-making, intensive care monitoring, kidney-matching and other transplant procedures, blood transfusion systems, vaccination and immunisation call-up, cancer registration and follow-up); those with direct consequences for patient services (eg menu planning, pathology systems, nurse scheduling, in-patient and out-patient administration); and those with no immediate consequences for care or services (eg payroll and accounting, manpower and other statistics, stock control).

5.   Computing staff Other than data-preparation staff, who are mainly locally-recruited, young school-leavers, most NHS computing staff are professionals ie computing rather than health services is their intended career. A few health professionals, notably doctors, nurses and pathologists, have added computing competence to their health qualifications; and some career administrators have either moved into computing or spent a spell of their careers closely associated with computing developments - often administrative staff who have worked in other parts of management services.

6.   Thus, although some computing staff, mainly at the directing and development level, have become fully integrated with other members of multi-professional health care teams, for many system designers, programmers and operators the NHS tends to be primarily an opportunity to widen their experience in an area of work that - so far as true "medical" computing is concerned - is unique, innovatory, and varied. Their commitment is generally more to computing per se than to health services or patient care (from which they are in any case often remote). That is not to say that they are indifferent to the social service element in many medical computing applications: rather that when they accept, as they often must, some of the "kicks" of a state-financed service, they do so because of the compensating advantages to their computing careers, not from dedication to a public, social service. This is not a criticism but a fact relevant to industrial relations.

7.   Their relations with other health service staff are usually good, if a trifle distant. Many staff still regard computing as a discrete, esoteric profession and its practitioners as technologists with only a marginal commitment to patient care, sometimes a potential threat to their own work and security; notably clerical staff in patient administration, filing and retrieving medical records, making appointments, pay salaries and keeping accounts, and so on. There is rarely any explicit antag-onism, but the lack of empathy is yet another relevant factor in industrial relations.

8.   NHS computing salaries are rarely competitive with comparable market rates in the industrial/commercial sector, particularly as seen by staff, who seldom quantify such intangibles as job security and conditions of service. Health computing staff, are a very small percentage (probably about 2%) of the UK computing workforce; and the

computing press regularly shows them that - except during severe recessions - in the outside world salaries are higher, there are many jobs available and promotion by frequent movement from job to job is usually faster than in the public services.

9. Forms of industrial action Industrial action by computing staff can vary greatly. In terms of withdrawal of services, the available action is not different from that available to other staff, ranging from a refusal to work overtime, an insistence on "working to rule", token strikes of an hour or a day or whatever, to a complete and indefinite strike. Additionally the complexity of computing systems and procedures offers computing staff the chance of more subtle impediments. Programs for the payment of bills or fees can be halted at the point at which a schedule of payments or perhaps a run of cheques would otherwise appear. Patient administration programs can be arranged to make appointments but fail to retrieve relevant medical records. Stock control programs may be manipulated to continue to itemise scarce items but not print out reordering details. System design work may suddenly encounter problems that delay programming to a point at which new equipment is lying idle. The distinction between the avoidable and the unavoidable in such circumstances is - if undeclared - hard to prove, Consequently industrial action by computing staff is not always readily detected, and both appropriate remedial action and appropriate penalties - which may be easy to apply and are often prescribed by agreed rules, when the action taken is the withdrawal of services - are hard to determine.

10. Likelihood of industrial action Some reasons why staff in public services may take industrial action were outlined in paragraph 8: slow promotion; slow salary increases and low salaries compared with industry and commerce. Other motives are more complex. One example is frustration at the apparent inadequacy of public funding of health services; and as a sub-category, frustration at the apparently low priority given to medical computing facilities, particularly when they fluctuate frequently and the same variability is communicated to the priority of, and resources for, computing. Computing developments need a steady and assured input of money and skills for long periods - but are often seen by management as an activity from which at times of financial stringency savings can easily be made by deferring capital expenditure or, more modestly, failing to recruit staff.

11. Another problem is the inhibiting effect of standardisation of computing systems. System designers in particular get most of their intellectual and job satisfaction from the development of new and preferably complex computing processes. Developing a standard system offers wide scope for innovation but its introduction into a different environment, with major constraints on its adaptation to the new situation, provides much less of a challenge. Enthusiastic and talented system engineers do not take kindly to installing systems invented elsewhere.

12. However, senior computing staff are a high-IQ group, highly involved in and stimulated by their work; and in the NHS they have so far had little resort to industrial action. High-IQ groups are of course not necessarily less prone to taking industrial action; but computing staff are often an isolated, almost monastic group and,

if unionised at all, likely to be members of professional associations. Their prone-
ness to industrial action is more influenced than that of many other workers by the
strength and attitude of local union organisers, and by the attitudes and aspirations
of local management. But in centrally-directed and nationally-organised health services, as in the UK, they are nonetheless sensitive to the conflicts inevitable in
national negotiations of pay and conditions of service.

13. <u>Effects of industrial action</u> Paragraph 4 above categorised the effects of industrial action by health service computing staff. The effects of an interruption or
withdrawal of computing services from any given application may be inferred from the
category into which it falls. Some examples follow.

14. <u>Patient care applications</u> A radiotherapy department dependent on a computer and
computer staff (as opposed to a small computer operated by scientific or clinical staff)
for its treatment programme will need to stop treatments: the substitution of cruder
manual methods of calculation and treatment planning will take a long time to achieve.
On the other hand an intensive care unit using an on-line computer link to aid patient monitoring will not have left itself defenceless against the more likely computer
failure, and readily-available substitute manual methods will maintain an adequate
level of care. A kidney-matching unit, if dependent on computer staff at all, will
usually have standby computing facilities eg in a nearby commercial or industrial
installation. Computer-based patient record retrieval at ward locations can rarely
be substituted at short notice: clinical decisions and treatments may be impeded but
will not be impossible. Systems for the call-up and vaccination and immunisation of
children will, if suspended by industrial action, defer those treatments; but they
are rarely time-critical.

15. <u>Patient service applications</u> Failure of computer-based menu planning will obviously not stop meals being prepared and served - dissatisfaction but not starvation
of patients is the likely effect, with some immediate dislocation of catering services, including re-ordering procedures; but manual methods will be rapidly resumed
by experienced catering managers. Pathology laboratory instrumentation is nowadays
rarely dependent on extramural computing facilities and staff, but where it is blood-
testing will be halted with little chance of substitution by manual methods. Communication of results to wards is more likely to be impeded but is readily substituted
since simultaneous laboratory print-outs of results and the transmission to wards is
the norm. Nurse scheduling by computer is an efficient method of allocating nurse
learners for their training programmes and its failure would cause inconvenience to
nurses at all levels and might affect individual treatment programmes. And reversion
to manual methods is disruptive, complicated and costly. Computer-based out-patient
organisation, which normally includes registration, making appointments, patient
scheduling and routing, and discharge procedures, will be impeded by the sudden
withdrawal of computer services: patient treatments will be deferred, waiting lists
will grow and only the availability of emergency admission procedures may prevent

serious risk to the health of at least a minority of out-patients. In many respects failure of in-patient organisation systems is less serious, since the organisation of the care of already-admitted patients can be diverted to manual procedures with only inconvenience and delay, while emergency admissions can substitute for planned waiting-list admissions in acute cases.

16. Financial and administrative applications The withdrawal of a computer-based payroll system is the most serious immediate threat to be faced: the usual standby method for the payment of wages is to pay staff by cheque or other instrument using a convenient past payment or average of payments as the benchmark sum and failure to provide such substitutes will obviously lead to withdrawal of the services of most unpaid staff. Substitute manual methods of accounting and audit are needed to back up manual payments. Impedance of computer-based payment of suppliers of goods - especially those needed daily, such as food - will have medium-term but disastrous effects on services (as suppliers refuse to extend credit) unless substitute payment methods are quickly found.

17. These examples illustrate the potential damage to patient care and services that withdrawal of computing facilities may cause. Where they have not been used as weapons of industrial dispute - and, so far, in the UK NHS they have not - despite the pursuit of industrial action by other measures, it may be because the sense of responsibility of the unions concerned has led them to draw back from actions clearly likely to have effects on patients. But it would be unwise to assume that that will always be the case. So what shall we do to be saved? Two answers are: avoidance and remedy.

18. Avoidance of industrial action The counsel of perfection is of course impeccably good industrial relations. But perfection is out of the reach of most organisations - and particularly of publicly-financed health services. However, an important element of good industrial relations is the consultative machinery. Particularly where unions are strong, the machinery of joint management-staff consultation is easy to establish; but both sides must know how to use it. Joint consultation is most effective at local levels, where it may avert conflict by its availability for discussion of problems at an early stage. At national levels it is too cumbersome to be rapidly available; and in any case problems that have reached, or originate at, national levels are often fundamental, long-standing or already subjects of intransigeance and attitude-striking.

19. However, national consultative machinery is not to be despised or ignored: better to improve it. One improvement might be the participation of some disinterested third party in all national and local consultative machinery. At the least a neutral presence may enhance the collective bargaining and consultative processes by taking some heat and unreasonable argument out of the discussion: at best a neutral may have constructive and acceptable solutions to offer.

20. But to consider the role of neutrals in any disputes is to imply that disputes are inevitable. They may be; but aids to their avoidance are available. One is to

reduce the isolation of computer staff by integrating them into wider staff groupings. With the advent of mini-computers, desk computers and now microcomputers computing has become less esoteric and remote a specialism. In health care many applications directly affecting patient services have two features in common: they use patient data and they involve rapid, frequent communication of those data. The staff involved include many clerical staff operating medical record, in-patient and out-patient systems, statisticians and operational research staff, management services staff. All may be subsumed within a generalised discipline: information-processing. And computer staff and facilities are the kernel of the services they provide and so are part of the same organisational unit. Making this explicit, by organisation charts and job titles, and by common management at middle-management levels, would be one move towards integration of computing staff into a wider hospital occupational group, and to common pay, gradings and conditions of service for that group. That in turn could give "professional" computing staff a greater sense of commitment to patient care and to health services as a career but it would also mean that a dispute concerning one specialism in the group might involve the whole group in industrial action.

21. Other conventional methods - such as "no-strike" agreements - of averting the disruption of patient services are not specific to computer staff, and indeed they often depend on the acquiescence of all staff. Expositions of the philosophy and practice of such wider agreements can be found in industrial relations literature.

22. Some organisational and technological measures can help to minimise the effects of industrial action by computing staff. One prospect is to maximise the use of the growing micro-technology. Thanks to this development a growing range of medical equipment has an integral micro-processing facility requiring no external intervention by computing staff. Advanced desk computing facilities - particularly programmable terminals - may change the character of multi-access hospital computing. Their growing 'intelligence', and their versatility suggest there will supplant terminals demanding control by a master computer and with virtually no self-programming facility. Before long systems of mutually linked desk computers, operated and perhaps even programmed by non-computing staff as part of their normal work, may displace the older form of multi-access computing for at least administrative and finance work, including, in hospitals, patient administration procedures.

23. Another way of avoiding industrial action by health service computing staff would be to use commercial health care computing systems provided to hospitals on an agency basis. Private sector computing companies offer advantages to publicly-financed health services but, as substitutes for in-house computing facilities, they also have disadvantages. They suffer their own industrial action; they go bankrupt at short notice; they are less sensitive than in-house staff to a hospital's needs; they find it harder to get on good working terms with the hospital's own staff and occasionally their contributions may be "blacked" by other staff; and they are usually more costly.

24. The other extreme would be to seek to employ no 'professional' computing staff at all but to train and use other health professionals - administrators, scientists, finance staff - for part of their careers in the development of hospital systems. They have the right relationship with other hospital staff and a commitment both to patient care and to health services as a career. An objection is that computer system design and development has grown rapidly in complexity and consequently training to the necessary degree of competence for the development of efficient systems is long and costly. It is unlikely that that expenditure of time and resources would be recouped in terms of effective computing systems in less than five years; and health service staff originating in other professions and occupations might well feel that so long a period out of their chosen profession was unacceptable. Finally, it could reasonably be argued that for cost-effectiveness most health care professional staff are better employed on their own professional work.

25. To summarise, the best prospect of avoiding industrial action by hospital computing staff, and of minimising its impact if it does happen, lies in technological advances that will substantially reduce, if not altogether avoid, the dependence of functioning computing facilities on such staff.

26. Remedial action All computing systems providing a real-time service (other than aerospace and defence) - whether on-line or not - require some kind of manual standby facility, justified by the possibility of serious technological failure. However, the use of manual alternatives to computer-based hospital systems in times of industrial action by computing staff raises some special problems. The major problem is that even if other hospital staff are not positively supporting the computing staff in their industrial action, many will be unwilling to provide substitute services that would have the effect of undermining or aborting the action that the computing staff are taking. For doctors and nurses, in particular, loyalty to other staff may in the last resort have less force than loyalty to patients. But that decision entails for each affected individual an informed assessment of the merits of the case for industrial action by their colleagues; and that in turn requires management to be willing and competent to communicate its side of the case to all staff - the case for those taking action will certainly be put forcefully by their unions or local organisers. Nevertheless, successful remedial action during impedance of computer-based services by computing staff will usually be mainly confined to those services directly provided to patients and, mostly likely, within the competence of doctors and nurses.

Conclusion

Health service computing staff are, if anything, less prone than many staff to take industrial action in pursuit of their aims. Nevertheless, where they do, and particularly where a hospital has become heavily dependent on computing for its operational efficiency, the effects of their action can, at worst, lead to a deterioration in patient services. The avoidance of such action by impeccable industrial relations (which would mean satisfying all the staff all the time without unreasonable cost to management) is unattainable, and hospitals must take such avoiding action as they can while being prepared to take measures to ameliorate the effects when it happens. Fortunately technological progress in computing is increasingly offering facilities that will reduce the direct dependence of computing systems on computing staff on site.

Note

The opinions expressed in this paper are those of the author and are not necessarily shared by either the Department of Health and Social Security or the National Health Service.

References

1.   "Synopsis of National Health Service Computing 1977"
          - Department of Health and Social Security, London. 1978

2.   "Impact of the 1974 Health Care Amendments to the National Labour Relations Act
          on Collective Bargaining in the Health Care Industry" - US Department of Labor,
          Labor-Management Services Administration; and Federal Mediation and
          Conciliation Service, Office of Research, 1979

3.   "Pay Negotiations in Six Overseas Health Services"
          - D White, Department of Health and Social Security, London.   1980

D White
Department of Health and Social Security
Hannibal House
Elephant and Castle
LONDON
SE1 6TE
England

The design of a National Information System for Thalassemia.

A.Rossi-Mori, F.L.Ricci, A.M.Bocchi, A.De Blasi, R.Gaviano, B.Rossi
Group on Health Information System, Inst. for Biomedical Technology,
National Research Council. V.Morgagni 30/E 00161 Rome (Italy)

ABSTRACT: The control of thalassemia, a genetic disease, depends upon
preventive and therapeutic   programs, that are planned at Regional
level and carried out by a large number of autonomous health services.
On this structure, a specialized hierarchic Information System was designed, as a part of the whole Health Information System now under development in Italy.
No specific I.S. for thalassemia was available before, so that the design was planned following a preliminary study to obtain a reference
framework and to identify precise objectives.

INTRODUCTION

The general term "thalassemia" stands for a wide set of genetic disorders in the production of hemoglobin (1).
A serious form of thalassemia is the "mediterranean anemia": affected
people require constant and heavy care to reach an average age of 20 -
- 30 years.
The control of thalassemia is attained by adding a preventive program
on the population with therapy, in every area where the high incidence rate makes this disease an evident local public health problem.

Current scientific advances allow an effective control of the disease
to be truly realized, since the model of the intervention is defined
and clear.

METHODS

Before the present work, no permanent Information System (IS) was effectively implemented for the collection and the processing of thalassemia data. There were of course various nuclei of aggregated information (health services, regional health authorities, patient associations, etc.), however their approach was not systematic and there was no
integration among them.

The study was carried out in three steps:
(i) the set up of a reference framework for the problems related with
     thalassemia;
(ii) a parallel analysis of the program organization (2) and of the
     old implicit IS, which has been summarized in a list of relevant
     information subjects, together with the related sets of data (3);
     the few available files -usually on paper support- were described
     by means of standard techniques (4,5);
(iii) the analysis of the institutional tasks of each involved subject,
     the determination of its information needs and the design of a pi-
     lot IS.

RESULTS

Many studies existed on narrowly related topics, with differences in
aims and thus in subjects and procedures. In spite of these difficult-

FIG.1 An example of the information changes at the different functional levels; only the most relevant items related to blood transfusions are shown.

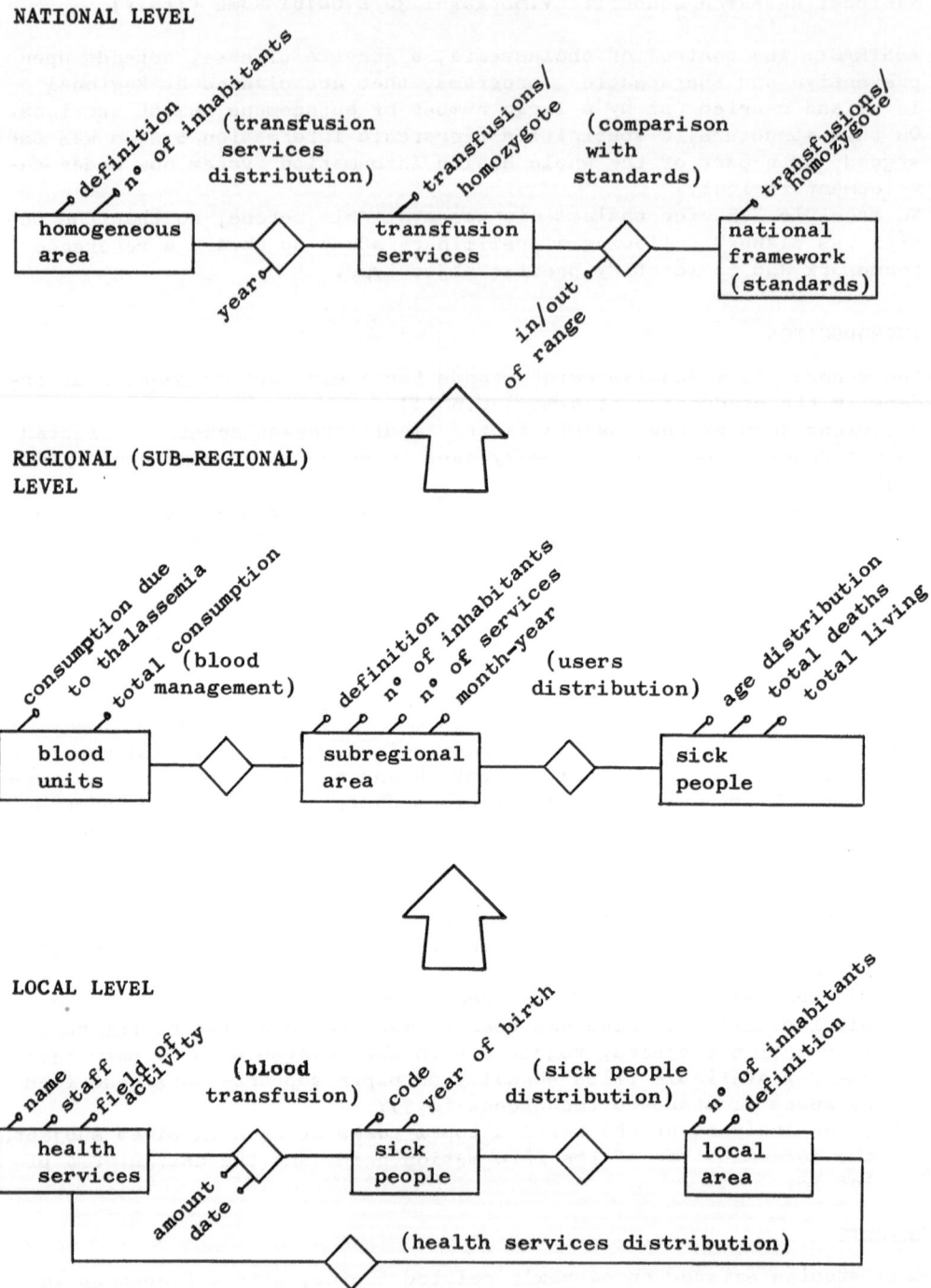

ies, the integrated processing of this data gave a careful evaluation (6,7,8,9,10,11) of:
- geographic distribution of the disease (carriers and sick people);
- indicators of therapy effectiveness, in various areas;
- indicators of activity for the programs on therapy and prevention;
- possible evolution in resources requirements.

A hierarchical structure was outlined for the IS, and its main features were pointed out (see tab.1 and fig.1).

The parallel implementation of the pilot IS is still in progress:
1. national level. In order to fulfill the most urgent necessity (i.e. predicting the need of blood and drugs) a national census of the 6000 treated sick people and the 400 involved health services was done. This data is now becoming the nucleus of the various Regional Registers for monitoring services.(12,13).
2. Regional level. In few Regions, sets of additional data are collected. The objective is to study problems of importance, such as:
   - reproductive behaviour of at-risk couples;
   - direct purchasing of drugs by the Regional Health Authorities;
   - optimization of transfusion services and blood stocks;
   - effect of internal migrations.
3. local level. In different services, information subsystems are being tested, to experiment appropriate tools: a) in care units, to support the standard case sheet; b) in clinical laboratories, to standardize the registers; c) in transfusion services, to make the matching with donors easier.

DISCUSSION

The non-complexity of the intervention model allows to experiment on a methodology for the evaluation of each local program. The main (information) problems of the control programs are the difficulties in putting together -in a comprehensive frame- actions taken by different autonomous services and in obtaining constant information about the effectiveness of a program (14,15,16).

The main features of the designed IS are:
1. the strong selection of "flowing" information that guarantees the realization and the updating of the higher levels of the IS;
2. the feedback of processed information to local services that involves the operators and rises the reliability of the data;
3. the items reside at the level at which they are generated or immediately used. As a rule, the needs of higher levels are fulfilled by appropriate processing of these items. In this way the possibility to repeatedly collect the same data -used for different purposes at each functional level- following independent procedures, is excluded.
4. the data is organized into indicators, designed to express the time evolution of the programs and to allow comparisons with intermediate or final pre-established goals (17).
5. the "routine framework",produced by the IS,aims at pointing out problems, which are to be solved by means of ad hoc studies.

CONCLUSION

The IS for thalassemia is implemented with a hierarchic organization.

The objective is to fulfill three kinds of requirements: (i) the proper operation of the involved services; (ii) the planning of a whole local program and (iii) coordination among different programs.
These three functional levels correspond to the local, regional and national levels of the whole Health Information System, now under development in Italy.

Thalassemia is only a small scale problem, for the National Health Service; accordingly, it deserves -as a rule- only "attention" by the Health Information System. Thus earmarked resources are not requested, and the cost of the IS is low, limited mainly to this phase of design.

This work was partially supported by "Progetto Finalizzato Medicina Preventiva" of the National Research Council (sottoprogetto Malattie Ereditarie dell'Eritrocita).

REFERENCES
(1) D.J.Weatherall, J.B.Clegg: The Thalassemia sindromes. Blackwell Publications, Oxford 1972
(2) J.L.Peterson: Petri Net theory and the modeling of systems. Prentice Hill, 1981
(3) F.L.Ricci, A.Rossi-Mori: Definizione delle caratteristiche di base di un Sistema Informativo per le Talassemie. (unpublished)
(4   P.Chen: The Entity-Relationship model: toward a unified view of data. ACM TODS, 1976
(5) C.Batini, G.Santucci: Top-down design in the Entity-Relationship model. Int.Conf. on the E-R approach to system analysis and design, Los Angeles, dec. 1979
(6) E.Attanasio, A.Rossi-Mori, G.Ansuini: La prevenzione della talassemia in Sardegna. in Atti del Simposio "Analisi Costi Benefici nei Sistemi Sanitari" Bellagio, 1979; Fondazione Smith Kline ed.
(7) E.Attanasio, R.Galanello, A.Rossi-Mori: Analisi costi benefici di un intervento preventivo per la talassemia. in Atti del VI congr. Int. sulla Prevenzione delle Malattie Microcitemiche, Roma, 1980
(8) G.Modiano, A.Rossi-Mori: Distribuzione teorica e frequenza del morbo di Cooley in Italia. in Atti del VI congr. int. sulla Prevenzione delle Malattie Microcitemiche, Roma, 1980
(9) B.Rossi, A.Rossi-Mori: L'anemia di Cooley in Italia. Una analisi di alcune fonti di dati. III congr.naz.AICM, Ferrara, 1980
(10) B.Rossi, A.Rossi-Mori: La prevenzione della talassemia. Stime di alcune grandezze rilevanti per la pianificazione degli interventi. III congr.naz.AIGM, Ferrara, 1980
(11) A.Rossi-Mori, B.Rossi: La talassemia beta in Italia. Dati statistici e prime elaborazioni. (unpublished)
(12) J.M.Weddel: Registers and registries: A Review. Int.J.Epidemiology, 2, 221-228, 1973
(13) Emery et al: A Report on Genetic Registers. J.Medical Genetics, 15, 435-442, 1978
(14) G.S.Stamatoyannopoulos: Problems of screening and counseling in the hemoglobinopaties. in Birth Defects (A.G.Motulsky, W.Lenz ed.) Excerpta Medica, 1974 pag.2Ø8-276
(15) - : Population screening of recessively inherited disorders. Lancet, ii, 679-680, 1980
(16) F.L.Ricci, A.Rossi-Mori, B.Rossi: The role of the Information Sy-

stem in planning the control of a genetic disease. in Medical Informatics Europe 1981, Lecture Notes in Medical Informatics, Springer Verlag, 1981 (D.A.B.Lindberg and P.L.Reichertz eds.)
(17) A.Rossi-Mori: Criteri per la valutazione dei programmi di screening. III congr. naz. AIGM, Ferrara, 1980

TAB.1 List of identified tasks for the three functional levels of the Information System for Thalassemia.

NATIONAL LEVEL:

- to help the coordination among Regions;
- to avoid duplications in sick people census;
- to allow epidemiological investigations of general interest.

REGIONAL (sub-regional) LEVEL

-to support the planning of interventions (therapeutical and preventive);
- to evaluate the effectiveness of the programs (retrospectively and prospectively).

SERVICES LEVEL

- to handle the routine operation;
- to produce data for upper levels.

THE REGIONAL ONCOLOGICAL CENTER IN UPPSALA.   DEVELOPMENT, FUNCTIONS AND INFORMATION PROCESSING.

Leif Gustafsson (1), Inge Hesselius (2), Alf Lycksell (1), Bengt
Sandblad (1,3) and Werner Schneider (1).
1) Uppsala University Data Center, Box 2103, S-750 02 Uppsala,SWEDEN.
2) Uppsala University Hospital, S-750 14 Uppsala, SWEDEN.
3) Dept. of Automatic Control and Systems Analysis, Inst.of Technology,
    Uppsala University, Box 534, S-751 21 Uppsala, SWEDEN.

ABSTRACT.

In each of the seven Swedish health care regions, each with
1-1.5 million inhabitants, work is in progress to develop regional
oncological centers.   These centers do not take a direct, active part
in the clinical or planning activities of the total care process, but
act as service functions to such activities.   Outgoing from general
directives, specifications for functions of a regional center in Uppsala
have been formulated.   From these the needs for information and information processing have been derived.   The formulation of care programs
for different types of tumour diseases are fundamental.   Finally
specifications for an information system have been made, and parts of
this system are today developed and implemented.   The basis of the
system is a distributed, database-oriented structure of registers.

A COMMUNITY CARE INFORMATION SYSTEM

Michael McLoone,
Programme Manager,
Community Care Services,
North Western Health Board,
Ireland.

Andrew Hunter,
Management Consultant,
Arthur Andersen & Co.
Ireland.

SUMMARY

This paper describes the development of information systems for the community health and social services programme of a regional health authority. The objectives and background to three projects are explained and each project - user training programme; management reporting system; community index system - is described.

1. INTRODUCTION AND OBJECTIVES

1.1 Background

Work is currently being carried out by the North Western Health Board - one of eight regional health boards in Ireland - in the development of systems for its community care programme. The North Western Health Board is a statutory body set up under the Health Act 1970 with a responsibility for the provision of health services in the counties of Donegal, Leitrim and Sligo. The services are divided broadly into two programmes - hospital care and community care. Line management in these programmes are supported by specialised departments of finance, personnel, planning and evaluation, and systems.

The community care programme of the Board covers a very broad range of community health and social services - including residential services for the aged and the handicapped. The programme is organised in two community care areas, each headed by a Director of Community Care/ Medical Officer of Health (the population of the Donegal community care area is approximately 124,000 and of the Sligo/Leitrim area approximately 80,000), and the primary professions in the community care service are:

- Medical
- Public Health Nursing
- Social Work
- Dental
- Health Inspectorate

- Community Welfare
- Mental Handicap Nursing
- General Nursing (Units)
- Paramedical
- Administrative

1.2 Organisation/Systems Environment

1.2.1 Senior Health Professionals

The evolution of the structures and systems in the regional health
services has resulted in the situation where many of the health
professional users have little experience in:

- using management information reports that have not been prepared
  manually by themselves

- reviewing regular reports to monitor and plan service developments,
  or

- defining their own (financial and service) information requirements
  for a new system.

1.2.2 Budgetary Control

Senior professionals are not responsible for preparing their own
estimates, and are not in receipt of regular information on expenditure
within their specific area of responsibility. Consequently senior
health professionals are not in a position to manage service
expenditure in the context of an annual plan and budget for their
specific areas.

1.2.3 Client Indexing, Service Information and Case Records

- Case records are maintained on a service by service basis i.e.
the same client is registered under several numbers by reference to the
service or allowance being received. Therefore the record keeping and
potential information does not support the integration of community
care client services.

- Standards, policies and procedures for record keeping are not
uniform.

- Information on the client care base to support management control
and service planning is difficult to extract from existing manual
records.

1.3 Objectives

The objectives of the projects described later in this paper are
briefly as follows:

a. Health Professional Training

To enhance the managerial role of senior health professionals in the
development and use of management information systems.

b.   Management Reporting

To develop and refine the Board's existing financial reporting system
for use by Community Care managers.

c.   Community Index Project

To design and install a registration and management information system
covering all Community Care clients: and to index case records by
reference to a common client index number.

2.   TRAINING AND INVOLVEMENT OF SENIOR HEALTH PROFESSIONALS

A major training programme was carried out recently for the future
users of the new information systems.   It consisted of ten one-day
sessions and on-site intersession work projects for the two Community
Care Programme Area Teams.

The objectives of the training programme were to prepare the users of
new, comprehensive information in; a) their role in the development of
the systems, b) their role in the design and use of management
information reports, c) their role in dictating the requirements and
shaping the design principles of the Index systems.   The major
components of the training programme were:

a.   Policy Development

Policies for many of the community care services were documented during
the course of the programme.   These policies set out service levels as
well as attitudes and approaches to particular service situations.

b.   Annual Planning and Management Reporting

Specific responsibility for elements of the annual planning process
and responsibility for budgetary preparation and expenditure control
were identified.   This work was obviously a pre-requisite to designing
the responsibility, statistical and expenditure reports identified in
the management reporting project.

c.   Computer Appreciation

The users only experience in the area of computers had been a) in
preparing batch inputs and b) using batch outputs.   The functions of
computer hardware components were explained to the users and there was
an introduction to on-line systems.   Practical problems were solved by
users using VDU screens.

d.   Systems Development

The difference between developing information systems and installing

computers was emphasised. User involvement in the development of the
two main systems was incorporated through the training programme into
the actual design and installation process. The user role was put in
context of a complete systems development life cycle.

Other topics covered were in the area of general management techniques,
leadership and effective group work.

The training programme was action-based concentrating heavily on
practical instruction and good documentation for the installation of
new management processes using the management reporting and index
information systems.

3.   MANAGEMENT REPORTING SYSTEM

3.1 General Introduction

This system is a second phase development of the general accounting and
management reporting system for the Board. For the Community Care
programme the phase one system was providing monthly expenditure
reports against budget using sub-cost centres as the reporting head.
These sub-cost centres reported expenditure by service and allowance
activities across professional responsibility boundaries, e.g.
expenditure on all medicines and appliances was reported as a total
irrespective of whether nursing, medical or paramedical staff
requisitioned the item.

The second phase therefore has resulted in regular management information
reports showing planned versus actual expenditure on a monthly cycle
with appropriate statistical support for the following users:

-    Chief Executive Officer   -   Superintendent Community
-    Community Care Programme   Welfare Officer
     Manager   -   Senior Area Medical Officer
-    Director of Community Care/   -   Senior Health Inspector
     Medical Officer of Health   -   Director of Nursing, Mental
-    Principal Dental Surgeon   Handicap
-    Superintendent Public Health -   Community Care Administrator
     Nurse   -   Residential (Nursing) Units
-    Senior Social Worker

3.2 Structure of the Information Reports

The reports are divided into three categories, as follows:

-    Responsibility Reports which measure actual expenditure against
planned expenditure in such a way that variations from the plan can be

related to the individual responsible for controlling them. The annual budget is based on planned payments so control (rather conservatively) measures actual payments plus commitments against month and year-to-date budget.

-   Statistical Reports which act as a back-up to the responsibility reports in clarifying the expenditure variations; for example, average cost figures and activity volumes in particular areas of expenditure are reported for the current month, year-to-date and this month last year. Actual is reported against budget for year-to-date average costs.

-   Expenditure Reports which assist primarily the Programme Manager to discharge his responsibility as a member of the Management Team: and assist the Finance Function to discharge their role in a) the overall management of the finances and b) advise to line management. These reports use the same control headings as the responsibility reports and provide a total programme summary facilitating a senior manager review of the overall financial position.

The reports assist the programme headquarter staff in the collection of data for Department of Health returns and Health Board reports. The expenditure reports also assist the Community Care Area Teams in co-ordinating Community Care professional and unit services.

4. COMMUNITY INDEX SYSTEM

4.1 General Introduction

A project is currently been undertaken to design a Community Index System for the Board. The system will register all Community Care clients and provide management information on Community Care services. A unique number will be assigned to each client registered and this number will be an index to manual case notes and a common client index for all services. It is planned that this system will operate on the Board's own computer and interface with other applications running on this computer and a central mainframe operating in Dublin. The overall objective of the system is to support Community Care professionals and administrators in the management of a comprehensive - multi-service/multi-professional - client service and to support the co-ordination of services and professionals to each client. The system will also report data to the Community Care programme which will be of value in the planning of future services.

4.2 Design Approach and Principles

1. The system will not be a mechanisation of existing manual case

records however, we recognise that such options as the mechanisation of case notes, in certain areas which would lend themselves to computer input and retrieval, do exist.

2.   In the design we are recognising that in the future, operational (transaction) systems for particular functions will be installed which have an interface to the system; for example, a system for the recording of Immunisations and Vaccinations, the scheduling of Child Developmental Clinics, data collection for research into particular adult problems, data collection for other epidemiological research, etc.

Our design approach therefore has involved a comprehensive analysis of existing manual procedures in all of the major areas of Community Care 'services, such as Public Health Nursing, Social Work, theprovision of financial allowances and services, Mental Handicap Services etc. This analysis has enabled us to:

-    Detail how the mechanised procedures will interface to the future manual procedures

-    Examine the change to be imposed on the day-to-day routines of the Community Care staff

-    Identify the opportunities to mechanise existing manually prepared information

-    Identify the business functions and information needs of the programme.

4.3 System Functions

The system will be designed on a modular basis which recognises software routines which are common across the professional services: for example, client registration and application/referral control processes are primarily similar for every service. Another example is that every service sets a review data to initiate a client care procedure in the future. In this way we will meet two objectives which are:

a.   To have software modules which can be installed on a phased basis;
b.   To have software routines within modules which are generalised to avoid having the repetition of these routines in various sub-systems for each professional discipline.

Seven major functions have been identified for the Community Index system which are described below:

Client Registration:

.   Add, Delete and Maintain I.D./Demographic Client Information
.   Print/Display Client Information

Service Information Maintenance:

- Add, Delete and Maintain professional descriptions
- Add, Delete and Maintain service descriptions
- Print Display professional and service information.

Application Processing:

- Add, Maintain applications or referrals
- Print control reports
- Display outstanding applications and referrals.

Client Service Control:

- Add, Close and Maintain approved cases and services
- Maintain record of client service statae (medical, nursing, social, dental etc. classifications)
- Maintain record of target group classifications (children at risk, handicapped, elderly at risk).

Client Service Planning:

- Print master lists of client by service
- Print master lists of client service status
- Print summary statistics by service and client service status
- Display client lists by target group classification.

Professional Planning:

- Print case loads list by professional
- Print case load lists by service.

Index Analysis:

- Print selective analysis of the services and client characteristics on various parameters:

a. by service
    by district electoral division
    - numbers in receipt with a distribution by age, client service classification, marital status, GP etc.

b. by target group
    by public health nurse
        numbers in receipt with a distribution by age, client service classification, marital status etc.

IRISH PSYCHIATRIC CASE REGISTERS, THEIR
CONTRIBUTION TO COMMUNITY HEALTH CARE

Aileen O'Hare,
Medico-Social Research Board
73 Lower Baggot Street
Dublin 2   Ireland

SUMMARY

Three psychiatric case registers were established in 1973 by the Medico
Social Research Board in counties that were reflective of the range of
hospitalised morbidity in Ireland. Findings from these registers can
contribute to community health care not just for the three counties
concerned but for the country as a whole by providing information on
reported psychiatric morbidity, its social and demographic concomitants
and the use of available treatment services. The limitations and
further scope of the register is discussed.

1.   INTRODUCTION

Prior to the setting up of Psychiatric Case Registers in Ireland the
only source of information on mental illness was mental hospital
statistics. These showed that Ireland in 1971 had almost double the
hospital admission rate of, for example, her nearest neighbours England
and Wales[1][2] and the highest number of mental health facility beds,
7.3 per 1,000 population, of the WHO member countries, as the following
Figure illustrates:

Figure 1.   Reported number of mental health facility beds per 1,000
population*

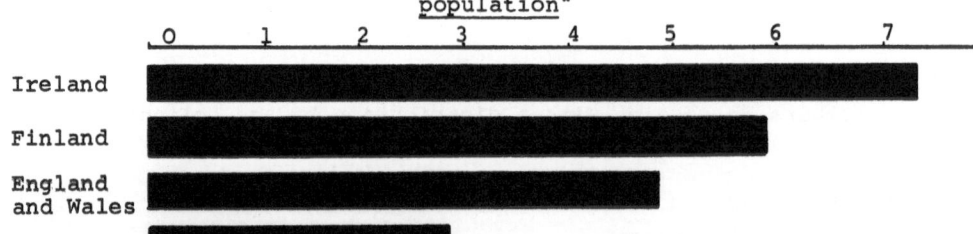

* Adapted from Mednick SA, and Baert AE, eds. Prospective Longitudinal
  Research: An empirical basis for the primary prevention of
  psychosocial disorders. (3)

Apart from the fact that the high number of mental health beds in Ireland are a legacy from the past, a measurement of mental illness in terms of mental hospital bed occupancy is no longer valid today, when so many patients are now treated in the community.

Accordingly three psychiatric case registers were established to obtain a more reliable measurement of reported prevalence and incidence in the counties and in the country as a whole of which the counties are representative.[4] Data from the registers could also provide essential information for community health care programmes on, for example, the pattern of service use and the characteristics of the patient population.

2. METHODOLOGY

The choice of register areas was determined by the available hospital statistics at the time of planning.[5] County Roscommon was selected as typifying an area of high hospitalisation, Carlow an area of low hospitalisation and Westmeath an intermediate area, as Table 1 illustrates.

Table 1. One-day prevalence 1971. Hospital rates per 1,000 population

Carlow *	Westmeath *	Roscommon
3.4	6.3	7.0

*Estimate, not co-terminous with study areas.

Each of the three counties have a defined catchment area and a population of approximately 50,000. Psychiatric case registers commenced in each of these areas on March 31st 1973 with a census of patients in all forms of psychiatric care. After this date as new patients came into care they were added to the register and information up-dated as former patients returned to care. Hence our definition of the mentally ill was persons who on contact with a psychiatric service were given a psychiatric diagnosis.

A register is simply a list of names of people with common characteristics like a school or medical register. Our psychiatric registers contain the names and specified characteristics of people from defined catchment areas who are given a psychiatric diagnosis. However unlike the old school register with its manual limitation the considerable scope, flexibility and output of these registers is possible because of advanced technology and the sophisticated use of computers. Computerisation of these sensitive records also ensures maximum

confidentiality of the information. The following flow-chart gives an
outline of the input data which is collected, the computer process and
the available output statistics.

FIGURE 11

INPUT FORMS

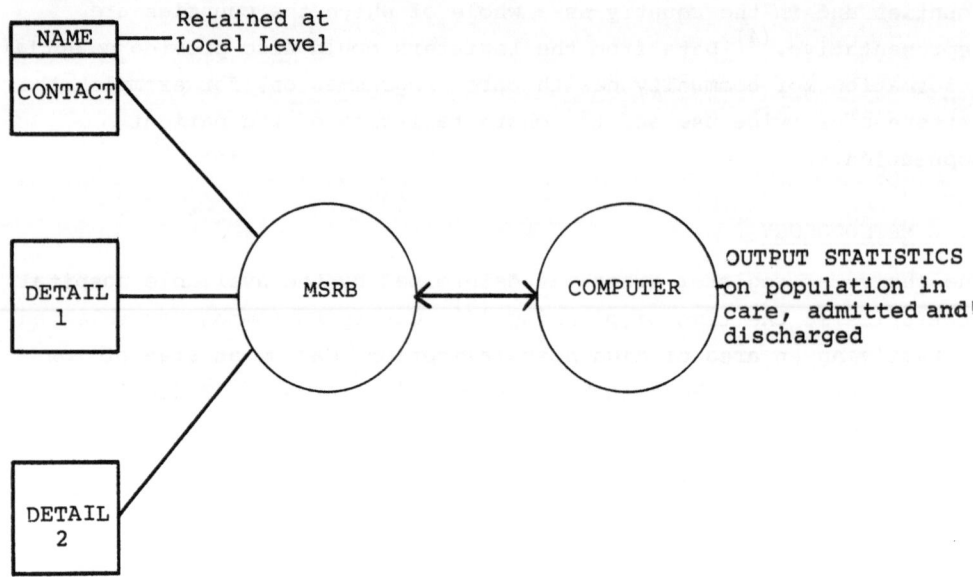

Considerable bio-social and medical information is collected by trained
interviewers on Patient Detail 1 and 2 forms from persons in the
defined areas who through their use of a psychiatric service are
entered on the register. The Contact Form, with an admission and
discharge section, monitors the patient's use of the different types
of care, such as, in-patient, hostel and out-patient care. It should
be noted that patients' names and addresses are retained on a rotadex
at local level by the register controllers. A unique number is used
for identification purposes. All information from the areas is checked
at the Medico-Social Research Board (MSRB) before going to the Computer,
an ME29 located in the Eastern Health Board, Dublin.

3.   FINDINGS

Output from the register is considerable so this paper will focus only
on data relevant to community health care. The concept of psychiatric
community care used is that of a range of psychiatric services which
in the case of our registers include in-patient, out-patient, day

715

hospital, day centre, hostel, domiciliary visits and consultations in wards of general hospitals catering to the needs of people in a defined geographical area. The following table gives the rates for one-day prevalence for persons on the register on the 31st December 1974.

Table 2. One-day prevalence 1974. Register rates per 1,000 population

Carlow	Westmeath	Roscommon
19.2	11.7	11.8

The table shows that contrary to the situation revealed by hospital statistics Carlow and not Roscommon had a higher reported one-day prevalence rate. Some interesting differences emerged between the counties as follows:

Table 3. One-day prevalence 1974. Selected inter-county differences

	Carlow %	Westmeath %	Roscommon %
Out-patient (all forms)	73	47	41
Female	54	51	48
<45 Years	36	35	27
Neurotic/Personality Disorder	39	9	10
Schizophrenia	35	35	49

As the table shows Carlow had a higher percentage of out-patients, women, persons aged under 45 years and those with a neurotic/ personality disorder than the other two counties. The schizophrenic proportion was highest in County Roscommon.

The higher one-day prevalence rate in Carlow can largely be accounted for by the high percentage of out-patients in care, 73, of which 51 per cent were neurotic or had a personality disorder and 68 per cent of whom were women. The same emphasis on out-patient care existed for schizophrenia as seen from Table 4 where 60 per cent were in out-patient care in Carlow, in contrast to 40 per cent in Westmeath, and 32 per cent in Roscommon.

Table 4. One-day prevalence 1974. Schizophrenia by type of care

	Carlow %	Westmeath %	Roscommon %
In-patient	40	60	68
Out-patient (all forms)	60	40	32

This pattern of service provision and use is probably typical of
Ireland as a whole where inter-county demographic differences of
population density, age and sex structure, often determine such
variation. Further analysis of register data over time should enable
us to make firm statements concerning the advantages of the differing
provisions of care and the community's response to them. When data
from the three counties are combined the rates were approximately
double those of the English registers in Camberwell and Salford.[6]

Table 5. One-day prevalence 1974. Register rates per 1,000 population

Three Counties	Camberwell	Salford
14.1	7.7	5.4

These findings concur with data from an earlier register paper by Walsh
et al.[4] Some of the explanations considered for the raised rate
include "historical-cultural characteristics such as an over-generous
provision of in-patient facilities, a passive/submissive tendency on
the part of patients to accept and protract hospitalisation and other
forms of care... and a lack of involvement of primary health care
personnel in psychiatric care".

When first-ever contact with the register is analysed for 1974 and
compared with Camberwell and Salford data the following picture emerges:

Table 6. First-ever contact 1974. Register rates per 1,000 population

Three Counties	Camberwell	Salford
2.4	3.4	2.1

This important finding, albeit for one year, that the three county
rate is lower than that of Camberwell and marginally higher than
Salford suggests that whereas psychiatric prevalence rates are high in
Ireland this is not so for incidence. On this basis community care
programmes could plan for a predictable number of new cases occurring
annually while at the same time guarding against an accumulation of
new long-stay patients. Further register data is required over time
to ensure the stability of this rate, although findings from a recent
study also suggest that first contact rates in Ireland are lower than
expected.[7]

4.   CONCLUSIONS

On the basis of one year's information presented in this paper one-day reported prevalence of mental illness is raised in our three research counties in comparison to that of registers outside Ireland, but not one-year incidence. Additional longitudinal register data is required to validate this position.

One of the limitations of the three county register's contribution to community health care is that it deals with reported rates of illness to the specialised services only. It is essential to extend the scope of the Irish registers to determine the extent to which general practitioners diagnose and treat mental illness within the defined community catchment areas. Only then will a true measure of reported community psychiatric morbidity be possible. A recent WHO Report on "Changing Patterns in Mental Health Care" points out that in the planning of community mental health services few serious attempts have been made to achieve an effective balance between specialist and generalised (primary care) facilities within the mental care system.[8]

A much neglected aspect of community care is the role of patients' relatives and as Wing observed the success of a community care system depends upon relatives who provide most of the domestic supervision that would otherwise be given by trained staff in hospitals or hostels.[9] The relatives of patients currently on the Irish registers could be contacted and their definition of the problem sought.

The fundamental principle behind the concept of community care is that "planning should be based on the needs of the people for whom the services are designed, rather than on the organisation of institutions where they receive care and treatment".[10] Case registers as a tool of investigation make a positive contribution to such a principle. However, central and local administration must also play their role in making use of these data. Community health care planning must be based on available facts and not proceed from irrational political motivation or ad hoc short-term considerations.

5. REFERENCES

1. O'Hare A, Walsh D. Activities of Irish psychiatric hospitals and units 1971 and 1972. Dublin: Medico-Social Research Board, 1975.

2. Department of Health and Social Security. Psychiatric hospitals and units in England and Wales. Inpatient statistics from the Mental Health Enquiry for the year 1971. London: HMSO, 1973.

3.   Mednick SA, Baert AE. eds. Prospective longitudinal research: an empirical basis for the primary prevention of psychosocial disorders. Oxford: Oxford University Press, 1981.

4.   Walsh D, O'Hare A, Blake B, Halpenny JV, O'Brien PF. The treated prevalence of mental illness in the Republic of Ireland - the three county case register study. Psychol Med, 1980; 10:465-470.

5.   O'Hare A, Walsh D. The Irish psychiatric hospital census 1971. Dublin: Medico-Social Research Board, 1974.

6.   Wing JK, Fryers T. Statistics from the Camberwell and Salford psychiatric registers 1964 - 1974. London: Institute of Psychiatry, 1976.

7.   Walsh D, Butler S, Starks S. The St. Loman's psychiatric service: an exercise in parsimony. Ir J Psychiat. 1981; 1:9-22.

8.   Report on a WHO Working Group. Changing patterns in mental health care. Copenhagen: WHO, 1980.

9.   Wing JK, Hailey AM. Evaluating a community psychiatric service: the Camberwell register 1964-71. London: Oxford University Press, 1972.

10. Report on a Conference convened by the Regional Office for Europe of the WHO. The development of comprehensive mental health services in the community. Copenhagen: WHO, 1973.

REGISTER OF TREATED ALCOHOLICS
IN THE SOCIALIST REPUBLIC OF CROATIA

Vladimir Hudolin, Petar Mačašović* and Slavko Sakoman

University Department of Neurology, Psychiatry, Alcoholism and Other Dependencies

"Dr Mladen Stojanović" Clinical Hospital

*University Computing Centre (SRCE)

Zagreb

Yugoslavia

SUMMARY

The World Health Organization considers that by the year 2000 basic health protection will have been ensured for every inhabitant of this planet. Chronic diseases tend to play an even more important role among the health problems. One of these is the dependence on alcohol which, in view of its prevalence, has been listed among the 3 or 4 leading socio-medical problems in the world.

The most important source of data on alcoholism in the Socialist Republic of Croatia has been provided by the Republican Register of Treated Alcoholics. This paper describes the evolution of the Register and its present usage.

1. INTRODUCTION

The Register might generally be described as a collection of documents, containing uniform medical or socio-demographical data on individual subjects, compiled in a systematic and preconceived way for the purpose of serving a predefined certain goal (1). In the eleventh report by the Professional Committee of WHO dealing with health statistics, it was mentioned among other items that the Register ought to be an instrument for the permanent compilation of data necessary for statistical elaborations and for the follow-up of every individual case. It was also mentioned that the patients whose names have been entered in the Register ought to be the subject of a separate series of studies (2). Gorwbtz (3) describes the Register in a similar way, i.e. a data dollecting system in which information about individuals is compiled in one central spot. Subsequently the information is studied by a specific group of institutions, organizations or professionals for the purpose of obtaining data on a certain disease. In order to obtain data about the development of the disease, every episode of the disease is followed for each registered patient and connected longitudinally. The Register is, accordingly, a dynamic statistical instrument, very suitable for the mass observation of chronic diseases, which are beginning to fill an ever more important place in the total national morbidity.

Contemporary health prevention, especially in the sphere of socio-medical diseases indicates the need for an increasingly greater use and dissemination of information. The information is required as accurate as possible. Data about mental diseases and diseases of dependency, particularly those dealing with alcoholism, are in the focal point of interest. It is not only important to know the number of subjects suffering from the disease in the entire population or in specially defined groups, but even more important is the need for the observation of the regular work of the health services, of the quality of this work, the justification for the expenditures involved and the efforts invested and of the economics of the whole business. All this information supplies the basis for contemporary long-term planning (4)

Since alcoholism is one of the most serious socio-medical problems in this world, because of its prevalence and equally because of the very characteristics of the disease (uncritical, disturbed behaviour of the patient (5)), and taking into account the fact that adequate measures may considerably affect this problem, the Republican Register of Alcoholics of the Socialist Republic of Croatia was established in Zagreb. Data about all alcoholics treated for alcoholism in any of the psychiatric or specialized institutions dealing with alcoholism in the Socialist Republic of Croatia have been entered in this Register. Earlier statistics on alcoholism, relying on data supplied by individual psychiatric institutions mainly about the number of hospitalized cases, did not reveal much about the number of subjects suffering from the disease and their movements with regard to time and space.

This is basically due to the fact that alcoholism is a chronic, life-long disease in which relapses are one of the main characteristics. Only 50% of all alcoholics undergo treatment for the second time in the same institution where they were treated for the first time and where all the medical documentation pertaining to their case is kept. The great advantage of the Register lies in the possibility of longitudinal observation and following of each individual case over an extended period of time. Although the Register provides data only for one (alcoholics undergoing in-patients treatment) category of alcoholics, the great advantage over other epidemiological instruments lies in its accuracy and on the other hand in the manner the services for the controlling of alcoholism have been organized in the Socialist Republic of Croatia. One has to bear in mind that, with regard to territory and population, the Register entirely covers a clearly defined region of the Socialist Republic of Croatia within the framework of the Federation of Yugoslavia. According to the Census of 1971, the Socialist Republic of Croatia numbered 4,420.000 inhabitants. The entire Republic is divided into 10 regions, 113 communes and 1950 local communities.

2. ORGANIZATION OF WORK WITHIN THE REGISTER

Statistics containing information on cases of disease or about treatment only, can no longer satisfy the requirements of the contemporary health services. A qualitative study of many diseases and particularly of alcoholism is impossible without information about the individual, mostly life-long patient. Comprehensive observation and follow-up of the alcoholic was possible only with the help of the national Register, closely connected with other health, statistical and demographical systems. One and the same alcoholic may report several times to the Register (there are individuals treated more than 50 times over a 10-year period but still followed as an individual).

The registration of treated alcoholics was started on 31 December, 1964, by compiling a list of names in all psychiatric institutions where the individual alcoholic happened to be on that day. A separate form was devised, on which along with the identification date and the domicile, data about the disease were entered, possible compilations and some general data about the patient. Only those cases were entered in the Register where hospitalization because of alcoholism or alcohol related psychiatric complications were involved. It was considered that this was the only way to determine with sufficient reliability whether in fact alcoholism was involved. Accordingly, the first registration of an individual had to come after the diagnosis, given by a psychiatrist. Subsequently it became possible to add information obtained from other sources to the data of these registered individuals (e.g. about their treatment in other departments for various complications). During the first year of work the material in the Register was sorted out and elaborated by hand. The bulk of data increased rapidly and its exploitation was made more difficult by the need of processing by hand. The speed, volume and quality of the data obtained were unsatisfactory in spite of the great amount of time spent on it. The computerization of the Register was introduced as a solution and, with a fair amount of difficulties, completed in 1974 for the material collected until that time (6).

Due to the state of the data processing technology at that time the Register of Alcoholics was organized as a sequential file. Problems began to appear when, with the passing of time, the system began to develop and with regard to the great amount of cases registered, outgrew such a technology. At the present moment some 70.000 subjects and about 110.000 of their hospitalizations have been registered in the Register. Work has therefore begun for the purpose of establishing a data base for this Register and one of the existing techniques of the Data Base Management System (DBMS) will be used.

It is difficult to omit the medico-legal aspect of the work in the discussions about the Register. The secrecy of data concerning an individual is guaranteed and nominal data can be used only by the health service of the institution or region where the patient has been treated or where he was referred to for further post-hospital treatment and observation. All data on an individual case are registered under a current number, taken from a separate book of current numbers and entered for each individual on his first appearance in the Register. Moreover data are not made public nor are data published about the work of individual institutions if these data could present a danger to their reputation (7).

3. USAGE OF THE REGISTER

In view of the fact that the Register has ample programmatic support, it is in practice possible to process easily and rapidly every existing variable, following whatever criterion, in the Register, especially by using prepared software packages. On the level of every individual commune (by adding data of individual groups of communes, the data for individual regions are obtained) several basic data longitudinally followed over all the years of the Register's life cycle are routinely processed. These are data about the number of newly detected cases, about the age at which the patients are admitted for their first treatment, about the number of cases suffering from alcoholic psychoses, the number of patients who died in the course of treatment, the number of hospitalizations and the relevant days of sick-leave, and the proportion of active health insurance beneficiaries, retired subjects and agricultural workers. All these data are also processed in respect of sex, observation of the inter-relations of the signs listed and finally by longitudinal following from year to year of changes in individual signs, especially after a comparison of characteristics between individual communes. This, however, is more frequently carried out on regional level. Finally possibilities have opened for practically continuous evaluation of the communal programmes for the control of alcoholism and alcohol related problems.

Every interested institution may on request receive processed data about their patients. The criterion usually applied is that the patients received their first treatment in that institution. The institution may, naturally, use data about these subjects from all of their repeated treatments, regardless of the institution in which treatment was administered.

A special advantage of the computerized Register is the speed at which the Register prints lists of patients with all information collected about them. These, very clear transcriptions sorted in alphabetical order are most frequently made on the level of an individual commune or institution. Lists on the level of the individual commune are sometimes indispensable to the health service in establishing Clubs of Treated Alcoholics, which following field visits may motivate a certain number of treated alcoholics and their families to join or to form a club.

4. CONCLUSION

The Republican Register of Treated Alcoholics of the Socialist Republic of Croatia, which is kept by the University Department of Neurology, Psychiatry, Alcoholism and Other Dependencies in the "Dr Mladen Stojanović" Teaching Hospital at Zagreb (data processing is performed by SRCE, the University Computing Centre in Zagreb) is a dynamic statistical and epidemiological instrument which with regard to the multiplex possibilities of its usage has considerably advanced the development of the study of alcoholism and the relevant services in the Republic. This development did not proceed uniformly in all regions of the Republic (and communes respectively), just like the contemporary conception of combating alcoholism set down by the School for the Study of Alcoholism within the scope of the previously mentioned Clinic, has not been uniformly accepted everywhere. Equally the approach to the very treatment of alcoholism in individual institutions did not comply with the contemporary conceptions and methods including the necessity of long-term observation of every individual patient by means of groups practicing self-help and by Clubs of Treated Alcoholics respectively, of which about 400 have been formed in the Socialist Republic of Croatia. It was precisely the Register that made possible the dynamic conceptions about all positive and negative trends on republican, regional and communal levels, thus creating a prerequisite for taking efficient actions where this is most necessary.

REFERENCES

(1) Brooke, E.M.. The current and future use of registers in medical information systems. WHO/HS/NAT.COM./71.280,1971

(2) WHO. Epidemiological Methods in the Study of Chronic Diseases. WHO Techn. Rep. Series, No. 365, Geneva, 1967

(3) Gorwitz, K.. Psihijatrijski registar države Maryland. Lij. Vijes.. 12:1211, 1968

(4) Skupjak, B.. Zdravstveno planiranje, preduvjet razvoja samoupravno organiziranog zdravstva. Soc. med. Sarajevo, 2:119, 1974

(5) Hudolin, V.. Bolesti ovisnosti. Klinika za neurologiju, psihijatriju, alkoholizam i druge ovisnosti. K.B. "Dr M. Stojanović", Zagreb, 1977

(6) Sakoman, S., Maćašović, P., Lazić, G.. Informatika u psihijatriji i alkohologiji. U knjizi: Problemi i perspektive interdisciplinarnog rada i obrazovanja, II dio, Društvo psihologa SR Hrvatske, Zagreb, 1979

(7) Hudolin, V., Skoman, S., Maćašović, P.. Rukovanje zdravstvenim podacima i medicinska etika. Anali K.B. "Dr M. Stojanović", Vol. XVI, Br. 3, Zagreb, 1977

SPANISH NATIONAL CHILD CANCER REGISTRY (NCCR)

R. Peris-Bonet, E. Casaban
Centro de Documentación e
  Informática Biomédica
Avda. V. Blasco Ibáñez, 17
  Valencia-10, Spain

J. Donat
Departamento de Pediatría
Hospital Clínico Universitario
Avda. V. Blasco Ibáñez, 17
  Valencia-10, Spain

The NCCR has been set up following the WHO and IARC recomendations.

The philosophy, organization, coverage and items of information are briefly described, and the computer instrumentation is outlined. It covers the automatic creation and management of a master file of tumor patients and secondary files, the statistical process and the production of reports of diverse types.

1. INTRODUCTION

The National Child Cancer Registry (NCCR) is a project of the Oncology Section of the Spanish Pediatrics Association, and is carried out by the Centro de Documentación e Informática Biomédica (Center for Biomedical Documentation and Informatics) of the University of Valencia. It consists in an information system of cancer patients of less than fifteen years of age.

In Spain up to-date information about cancer can be obtainend from vital statistics (1), but general information about morbidity is only obtainable from the Hospital Morbidity Survey (2), whose first results, corresponding to 1977, have just been published, and presents all malignant tumors in a single group.

The population-based registries of Zaragoza and Navarra send their data to the IARC, but these data are not published jointly with the ones of the National Institute of Statistics.

The NCCR is dedicated to bettering the knowledge of the dimensions of cancer among children, and to make possible the active follow-up of the patients, to facilitate the study of preventive mesures, the rate and quality of survival, and to contribute to clinical investigation and the improvement of medical care. It is based on the following philosophy: 1) voluntary participation of highly motivated collaborators; 2) notification of all cases to a central register; 3) useful feedback to the collaborating centers; 4) control of the quality of diagnosis; 5) preservation of the personality of each collaborating center; and 6) all these patients should obtain medical care in higly specialized centers located in the regional hospitals.

2. GENERAL SCHEME AND COVERAGE

The NCCR works as a set of hospital-based registries (one for each collaborating center) that are integrated in a central registry. The collaborating hospital departments look after the notification and the follow-up. The data processing is central.

The NCCR should obtain notification of all cases that are carried for at those collaborating centers that are represented in the Section of Oncology of the Spanish Paediatric Association. At the moment these centers are the following: the pediatric oncology units of the Social Security hospitals of Spain (except Asturias, Galicia and Extremadura), the teaching hospitals of Barcelona, Sevilla and Valencia, the Red-Cross' hospital of Madrid and some private centers. To be a member of the Section of Paediatric Oncology standards must be guaranteed.

The International Classification of Diseases for Oncology (ICD-O) (3) has been used up to now as reportable list.

2.1. Items of patient information

The set of data to be collected has been based on the recomendations of the WHO Handbook for Standardized Cancer Registries (hospital-based) (4).

The items collected are: registration number, identification of the collaborating center, change of center, medical record number, name of the patient, sex, date of birth, place of birth, usual residence at the moment of registration, last address for contacts, telephone number, age at incidence date, date of first diagnosis, date of first consultation to the collaborating hospital (incidence date), previous diagnosis or treatment elsewere, investigations previous to initial treatment, most valid basis of diagnosis cancer, topography, laterality, morphology, differentiation, multiple primaries, clinical extent before treatment, site/s of distant metastases, staging of lymphomas and leukemias, initial treatment, protocol code, surgical-cum-pathological extent before treatment, metastases, lymphomas and leukemias staging, date of death, cause of death, coincidence between cause of death and tumor, results of autopsy, last date of follow-up, number of last anniversary followed-up, status at annual follow-up. The 37 items are represented by 82 fields on the magnetic disk.

Most of these items are identical to the core ones in the WHO Handbook and they follow its definitions. Some may be slightly different in coding but the compararability of results has been preserved. The registration number is assigned automatically by the computer program. The hospitals and patient's addresses are coded according to administrative standard boundaries and census units. The anatomical site, morphology and differentiation are coded with the ICD-O.

2.2. Notification and follow-up

Each collaborating center notifies each new case to the central registry by means of a special form (initial data sheet). As the anniversaries arrive follow-up is done and another form (the anniversary or update sheet) is sent to the central registry. Active follow-up is made for the anniversaries of the incidence date. A tumor may cause up-dating in between anniversary contacts too.

The initial data and anniversary sheets are self-explanatory and have been designed to be completed directly by the clinician without any coding.

2.3. Outputs and reports

1) Auxiliary reports: list of tumors that should be contacted (follow-up reminders), list of patients with incomplete data, letters for patients, etc.

2) Selective retrieval of tumors: The central registry will retrieve selectively sets of cases for investigation on its medical records, surveys or direct statistical processing.

3) Reports: The NCCR plans to produce its reports according to the recomendations for annual reports made in the International Agency for Research on Cancer Scientific Publication nº 21. (5). Reports for ad hoc requests would also be made. On the 24th of May a first draft version of a statistical report was presented to the Annual Meeting of the Section of Oncology.

3. INFORMATICS SUPPORT

The computer instrumentation of the NCCR can be summed up in the following points: 1) Automatic creation and management of a masterfile of tumor patients and secondary files. 2) Statistical process. 3) Production of reports of diverse types.

The application is processed by an IBM 4331/1 computer of 1024 KB. It utilizes a peripheric storage of 70 MB in IBM 3370 disks, and futhermore makes use of one or various IBM 3279 polychromatic screens. For the output an IBM 3262 printer is used.

With regards to software, the application makes use of IBM DMS/CICS/VS software (6), of statistical package SPSS (7) and batch programming in COBOL ANS, as well as VSAM files (8).

The information unit which constitutes a master file record is made up of the eighty-two fields which describe a patients' tumor. This master file is of the type KSDS/VSAM, which is indexed by two different keys, the principal, a number key, is formed by the system itself from the current date and current time, at the moment a new record is introduced, the other is a key made up of the patient's first and last names.

The creation and management of the master file has been accomplished with the design of the DMS/CICS panels and their programming. Ten different panels have been used, which, when combined, outline fourteen panels in the complete course of the program, this owing to the various functions invoked through the use of the screen. With this type of programming it is possible to resolve in real time the visualization functions of the patient's names and tumors, the addition of new records, the updating and deletion of existing records and the visualization of any particular record.

The figures 1 and 2 are taken from representative panels.

In considering the details of operation, in the case, for example, of the addition of a new record, the following steps would be performed: In the initial panel (fig. 1) is entered the name of the patient whose tumor is to be registered (it may be entered incompletely if necessary). By means of a screen's function there then appear, in an ordered fashion and from the name in question, the secondary keys of the file, which are nothing more than the names of distinct patients (fig. 2). In this way it can be observed whether a patient with a specified tumor already exists and if not, whether it is thus proper to add the case to the file. As was stated, the system itself appropiates an unmistakeable number, and as a main key, for each record.

Special care has been taken in the treatment of errors. From the standpoint of the storage of the values of the distinct items which constitute a record, the two types of errors which can happen, intra-item (values outside the order) and inter-item (contradictions between values of different items) have been solved. In the latter case, some of these errors are only detected when comparing the historical file with the on-line file.

The master file is treated with statistical package SPSS. Futhermore a battery of Cobol ANS programs has been formed to be batch-processed, which produces the auxiliary reports and selective retrieval previously mentioned.

4. REFERENCES

(1) Instituto Nacional de Estadística. Movimiento Natural de la Población Española. Año 1976. Tomo III: Defunciones según causa de muerte. Madrid. Ministerio de Economía, Instituto Nacional de Estadística, 1979.

(2) Instituto Nacional de Estadística. España. Anuario Estadístico 1979. Madrid. Ministerio de Economía, Instituto Nacional de Estadísti-

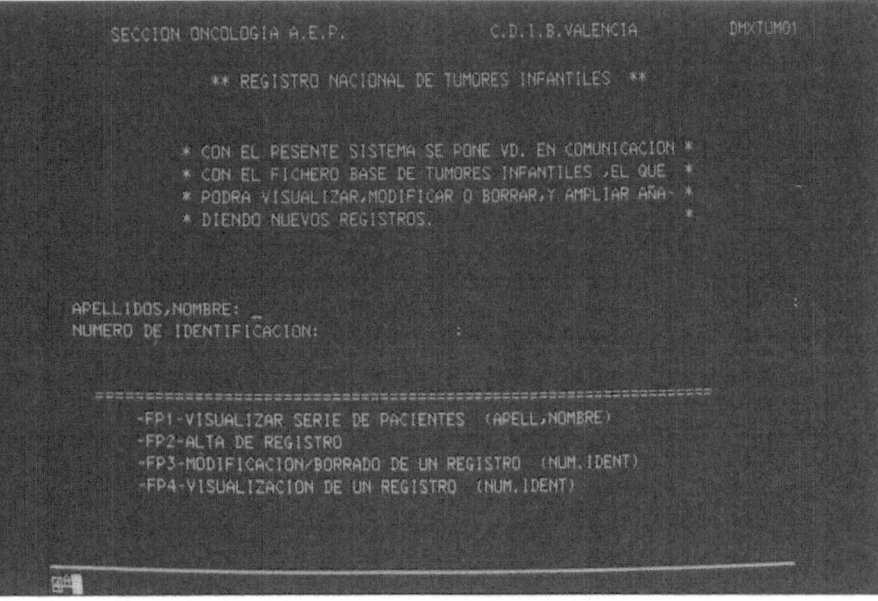

Figure 1

SECCION ONCOLOGIA A.E.P.   C.D.I.B. VALENCIA   TUMPED02

** REGISTRO NACIONAL DE TUMORES INFANTILES **

	N U M E R O	APELLIDOS Y NOMBRE	TOPO	L	MORFO	D
1	813021137491	ARENCIBIA URIEN, ISABEL	1890	1	89600	0
2	813021128550	BARROS ALFONSO, ROBERTO	1954	1	08901	0
3	813021123326	GARCIA ROMAN, DANIEL	1642	1	08580	0
4	813021116524	GIMENEZ SITGES, JUAN ENRIQUE	1915	3	00000	0
5	813021134507	GRACIA VSIETO, CARLOS	1901	1	08901	0
6	813021029567	HIDALGO MARTINEZ, MANUEL	1968	0	96203	1
7	813021141026	ONANDIA PASTOR, MARIA ARANZAZU	1890	1	08960	0
8	813021146103	PALOMAR CLUA, RUBEN	1890	1	08960	0
9	813021143542	PUJOL MAESE, MARC	1890	2	08960	0
10	813021002558	VIDIELLA MARTORELL, ROSA MARIA	1917	3	00007	0

FP1 ... PAG.ADELANTE FP2..PAG.ATRAS   FP3 ... VOLVER A PANEL PRAL.
FP4 ... CONSUL.REG.   FP5..MOD/BORRAR REG.   FP6 ... OTRA PAGINA

NUM

Figure 2

728

ca, 1979.

(3) Organización Panamericana de la Salud. CIE-O. Clasificación Internacional de Enfermedades para Oncología. Washington. OPS Publicación Científica nº 345, 1977.

(4) Organización Panamericana de la Salud. Manual para la Estandarización de Registros de Cancer de Hospital. Washington. OPS Publicación Científica nº 349, 1977.

(5) Maclennan R et al. Cancer Registration and its Techniques. Lyon. International Agency for Research on Cancer, IARC Scientific Publication nº 21, 1978.

(6) IBM. VSE/VSAM General Information. Program Number 5746-AM2. 2nd ed. New York. IBM Corp., 1979.

(7) IBM. Development Management System/Customer Information Control System/Virtual Storage: Program Reference Manual. Program Numbers 5746-XC4 and 5740-XC5. 4th ed., New York. IBM Corp., 1981.

(8) Nie NH et al. Statistical Package for the Social Sciences (SPSS). 2nd. ed. New York. McGraw-Hill, 1975.

AN ANALYSIS OF SHORT-STAY CASES
IN AN ACUTE GENERAL HOSPITAL

Rosemary Hamill,
Medico-Social Research Board
73 Lower Baggot Street
Dublin 2   Ireland

SUMMARY

The reason for admission to hospital of 1181 patients who had lengths
of stay of three days or less were analysed. More than 50% of the
patients were admitted for three principal reasons - for investigations, for minor procedures or as a result of injuries.

1.   INTRODUCTION

1.1 Financial restraints demand that consideration be given to ways
of reducing the cost of treating the sick without in any way
compromising standards of medical care. This is particularly
relevant in the area of general hospital services which receive a
large portion of the health service budget.

Two facts stand out as problems in the provision of hospital services.
First, the number of in-patients has almost doubled in the years 1961
to 1979[1] although the population of the country has only increased by
about 20%[2] in the same period. Secondly, a large proportion of in-
patients spend less than four days in hospital (37% in 1979[3]).
The fact that most of these patients have stays of two days or less
suggests that at least some of the conditions for which patients are
admitted could be treated without the expensive facilities of an
acute general hospital.

The aim of this study is to identify those conditions for which
patients were hospitalized for three days or less in one particular
hospital.

2. METHOD

2.1 The Hospital In-Patient Enquiry Scheme (HIPE).

The HIPE scheme is a reporting system which is organized by the Medico-Social Research Board (MSRB) to collect medical, social and administrative information on all patients discharged from general hospitals (excluding psychiatric and obstetric units). The administrative and social data include age; sex; marital status; area of residence (eg: county); date; method (booked or immediate) and source of admission; date of discharge; place to which discharged (eg: home, other hospital) and the hospital discharge number. The medical data includes main and secondary diagnosis, any surgical operations performed and the consultant code. The diagnoses are coded using International Classification of Diseases (ICD) and the operations are coded using the Classification of Surgical Operation codes, produced by the Office of Censuses and Surveys in London (OPCS).

2.2 The study is based on HIPE returns from one acute general

hospital in 1979. A hospital typical of most general hospitals in terms of size, catchment area (urban-rural) and range of specialties was selected. It treated approximately 9,000 in-patients in 1979 and had 95% coverage by the HIPE.

A systematic sample of 1181 discharges was drawn from all discharges with lengths of stay of three days or less. To avoid the possibility of drawing a sample from one particular reason, discharges were arranged in sequence by month of admission prior to drawing the sample.

Discharges were assigned to specialties according to the consultant code. The specialty, general medicine, includes paediatrics and geriatrics. Length of stay was divided into 1 day, 2 days, 3 days. If a patient was admitted and discharged on the same day this was counted as one day. The principal diagnosis or principal operation on the summary sheet was taken as the reason for admission.

3. FINDINGS

3.1 Table 1 shows that 38% of all in-patients spent three days or less in hospital. Of these 75% (876 out of 1181) were discharged within two days. Deaths accounted for less than two per cent of the short-stay cases.

Table 1

Total number (no.) of patients	9314
Total no. with stays of three days or less (short-stay)	3549
No. in sample	1181
No. of deaths in sample	22

3.2 Almost half of the cases were treated under General Surgery and roughly one-third under General Medicine.

Specialty	No. of cases	% of cases
Surgery	551	46.66
Medicine	381	32.26
Obstetrics and Gyaecology	134	11.35
Otolaryng- ology (ent)	94	7.96
Miscellaneous	21	1.78

Table 2 : Short-stay cases by Specialty

3.3 Conditions dealt with by each specialty. Surgery (551 cases) shown in Table 3. Injuries, the larges group consisted of fractures (44%), non-fracture injuries (26%), observation of injuries (29.6%) and overdoses (0.4%). Most fractures were of the arm (62%) mainly Colles fracture and dislocated shoulders.
Most non-fracture injuries consisted of lacerations and bruising. Observation of injuries were almost all observation of head injuries and 68% of these were discharged within 24 hours.

Condition	No. of cases	% of cases
Injuries	234	42.47
Minor Pro- cedures	90	16.52
Investigat- ions	55	9.98
Symptoms	137	24.86
Other oper- ations	35	6.17

Table 3 : Short-stay surgical cases.

Symptoms, the next largest, is a very broad group and includes
diagnoses such as enlarged tonsils, diarrhoea and prostatism, but
more than half of this group consisted of"abdominal pain"without
mention of procedure or treatment.

The minor procedures preformed were:- removal of cysts, lipomatas,
abcesses, foreign bodies, etc. (65 cases), circumcisions (17 cases),
and removal of in-growing toe-nails (8 cases).

Medicine (381 cases)

		No. of cases	% of cases
One-fifth of the medical	Investigations	77	22.21
cases were admitted for	Overdose	20	5.25
investigations. The group	Respiratory system	69	18.11
"other" consisted of skin	Gastro-Intestinal	53	13.91
conditions, infectious	Central Nervous		
diseases and ill-defined	system	36	9.45
conditinns eg: backache,	Cardio-Vascular		
allergy. pyrexia of	system	30	7.87
unknown origin. There	Haematology	11	2.89
was a slight preponderance	Endocrine	27	7.09
of respiratory conditions.	Ordinary tract	2	0.52
	Other	56	14.7

Table 4 : Short-stay Medical cases

Obstetrics and Gynaelocology (134 cases)

		No. of cases	% of cases
More than half of these			
patients were admitted	Investigations	11	8.12
for investigations	Procedures	62	46.27
(mainly hysterosalpingrams)	Observations, PET,		
and minor procedures. The	Etc.	61	45.52
commonest procedures			

preformed were:- dilation and curettage (D&C), biopsies, vaginal dilations and laparoscopies. 13 out of 62 procedures were

Table 5 : Short-stay obstetric and
                gynaecological cases.

admitted as emergencies. Nevertheless, investigations and elective
minor procedures accounted for 48% of the short-stay obstetric and
gynaecological patients.

The remaining cases were admitted, most frequently, for observation of pregnancy, false labour, pre-eclamptic toxaemia (PET).

ENT (94 cases)

Injuries (mainly fractured nasal bones), investigations, and minor procedures together made up 54% of the cases. The commonest procedures preformed were antral wash-outs, myringotomy and ear toilet.

	No. of cases	% of cases
Investigations	3	3.19
Injuries	8	8.15
Minor procedures	38	40.43
Sinusitis, Tonsill-tiitis, etc.	35	37.23
Oscopies	10	10.64

Table 6 : Short-stay ENT cases

3.4 Table 7 lists the type and number of investigations which were carried out (all specialties). The two commonest were intravenous pylography (IVP) and sigmoidoscopy together amounting to 50% of investigations.

Investigation	No. of cases	% of cases
IVP	52	35
Sigmoidoscopy	22	15
Cyst o graphy	6	4
Unspecified gastro intestinal	15	10
Unspecified urinary tract	9	6
Respiratory	3	2
Barium Studies	10	7
Lumbar puncture	2	1
Glucose tolerance test	10	7
Hysterosalpingrams	7	5
Other (shilling, thyroid, liver, etc.)	11	8

Table 7 : Investigations including all specialties.

3.5 Taking all specialties together, Table 8 shows that 52% of the short-stay cases were admitted for three principal reasons:- for minor procedures (17%) for which 80% had stays of at least two days; as a result of injuries (23%) of which half were discharged within 24 hours or for investigations (12%).

Condition	No. of cases	% of cases
Injuries	267	23
Minor procedures	199	17
Investigations	147	12
	---	--
	613	52

Total no. of short-stay cases 1181

Table 8 : All specialties. Principal reasons for admission.

4.   DISCUSSION

There is evidence from Great Britain and elsewhere that most, if not all of the minor procedures described - general surgical, gynaecological and ENT [4,5,6,7] - can be successfully treated on a short-stay or day care basis. In fact it is estimated[8] that 39% of all surgical admissions can be dealt with in short-stay (5 day) units.

As previously stated more than half of the injuries (57%) were discharged within 24 hours. It is reasonable to assume that these could have been treated in an Accident and Emergency Department given suitable facilities and accommodation. Accordingly, if injuries detained longer than 24 hours are excluded, the three groups listed in Table 8 - investigations, minor procedures and injuries - were suitable for treatment in some kind of alternative care unit. Altogether these accounted for 42% of the short-stay cases.

Long travelling distances from rural areas may explain why some patients were admitted. It was not possible, in this study, to look at the distances patients lived from the hospital. Place of residence, given as County, was not useful in this instance. However, overnight accommodation for these patients could be more economically provided in a short-stay unit.

Where there is pressure on beds with waiting lists for certain conditions and, in some general hospitals, overcrowded wards, the provision of extra beds in short-stay or day units for selected conditions and investigations should reduce the cost and difficulty of treating these patients who do require general hospital facilities.

In conclusion, the study shows that at least 40% of the conditions for which patients were hospitalized for three days or less could have been treated in an "alternative care" unit rather than an acute hospital bed.

5. REFERENCES.

1. Planning Unit, Department of Health, Dublin. Personal communication.
2. Cencus of Population of Ireland 1979 Vol. 1, Stationery Office, Dublin.
3. Hospital In-Patient Enquiry Scheme 1979, Medico-Social Research Board, Dublin.
4. Rainey J. B., Ruckley C. V., Work of a day-bed unit 1972-8, British Medical Journal, 1979,2 714-717.
5. Atwell J. D., et al Paedietric Day-Case Surgery Lancet, 1973, 2 895-897.
6. Berill T. H., A year in the life of a Surgical Day Unit. British Medical Journal, 1972, 4 348-349.
7. Bevan J., Newton J., Eight years' experience with a weekday gynaecological ward. Lancet 1979, 2 137-139.
8. Cliff K. S., The use of hospital activity analysis data in accessing operative procedures suitable for five-day care. Health and Social Services Journal, 1979, A 29-32.

A DATA BASE FOR THE STUDY OF THERAPEUTICAL STRATEGIES FOR HAEMOPHILIACS

Klonk,J., Hoffmann,W.D.

Institute for Medical Informatics
(Director: Prof. Dr. P.L. Reichertz)
Medical School Hannover
3000 Hannover, W-Germany

ABSTRACT

Fifteen treatment centers for haemophilia in northwestern Germany are conducting a multi-center study for monitoring and documenting the ambulatory treatment of this severe bleeding disorder. The data from this study are collected in a hierarchical data base under the data base management system IMS and retrieved using a descriptive query language. The DBMS proves to be a valuable tool to support such a study. The design of and the requirements for specialized DBMS for statistical studies are investigated.

1. MEDICAL BACKGROUND, GOALS AND DESIGN OF THE STUDY

Severe haemophilia is a rather rare hereditary bleeding disorder where the patients suffer from a deficiency of a certain clotting factor. haemophilia A (classic haemophilia), due to a deficiency in clotting factor VIII, is the most common type and accounts for about 70 - 80 %. haemophilia B (christmas disease), due to deficiency in factor IX, accounts for another 10 - 15 % of patients. The remaining 15 % are cases of Willebrand's disease and other seldom types of haemophilia.

PARTICIPATING CENTERS

Dr.Beck, Universitaetskinderklinik, Berlin; Dr.Bock, Staedt. Krankenanstalten, Bielefeld; Dr.Fenne, Kinderklinik, Braunschweig; Dr.Holzhueter, Bremen; Dr.Leithaeuser, Allgemeines Krankenhaus, Celle; Dr.Moesseler, Universitaetskinderklinik, Goettingen; Prof.Tilsner, Chir. Universitaetsklinik, Hamburg; Dr.Kurme, Hamburg; Dr.Skrandies, Dr.Kramarz, Krankenhaus St. Georg, Hamburg; Dr.Barthels, Medizinische Hochschule, Hannover; Dr.Schulz, Kinderklinik St. Bernward, Hildesheim; Dr.Lasson, Universitaetskinderklinik, Kiel; Prof.Asbeck, Medizinische Universitaetsklinik, Muenster; Dr.Mertner, Muenster; Dr.Bartsch, Sarstedt; Prof.Barthelmai, Rehabilitationsanstalten Volmarstein;

Approximately 4270 haemophiliacs live in the Federal Republic of Germany, 3500 suffering from haemophilia A and 770 from haemophilia B (1).

Thirty years ago bleeding to death, mutilation and pauperization was the fate of most haemophiliacs (2). Since the early seventies the production of high quality coagulation factor concentrates in larger amounts is possible. Treatment with this factor concentrate is very succesfull, but extremely expensive (in Germany several 100.000 DM per patient per year) and the general necessity to lower the cost of health care is notorious. In this situation several haemophilia treatment centers in northwestern Germany decided to conduct a common prospective study. 'The value of a prospective survey recording the ambulant treatment of patients suffering from haemophilia consists in the description of the factual conditions: An account of medical attendance can be given, the administration obtains data for planning and hypotheses for future clinical experiments can be generated' (3).

Because of encouraging results from a pilot study in 1977, the participating centers decided in 1979 to establish a longterm study for documentation of therapeutical data and as a multi center study for monitoring ambulatory therapy of haemophiliacs.

Such a documentation-oriented longterm study requires a high degree of flexibility in the management and processing of this data:
- complex data structures have to be handled,
- data arrive in differing time intervals and quantities,
- reports for study-monitoring and for feedback to the participants must be produced,
- unforeseen requests for data-extraction and -evaluation must be served.

2. REALIZATION

2.1 DATAFLOW

Fig. 1 shows the flow of data:
- For every treatment episode the patient fills in the 'Treatment Documentation Form'. This form is printed on NCR-Paper and containes fields describing the indication for the treatment, the dosage, date and time of day for every single injection, and the

outcome of the treatment episode. For longer episodes with many injections an arbitrary number of continuation forms can be used.

- The centers collect the forms from the patients during their visits, check the forms for validity and completeness, compare the sums of prescribed concentrate and documented usage, and send the copy to the central documentation group.
- The documentation assistant types the data into a terminal and initiates computer runs for plausibility checking and for insertion of the error-free data into the data base.
- The study coordinator prepares and initiates computer runs for yearly evaluations, quarterly summary reports on every patient, and ad hoc evaluations as requested by the centers. Other reports are printed for study control and monitoring.

In addition to this treatment documentation form a 'Basic Documentation Form' is filled in for every patient on a yearly basis. This form contains the parameters which change slowly or not at all, like body weight and type of haemophilia, and the results of a yearly assessment of the patients' disablement status.

2.2 THE HAEMOPHILIA DATA BASE

The pilot study showed that effective management of the data from these forms was difficult due to its complex structure and the goals and set-up of the study (3). This situation lead to the decision to use a data base management system (DBMS) and establish a data base.

A semantic analysis (4) of the data acquisition forms described in the preceding paragraph shows:
- There is a number of patients.
- An arbitrary number of basic documentation units belong to every patient.
- An arbitrary number of treatment episodes is related to every basic documentation. (Note that this entity is not identical to the respective form because of the continuation forms.)
- In every treatment episode an arbitrary number of medications is applied.
- The forms do not contain information which is specific to centers and therefore there is no need for entities 'center' in this data base.

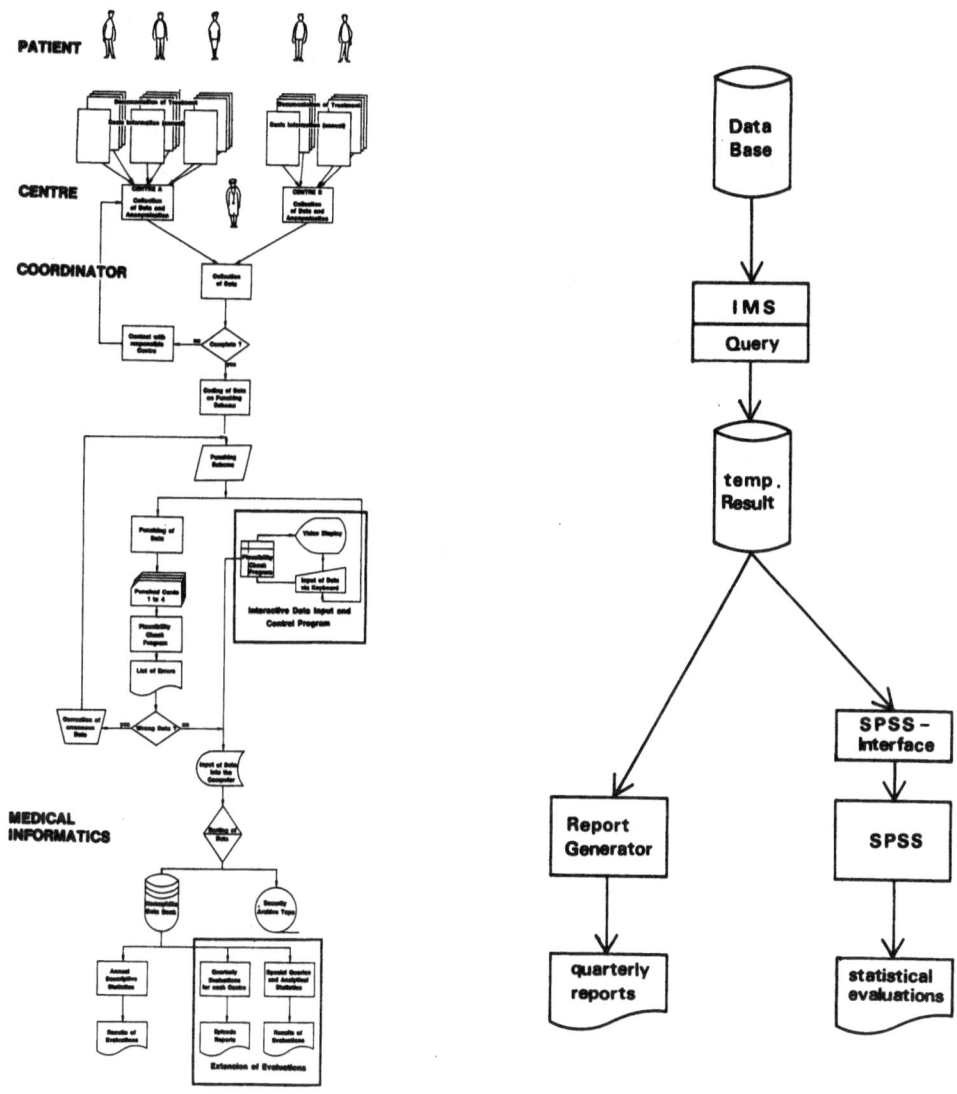

Fig. 1: Data Flow   **Fig. 2:** Data Base Retrieval

The data structure which results from these observations is a linear four-level hierarchy of the 4 entities PAT - BAS - TREAT - MED. It can be translated directly into a data base description for the data base management system (DBMS) IMS (5), which is in use in the Medical System Hannover (6).

The program which was written to load and update this IMS - haemophilia - data base operates in batch as a sequential merge. Fig. 2 gives an overview over the retrieval from this data base. All retrieval is done using the query - system (7) which was developed for the

hierarchical data bases of the Medical System Hannover. This query system permits the descriptive formulation of retrieval requests in a flexible, concise and easy-to-use way.
The query processor passes the data either to a report generator program (for the quarterly reports) or to the statistical program package SPSS (8). As much as possible of the data description for SPSS is generated by the query processor.

3. DATA BASE SYSTEMS FOR STATISTICAL STUDIES

The haemophilia study can be viewed (apart from its medical goals) as an example-study of a data base management systems in longterm statistical or epidemiological studies.

This usage of a DBMS in such a study introduces an additional level of complexity. The usual way of directly submitting the data cards (or card-image records) to the statistical package appears to be much simpler. There is, however, a growing recognition that a DBMS can solve a number of data management problems in studies of the type of haemophilia project (9,10). One of the most important of these is the data structuring problem. The standard input data structure for statistical programs is 'rectangular'. The data structure of the haemophilia study however was shown to be much more complex, and the same applies to many other studies. For the haemophilia data base this problem is solved through the combination of IMS and the query processor: For every type of evaluation the appropriate query generates the data matrix for the statistical evaluation.

Schneider (10) emphasizes that in most studies 'the problems of data-handling, data manipulation and data description are predominant over the problems of analysis', and that statistical packages should be designed modularily, with several autonomous modules. The experience with this study can be summarized in the following list of requirements for the data management module:
a.) Support of complex data structures
b.) No upper limit for the number of record types and occurences, of fields and repetitions
c.) flexible and easy to use data extraction facility
d.) application independent data description
e.) data security
f.) no professional DBMS - knowhow or full-time data base

administrator
g.) support for online data entry and update without programming in a normal general purpose language
h.) support for plausibility checks
i.) support of checks for consistency and completeness

IMS was chosen for this study because this DBMS and trained staff were available. Clearly requirements a.) to e.) are fulfilled by IMS and the query processor, but at present not requirements f.) to i.). Since the design phase of this study specialized DBMS for statistical purposes such as SIR (11) have appeared on the market. SIR is presently beeing installed into the MSH, and conversion of the haemophilia data base to SIR is under investigation.

4. FIRST RESULTS AND CONCLUSIONS

In 1979 and 1980 fifteen centers participated in this documentation project. The number of patients increased from 180 with 2660 treatments in 1979 to 208 patients with 3242 treatments in 1980. One of the preliminary results of the study is shown in Fig.3. There seems to be a relationship between the 'positive' stress on weekends and the occurence of bleedings.

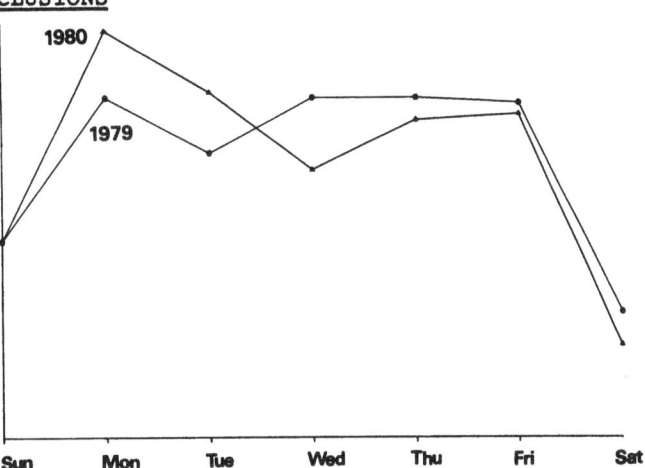

Fig. 3: Frequencies of bleeding episodes over the days of the week

A study on haemophilia with similar goals is in operation at the St. Thomas Hospital in London (12). Compared to the more conventional approach in (12), our approach has the following advantages:
- Only a limited programming effort was needed for the data base update program (approximately 2 man-months), and no special programming for data base retrieval.
- There is no predefined unit of evaluation; 'Patient', 'Basic documentation', 'Treatment episode' or 'Medication' are equally

feasible as cases of the statistical analysis.

- The query system offers the ability to respond to unforeseen requests for reports or statistical evaluations without too much effort. This is particularly important in a documentation study, where there are only global goals.

The major drawbacks of the system are:

- The batch update of the data base is not very elegant. (In the next phase of the study one of the generalized systems which are in use in the MSH for online data checking and data base update will be used.)
- The data base management system requires a qualified data base administrator

Data base management systems prove to be a valuable tool in the conduct of a statistical or epidemiological study, solving the data structure- and data extraction-problem. The integrated design however of an data management system for online data acquisition and checking, for controlling and monitoring the progress of the study and for interfacing to statistical packages and programs remains a topic of research.

REFERENCES

(1) Schimpf K. Die Bedeutung der kontrollierten Selbstbehandlung fuer den Haemophiliepatienten. Blut 1978; 36: 63-71
(2) Marx M, Lechner, K. Zur Prognose der Haemophilien. Lebensversicherungsmedizin 973; 25: 59-65
(3) Reisch A, Reisch G. Northwest German Trend-Study on the Therapy of haemophilia 1977. 1st International haemophilia Conference, Bonn, 1980
(4) Chen PPS. The Entity-Relationship-Model - Toward a Unified View of Data. ACM Trans Database Systems 1976; 1,1
(5) McGee WC. The Information System IMS/VS, Parts I - V. IBM Syst Journ 1977; 16,2
(6) Reichertz PL. The Medical School of Hannover Computer System. In: Collen MF.(ed), Hospital Computer Systems, Wiley, New York 1974
(7) Klonk J, Sauter K. Erfahrungen mit dem Einsatz einer relationalen Datenbankabfragesprache. Angew Informatik, Dez. 1979
(8) Nie NH. SPSS - Statistical Package for the Social Sciences. McGraw-Hill 1979
(9) Kuhner A. et al. Moeglichkeiten der Realisierung einer Schnittstelle bei Datenbanksystemen und statistischen Auswertungssystemen. Statistical Software Newsletter, Vol 6. No.1, (1980)
(10) Schneider B. Statistical Packages for the Analysis of clinical Studies. MEDINFO, 3d World Congress on Medical Informatics, Tokyo 1980
(11) Robinson BN et al. SIR - Scientific Information Retrieval User's Manual, Version 2, Sir Inc. Evanston, Ill. (1980)
(12) Porter DM, Ingram GIC. Computer Monitoring of Haemophilic Bleeds and their Treatment. Medical Informatics Berlin, Springer Verlag, 1979. 427-434

This study is supported by Travenol, Muenchen

COMPUTER SUPPORTED INTERACTIVE DEVELOPMENT OF INFORMATION FLOW SYSTEMS

Roland Lindvall, Hans Karlsson, Olle Rosin, Ove Wigertz
Department of Medical Informatics
Linköping University
S-581 85 LINKÖPING
Sweden

Summary

This paper presents a new method for computer interactive development of information flow systems (rapid prototyping). The basic strategy for this method is to develop a new system in two stages:
- The first stage is to develop a prototype of the intended system in a highly interactive programming environment, using a graphic description language.
- When the prototype is working properly, it can be converted (partly automatic) into a production system, running in a distributed computer environment.

This system offers a promising method of supporting the development of data processing systems, in medicine and elsewhere.

Introduction

Development of computer based information handling systems can be a time consuming process. The result of the process is a production system. When the production system has been running for some time, the user usually finds that his ideas of the system and the system designers interpretation of the system specifications have some discrepancies. Changes in the system at this point are very time and cost consuming.

To facilitate this process a method for rapid prototyping can be used. In available reports on rapid prototyping projects, a general-purpose programming language has been used as the major software tool, for example APL (1). Sometimes the idea of rapid prototyping inspired the design of new generalpurpose languages, for example CS4 (2), whose good facilities for interactive use and for an entity-oriented data base, are particularly suitable for rapid prototyping.

744

Although such languages are probably more suitable than conventional, compilation-oriented languages for rapid prototyping purposes, we believe that special-purpose languages are even better. Some of the most important requirements on software tools for rapid prototyping are:

- they must make it possible to create an initial, simple prototype very quickly
- they must facilitate interaction between the end user and the system designer, not only about unimportant details in the designed system, but also about the essential characteristics of the design
- they must make it possible to incorporate additions and changes into the prototype rapidly, without causing chaos in the structure of the software

It was our hypothesis that special-purpose languages which use the terminology of the application domain have significant advantages in all these respects. We have chosen to work with one particular modelling language, namely for information flow (3,4), where information from administrative routines are modelled as packages of information which flow between workstations in the organization.

The basic overall strategy for this special-purpose language is to develop a new system in the following two stages:

- The first stage is to develop a prototype. The prototype version of the intended data processing system is developed in a highly interactive programming environment. The prototype is a model of the information system, which contributes to documentation and to the flexibility of the system, but it is also a running system which can be used for demonstrations and trial use by the end users of the intended system.
- When the prototype is working properly it can be converted into a production system running in a distributed computer environment, including minicomputers. The conversion procedure is partly automatic.

Method

The intended information handling system is initially described by the end user and the system designer by means of a graphic description method, using special symbols (5) for different operations on the information packages (records). To realize a prototype system the description must be entered into the computer. To accomplish this the graphic language is converted into a formal language (Figure 1) (3) which is entered by means of an interactive computer program. The computer program contains powerful tools for correction and modification of the model.

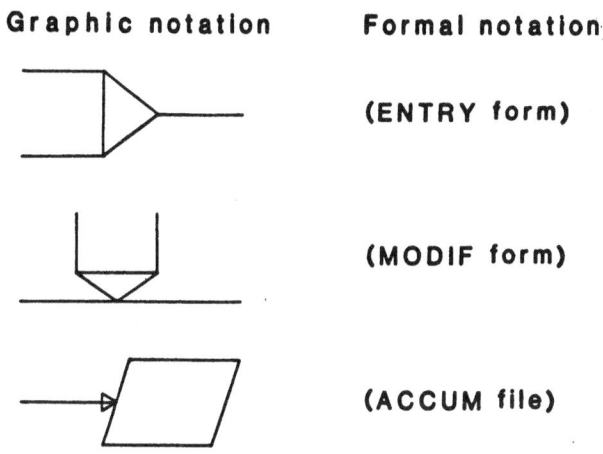

Figure 1

ENTRY - enters record from the user screen using the layout called "form"
MODIF - enters additional information into the current record using the layout "form"
ACCUM - accumulates the current record to the sequence called "file"

The information flow network consists of:

- work stations (e.g. wards and laboratory stations)
- channels, which connect the work stations
- files for information storage
- operations that should be supported at the work stations

The forms for information input (6) and output are built up by means of an interactive computer program, which allows the user to specify type of data and control functions to be executed.

Every form shows a subset of a record. The program allows the same information to be entered (or presented) by different form layouts. For example, different wards can have the same laboratory results presented on different forms, suitable for their needs.

The system was originally developed on a DEC 20 mainframe computer using LISP. Today the model interpreter is also implemented on a PDP 11/44 minicomputer, coded in MUMPS.

Work is in progress to enable a semi-automatic convertion of the prototype into a production system coded in some high level language, probably FORTRAN or PASCAL (7). This production system can be downloaded to a smaller computer, for example a PDP 11/03.

The application

The model and the tools have been used for prototyping in the DASIS project for the development of a comprehensive computer supported information system for medical care. The project was initiated by the Swedish National Board for Technical Development, with the participation of five provincial governments, as well as domestic producers of computer systems and services.

The DASIS system is intended to handle medical information about individual patients in a typical Swedish medical care district with more than 100 000 inhabitants. It will be possible to implement new functions step by step and to tailor the different modules to different specifications in different districts.

The DASIS system can be described as four additive main modules.

MODULE 0 keeps track of when, where and why a person has received medical care.

MODULE 1 contains procedures for the paper-based medical record archives.

MODULE 2 handles the communication between medical care units and service units as chemical laboratories.

MODULE 3 includes input of ordinary text to the medical record by means of word processing facilities.

Example

The method described above has been used to model module 0,1 and 2 of the DASIS system. Figure 2 shows an example from that model, containing wards and the clinical chemical laboratory in a large hospital.

In the wards information about new patients is entered via a form generated on the CRT. The information is stored in a patient record. Laboratory requests are entered via another form. The requests are stored in a check file and are also automatically sent to the laboratory.

In the laboratory, test samples are pro-cessed according to the instructions on the request forms. The analysis results are transferred to the forms, which after approval are returned to the clinic.

In the ward the results are inspected for abnormal results, or processed automatic-ally in the computer to give support for interpretation. The results are then trans-ferred to a cumulative list containing the analysis results for the patient over a period of time, using a layout that the specific user has designed.

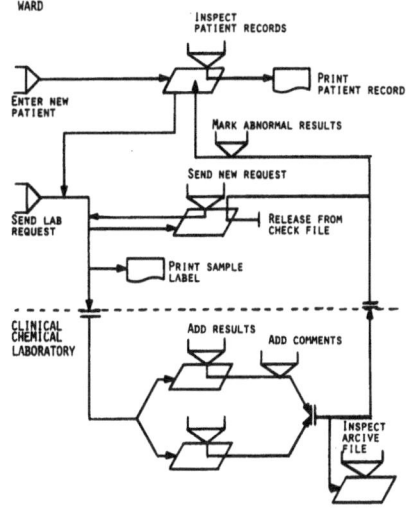

Figure 2

The ward keeps copies of the requests and action is taken if the results are delayed. The laboratory keeps back-up copies of all results.

Discussion

This method, using an information flow model and supporting software tools, has proved to be an effective tool for rapid prototyping, as long as the target system can be described in terms of information flow. So far, this has been no limitation on the system. A certain amount of program code has to be written for each new appli-cation, but several advantages are obtained as compared to conventional programming techniques, for instance, the amount of code is quite small, and restricted to those things which are really specific to the application.

The standard models in the system (that is for forms, information flow, etc.) are not final. The characteristics of the programming system makes it easy to modify these models.

The approach and the system described here offer a promising method of supporting the development of data processing systems, in medicine and elsewhere, and to meet e.g. the objectives:

- cut manpower costs for programming
- cut system development time
- increase the flexibility of the developed system.

References

(1) Gomaa, Hassan, and Scott, Douglas B.H.: "Prototyping as a Tool in the Specification of User Requirements". Proc. of the 5th Int. Conf. on Software Engineering, San Diego, 1981, published by IEEE.

(2) Berild, Stig and Nachmens, Sam, "CS4 - A Tool for Database Design by Infological Simulation", Proc. of the Third Int. Conf. on Very Large Data Bases, Tokyo, 1977, published by IEEE.

(3) Sandewall, E., "A Description Language and Pilot-system Executive for Information-transport Systems", Proc. Fifth Int. Conf on Very Large Data Bases, Rio de Janeiro, Brazil, October 1979, published by IEEE.

(4) Ellis, Clarence A., and Nutt, Gary J.: "Computer Science and Office Information Systems". Computing Surveys, Vol. 12, No. 1, pp. 27-60, March 1980.

(5) Karlsson, H., Kågedal,B., Sandewall, E., Sörensen, H., Tegler, L. and Wigertz, O., "A Notation for Information Flow Models and its Application within Medical Care", Research Report, Dept Medical Informatics, Linköping University, 1981.

(6) Sandewall, E., Strömberg, C. and Sörensen, H., "Software Architecture Based on Communicating Residential Environments", Proc. Fifth Int. Conf. on Software Engineering, San Diego, Calif., March 1981, published by IEEE.

(7) Rosin, O., "Medical Simulation with a Mainframe or Micro. A Case Study of Program Transfer", Proc. 5:th NMMBE Conf., Linköping, Sweden, June 1981.

MICROCOMPUTER AND MUMPS BASED REFERENCE VALUE SUPPORT IN LABORATORY

Vesa Kuusela   Heikki Lang   Liisa Nordman

Department of clinical neurophysiology
University Hospital of Turku
20520 Turku 52, Finland

1.   SUMMARY

In order to achieve a more reliable clinical decision making procedure Kuusela and
Lang (1) suggested that a statistical reference model should replace the conventional
reference values. The adequate usage of the system requires, however, a computer.
This paper deals with the implementation of the model on a microcomputer connected to
the central computer of a hospital running under MUMPS. In this way adequate data
maintenance and computations fast enough were achieved.

2.   INTRODUCTION

The variability of laboratory measurements has been approached from several aspects.
The standardization of the measurement procedure has been found necessary in numerous
situations. Kuusela and Lang (1), however, suggested a new statistical method in order
to achieve more reliable clinical decisions by eliminating part of the variation from
unstandardized measurements. The method is based on a reference model, which replaces
the conventional usage of the reference values.

The suggested method invloves the elimination of the systematic variation from the
measured values through a multiple regression model. The systematic variation means
the part of the total variation which may be explained by known human characteristics
such as age, sex, body temperature, body length, diet etc. Every single value is
compared to the regression model based on the reference sample group, in order to
estimate whether the observation belongs to the reference model (i.e. is "normal").
The independent variables in the regression equation are those causing systematic
variation, and the dependent variable is the one which is measured in the laboratory.

The reference regression model is calculated from so called "normal subjects" thus
reflecting the state of relatively healty persons. The result of the comparison is
given by a probability value, the P-value. The P-value thus gives the probability that
the examined patient is "normal". To be more precise it gives the probability that
the patient belongs to the reference sample group.

The method provides several desirable features and makes the clinical   decision-making
more accurate. On the other hand it requires computing facility to achieve to the best
results. The model has been implemeted in a pocket calculator with a printer, but this
application is quite cumbersome.

A hospital computer system supported by a MUMPS stand-alone system gives adequate means for storing and retrieving of data, but the arithmetic ability of MUMPS is not good for the presented reference model. The fact is that the model requires some fairly complicated calculations (matrix operations, square root, trigonometric functions ets.) for each determination of P-value. It is impossible to use MUMPS for this purpose.

On the other hand a desk-top computer is fast enough for frequent computations of the P-values but its capability of data maintenance is limited. Especially the time needed when data is search from floppy disk or magnetic tape makes the system too slow for routine use in the laboratory in such form which shall be described in next chapter.

We solved the problem by combining the features of the two computer systems. This was done by connecting the desk-top computer of the laboratory as a terminal to the central computer. The laboratory computer can be attached to and detached from MUMPS through a program. In the system implemented the central computer takes care of the data maintenance and the desk-top computer (i.e. the terminal), after receiving the required parameters, takes care of the computations.

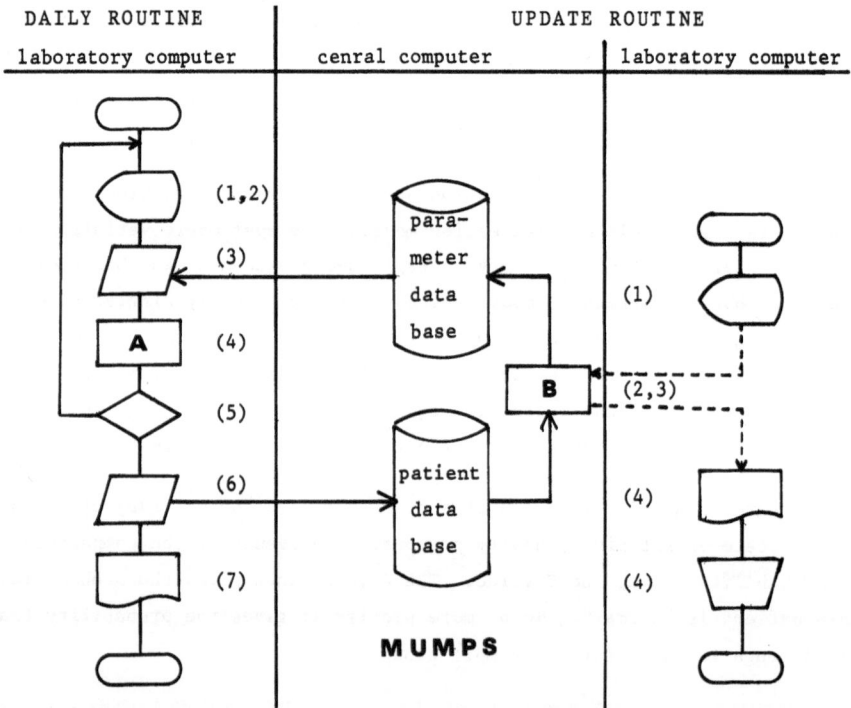

Figure 1: System flow chart of the reference system presented. The numbers refer to the text.

3.   DESCRIPTION OF THE SYSTEM

Two separate routines were built to meet the goals set to the system by the personnel
of the laboratory (see figure 1). It should be noted that both routines involve some
computation procedures: In procedure A (in the daily routine) the P-value for a single
measurement is calculated on the desk-top computer. In procedure B (in the update
routine) the parameters of the reference model are computed by MUMPS. In addition a
procedure for the definition of the new models for new groups of laboratory measurements
is needed.

In order to hinder the reference model from sliding into unreasonable reference range
the results are checked by a doctor after each update run. If evident faults appear
the reference sample group in the patient data base is scanned for the reason. The
functioning of the system is monitored with the help of so called standard patients:
When the new parameters are calculated in procedure B, they are first applied to a few
patients whose data has been analyzed before and trend indicates systematic change.

3.1.   Daily routine in laboratory

The purpose of the system implemented is to give support to the decisions which the
doctor makes concerning the diagnostics, terapy, and prognosis of a patient.   In
addition it does a part of the typist's work and stands as an archieve.

The daily routine in laboratory consists of similar procedures for each patient (see
left side of figure 1).

> (1) Information of the patient is fed into the laboratory computer from data
>   collection sheets. The input routine is highly structured.
>
> (2) Information concerning the measurement is fed in. It is composed of
>   > (a)   the value of the characteristic which is measured,
>   > (b)   the values of the systematic factors included in the model,
>   > (c)   other relevant information (initials of doctor, information
>   >   of other diseases, reference validity etc.)
>
> (3) Parameters required for the elimination of systematic factors and for the
>   computation of P-value are read from the parameter data base of the central
>   computer.
>
> (4) The P-value for the measurement is computed by a program coded in BASIC.
>
> (5) Steps (2) - (4) are repeated until all measurements are analyzed.
>
> (6) The laboratory report is stored in a packed format by MUMPS in the patient
>   data base in central computer.

(7) The laboratory report is printed for the clinician. (Common practice, however, is to use a separate output routine and print all reports of a day at the same time.)

3.2. Updating of the parameter data base

The reference sample group is of crucial importance in all reference models or reference values. Therefore it should not be a fixed set of observations but reflect changes in the population which it represents. In addition the growth of the reference material shortens tolerance intervals if the measurement procedure is reliable.

To allow changes in the reference model we update the parameters of the reference model frequently. This is done simply by computing the parameters from updated patient data base. The suitable cases for the reference sample group are marked in the data base after careful evaluation. A case may be excluded from the reference group, too.

The update routine is as follows: (See right hand side of figure 1)

(1) Information for identification of the measurement for which the parameters are calculated is fed in from terminal.

(2) Parameters for reference model are calculated as follows:

   (a) The data base is scanned for the reference cases,

   (b) the cross product matrix is calculated and

   (c) regression parameters are estimated through an upper triangular SWEEP operation by MUMPS (The SWEEP operation is described by Goodnight in (2)).

(3) Standard patients are analyzed by the new model.

(4) Results are printed and checked before furher use.

The SWEEP operation works well and is fast enough although MUMPS is not at its best with arithmetic operations.

3.3. Furher development of the system

The system presented allows an insertion of new measurements of similar form (i.e. the model consists of same number of variables and they form a linear structure), but the reference model vary between different measurements. The flexible insertion of varying reference models requires a model data base in which each measurement is defined.

4.   TRANSFERABILITY

Only one laboratory was in mind when the system was designed and in addition it is a rather specialized one (neurophysiological). Therefore the system is not directly applicable to other kinds of laboratories. The principle (reference model and P-value) on the other hand is applicable to most laboratory measurements because its generality. In fact we have suggested (1) that the P-value should replace the reference values in many cases.

The system presented is running on PDP 11/44 MUMPS stand-alone system and it requires a minor memory space except the patient data base, which takes 1200 bytes/patient in average. This part of the system fits to all MUMPS applications. The laboratory computer is Tektronix 4051 with 32 Kbytes of central memory and a floppy disk system. The program of the daily routine (A in figure 1) in its present form needs almost all available core memory. This program is coded in BASIC, which has some machine-dependent features.

5.   DISCUSSION

The greatest difficulties in the usage of the system have been in the attitudes: The decision making has been experienced more laborious when the dichotomous division of normality is replaced by a continuum. This and other matters involving the principle are discussed in (1) and we shall not deal with them in this context.

The experience of the system implemeted have been very satisfactory as to our lab. The benefits of the system are most apparent when new measurements are included in the repertoire of the laboratory. The reference material grows at the same speed with the knowledge of the measuremet. On the other hand the patient data base is all the time available for research purposes or e.g. for quality control. One obvious gain is that the daily routine has become more rationalized as before.

The greates difficulties in the implementation was the training of the laboratory personel to accept and use the computer as a component in the daily routine. Besides a typist was changed to a computer operator who partly took care of the programming. When the system was ready it was easy for e.g. nurses to learn to use it.

6.   REFERENCES

(1) Kuusela V, Lang AH. Elimination of systematic variance in laboratory measurements and P-value; A method for reporting laboratory results. In: Lindberg DAB, Reicherts P (eds.) Lecture Notes in Medical Informatics 5, Springer-Verlag, Berlin, 1979, 435-444

(2) Goodnight JH. A tutorial on the SWEEP operator. The American Statistician 1979,33,3

Data Dictionaries in the Software Engineering Environment

G. Klementz and J. Timm
Institute for Medical Informatics and Health Services Research
Department 3: Information Systems
MEDIS-Institut der Gesellschaft für Strahlen- und Umweltforschung, München
Ingolstädter Landstrasse 1, D - 8042 Neuherberg

ABSTRACT

This paper discusses aspects in the realization of project libraries using data dictionaries. Concepts of project libraries and data dictionaries are introduced. The internal structure of the project library is directly related to structuring principles of the software development process. Capabilities of the dictionaries are extended to include the project, the unit, and the library object-type. Additionally, functions to handle instances of these new objects are defined.

1.   Introduction

Massive research in the field of software technology is in progress to curb the rising costs of software development. Three areas of interest have evolved in this endeavor: high level programming languages, software development methodology, and the software engineering environment (1) A result of the research in the software engineering environment is the concept of   project libraries.   Simultaneously, research in the data base management systems brought about the evolution of data dictionaries.

The functional capabilities of data dictionaries, when modified and extended, encompas many of those required by project libraries. This paper will not present new project library concepts rather their realization using data dictionaries.

2.   Software Development

Modern methodologies support a structured approach to software development. The project library as a tool of the software engineering environment eases the practical application of these methods.

2.1 Software Engineering Methodology

Many of the development methods use a top down approach. Following systems analysis, the requirements having to be fulfilled by the completed product are defined These go as input into the product specification phase where the product's interface to the outside - either to a user or to other system components - is defined. This is followed by the decomposition - generally according to functional classes - of the product into components. The components are then specified and if necessary, further decomposed until a continuation of this process is no longer necessary. This defines the modular level where specification is directly followed by coding. It is the lowest level in the hierarchy resulting from the top down approach. Module implementation is followed by module validation and integration. Validation and integration of components follow in a bottom up manner until the highest level i.e. the completed product, is reached.

2.2. Project Libraries

A project library is a set of files containing a project's documents or at least references to those which cannot be stored in the computer. An overview of existing realizations is given in (2), and a discussion of project libraries' usage in (3) and (4). Objectives to be fulfilled by project libraries include centralized storage of a project's information, establishment of guidelines for all stages of production, concurrent development of documentation and product, increased visibility of the production process, and the existence of the current product version at all times. The structuring principle and the operations introduced are similar to those presented by Denert in (5).

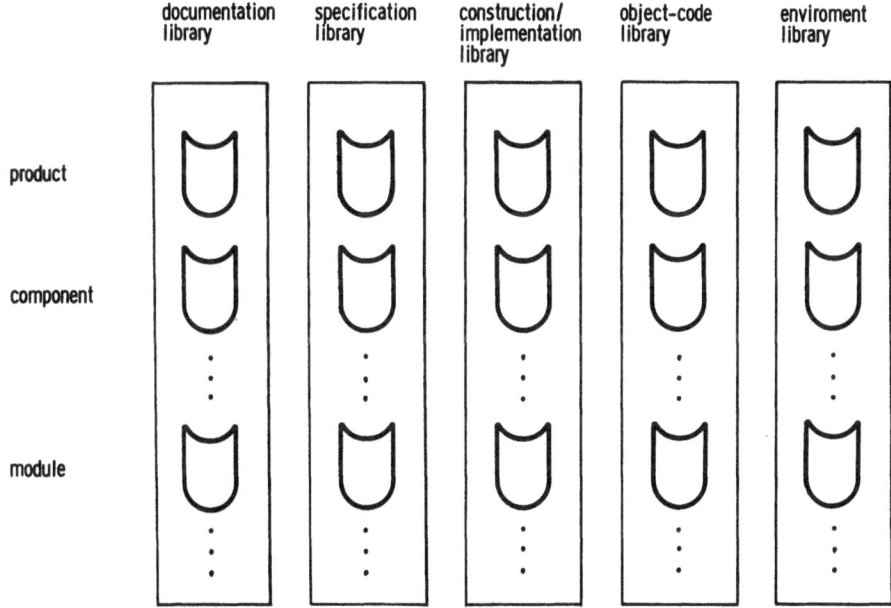

Figure 1: Structure of the project library.

The documents of a project are divided into five classes, each associated with a sublibrary and distinguished by their type of contents. Each sublibrary is logically further subdivided in correspondence to the product's decomposition into units (Figure 1). The documentation library contains general information i.e. overview, conventions, references etc. Additionally, the results of a product's requirements analysis phase are included. Specification, construction / implementation, and object code are stored in corresponding libraries. Test frameworks, compiling, and binding information belong to the environment library. Since the project library includes the documents of all phases of the project, a separation between those that are still evolving and those that are completed is made.

A project is not a static object. This necessitates the existence of functions which allow to manipulate the library's contents. Operations which add and modify documents in the library must be available. A reporting facility must be foreseen to aid project administration The support of programmers and systems designers is realized by providing copying functions.

3. Data Dictionaries

Traditionally, the data dictionary was a repository of data about an organisation's data. Every data item was defined there along with a list of its attributes. Data dictionaries are generally used in conjunction with data base management systems to assist in the administration of data. Further information on data dictionaries is presented in (6) and (7).

3.1. Entry Types

All data dictionaries contain data structure and processing entries. Data structure entries generally include definitions for: data bases, files, and fields. Attributes of these categories can be: object type, length, access rights etc. Processing entries define systems, programs, modules, and procedures. Attributes here include: programming language, access rights, parameters etc.

3.2. Functions

A data dictionary is useful in increasing the transparency of the data processing environment. All objects defined in the dictionary are cross-referenced enabling questions of the following type to be answered:
- Which files are accessed by program B ?
- Which files belong to data base C ?
- Who is the author of program B ?
- Which users have access rights to field D ?

An online query facility should be part of every data dictionary system enabling immediate access to all information. Reporting and maintenance should be possible in both batch and online mode.

Most dictionary systems include a utility for the creation of copy code. This supports the one-time definition of a data item in adherence to the organization's standards. Code for the copy libraries is created for use in applications development.

4. Enhancements to the Data Dictionary

4.1. Entry Enhancements

The dictionary is extended to include four new entry-types defining the project and the project library as objects of the environment:

```
ENTRY   project;                        ENTRY library;
projectname     : identifier;           librarytype   : ONE OF (documentation,
description     : text;                                         specification,
commissioned_by : LIST OF person;                               construction /
date_started    : date;                                         implementation,
date_due        : date;                                         object-code,
personell       : LIST OF person;                               environment);
structure       : TREE OF unit          libraryfiles  : LIST OF projectfile;
ENTRYEND                                relationships : LIST OF link
                                        ENTRYEND


ENTRY unit;                             ENTRY project-file;
unitname        : identifier;           filename      : identifier;
unittype        : ONE OF (product,      owner         : LIST OF person;
                          component,    version       : ONE OF (accepted,
                          module);                              work);
personell       : LIST OF person;       relationships : LIST OF link
date_due        : date;                 ENTRYEND
relationships   : LIST OF link
ENTRYEND
```

The project-entry is used to characterize a software project. "description" contains a short explanation of the project and its goals, "personell" is a list of persons involved in the project, and "structure" represents the hierarchical ordering of the project's units.

The five different library types comprising a project library are characterized by the library-entry. Each library is of one of the above indicated types and contains a number of project-files. The entry has a list of the names of these files. The field "relationships" in this entry as well as in the other entries cross-references objects.

The units (i.e. components and modules) into which a product is subdivided are all characterized by the unit-entry. "unittype" indicates, whether a product, a component, or a module is represented.

Each file in the system belonging to a project library is called project-file. This name is used to distinguish it from the standard-file category of the system. A project-file occurence is associated with a project-file-entry in the dictionary. The "version" of a project-file-entry indicates the project-file's status. Files that have been reviewed and approved are marked "accepted" while those still being developed are marked "work".

4.2. Operations Enhancements

The operations on a project library can be divided into two classes: one containing those that operate directly on the dictionary and the other containing those operating directly on the project-files For the purpose of this paper, only the operations of the first class will be discussed.

CREATE_PROJECT, MODIFY_PROJECT, DELETE_PROJECT:
A project-entry and the library entries are created in the dictionary with CREATE_PROJECT Additionally a unit-entry of type "product" is generated and registered in "structure" of the project-entry. MODIFY_PROJECT allows the alteration of the contents of all fields in the project-entry except "structure" (cannot be explicitly modified). DELETE_PROJECT deletes all entries in the dictionary and all project-files belonging to a project after being archived.

CREATE_UNIT, MODIFY_UNIT:
CREATE_UNIT creates a unit-entry which is noted in the project-entry's "structure". MODIFY_UNIT allows the changing of the contents of all fields in a unit-entry. An alteration of the "unittype"-field results in the modification of "structure" in the project-entry.

CREATE_PROJECTFILE, MODIFY_PROJECTFILE:
By invoking CREATE_PROJECTFILE, a project-file-entry in the dictionary is created, a file in the system is generated, and the appropriate library-entry is updated. The entry's fields are altered with MODIFY_PROJECTFILE. A programmer will lose access rights to a file if it belongs to a module-unit and "version" is changed from "work" to "accepted". This prevents the modification of the file's contents without project management's approval.

COPY_DATA_DESCRIPTION, COPY_PROCESSING_DESCRIPTION:
These operations copy data or processing descriptions from the dictionary's data and processing categories into project-files.

5. Usage of the Enhanced Data Dictionary

When initiating a project, CREATE_PROJECT is issued by the project management to generate the basic dictionary entries upon which the ensuing phases are built. After having filled these entries with the necessary data, information pertaining to the systems design stage is written into appropriate project-files (each generated by CREATE_PROJECTFILE). This includes the formulation of requirements and the decomposition of the product into components.

The development of each component starts with the CREATE_UNIT operation ("unittype" is set to "component"). This is followed by invoking CREATE_PROJECTFILE, allocating the necessary project-files to the unit. The generation of new unit-entries for components and their associated project-files continues hand in hand with the product's decomposition. At the lowest level of the hierarchy, CREATE_UNIT is invoked with "unittype" = "module".

The programmer assigned to a module uses the information in the specification library associated with the module as input for its implementation. Data structures required for coding are written into copy libraries with the dictionary's copy-code facility. The object-code of the completed module is stored in the object-code library. Testing and binding information is written into the environment library.

Definitions of data structures and procedure headings representing parts of specifications can be made in all phases of a product's decomposition. This is done directly in the data dictionary where an indication of their incomplete nature must be set. These specification-parts may then be copied into appropriate project-files with the COPY_DATA_DESCRIPTION and COPY_PROCESSING_DESCRIPTION operations. These functions are required since the standard copy-code capability generates only code (in copy libraries) for data structures and not for procedures.

The implementation of a module is followed by its validation. Project management accepts the project-files associated with each module with the MODIFY_PROJECTFILE operation, changing "version" from "work" to "accepted". The integration of a component's modules can begin when all have been accepted. A project-file to store the bound object code is created for each component. Integration, validation, and acceptance proceeds in each level of the hierarchy in an analog manner until the highest level, i.e. the completed product, is reached. This marks the end of the project and results in the archiving followed by the deletion of all of the project's entries and files with DELETE_PROJECT.

6. Conclusions

The concepts presented in this paper represent ideas which are to go into a first realization of a project library using a data base system and a data dictionary available at the MEDIS institute. The dictionary enhancements are by no means complete. Additional functions and modifications of entry-fields will evolve with the further development of these concepts. This approach to project libraries is practical for those data processing installations already having data dictionaries.

REFERENCES

(1) Hesse, W.: Methoden und Werkzeuge zur Software-Entwicklung: Einordnung und Überblick. Proceedings, Werkzeuge der Programmiertechnik, GI-Arbeitstagung (Karlsruhe 1981), Springer 1981, 113 - 153.

(2) Denert, E.: Projektmodell und Projektbibliothek: Grundlagen zuverlässiger Software-Entwicklung und Dokumentation. Informatik-Spektrum 1980, Heft 4, 215 - 228.

(3) Schnupp, P.; Floyd, C.: Software - Programmentwicklung und Projektorganisation. Walter de Gruyter 1979.

(4) McGowan, C.; McHenry, R.: Software Management. Research Directions in Software Technology. MIT Press 1979, 207 - 253.

(5) Denert, E.: The Project Library - A Tool for Software Development. Proceedings, IEEE 4th Int. Conf. on Software Engineering 1979, 153 -163.

(6) Reusch, P.: Informationssysteme, Dokumentationssprachen, Data Dictionaries. BI Wissenschaftsverlag 1980.

(7) Uhrowczik, P.: Data Dictionary/Directories. IBM Systems Journal, Vol. 12, Num. 4 1973, 332 - 350.

THE DEVELOPMENT OF A LOW COST LABORATORY INTERFACE UNIT.

J. Ryan. H.C.I.L.
Dublin.

This paper describes the development of a low cost
microprocessor based laboratory interface module.   The
design strategy of reducing the complexity of the circuit
to gain low cost of maintenance, low mean time to repair,
and low unit cost without sacrificing flexibility is
presented.

INTRODUCTION

The main objective in developing the interface unit described
here was to reduce the cost of a MUMPS based laboratory system.[1]
The system was to support on line several Technicon and LKB
analyers of various types and ages.   The interfacing methods
employed in the MUMPS system required PDP 11/03 micocomputers
as interface controlers.   The cost of the necessary interfacing
equipment was almost one third of the total cost of the system.
While reduction of the unit cost was of prime importance, the
opertunity was taken to design into the units features that
would make them both flexible and easy to maintain.   Experience
has shown that intermittent faults on interfaces can be the
most costly, with each service engineer claiming the fault
is not on his machine.   It should be possible therefore
to break the link and monitor the data transmission using
simple equipment thus speeding up the diagnosis of the
fault.   As the commonest device on a MUMPS system is a
VDU the maintenance procedures were based on the use of a
VDU as line monitor and mainframe/interface emulator.
Thus with a working interface and a VDU it would be possible
to locate the source of an error.   Instead of building
into the interface complex self test features it was decided
to reduce the circuit complexity to a level that made
replacement of the whole unit possible.

[1] O'Moore, R.R., Love, Wm. C., Ryan, J., Ratcliffe, J.,
Mc Sweeney, J.R., Cranny, A., Field, L. Experience with a
MUMPS based system for clinical chemistry. Medical Informatics
Europe Dublin 1982, pp. 82-88. Ed. R.R. O'Moore, Barber, P.L.
Reichertz, F. Roger, Springer-Verlag Berlin Heidelberg New York.

DESIGN OBJECTIVES

LOW UNIT COST

The unit cost should be low enough to justify:
a)   total replacement as the prefered method of repair.
b)   the use of the unit on analysers with their own control
     computers.

ONE STANDARD MODULE

The unit electronics should be electrically and mechanicaly
identical.   All function configuration data should be held in a
"personality PROM"

INTERFACE TO MOST ANALYSERS.

Thus must accept as input:
a)   RS232 (Minimum subset)
b)   20 mA current loop.
c)   SERIAL BCD.
d)   PARALLEL BCD.
e)   PARALLEL BINARY.
f)   STROBED OR TIMED DATA.
g)   ANALOG (8 channels)

SUPPORT A CONTROL VDU

The VDU should be software switchable to act as a terminal for
the mainframe.

SUPPORT A CONTROL MICROCOMPUTER

The microcomputer could be one attached to a analyser or one
used for statistics or data reduction.

LINK TO THE HOST AS A CONVERSATIONAL TERMINAL.

The linking protocol must have full error checking and recovery.

PROVIDE ALARM OUTPUTS.

HARDWARE.

The hardware configuration decided upon was:

a)   8085 Micro processor.
b)   8K static RAM.
c)   8k EPROM.
d)   3 x programable USARTs.
e)   66 buffered programable I/O lines.
f)   DATEL MDAS-8D 8 channel A/D converter.

This was constructed on a printed circuit board approximately
150 mm. X 250 mm. in size.   The USARTs, under software control,
can handle both asynchronous and synchronous transmissions up to
56k baud.   The I/O lines are arranged into six eight bit ports and
three six bit ports.   Each line is individually addressable and
may be programed to be input or output.   The DATEL a/d converter
was kept as a separate board due to the fact that it need special
power supplies and also because the majority of analysers do not
need an analog interface.   Thus the laboratory interface unit
contains three modules.

1)   Main circuit board.
2)   Connector harness and analog board.
3)   Power supply.

SOFTWARE

It was decided to use Assembler rather than BASIC as the
programing language in order to reduce the size of the
routines in ROM and to gain the maximum speed from the 8085.
The software has been written as a library of Assembler routine
on a CP/M based system running microsoft MACRO.   Standard routines
are available to handle the prompt/response sequence with the
mainframe, to calculate checksums, to monitor status lines and other
such common tasks.   Although program development in Assembler
tends to be slow, with a well maintained routine library and
orthodox programming technique, it can rival BASIC for this type
of application.   For diagnostic and developmental use 2K basic
is available.

EXAMPLE HARDWARE CONFIGURATIONS (SMAC ON LINE)

SERIAL PORT 1   TO PDP 11/44 (RS232)
SERIAL PORT 2   Input from SMAC
INPUT PORT 1 (8) Control/Reset
OUTPUT PORT 1 (8) Alarm/Status

This configuration would act as a basic resetable data rate buffer and would prevent data loss due to any extended response time on the PDP 11/44.

SERIAL PORT 1   TO PDP 11/44 (RS232)
SERIAL PORT 2   Input from SMAC
SERIAL PORT 3   Control VDU
INPUT PORT 1 (8) Reset.

This configuration would provide improved control such as batch editing, scheduling and basic quality control.

HARDWARE CONFIGURATION (IL 543 FLAME)

SERIAL PORT 1   TO PDP 11/44 (RS232)
INPUT PORT 1 (8) Bit 0x8
INPUT PORT 2 (8) Bit 1x8   IL 543 flame.
INPUT PORT 3 (8) Bit 2x8
INPUT PORT 4 (8) BIt 3x8
INPUT PORT 5 (8) Read strobe.
OUTPUT PORT 1 (8) Hold data.

This configuration could provide data logging from an IL flame (//BCD), data buffering and transmission to the PDP 11/44.

HARDWARE CONFIGURATION   (LKB RACKGAMMA)

SERIAL PORT 1   TO PDP 11/44 (RS232)
SERIAL PORT 2   TO LKB Rack Gamma
INPUT PORT 1   (8) Data in from Apple.
INPUT PORT 2   (8) Control in from Apple.
OUTPUT PORT 1 (8) Data out to Apple.
OUTPUT PORT 2 (8) Control out to Apple.

This configuration would interface an Apple microcomputer to the LKB providing the control terminal needed for the LKB.

DISCUSSION

The unit described provides interfacing facilities for most laboratory equipment while making as few assumptions about the nature of the output date from the analyser as possible. Although the unit is very flexible it is, most importantly, simple and cheap. The costs have been switched for hardware to software allowing the inventory cost of the processor board to be kept below $100. This simplicity provides for low cost maintenance. Any failure in the unit itself can be quickly rectified by replacing the entire unit. If the failure is in either the analyser or mainframe or is intermittent in nature then the unit can be used to isolate the two machines from each other and thereby cut short the arguments between the service engineers as to which machine is failing.

Although the unit was designed to interface to a MUMPS system the hardware and methods are generally applicable to any system that supports standard interactive VDUs. The ability of the unit to tolerate very long response times from the mainframe allows the system to be loaded to its maximum capacity without the fear of data over run.

Although the hardware described was custome built system boards with similar functional specification are available from :-

1)   INTEL CORP. 3065 Bowers Avenue, Santa Clara CA.
2)   RCA Solid State Sommerville New Jersey U.S.A.

A SYSTEM FOR ON-LINE DETECTION AND ANALYSIS OF SACCADIC EYE MOVEMENTS

Mladen A. Vouk
University computing centre
Engelsova bb, 41000 Zagreb
Yugoslavia

Ljiljana Kaliterna
Institute for Medical
Research and Occupational Health
M. Pijade 158, 41000 Zagreb
Yugoslavia

A mini computer based system for real-time aquisition and analysis of saccadic eye movements is described. The system incorporates a module for calibration, data aquisition, identification of saccades and extraction of the basic saccade parameters and a module for graphic display of the collected information. The software was developed and tested on a DECLAB PDP 11/03 minicomputer system (A/D converters, diskettes, 32 kB memory, kW 11 clock). All programs (including the basic signal identification routine) are written in FORTRAN while the communication with the A/D converter channels is achieved through DECLAB 03 FORTRAN Extensions Library subroutines (1) which greatly facilitates software installation and maitenance.

The saccade identification algorithm is based upon the Baloh et al (2) model and has the following characteristics:

Saccade analysis is passive in the sense that the generation of exciting impulse is completely independent of the reaction analysis procedures (i.e. exciting pulses are not generated by program). Duration of the experiment is not limited, however, after a preset maximum number of accepted excitation pulses and eye responses, analysis of the acquired data is discontinued. Frequency of saccade excitation pulses is not greater than about 30. Hz. Sampling frequency is 200 Hz but can be varied if necessary. Calibration and initial triggering of the sampling process are semi-automatic operations i.e. activited by the operator. For data acquisition and signal identification the following strategy was employed. Data are collected (sampled) from three A/D channels, a channel carrying excitation pulses and two channels carrying eye reactions, however most of the time, analysis is performed for the data from the excitation pulses channel. Once a saccade is identified on a reaction channel monitoring and analysis of this channel is dicontinued. When saccades are identified on both reaction channels reaction monitoring is finished and monitoring of the control channel is resumed. Monitoring of the reaction channel data is performed only for periods not exceeding maximum latency of the saccade with respect to the exciting pulse, after that if a saccade has not been detected analysis switches to control channel data only.

767

Sampled data are processed asynchronously in a "circular" buffer subdivided into three
sub-buffers consisting of intermeshed grids each of which stores the data for one of
the A/D inputchannels. The average sub-buffer processing frequency must be greater
than the data input frequency.

To reduce the sensitivity of the identification algorithm to noise the input data
are prior to analysis filtered by a simple moving digital filter of the type (e.g.
2,3)

$$Y_i = Y_{i-1} \ 0.25 + Y_i \ 0.5 + Y_{i+1} \ 0.25$$

Additional immunity to noise, anticipatory saccades and eyeblinks is achieved through
the fact that reaction channels are analysed only within the "window" defined by the
minimum and the maximum saccade latency with respect to the exciting signal. Resulting
noise immunity is quite high and saccades are correctly identified for signal to noise
ratios as poor as 7 db. Outputed information is the ordinal number of the registered
exciting pulses, channel number, the time (after sampling has been started) at which
the pulse was registered, reaction saccade latency, saccade amplitude and deflection
direction, saccade accuracy, maximum recorded eye velocity, time of the maximum velocity with respect to the begining of the saccade, saccade duration and the average eye
velocity. A warning is issued if, for an excitation-reaction set of data, target deflection and reaction deflection directions do not match or no reaction corresponding to
saccade specifications was detected. If a warning is issued results for that set have
to be compared with the analogue picture of the data (e.g. poligraph tracing) in order
to determine whether the reaction is an artifact or an actual subject reaction.

Reproducibility of the calculated saccade parameters is quite satisfactory even in the
case of poor signal to noise ratio. For instance for an average peak noise of 3 degrees
setting discrimination threshold to three degrees produces parameter reproducibility
(e.g. for saccade amplitude, average eye velocity) of about 99% for excitation pulses
and reactions have amplitudes six degrees or larger. The choise of an adequate discrimination threshold is very important since too low a threshold results is acceptance
of false signals while too high a threshold results in the loss of information. Experience shows that best results are obtained when the detection threshold is aproxima-
tely equal to the average peak to peak noise on the channel. Accuracy of the parameters
determined by SAKADA depends on the signal to noise ratio and the discrimination threshold used for the analysis. The system was used for investigation of saccadic eye
movements of persons exposed to low concentrations of pesticides (4).

(1) DEC (Digital Equipment Corporation - Massachusetts), 1977,
    "DECLAB 03 FORTRAN Extensions User's Guide", DEC Order No.
    AA-4951A-TC.
(2) Baloh R.W., Sills A.W., Kumley W.E. and Honrubia V., 1975,

"Quantitative measurement of saccade amplitude, duration and velocity",
Neurology (Minneapolis), Vol. 25, 1065-1070

(3) Lehtinen I., Lang A.H., Jäntti V and Keskinen E., 1979,
"Accute effects of alcohol on saccadic eye movements", Psychopharamacology,
Vol. 63, 17-23.

(4) Elsa Reiner (principal investigator), 1980., Behavioural studies in workers
chronically exposed to pesticides, Toxicology of Pesticides (EPA Grant R
804530919) Final report June 1980., Institute for Medical Research and
Occupational Health, Zagreb, pp 80-97.

THE DEVELOPMENT OF A DISTRIBUTED SYSTEMS APPROACH
IN A TEACHING HOSPITAL

P. Drury
Project Officer
Sharpey-Schafer Centre
St Thomas' Hospital
LONDON SE1 7EH

1. INTRODUCTION

This paper discusses the development of proposals for a distributed system of
computing in St Thomas' Hospital to replace an old centralised mainframe. The
results of a survey of current information processes in the hospital suggested that
a distributed system would be more congruent with the reality of a set of semi-
autonomous departments and activities, and have other merits besides. The principles
of the proposed solution to meet the objectives of such a system, and its initial
configuration, are discussed. Finally, some of the implications for management in
the development of a distributed system are considered.

2. THE DEVELOPMENT OF COMPUTING IN THE HOSPITAL

In 1971, St Thomas' formed a consortium with three other teaching hospitals in an
experimental 'Coordinated Project', funded by the DHSS. The overall aim of the
St Thomas' computer system was to function as an inter- and intra-departmental
communication network, based on a centralised store of patient-oriented data that
could be easily accessed, maintained and manipulated by staff in any department
provided they had the appropriate authority. The main technical goal was integration
of all relevant data within a single centrally maintained store. However, it became
clear, in 1978, that neither the DHSS nor the Regional Health Authority would be able
to continue to support the project in the future and that the suppliers' maintenance
of the Sigma 6 would stop in 1983. As a result, the District began to develop a
Strategic Plan for a new computing system.

3. UNDERSTANDING THE NATURE OF THE HOSPITAL'S REQUIREMENTS

Although the users were not completely satisfied with the Sigma 6 based system (e.g.
because it was only available five days a week, was not as reliable as requirements
dictated, and developments were slow) it was tacitly accepted that a large centrally
integrated type of system architecture would be best suited to the District's needs.

Because of the potentially strong interactions between applications in this kind of
design, it was necessary to adopt a global approach to planning the functional
requirements of the system. In an attempt to get a picture of information processes
across the Distirct, about fifty 'Interest Groups' were set up, comprising computer
staff and representatives of the users in each department (and some of the users
with whom they shared their information). They were asked to respond to a questionnaire which was designed to provide information about their activities, current
information processes and their current information problems. They were asked to
report within six weeks. This short time was imposed because of the timetable's
requirements for phasing out the Sigma 6 and the introduction of its replacement.

The results of this exercise, which was the first recent attempt to find out systematically how the hospital actually generates, stores and uses information raised
doubts about the wisdom of pursuing the objective of a totally integrated whole-
hospital system. It quickly became evident that the scope of the survey was much
too great to be accomplished fully in the six weeks. Some groups did not meet, others
could not produce a report in time. It also became clear that whilst some users with
Sigma based systems were happy with them, others were not. The extent of user enthusiasm for developing computer applications also varied widely.

From consideration of the seventeen groups who did submit a report and a detailed
analysis of some of them, a picture developed of the hospital as a large number of
semi-autonomous operational units each of which have about five distinct centres of
activity within them. Types of activities involved included the primary processes
with which the unit is concerned e.g. providing care on a ward, analysing specimens
or registering patients. Another group of activities were concerned with patient
information in a more aggregated sense, e.g. maintaining record storage and retrieval
systems or producing various patients' statistics.

A third group of activities concerned resource management and involved the monitoring,
planning and controlling of resources necessary to perform the primary process. The
number of other operational units which provided, or were provided with, information
averaged about nine per Interest Group.

The way the activity centres interact with each other within each operational unit
is extremely complex, as is the way the units interact with each other. Not surprisingly, communication problems are very common. It became increasingly clear that a
major objective in any new strategy must be the provision of an effective, flexible
and reliable vehicle for the transfer of information between units.

4. OBJECTIVES OF THE PROPOSED SOLUTION

Soon after the Interest Group exercise was completed, the Computer Steering Committee began to consider the merits of a Strategic Plan in which the overall design was based on the controlled decentralisation of computing. Bearing in mind the increasing turbulance of the hospital's environment (e.g. the 1982 reorganisation, and the increasingly severe resource constraints) the objectives of this approach were to design a system which would:

a) enable users to assume a direct and responsible role in the operation and development of their information systems

b) allow relatively independent development in each application area in terms of timing, design features, interfaces to non-computing devices and equipment chosen

c) provide a highly secure, reliable and available communications service to allow users to request or provide information to other users (both on and off the hospital site) either directly or via message store and forward/collect systems

d) minimise the cost and commitment required for the systems infrastructure which supports the various applications

e) allow incremental and 'organic' development so that advantageous developments in computer technology can be incorporated as resources permit

f) develop modules which can be transferred efficiently from one application to another, and to allow application systems to be transferred to other Districts.

The outcome from these proposals and discussions was a broad agreement, endorsed by the District Management Team, that the new system should, in principle, be decentralised, highly modular and supported by a passive communication and information network.

5. DESIGN PRINCIPLES OF THE PROPOSED SOLUTION

The term Shared Service Network (SSN) was coined to describe the communications network and the central facilities it provides to users, whilst it is through this network that users share their information. The design principles of the SSN are outlined below.

The communications network is to be transparent to the user, be available 99.95% of the time and control access (and security) to itself, other SSN facilities and other users both on and off the hospital site.

Attached to the communications network are to be a number of commonly shared facilities:-

a) a 'bulletin board' will be used to provide access by all users, or a subset of
    users, to files of information which do not change every few minutes. An example
    might be a patient location file, which was changed on a regular basis by admiss-
    ions and wards, and was accessed by many users. It may consist of one or more
    small computers with associated software for file handling and transaction manage-
    ment, and requires a response time averaging two seconds

b) a message handler will accept both structured and unstructured non-urgent messages
    to be passed between users in a 'store' and 'collect' (and possibly a 'store and
    forward') mode. As with the bulletin board, it will require a 99.5% availability
    and be able to handle files and manage transactions with a response time averaging
    two seconds

c) a patient identification system will allow users to access patient data to deter-
    mine whether or not a particular patient had been in contact with the hospital
    before, or to verify or obtain relevant identification details. It requires a
    response time of less than two seconds, 99.5% availability and transaction manage-
    ment facilities

d) system development aids will be available to all authorised staff who wish to
    develop application systems running on a range of different equipment hardware
    and software.

To allow subscribers the maximum freedom to choose equipment, whilst also establishing
the discipline essential for effective use of the SSN, four classes of service are
proposed, which are not mutually exclusive. The first assumes no direct contact with
the SSN, i.e. data has to be transferred in by magnetic tape, re-keying, etc. For
those occasional users who want, for example, to identify single patients or users
remote from their own system a second class of service offers a simple two-way transparent transmission capability. A 'do-it-yourself' class offers access to all the
facilities of the SSN but no communications software routines, and may be useful to
those for whom a particular packaged system justifies the cost of writing them. All
major users are recommended to use the full class of service which offers all the SSN
facilities, communication software routines and comprehensive hardware and software
support. A centralised network diagnostic facility is also required to monitor, test
and reconfigure the network.

6. THE INITIAL CONFIGURATION

The initial configuration that has been chosen is shown in Figure 1. It has had to match objectives and design principles with a number of uncertainties. For example, in such a new environment it is difficult to estimate the peak loads that may be required of the shared services. Also the availability of proven hardware and software products over the next couple of years is uncertain. The sources of funds, and the levels likely to be available are restricted, as is the financial planning horizon. The policy of incrementalism has guided the development of an implementation plan both for the network and the shared services.

The choice of the Ungermann-Bass Net/One system, rather than a more conventional PACX switch was made on the grounds that it gives a more acceptably transparent and fast service to users, and offers significantly greater functionality e.g. few restrictions on the types of devices that can be connected since varying transmission speeds and signalling procedures can be handled. It is, however, more costly and less proven than a PACX. A minimum network of two Network Interface Units will be installed on a trial basis for a period of six months. In the event of it not proving to fulfil adequately all needs, a more conventional device such as an intelligent PACX will replace the Net/One.

The decision to use DEC hardware for the shared services was made as it gives a very wide range of development hardware and operating environments, and because it is also a solution chosen by many other hospitals. MUMPS was chosen as the major operating environment for the SSN primarily because it allows applications to be developed very quickly. The decision to begin the shared services' development on PDP-11/44s rather than the larger VAXs was taken in part because the MUMPS on VAX is not yet as efficient in its file handling as PDP-11 MUMPS, and also because the size of the PDP-11s may be sufficient to cope with actual loads in the immediate future. As new VAX machines are announced, their price-performance ratios are likely to become more attractive and a migration to them at a later stage is possible, as is expansion within the PDP-11 family. A mixed VAX/PDP-11 solution for the SSN, however, presents unattractive backup (and compatibility) problems.

Although MUMPS is to be used to develop the patient identification system on one PDP-11/44 and a message handler/bulletin board on another (which will also be used as a backup system), a third PDP-11/44 is planned for use as a development machine. This would support non-MUMPS developments, probably using UNIX.

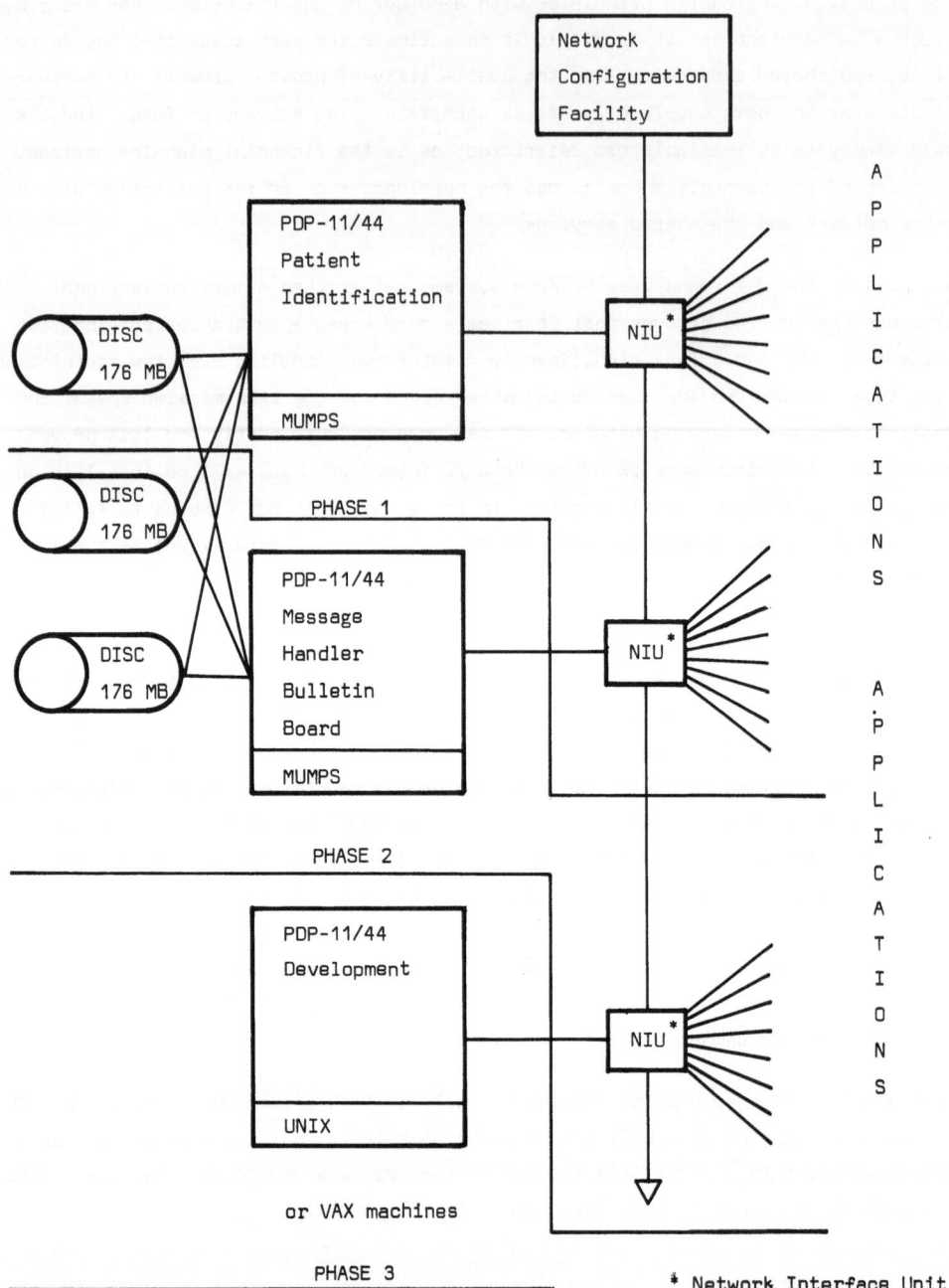

FIGURE 1   SHARED SERVICES NETWORK

                  INITIAL CONFIGURATION

Network
Configuration
Facility

A
P
P
L
I
C
A
T
I
O
N
S

PDP-11/44
Patient
Identification

MUMPS

DISC
176 MB

NIU*

PHASE 1

DISC
176 MB

PDP-11/44
Message
Handler
Bulletin
Board

MUMPS

DISC
176 MB

NIU*

A
P
P
L
I
C
A
T
I
O
N
S

PHASE 2

PDP-11/44
Development

UNIX

NIU*

or VAX machines

PHASE 3

* Network Interface Unit

7. SOME MANAGEMENT IMPLICATIONS OF A DISTRIBUTED SYSTEM

The development of a distributed systems approach in a hospital with no computing facilities may be easier than when it replaces a centralised system. Adjusting to the requirements of an unfamiliar computing system may create great stress for computer staff, particularly if they have doubts about the provenness of the technology or the wisdom of dispensing with a single centrally integrated store of information. For users too, there are new responsibilities to be taken on and realities to be appreciated about the complexities of computing from which they may have been protected in the past. For example, if they want very rapid access to current patient identity files they may need to hold them locally. Also, users become responsible for answering requests for management information. For District level managers there is a delicate balance to be struck, or continually negotiated, between the demands on available resources made by users whose power is not commensurate with the relative importance of their application. If users are required to find their own resources to purchase systems some may find it very much easier to attract funds than others whose need (e.g. for their own activities or because of the information they provide to others) is greater. These dilemmas are not peculiar to distributed systems, but they may be more apparent.

8. CONCLUSION

St Thomas' experience of computing and its internal organisational environment may be unique, but other hospitals face the same external organisational environment of the NHS and the same opportunities offered by developments in computer technology. Stand-alone mini and micro-computer systems are beginning to be introduced in many hospitals, and this trend seems likely to continue. Whether the perspective is that of hospital user or a Regional Health Authority, the spectre of incompatible systems is as disagreeable as the vision of transferable systems is attractive. The potential to interface incrementally different applications using common communication systems specifications may prove to be the most cost-effective way around the difficulties posed by the complex and changing requirements of hospital information systems.

9. REFERENCES

CLARK DD, POGRAN KT, REED DP. An Introduction to Local Area Networks. Proceedings of the IEEE. 1978;66,11: 1497-1517.

REPKO, M. Network Assessment. Systems International 1981; Oct:21-26.

CO-ORDINATED DECENTRALISED COMPUTER SYSTEMS

N. Harris, C. Horn, S. Baker, P. Duggan, D. Lyons,and B. Tangney
Department of Computer Science,
Trinity College, University of Dublin,
Dublin 2, Ireland.

— — —

Due to the decreasing cost of computer hardware the trend in computer development
has been away from the large centralised computer systems and towards a large number
of autonomous microcomputer systems. This development has had many benefits not
least the local departmental control over the operation of the system and also the
increase in availability. But it also has its disadvantages, the main ones being
the difficulty in exchanging information between autonomous systems and secondly the
inability to share underutilised and expensive resources. Local networks provide a
high speed communication facility between computers within a radius on one or two
kilometres. The communication media is usually coaxial cable and the transfer speed
is comparable with disk transfer rates. The local network provides the ability to
exchange information rapidly and easily and also the ability to share resources.
The next stage in the development is to weld the loosely connected systems into a
coordinated decentralised computer system by a distributed operating system. This
paper discusses a project in this area.

1.   Introduction

Although the computer industry is in its infancy compared to most other industries,
it has already progressed through several phases. Initially computer systems were
highly localised and usually within a large single room. A University or medium
sized Company might have one or two such "computer centres" if it was lucky. However integrated circuit (IC) technology was advancing behind the scenes and the IC
manufacturers quickly realised that the advantages of mass production of their products could only be obtained if the purchasers of a "chip" could configure it to
their own particular needs. Programming and silicon chips were united to give birth
to the microprocessor and since the beginning of the last decade more microprocessors
have been manufactured than all other computers combined. The widespread use of these devices in process control, instrumentation, automation and data analysis has led
on to further applications in text processing systems in the office, and to teaching the fundamentals of Computer Science in schools and to information systems in the
hospital. The computer epidemic at work has begun to make new microprocessor users
realise the inevitable need to exchange information between two different machines.
This is particularly true as the hardware cost of computers diminishes and more and
more groups within a given organisation are able to purchase their own machines.
Information exchange may happen when one system is being replaced with another or

when one machine has failed but more routinely so that a program written on one machine can be used on another or data that someone has produced on another machine elsewhere can be further processed. Shipping files from one computer to another can be
done by transferring, for instance, floppy discs. A more obvious and possibly faster
transfer would conceptually be possible if the machines were directly connected; with
the further advantage that once the transfer started it should be automatic and require no further human intervention.

Connecting computers together has additional possibilities. While IC technology has
reduced the cost of a processor and its memory, the electromechanical peripherals
such as printers and floppy disc drives remain relatively expensive. The cheapest
peripherals can be unreliable; for example, a reasonable quality floppy disc drive
with moderate capacity might cost 50% more than one at the lower end of the market.
Conceptually it would be advantageous if two or more processors could share common
peripherals rather than having a full set of peripherals each. Developing this further, it should be possible for an individual at a computer terminal to select one
of several machines available to him in his institution to use. One can also appreciate the benefits of being able to purchase a new processor without necessarily having to obtain peripherals for it as well. This multi-machine communication not only
allows sharing of information, but also sharing of hardware resources.

To the Computer Scientist, these ideas can be summarised to the notion of interconn-
ecting previously autonomous computers together so that essentially they still function independently, but data can be shipped between them when necessary. If several
different types of computers form this network, it may be desirable to design a common command for each machine so that someone using the system does not have to learn
a different set of commands for each processor type in the network. Implicit too
would be the automatic conversion, where necessary, of the representation of data on
one machine type to that on another. A system such as this has been termed a Network
Operating System (NOS) (1) and many examples appear in present day Hospital Information Systems (2, 3).

The terms Distributed System or Distributed Operating System (DOS) have led to considerable disagreement within the computer fraternity. We take them to imply a more
controlled system than a NOS as described above. We expect the machines in the network to function coherently together to perform the various tasks presented to them
all by the different individuals using the system. Thus the idea of someone sitting
at a terminal and selecting which machine he is going to use is replaced with that
of the same individual not caring which processor he is currently using: he is instead being served by the network system as a whole. In a hospital environment this
might mean being able to access data stored on another machine within the area, but
without having to specify where this data is actually located. Internally the network

may select different processors (and perhaps different peripherals) at different times to satisfy this individual's requests but at no time should he have to be worried or distracted by decisions made on his behalf by the network. The network should make global decisions about the complete system rather than highly local, independent and possible conflicting decisions made within a NOS. As an example, the network could attempt to balance the load imposed on it by all the various users, at possibly different locations, amongst its collections of processors and peripherals.

Inherent in our concepts of a distributed system are the issues of reliability and of incremental growth. By this we expect that should any portion of the network system fail or just be taken "offline" for service, the remainder should be able to continue to function normally, albeit with a possible reduction in performance. Similarly the total capacity of the system should be easily enhanced by simply "plugging" in additional units - processors or peripherals. The twin goals of graceful degradation in the event of any failure and of easy augmentation to increase capacity imply that the control of the network system should be decentralised and not specific to any individual or restricted group of processors. Systems with centralised control are vulnerable to the failure of the central controller - whether it be a critical hardware or software component - and supplementing the capacity of the central controller may be difficult (4). In summary we see a distributed system to not just include a physical separation of a collection of interconnected processors and peripherals but also to include decentralised communal control by which the whole system in a global sense is managed. With a Distributed Operating System all the component microcomputers together form a single logical system.

2.   The Subnet

Fundamental to a network of computers is a reliable method of communication between them. This "subnet" can be based on a number of communication technologies depending on the distances between the machines, the maximum throughput and minimum delay expected of the subnet and the amount of financial backing available! While long-haul computer networks - linking machines from several kilometres to hundreds or thousands of kilometres apart - have been in existance since the early sixties, so far they do not usually provide the performance necessary to support our ideas of a distributed system. Our attention has instead been focussed on smaller networks (say under a couple of kilometres) for which the shorter distances and subsequent lower transmission error rates have meant that high throughputs and low delays can be achieved. These local computer networks can presently achieve data rates of the order of 1 to 10 Mbits/sec but still with reasonable access delays. At least three classes of local computer networks exist: packet-switched (5), ring nets (6), and linear broadcast nets (7). The packet-switched nets use techniques similar to those in use in most long-haul nets while both the ring and linear broadcast nets in general only allow access to the subnet by one computer at a time.

We have incorporated a linear broadcast type subnet as a basis for our distributed
system. It allows peripherals and computers to be interconnected via a "black box"
to a coaxial cable on which data is transmitted at 3 M bit/sec.

3. Oghmos - an experimental distributed System

Over the past two years work has been performed at Trinity College Dublin on implementing a rudimentary distributed system "Oghmos". While one could attempt to build
a distributed system by imposing some sort of coordination on top of the software of
existing independent computer systems (8), we believe in the more fundamental approach
of replacing the existing operating systems with a distributed version. In this way
the autonomy of a processor is removed and it is no longer capable of making decisions on its own behalf which may be to the detriment of the network as a whole. Our
system is not built on top of an existing system; instead it only requires a kernel
on each processor to schedule the processes which form the distributed system. Our
prototype system has been designed to be portable and while it is presently being
run on a Vax-11/780 under VMS, it is our intention to modify the system to run on
'bare' microcomputers.

A characteristic of the Oghmos System is that it consists of many co-operating processes, each independent and only able to directly perform actions on objects within
its own address space. Sharing objects then entails creating a "guardian" (9) process to control access to objects and to maintain consistency in their value. To
maintain robustness and to exploit parallelism, guardians may be replicated (presumably on different processors) to perform their work concurrently. This leads to a
network system on which all resources have "proprietary" processes handling requests
for their own resources from other proprietors or from human users. The advantage
lies in the flexibility of control and of queuing for resources which is possible
within the proprietors, rather than the more restrictive "Monitor" (10) mechanism
where the operating system kernel usually makes all the queuing decisions itself
(normally first-come first-served or static priority).

Our Inter-Process Communication (IPC) facility is based on messages passed by links
(11, 12). Owning a link to a guardian can indicate a process's ownership of a resource and thus the link represents a "capability" or entitlement. Restricting the
links available to a process limit its dynamic environment and so both fence it in
and protect it form other processes in the system.

Links are unidirectional, but it is always possible to create a "full-duplex" connection by forming a link pointing in the opposite direction. Each process can choose
which link it wishes to perform an operation on by specifying a small integer value.
This together with the required operation and its parameters, are communicated to

the kernel, which uses the link number to find the destination process. Processes
which hold links merely have the link number to describe a communication path and
cannot, for instance, identify the process at the other end of the link.

To date we have successfully implemented the kernel of the Operating System using
Pascal and a minumum amount of assembly language. In addition, a distributed file
system and the functions to perform communication across a subnet have been written.
One uses the system via a command interpreter to load and run programs from the file
store. Each hardware resource (terminals, printers, storage units) has an associated guardian process to whom one applies to make use of the resource. Note that this
resource may actually be located "across the network", in which case all communication is performed automatically on your behalf. Software resources - such as a compiler or text editor - can also be similarly represented by guardians and thus usage
of resources is harmonised and virtually independent of what the resource in question
actually is.

The benefits of simple, standard usage of all the facilities available via the subnet, whether they be hardware or software, local or remote, must be balanced against
the overheads incurred in implementing such a system. The Oghmos System is now being
ported from the VAX computer to a number of microcomputers connected together by a
local area network. Future research will indicate the efficiency and robustness of
our implementation.

4.   Example Application

An example of a distributed operating system is identical to an example of a central
operating system. The difference lies not in the application but instead in the
topology of the system and its reliability and robustness. The processors and peripherals may be distributed around the hospital in locations most appropriate to
their function. The system still functions, even though at reduced efficiency, when
parts of the system are out of service. Hence an example of a network operating
system applied to a hospital information system is given and from it the distributed
operating system may be inferred by removing the visibility of the network and the
nodes from the users. Figure 1 shows a hypothetical hospital information system.

The financial section, admissions, patient management and laboratory have one or more
microprocessors. The file store contains the mass storage for the system but individual sites e.g. patient management, may have their own local discs. Access to the
system is by means of a common command language. The admissions operator updates
remote files in the file store for each patient admitted. File records are read over
the network from the remote disc just as if they were read from a local disc. At the
same time the laboratory operator may read and write to a different file in the central file store. The blocks of data are multiplexed on the network for the different

file operations and hence do not corrupt each other. The financial operator may execute a program to read records from the central file store and also read a local file in order to produce a billing statement for a patient being discharged. In addition, the financial operator may have a file which is stored at the central file store printed at the high speed printer site.

In this application the processor nodes and the network are visible to all the operators while a distributed operating system would make the system appear as a single unit just like a centralised computer system.

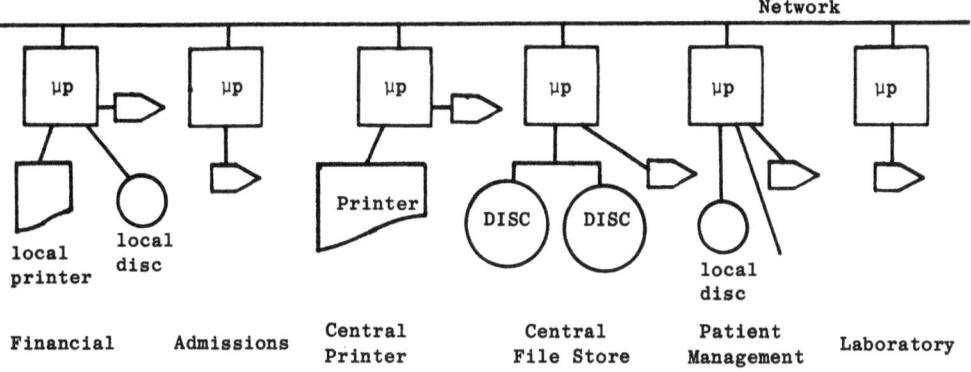

Figure 1

5. Summary and Note on Oghmos

We believe that a true Distributed System not only comprises a multi-processor system but also includes a mechanism for a global management of the system in a highly decentralised way. We have developed an experimental distributed system Oghmos with which we are gaining further experience of designing and implementing reliable, decentralised and co-ordinated multi-processor systems.

In Celtic Mythology, Oghmos was the most revered god of the people of Tuatha De Danann and patron of elegance and literature. He was normally depicted as a man drawing behind him a group of willing followers, attached to him by slender golden chains.

6. References

(1)   Kimbleton SR. The NBS experimental network operating system. Distributed systems - Architecture and Implementation: Lecture Notes in Computer Science No. 105, Springer Verlag 1981; 308-356.

(2)   Bakker AR. Centralisation and decentralisation aspects in hospital information systems. Lecture Notes in Medical Informatics, Springer Verlag 1981; 41-49.

(3)   James RM, Viale RO. The evolution of a data communications network in an university hospital. Lecture Notes in Medical Informatics, Springer Verlag 1981; 922-927.

(4)   Jensen ED. Distributed Control. Distributed Systems - Architecture and Imp-
        lementation: Lecture Notes in Computer Science No.105, Springer Verlag 1981;
        195-190.

(5)   Faldella E, Neri G, Salomon T. Cost effective station implementation in min-
        inet. Euromicro No.5 1979. 285-294.

(6)   Hopper A, Wheeler D. Maintenance of ring communication systems. IEEE Trans
        on Comm. Vol.27 No.4, April 1979, 760-761.

(7)   Metcalfe RM, Boggs DR. Ethernet: Distributed packet switching for local com-
        puter networks. Comm ACM Vol.19 No.7, July 1976.

(8)   Holler E. The National Software Works. Distributed Systems - Architecture
        and Implementation: Lecture Notes in Computer Science No.105, Springer Verlag
        1981; 421-442.

(9)   Svobodova L, Liskov B, Clark D. Distributed Computer Systems: structure and
        semantics. MIT LCS TR-215 1979.

(10)   Hoare CAR. Monitors: an operating system structuring concept. Comm ACM Vol.
        17 No.10, Oct 1974; 549-557.

(11)   Basket F, Howard JH, Montague JT. Task Communication in DEMOS. ACM Operating
        Systems Review Vol.11 No.5, Nov 1977; 23-32.

(12)   Solomon MH, Finkel RA. The Roscoe Distributed Operating System. Proceedings
        of the 7th Symposium of Operating System Principles (ACM Order No.534790),
        Dec 1980; 108-114.

FEATURES OF MICRO DATA BASE SYSTEMS

AND THEIR IMPACT ON APPLICATIONS IN HEALTH CARE SYSTEMS

by

F.J. Leven / Ch. Stoll

Studiengang Medizinische Informatik

Universität Heidelberg / Fachhochschule Heilbronn

D-7100 Heilbronn

SUMMARY

Database management systems on microcomputers (micro DBMS) are not degradations of mini or mainframe systems, but stress special principles to meet or bypass the bounding limitations set by typical microcomputer hardware configuration.

Besides more than 15 micro MUMPS systems there are also some other types of micro DBMS available eg CODASYL-oriented packages. Impact on medical application systems will be given by the availability of micro data base application programs for nonprogramming users to quickly form - in the sense of programmerless systems development - new applications meeting their requirements.

1. INTRODUCTION

According to many experts' predictions the computing scene in the 1980's will be dominated by two innovations: The development of microcomputers and the application of Data Base Management Systems (DBMS). These two innovations are combined together in micro DBMS now available for the most widespread types of microcomputers.

In the way the development of MUMPS belongs to the pioneer approaches in the history of medical data bases, a new generation of information systems in medicine is entered by the micro MUMPS approach which is now available or under development in more than 15 different implementations. This new generation of data management systems is furthermore characterized by CODASYL-oriented micro DBMS which thus try to intrude an area that until today has been reserved to mainframe systems. Indeed, most of the data base applications - especially in the area of medicine - follow conventional file management systems and the general mainframe concepts of eg the CODASYL, IMS, or, relational approach respectively appropriate modifications of them for minicomputers. The trend in the evolution of these general DBMS concepts over several generations leads to an ever increasing degree of data independence in that

784

the user does not have to know the storage representation of the data and access paths, but can concentrate on specifying his information needs. To characterize micro DBMS, questions have to be discussed with respect to

- the capabilities of micro DBMS,
- the differences between mainframe and micro DBMS,
- running or potential applications of micro DBMS (are micro DBMS "solutions looking for problems"?), and
- micro DBMS performance figures, regarding the limitations of microcomputers in processing speed and memory capacity.

2. FEATURES OF MICROCOMPUTERS

Microcomputers today can be classified into 8 bit machines (on the basis of eg Intel 8080 or Zilog-Z80 microprocessors), 16 bit machines (on the basis of eg Zilog-Z8000 or LSI 11/23 Microprocessors) with processing speeds a factor of ten times that of 8 bit CPU's, or, even 32 bit machines (like Intel iAPX432).

Main storage capacity of microcomputers is rather limited, for 8 bit machines eg usually to 64 KB. With the aid of additional memory management chips, however, for some machines the address space can be expanded, eg in the case of Zilog-Z8000 up to 48 MB.

As standard low cost mass storage devices floppy disks and hard disks are available in a variety of types (Figure 1).

	5$\frac{1}{4}$'' FLOPPY DISK		8'' FLOPPY DISK		HARD DISK
	one sided	double sided	one sided	double sided	
CAPACITY (KB) (unformatted) single/double density	110/220	220/440	400/800	800/1600	30000
AVERAGE ACCESS TIME (MS)	500	300	200	100	50
Purchase COSTS ($)	350	450	600	750	2500

Figure 1. Characteristics of floppy and hard disks

For producing back up copies one uses 2 disk units with one disk fixed and one removable or one hard disk with tape back-up device.

Portability between different types of microcomputers is provided by common operating systems – a quasi standard for various machines being CP/M, respectively its multi-user time sharing version MP/M - and high level languages like BASIC, FORTRAN, COBOL, PASCAL and PL/1 in defined subset form.

Despite these highlights "microcomputers are misunderstood by computer professionals. Because they are inexpensive they are assumed to be less valuable. Because they have limited storage capacity both in main memory and conventional (floppy disk) auxiliary storage, they are thought to have limited ranges of applications. Because they cannot effectively compile and execute the most sophisticated compiler systems running on larger computers, they are thought to be incapable of effective high level language computation .... The fallacy in each of the half-truths cited above lies in attempting to force large system computational concepts into admittedly smaller resources, then complaining about reduced performance." (1, pp22-25)

Microcomputers can in some cases outperform large computer systems that require special training, that have reliability and availability problems by unpredictable shutdowns, that are costly to obtain and costly to operate, and have difficulties to maintain data security. These are, by the way, some of the reasons why computers have been relatively under-utilized in medicine.

3. CAPABILITIES OF MICRO-DBMS

The capabilities of micro DBMS are limited by two boundaries:
The code must be small enough to be workable within memory contraints of eg 64 KB for an 8 bit machine: application program, database system, possibly an interpreter and a database buffer region must be memory resident at a time. Furthermore prices comparable to those for mini and mainframe database systems are untenable in the micro market, where most software packages cost at most a few hundred dollars.

This means that micro DBMS cannot be compared with mini or mainframe systems or be considered as mere degradations of them. They rather must stress special-probably new-principles to meet or bypass the bounding limitations mentioned above.

60% of the more than 20 micro DBMS available - a subset is characterized in Figure 2 - are micro MUMPS systems, the rest follows the CODASYL or other approaches.

3.1 CODASYL-oriented micro-DBMS

With more than 800 installations MDBS is one of the most widespread CODASYL-oriented micro-DBMS running under more than half a dozen operating systems, and interfacing with over a dozen host languages.

PROVIDER	DBMS-NAME	DBMS-TYPE	MICRO - HW (Bits/word)	OPERATING SYSTEM	MEMORY REQUIRED	PURCHASE COSTS
Micro Data Base Systems	MDBS	CODASYL-oriented	8080,Z80 (8bit) 8086,Z8000 (16bit) PDP 11 (16bit)	CP/M, MP/M CP/M-86,MP/M-86 UNIX	20 KB	1800 $ 2700 $
Microsoft	MICRO-SEED	CODASYL-oriented	8080, Z80	CP/M	48 KB	1500$
R.Walters	CP/M - Public Domain Version	MUMPS	8080, Z80	CP/M	56 KB	?
Medical Inform. Technol.	MIIS	MUMPS	LSI-11/23 (16bit)	MUMPS	64 KB	?
Hitachi Medico	Hitachi Micro MUMPS	MUMPS	8085 (8bit)	HIMEC 10/OS	64 KB	?
Tektronix	INGRES	relational	LSI-11(16bit)	UNIX	?	?

Figure 2. Micro Data Systems (1,2,3,4)

MDBS does not represent a CODASYL-subset implementation, but gains simplicity - as to the systems processing strategies, and to the definition and manipulation of a data base by the user - by introducing concepts even exceeding those defined in the CODASYL standard:
In strictly CODASYL systems, eg, a many-to-many relationship must be simulated by two conventional sets and an artificial "link record type". The resulting problem that such a data structure may be rather unnatural and complicate data manipulation programs unnecessarily, is overcome in MDBS by allowing n:m sets in the data base design.

A further extension with respect to CODASYL is the MDBS concept of recursive data structures. A completely new data structure in MDBS is the multiple Owner/Member-Settype. This means that a set may have many owner- and member record types, an owner record type also being a member record type in the set.

On the other hand the user interface is characterized by a formatted Data Definition Language and a rather tedious access path navigation in host language application programs by means of CALL-DML - commands. The subschema-concept has not been implemented. Management of the USER WORK AREA - a link between the application program and the data base - is a part of the interface and in responsibility of the user. Furthermore a special Storage Structure Language as proposed by CODASYL is not implemented.

However, additional software products are available allowing easier direct access to records, allowing a non-programmer to extract data from a data base by using a non procedural query language, or, allowing multiple users to share a single data base. Even utility programs for data base recovery and restructuring may be added to MDBS.

The restriction of program size by the main memory capacity of 64 KB can be bypassed by an overlay linking loader, a procedure, however, which needs some effort by the programmer: the program has to be divided into overlay segments which are loaded from the secondary storage device into the main memory when called.

The system uses a paging organization so that execution efficiency can be optimized by an adequate number of memory resident pages which is a function of both the page size and the amount of memory available. Experiments have shown (2) that the processing time may be reduced by a factor of 35 if the number of memory resident pages is increased by a factor of 6. This figures, however, could not be confirmed by our own experiments with MDBS, Version I, on a Z80-superbrain microcomputer using BASF minifloppies with 160 KB capacity.

Better performance, free-form DDL - specifications, etc. are some of the improvements that are claimed by the vendor for version III of MDBS available now.

3.2 micro-MUMPS

Whereas only 2% of the MDBS applications lie in the medical area the numerous applications of micro MUMPS need to be classified (1, pp 56-62) in order to keep survey (Figure 3).

Stand alone applications	Links to other systems	Transfer of large application systems to microcomputers
●Individual or small group practice support systems ●Research oriented summary data management	●Data entry validity checking ●Communication links between micro MUMPS interpreter and larger systems ●Development and testing of programs	●QUEST, a teaching program driver ●COSTAR (Computer Stored Ambulatory Record) ●Modules of an Hospital Information System

Figure 3. Micro MUMPS applications

15 of the 17 micro MUMPS implementations reported in (1, pp 36-40) - 8 for 8 bit - and 9 for 16 bit - microcomputers - comprise the ANSI - standard of MUMPS. Whereas all of the 8 bit implementations rely on existing operating systems and therefore

permit execution of other programming languages and access to external files, most of the 16 bit implementations are based on dedicated operating systems.

With respect to performance, MUMPS implementations on 8 bit microcomputers are primarily restricted to a single user running relatively simple tasks. The performance of 16 bit machines-rivaling and sometimes outperforming some of the 16 bit minicomputers - will allow complex MUMPS application systems to run in a multi user environment.

An example for such a large MUMPS application system is COSTAR (8), a package that seeks to provide comprehensive computer support for medium to large size ambulatory clinics and is now subject of several implementation approaches on microcomputers.

As described for MDBS a key performance problem in the usage of micro MUMPS is the slowness of floppy disks. This problem, however, has been significantly reduced in some implementations by using cache buffers (1, pp 34) or a buffer pool with an optimal number of buffers (1, pp 33,34), where this number increases as disk access times become greater. In (1, p 34) experiments have been reported showing that floppy performance with cache buffers is about twice as fast as hard discs without them.

Possible future developments (1, pp 26-32) for enhancing MUMPS performance on microcomputers are the availability of special purpose boards eg for string manipulation and conversion and new hardware architectures eg the "data flow" architecture (5). In data flow machines - opposite to the conventional v. Neumann computers the execution of an algorithm is not controlled by special instructions of a corresponding program, but implicitly by the data flow.

3.3 Relational micro DBMS

Though relational DBMS usually are reported as systems with CPU problems even on large mainframes a few relational micro DBMS approaches have been implemented following the philosophy "that for small or moderate quantities of data on smaller computer systems the efficiency of relational database systems is not so critical because the very long sorting times for very large files are not nearly as significant a problem with smaller files". (9) Nevertheless it will be usefull to check what is meant by "relational", if it is eg simply a renaming of flat file management: "a flat file is called a relation, a field is called an attribute, the merging of two files based on matching data values is called the joining of two relations, the exctraction of data values for one or more of the file's fields is called the projection on a relation, etc.". (10)

4. CONCLUSIONS

The importance of micro DBMS lies not only in the fact that low cost data management capabilities are available, but that a sort of "user independence" is achieved: The user is freed from constraints in a mainframe or minicomputer environment. Furthermore, the prerequisites for "programmerless systems development" (6) are provided, which means transferring development tasks from the computer professional to the end user who functions as his own developer and eliminates the programmer as middleman. Example for this trend are data base application programs, that can be interactively executed by non-programming users to quickly form new applications meeting their requirements: eg FILE MANAGER, or MEDUS/A (7), a MUMPS written high level DBMS designed for clinical research in medicine in public health which is being transferred to microcomputers.

REFERENCES

(1) Dayhoff, R. E. (ed), MUMPS User Group (MUG) Quarterly, Vol X, Nov. 1980.

(2) MDBS User's Manual, Micro Data Base Systems, Inc., Lafayette, In, 1980.

(3) Whinston, A. B., Holsapple, C. W.: DBMS for micros, Datamation, 4/81, pp 165-166, 1981.

(4) Krass, P., Wiener, H., The DBMS market is booming, Datamation, 9/81, pp 153-170, 1981.

(5) Giloi, W. K., Rechnerarchitektur, Berlin, Heidelberg, New York, Springer-Verlag, 1981.

(6) Johnson, M. E., Introduction to programmerless systems development in MUMPS, Proc. 4th Ann. Symp. Comp. Appl. Med. Care, pp 1643-1644, 1980.

(7) Goldstein, L., MEDUS/A, a high level database management system, Proc. 4th Ann. Symp. Comp. Appl. Med. Care. pp 1653-1660, 1980.

(8) Barnett, G.O., Justice, N. S., Somand, M. E., Adams, J. B., Waxman, B. D., Parent, M. S., van Densen, F. R., Greenlie, J. K., COSTAR, a computer-based medical information system for ambulatory care, Proc. IEEE, Vol 67, pp 1226 ff. 1979.

(9) Hamilton, P., Manuel, T., Relational data bases do it more easily, electronics, March 1981, pp 102-103.

(10) Holsapple, C., A path through the jungle of data management, data base focus (micro data base systems, inc.) Vol 1, No. 2, 1981.

ON INTEGRITY CONSTRAINTS AND CATALOGUES
IN RELATIONAL DATABASE SUPPORTING CLINICAL RESEARCH

Piotr J. JASIŃSKI, Bogumiła TALKOWSKA

Regional Computer Centre,
Technical University of Poznań,
pl. M.Skłodowskiej-Curie 5,
60-965 Poznań, Poland

Summary

Selected problems of integrity constraints within computer database
supporting clinical research have been discussed in this paper. The
concept of integrity constraints catalogues has been introduced,
through examples on certain data structures taken from operational,
cardiology-oriented relational database system. The limitations of
design proposed and trends of possible future investigations have
been examined in conclusions.

1. Introduction

One of the most important factors which highly influence users'
acceptance of computerized information system is the correctness of
stored data. For database designers, and also for experienced users
it is clear that it is not possible to develop a system which will
be completely proof against all kinds of errors. Consequently, the
pragmatic approach is to limit the amount of errors and exclude
those which seriously affect usability of database system. In this
paper we will discuss some problems of database protecting, known as
integrity constraints, using the relational database system CARDIO-
COD [1,2] as application scenario.

2. Controversy on updating within clinical user query language

In numerous, most often relational query languages, the end-user
may execute both retrieval and updating operations. Widely cited
language of such a type, Query-by-Example, includes powerful mechanisms for integrity constraints specifications, which are under
complete control of the end-user [3,4,5]. However, it seems for us
that in many applications the joining of retrieval and updating operations in the form of large, complex manipulation language is not
well-argumented and convenient, due to the principal execution difference between the two operations types and also heterogenity of
users groups, which groups mostly need only one type of operations.
Particularly, in research-oriented clinical databases there is no
need for instant updating of clinical events which occur with the
patients. As has been pointed out by Weyl et al [6], the day-to-day

clinical information system can be non-cumputerized as:

"A file of carefully structured sorted paper documents is an excellent source for answering questions related to an individual patient. If the record is at hand, information may be extracted directly from a patient record in less time than is required to initiate a computer search request."

Therefore, updating operations, together with embedded integrity constraints can be designed and implemented in the form of independent software module working in batch processing mode. In other words, all clinical researchers can retrieve and analyse the contents of database by means of query language (performing retrieval, read-only operations [7]), but only few adequately trained clinical secretaries are responsible for preparing and performing updating runs.

3. Nature of user errors and simple checking technique

User errors, which may occur in bulk input of clinical data can be divided into several groups (or categories).

A) Source wrong-writing errors: for example "digoxim" or "dugoxin" instead of correct "digoxin", which can occur due to the inaccurate or not intelligible handwriting in clinical paper forms.

B) Character or value misplaced errors: for example birth-date "1943" when the correct value is "1934" or systolic arterial blood pressure "510" when the correct value is "150". This kind of errors most commonly appears during preparation of input data medium (e.g. when typing punched cards in CARDIOCOD system).

C) Logical errors: occur when some restrictions resulting from using problem-orientation method are ignored by physician who deal with source paper documentation. In CARDIOCOD implementation this is the case when analysis-date of any laboratory test is later than the patient's discharge-date, or start-date of only one drug therapy administered due to a given problem is earlier than discovery-date of that problem.

D) Non-uniqueness of patient-no errors: each patient stay in clinic is given a unique value of patient-no identifier. The state when any two patient records have the same value of patient-no identifier is erroneous, even when those two records concern the same human being. Such assumption, and relatively small scale of CARDIOCOD system (actually less then 3000 patients) makes the control of uniqueness less critical and simpler than in the case of larger systems (e.g. two levels control in [8]).

It should be noted here that the above classification is not complete and in some places also not distinct. For example, the logical error may incidentally occur due to the wrong value of a date of a given clinical event, which failure results from wrong-writing or character-misplaced error in one or more digits in the date.

In CARDIOCOD updating software simple tests for single data elements are build-in for those attributes for which the permitted value range (or value set) is:

- <u>possible</u> to define explicite, with the appropriate level of certainty which, however, does not exclude changes in future;
- <u>independent</u> of the values of any other attributes for the same
  patient.

Examples of such constraints, or simply preprogrammed checks are:
- value set {F,M} for attribute sex,
- **value ranges** ⟨000;300⟩ and ⟨000;150⟩ for respectively systolic
  and diastolic arterial blood pressures.

However, such checking technique is of rather limited applicability; for error groups A) and B) we have shown examples of errors
which are practically not detectable, also by standard, most widely
used in today's information systems, <u>syntactic tests</u> [9]. More advanced method of detection, or protecting database against certain
types of errors are shown in next sections of this paper.

4. Complex conditional dependencies between attributes values

Let us analyse two examples of CARDIOCOD database relations, where
large variety of interferences between attributes values clinically
exist and - in our view at least - should be specified to some extend
for updating software. In Figure 1a relation LABORATORY is presented
diagramatically, with links representing interferences between attributes within relation (or more precisely, between given values of
one attribute and subranges or subsets of others). The same idea for
relation DRUG-THERAPY is shown in Figure 1b (note that only relevant
parts of both relations are illustrated).

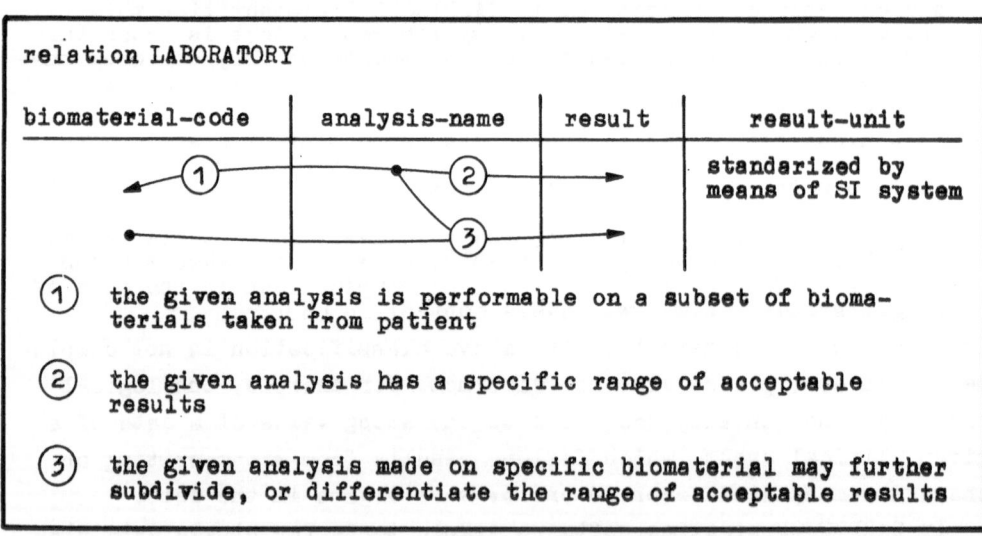

Figure 1a

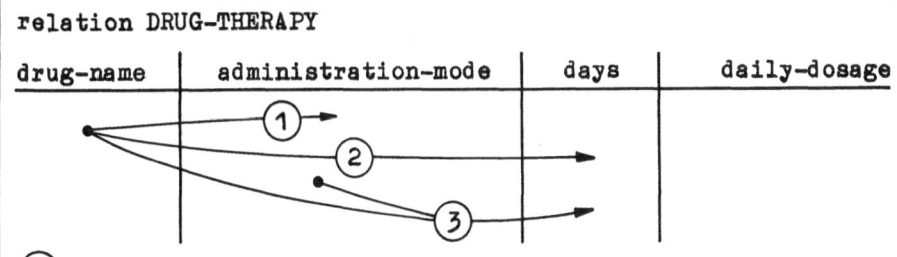

relation DRUG-THERAPY

drug-name	administration-mode	days	daily-dosage

① each drug has one or more administration modes

② some drugs have a limitation of days of administration, especially when therapeutical effects are negative

③ most of the drugs are characterized by maximum daily dosage, usually different for each possible administration mode

F i g u r e   1b

The idea to build-in constraints resulting from generalized conditions given in Figures 1a and 1b is rather simple. However, useful design needed:

- careful, clinically reasonable selection of limits of numerical, quantitive values;

- standarization, coding and relative constancy of laboratory and drug therapy terminology;

- proposals of adequate data structures and their maintenance.

5. Design of integrity constraints catalogues

The design concepts of <u>catalogues</u> for integrity constraints specifications discussed are shown in Figures 2a and 2b.

LABORATORY-CONSTRAINTS-CATALOGUE

analysis-name	analysis -code	biomaterial -code	patholog. limits lower	upper	
urea	urea	B	2.5	68.4	mmol/l
glucose	gluc	C	1.11	49.9	mmol/l
glucose	gluc	dU	0.05	50.0	g/l
serum potassium	spot	B	1.5	8	mmol/l
cholesterol	chol	S	2.5	12.7	mmol/l
creatinine	cine	S	22.1	504	μmol/l
protein	prot	S	40	97	g/l

extremal values actually stored in database

F i g u r e   2a

DRUG-THERAPY-CONSTRAINTS-CATALOGUE

drug-name generic	drug-code	administration-mode	days	maximum daily-dosage
procainamide	pide	intravenously	1	1
procainamide	pide	orally	-	6
chinidine	chin	orally	-	3.2
propranolol	plol	intravenously	1	0.005
propranolol	plol	orally	-	0.320

note: all maximum daily dosages are given in grams,
      sign '-' in days column stands for "empty" condition

F i g u r e   2b

   The first important question is how to select properly the upper
and lower pathological limits of laboratory analysis, as such data
are not obtainable from literature resources (contrary to so called
normal values). The solution is partly marked in Figure 2a. We assumed that extremal values actually stored in database would be
kept in LABORATORY-CONSTRAINTS-CATALOGUE and that both values could
change dynamically. That will be the case when a value not falling
into the permitted range appears in bulk input data. Such a value,
once detected as error will be once more externally checked and,
when entered repeatedly without correction, will execute updating of
given elementary data in constraints catalogue.

   Another problem is common to both 2a and 2b Figures and is con-
erned with terminology. During previous period of CARDIOCOD database maintenance we found high percentage of undetected errors similar to examples in group A) described in section 3 of this paper.
This errors have been quite frequent for drug-name and analysis-name
values. The primary reasons of those errors were:
- lack of clinically acceptable standarization of terminology,
- non-coded, free in format and variable in length entries of drug
  and analysis name which brings serious difficulties in achieving
  proper standarized nomenclature.
As can be deduced from Figures 1 and 2, proposal of constraints catalogues influence the structure of corresponding primary relations.
Formerly existed drug-names and analysis-names are substituted by
equivalent, fixed-length 4-character codes. Full names of drugs and
analyses are kept in catalogues however.

   At first sight our design can be seen as horizontal extension of
Wiederhold's relational lexicons [10,11]. In fact, different constraints must be specified for each clinically existing concatenation

of drug and possible administration modes, also analysis and bio-
materials which can be used. Therefore, the concept of constraints
catalogues lacks formal elegance of lexicon relations because of
redundancy of "name - code" pairs. However, it still posses some
lexicon properties-the important one is that the existence of tuples
is determined externally (e.g. introduction of a new drug) and deletion is constrained by existing references within the core of database. Another maintenance question is the ordering of tuples in constraints catalogues. Assuming sequential or jump table look-up,
tuples ordering should result from descending frequencies of use of
all drugs and analyses. The estimative cardinalities of currently
being implemented integrity constraints catalogues are as follows:
- for DRUG-THERAPY about 300 entries,
- for LABORATORY about 230 entries.

6. Discussion and conclusions

This paper can be treated as a re-examination of previous design
decisions in CARDIOCOD project and as a state report of works
currently conducted. Since the beginning of CARDIOCOD operation (1978)
we have used numerous syntactic and/or value tests (checks) for single
data elements, as described in section 3. The new concept of integrity
constraints catalogues, although   partly similar to constraints specifications in Query-by-Example language [4], stays beyond the direct
control of end-user of database system and offers more systematic
approach to input data quality guestions. Presented design of catalogues should reduce significantly the amount of previously undetected
errors, but some of them can still appear. The input data, when compared with source documents or clinical events can be erroneous but
still within limits given in catalogues. Therefore, we think that
developing users' motivation to prepare input data in highest achie-
vable quality is as important as sophisticated tools for constraints
specifications. It is also our opinion that two following topics are
still worth further efforts.

Firstly, any physician may conclude that integrity specifications
proposed for drug therapies are clinically primitive. Maximum of
therapeutical daily-desage of a given drug may vary highly depending
on diseases (problems) for which it is applied. Constraint maximum
of daily-dosage can be valid for therapy in one specific problem and,
contrary, much to higher (or even critically dangerous) when the same
drug is used in management of another problems. That means much more
complicated dependencies between diagnoses and sufficient therapies,

different loading and maintenance dosages, drugs interactions and so forth [12]. That may lead us directly towards higher models of integrity specifications, using e.g. methods of AI or fuzzy sets theory [13]. But how far should we go, having still in view archival, clinical database system?

Secondly, the importance of time-dimension should be underlined, known also as <u>temporal dimension</u> in database modelling. As has been pointed in [6], time plays a certain role in arranging an array of clinical data. It seems that the still open, general question is how to store correctly, and after that how to select properly the time-oriented sequence of patients' data concerning given (but usually not known in advance) "cause - effect" clinical study.

Acknowledgements

The authors wish to express gratitude to H.Krug, M.D. and S.Paradow-ski, M.Sc. for helpful explanations and preparation of examples which aided greatly to the completion of this paper.

References

[1] Jasiński P.J., Krug H., Zerbe F., Kierzkowski Z., Jasiński K.: Kardiologiczna Komputerowa Dokumentacja (KARDIOKÓD). Kard.Pol., 1979, 22:695-704.

[2] Jasiński P.J., Krug H., Talkowska B.: Relational database CARDIOCOD: a tool for clinical research in cardiology. Medical Informatics Europe 81, Lecture Notes in Medical Informatics 11, Springer-Verlag 1981, 512-519.

[3] Zloof M.M.: Query-by-Example: a database language. IBM Systems J. 1977, Vol. 16, No.4, 324-343.

[4] Zloof M.M.: Security and integrity within the Query-by-Example database management language. IBM RC 6982, Yorktown Hts., New York 1978.

[5] Ullman J.D.: Principles of Database Systems. Pitman Publ. Ltd, London 1980.

[6] Weyl S., Fries J., Wiederhold G., Germano F.: A Modular, Self-Describing Clinical Databank System. Computers and Biomedical Research, 1975, 8; 279-293.

[7] Vandijck E.: Towards a more familiar relational retrieval language. Information Systems, Vol. 2, 1977, 159-169.

[8] Sauter K., Juergen K., Rienhoff O.: Integrity problems within a database - supported patient information systems. Medical Informatics Berlin 1979, Lecture Notes in Medical Informatics 5, Springer-Verlag 1979, 570-579.

[9] Kent W.: Data and Reality. North-Holland Publ.Co., 1978.

[10] Wiederhold G.: Database Design, McGraw-Hill, New York 1977.

[11] Wiederhold G., El-Masri R.: The structural model for database design. Entity,Relationship approach to systems analysis and design (ed. Chen P.P.). North-Holland Publ.Co., Amsterdam 1980, 237-257.

[12] Forrey A.W.: Information and clinical pharmacology: role of the computer. Med.Inform. 1980, Vol.5, No.4, 245-252.

[13] Cerutti S.: Semantic models in medical record data bases. Med. Inform. 1980, Vol. 5, No. 3, 215-226.

DATA RELIABILITY IN LARGE DATA BASES

Ernst Risan
National Mass Radiography Service
Postbox 8155 Dep.
Oslo 1, NORWAY

Hartvig Opsjon
Unit for Health Services Research
c/o Plans and Systems Department
National Institute of Public Health
Postuttak
Oslo 1, NORWAY

SUMMARY

This study of data reliability is based on the creation of a 2.1 million records data file at the National Mass Radiography Service of Norway. Redundant information about 106.228 persons in the file gave an opportunity to study error situations and error rates in a medical information system.

Assigning data to wrong persons was estimated to occur in less than 0.05% of the cases. Errors in data elements that did not serve as identificators were also studied. Height and weight errors in the file were mainly due to misreading of handwritten figures in the punching operation.

The paper ends with a discussion of error liability and its consequencies for medical systems.

1. INTRODUCTION

Medical information systems are often characterised by the huge amounts of data to be handled. Hospital information systems and epidemiological systems are based on large files where the accuracy of data is crucial for the operation of the systems.

Data reliability concerns two major groups of data items, the identification elements and the various other data elements.

An epidemiological study that was carried out in Norway in 1981 gave some insight into the errors that are likely to occur in medical information systems. We will in this paper present a description of the errors we found in our data.

In Norway the National Mass Radiography Service (NMRS) has been carrying out examinations of the entire population since the early forties. There exist computer files with data from this work for the period since 1962. Based on these files there was carried out a study on the correlation between body height/weight and death rates.

Originally the data were spread on several files with different record formats. There was also a need for some corrections before the epidemiological analysis could be carried out. Thus the first stage of the study became the creation of one data file that could serve as a basis for the research work. This first stage will be denoted as "the creation of the height/weight file" and constitutes the basis for the data reliability analysis given in this paper.

2. THE CREATION OF THE HEIGHT/WEIGHT FILE

The original data files had approximately 4 million records covering the period 1962-75. There were four tape files for different subperiods. Not all of these records would have information of height and weight, and the first step therefore was to select all records from the original files that had height/weight information. This brought the number of records down to about 2.1 million.

The identification element in our files was the national birth register number (BRN), an eleven digit number in common use in Norway. This identifier is assigned to every person living in the country and is a unique identification. The BRN was designed by the Central Bureau of Statistics and was officially introduced in 1964. Several people have, however, later on got their BRNs changed. The Central Bureau of Statistics maintains a cumulative correction file. When we carried out our project, the correction file had 191.282 records.

Proper identification was crucial since the epidemiological project would require a match against the national death register file, a file whose identification element is the BRN.

The base material had previously undergone some corrections of the BRN. Our match against the updated correction file thus only resulted in 8.993 new corrections.

Sorting and merging the subfiles gave us a version number one of the height/weight file. A statistics run with some displays of dubious records gave us some insight into errors that still existed in our material. It is the study of this statistics run that is being discussed in the following chapters.

The height/weight file consisted of 2.059.304 records. For 106.228 persons we had from two to five measurements. For these persons we could examine error situations and estimate error rates. (Not all of these 106.228 had information about both height and weight. Thus table I shows height differences for a lower number of people than 106.228).

3. IDENTIFICATION ELEMENT RELIABILITY

In our analysis we investigated the height differences between the highest value and the lowest one for height and weight. If there was a difference of at least 10 cm and/or 30 kg, all records for a person were listed out. This resulted in some 1.800 records, all representing people aged above 19. To keep the work load within reasonable limits, we changed the conditions for listing out records, new limits were 30 cm and/or 40 kg. 82 records came on this new list.

4 of the 82 records were records that had been connected to wrong persons. We will give some detail to explain how these errors were created. To do this, we need to describe the routines used for the mass radiography screening at the time when our material was collected.

NMRS had several mobile teams touring the country. By mail people would receive a computer-printed message that they were to come for chest x-ray examination at a certain time. When people came for examination, they would be given a computer-printed examination card. On this card weight and height measures would be written down by hand. The same card was handed to the personnel operating the x-ray equipment. After x-ray examination the cards were sent to the main office of NMRS for punching and further checking.

The computer printed cards and the callings for examination were based on a census file from a regional computer centre. These computing centres have their own copy of the census file.

Registration of a wrong identification might basically happen in one of four ways:
1. There were errors in the register data.
2. A person was given another persons's examination card when he checked in at the counter to file up for x-raying. This reportedly mainly happened in case of close name resemblance.
3. In queueing just before the x-ray equipment some people put their examination cards down on whatever was at hand, and then hastily grasped a wrong card when it was their turn to enter the x-ray chamber.
4. There might be errors done at the main office of the NMRS. This includes punching and programming errors.

In three out of the four error situations mentioned above there was an error in the census data from the regional computer centre. The fourth error must have been entered somewhere in the processing at the NMRS office.

If the error checking routines of NMRS had functioned as they should, all the three errors in category one should have been detected at the x-ray examination. Both the personnel handing out examination cards and those operating the x-ray equipment should have verified both name and date of birth of the one coming for examination.

Occasionally these checking routines are not being used properly and some examination cards will refer to wrong persons. Such errors in identification may still be detected and corrected later on at the NMRS office. Some identification errors will slip through all normal checking routines and will then only accidentally be found later on.

Some x-ray photos have unclear spots that requires further examination. Before a person is called in for an extra x-ray, an experienced doctor will examine the questionable x-ray and possible previous x-rays to make sure that no one shall be alarmed unnecessarily. The experienced doctor acts as a referee. The referee may then come across cases where the photos cannot possibly belong to the same person. Correction of identification may then be done.

The error rate of identification error has to be estimated. Since identification errors are likely to create considerable height differences, we cannot use 4 out of 82 as an overall estimate of the error rate. Investigation of the checking routine at NMRS is likely to give a better estimate for the error rate in the person identification. Some 20.000 x-ray photos are annually presented to a referee for assessment. It is considered that there is a maximum of 10 cases pr. year where a wrong identification has been found. This means an error rate of 0.05%.

It is likely that the error rate for the complete data file is the same as for those records whose x-ray photos are being sent for special examination. This will mean that a maximum of 1.000 records in the 2.059.304 record file will have a wrong identification.

4. MEASUREMENT RELIABILITY

Data validation had been carried out in the original data entry to ensure a low punching error rate. Control programs had checked that the variables kept inside acceptable value ranges. In this way completely "wild" values had been taken out.

Body weight is fluctuating more freely than body height and errors are not as easily detected for weight as they are for height. The error sources were though considered to be similar, and the analysis of error sources for height should be valid for weight as well.

At an early stage in the work of creating the height/weight file, we found three records where extreme values had to checked against microfilm photos of the original x-ray examination cards. This revealed errors created by misreading handwritten figures (interchange of "0" and "1" in two cases caused a weight figure 100 kg off the true value).

Unclear handwriting turned out to be the major cause of the big height and weight differences for the 82 records mentioned before. We made 14 corrections on the 82 records, and 13 of the corrections were due to unclear handwriting. There was only one pure punching error.

Unclear handwriting will cause certain misrepresentations to occur more often than others. 10 out of the 17 errors mentioned above were caused by mistakingly reading a "5" for a "8", or the other way round. More rare a "4" and a "9" had been interchanged, this was detected 2 times. Interchange of "5" and "6" is also likely to occur, but since this would only create a 10 cm height difference, it would not occur in the list of 82 records.

<u>Figure 1</u> Measurement variations in a person's body height.

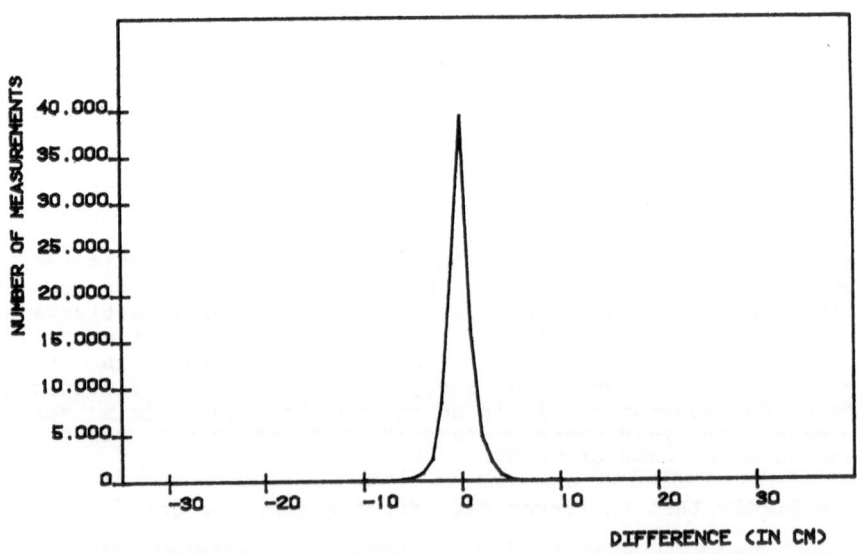

801

Table I Measurement variations in a person's body height.

Height difference in cm	Number of clients with their age distribution				
	20-29	30-49	50-69	70-99	Total
-50		1			1
-39 to -35			2		2
-34 to -30	2	3	1	1	7
-29 to -25	1	3	1	1	6
-24 to -20		2	1		3
-19 to -15	4	4	9	2	19
-14	1	1	5	1	8
-13	1	4	7	4	16
-12	1	9	15	3	28
-11	10	40	26	6	82
-10	15	42	42	8	107
- 9	20	29	27	10	86
- 8	6	17	25	6	54
- 7	6	19	39	19	83
- 6	25	50	72	44	191
- 5	31	84	188	83	386
- 4	80	254	452	182	968
- 3	232	792	1.097	322	2.443
- 2	1.040	3.416	3.311	559	8.326
- 1	4.568	10.732	7.164	969	23.433
0	18.512	13.359	6.447	965	39.282
1	5.872	6.873	2.964	525	16.234
2	1.559	1.714	1.256	367	4.896
3	326	636	817	313	2.092
4	118	253	302	98	771
5	43	90	70	27	230
6	16	40	20	7	83
7	14	20	18	8	60
8	11	21	13	4	49
9	11	51	47	10	119
10	26	50	41	8	125
11	14	36	20	5	75
12	1	9	11	7	28
13	2	2	7	1	12
14	2	1	4	1	8
15 to 19	4	7	8	5	24
20 to 24	4	4	5	2	15
25 to 29		4	3		7
30 to 34	1	4	3	1	9
35			1		1
Total:	32.581	38.677	24.544	4.576	100.378

Note: The differences are taken between the lowest and the
highest height measurement for a person. Age is that
which refers to the first measurement for a person
after the age of 19. A minus sign indicates that the
lowest measurement was taken later than the highest
measurement. Each of the 100.378 persons had from 2
to 5 height measurements.

Table I represents height differences for 100.378 persons who had
from 2 to 5 measurements each. Figure 1 displays in a graphical way
the distribution of the height differences.

Table I reveals height differences up to 50 cm. It is then timely to ask what an influence this gives on the reliability of the data from a statistical point of view. To answer this question we computed the mean and the standard deviation for the height difference for people measured for the first time in the age group of 30-69. It was believed that height in this group should be fairly stable and that deviations from zero for mean and standard deviation mainly would reflect the errors occuring in the material. Our computations gave a mean of -0.3 cm and a standard deviation of 1.9 cm. This probably reflects that there is a slight overall height reduction.

Figure 1 shows a graphical display of the height difference distribution. It shows a close resemblance to the Gauss distibution. It is therefore justifiable to say that roughly 2/3 of the measurements can be expected to fall within 2 cm of the true value. This is what is to be expected as a measurement exactness when people come for measurement at different times of the day, different socks, and so on. It is thus justifiable to say that from a statistically point of view stray erreanous measurements will have little influence if normal checking routines are applied.

For the individual the case is different. Undetected large errors in a medical journal may do severe harm if the figures are trusted fully as they are.

5. DISCUSSION

Our project has illustrated some of the error situations that are likely to occur in a medical system based on a large data base. We will in the following discuss further some of the consequences of such errors. We will limit the discussion to errors in the identificators, inasmuch as we think errors in other data elements have been properly dealt with in chapter 4.

We found that errors in the census files at the regional computing centres had caused errors in our files. The errors came into existence because there is not a complete identity between the register data at these centres and the census register at the National Bureau of Statistics.

This constitutes a general problem: data files received from various sources based on the same identification element may not have been updated to the same level. Erraneous identifications may have been detected and corrected at the institution that created the file, but these corrections will not help those working on previous versions of the file.

The problem reoccurs when the errors are to be corrected at our own computer installation. Unless we have a true database, thus avoiding data redundancy, the correction of an error will mean to correct all subfiles involved. Such an instant correction of all relevant files may not be feasible, and new errors may come into existence because we operate with files at various levels of update.

The need of a high degree of data reliability may be a major reason for introducing a data base system.

It is not possible to use the error rates found in this paper to estimate error rates in other large data materials. Data reliability

in a system is determined by the control measures that are
employed.But we have showed that even with fairly thorough control
measures an error rate of 0.5% is not an unrealistic measure. With
less rigorous control error rates will necessarily be much higher.

We have also shown that unclear handwriting is a major source of
wrong information. This may be of importance where doctors do the
main data entry, since the handwriting of doctors has a poor
reputation as far as readability is concerned. Figures are especially
liable to being misrepresented.

Many medical systems are based on interchange of information between
large computer-based data bases. Error situations are likely to occur
that may be very hard to detect and correct. It is advisable to pay
much attention to data validation before systems are put into
operation. Otherwise errors once introduced may exist forever in some
parts of an integrated system.

RECOVERY POSSIBILITIES IN THE PRACTICE OF
AN INTEGRATED HOSPITAL INFORMATION SYSTEM.

by P. Snitker and S.P.N.van Kampen
BAZIS, University Hospital Leyden
The Netherlands.

ABSTRACT.

In the Leyden University Hospital an Integrated Information System has been developed
on minicomputer equipment. The database, the operating system, and application
software are developed in house. The system is implemented in other Dutch University
Hospitals too, and in some General Hospitals. The total number of connected terminals is over 700. All the database-mutations are logged onto tape. Together with
the daily copy procedure of the diskfiles, this logtape guarantees an adequate
tool to protect the users against loss of data by accidental errors in the database.
This logging technique and the recovery procedure, (in case of loss of data) is
described. Results are given for the availability of the system and for the
Mean-Time-Between-Interruption of service.

INTRODUCTION.

The operational use of the Integrated Hospital Information System (HIS) was started
at the Leyden University Hospital in 1974. It has been developed for minicomputer
equipment and particularly for the PDP 11 series of Digital Equipment Corporation.
The configuration has been expanded to a double PDP 11/70 configuration (see fig. 1).
The one configuration is used for the productionsystem, the other for backup and the
development of application programs and operating systems. Six University Hospitals
and twelve General Hospitals have implemented this information system, where similar
configurations are also in use. The number of beds totals more than 10000, the number
of terminals connected with the various configurations is over 700. The largest
number of terminals is in the Leyden University Hospital (with 210 terminals).
At the start of this project it was concluded that there was no existing operating
system available which could fulfill the requirements with respect to conversational
ability, capacity availability and reliability. Therefore it was decided to develop
the system software, including the database software (and structure),in house.

805

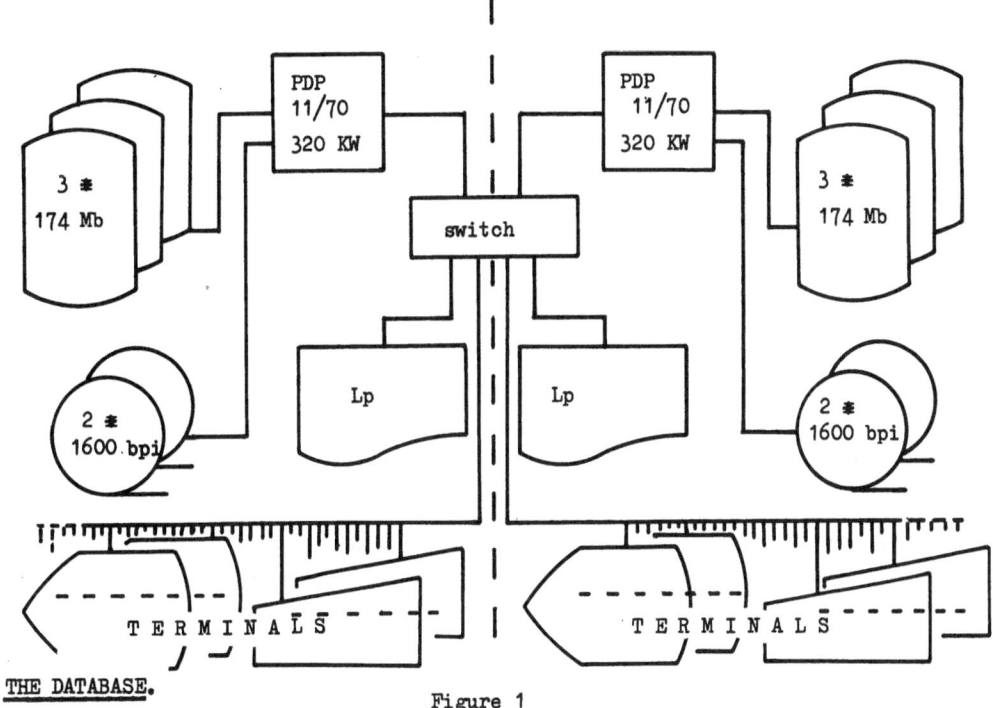

Figure 1

The structure of the database consists of two different parts. The one parts is a
number of multiple indexed random files, each called a "Thesaurus". The other part
is a chained structure of variable length subrecords. Every chain of linked subrecords is coupled to a record of a thesaurus and therefore called a Thesaurus Variable
Record (TVR).
The available call-functions which access the database are a search, read, write,
update and delete for both thesaurus records and TVR subrecords. A Thesaurus main-
file record is uniquely defined by the thesaurusnumber and the recordnumber. Therefore a single read-call covers the demands. There are however, several possible
occurrencies of a special TVR subrecord type connected to one thesaurusrecord,
which therefore are not uniquely defined by the thesaurusnumber and the recordnumber.
For this reason different selection possibilities are implemented for the TVR-
read-calls. To avoid the simultaneous update of the same record or subrecord by
different users, the update function is a critical region in the system, which is
semaphored, and the interface for the update-call requires both the old and the new
representation of the record/subrecord. The old representation is checked against
the actual contents of the record/subrecord, and if these are not identical, the
update is not effected. An error parameter is then returned to the calling program.
The capacity of the information system is large enough to serve a number of Hospitals
in a region, therefore several Hospitals sometimes share the same computer configuration. Data appertaining to different hospitals are flagged in the database to

enable the access-mechanism of the databasehandler,to check whether the requesting
user is allowed to access this data. Beside this one, there are several levels of
access-controll to assure that only qualified people gain entry to the system,and
that they are accessing only the data fore which they are qualified.

LOGGING AND RECOVERY ASPECTS.

In a large integrated HIS a number of interactive programs are using the same database simultaneously. Logging in such a system is primarily necessary to preserve
all the important mutations in the database. This is done by logging these changes
on magnetic tape. In the case of a total or partial loss of the data, this logtape
is then used to restore the data on disk.
Logging of all necessary information can be performed in two ways:
logical logging or physical logging. By the logical logging we understand both the
storage of the content of the parameters of the database-calls as well as the storage
of all terminal-input. An advantage of the logging of all terminal input is the
limited number of input characters ($\sim$1.3 M char. a day). Only a small storage capacity on magnetic tape or disk is necessary, and remote logging, (because of safety
considerations) is possible by means of a inexpensive telephoneline. During a
recovery action however, it is difficult to re-execute the programs from the terminal-input. Two programs that are mutating simultaneously the same file, may
influence each other in realtime. In a recover action all changes of this file have
to be synchronized thoroughly.
Another problem connected with the re-execution of the terminal-input is the necessity to log also all other program input. This input can consist of data from a
magnetic tape or of data sent to the central system by an external computer.
Physical logging of all disk mutations however gives a rather simple and reliable
recovery procedure. It is possible to recover data that is damaged by hardware
errors, but it is more complicated to restore the data when program errors have
destructed the files. A problem with physical logging is the large number of necessary logtapes (300000 discwrites a day will result in 7 logtapes (1600 BPI 3200 ft).
 The optimum situation is a compromis between logical logging and physical logging.
Database mutations, executed through the formal interface, are logged logical.
Accesses generated by the filesystem, which is not implemented in the operating
system but linked to the application programs, are logged physically.
A difficulty arises however since the description of the database is not contained
in the database itself. As a consequence the implementation of a new thesaurus is
neither logged nor recovered. This can cause difficulties in recovery-runs, if
these problems are not solved with proper procedures of the operating staff.

LOGGING.

In the information system, all the database mutations are logged on magnetic tape together with additional information. The logtape provides several facilities:

a. Recovery:
   The logtape contains the necessary information to restore the thesauri and TVR's in case of lost data on disk, or diskdamage.

b. Statistics:
   The logtape contains also the information, to enable system and program analysis. This information can be used for the examination regarding the system performance and for determining the workload per program.

c. Investigation:
   After a user-complaint or the detection of some error in the database, the logging of the terminal-input allows an investigation of the events that have happened. These errors can be a consequence of erroneous conversational input, or of course, faults in the system or application software.

The information on the logtape consists of three catagories: functions, events and additional information.
The functions consist of the mutating operations: the write, the update and the delete actions in the databank.
The events are logged to enable the non-recovery functions to be executed. These consist of the read and search actions on the database, user-logon acceptance, the completion of a database mutation, escape interrupts, etc. The additional information on the logtape, is required to recover or to analyse the data.
This is formed by the essential parameters of the functions and events, e.g.:
the old and new representation of the database (sub)records and the terminal input.

RECOVERY .

There are several levels regarding the loss of data whereby a recovery is required.
In the less severe situation only the current pointers of the datadescription of a file are erroneous. This situation can occur after a (hardware) system-down.
The procedure for the recovery of these pointers is started automatically by the system. This recover action is performed within a couple of minutes.
When data is lost of a define part of the database, e.g. one special thesaurus, a partial recover action is possible. Only the mutations of that thesaurus and the matched TVR's are recovered. The action lasts about half an hour and can be effectuated on the back-up computer while the production system is still running.
After the recover action, the restored thesaurus is loaded on-line in the production database.

A total recover action is required when the database or an unknown part of it is destroyed (e.g. in case of a diskhead crash). The recovery is performed by means of the most recent copy of the disks and the logtapes since the diskcopy. A total recovery requires two to four hours, during which there is no production system available.

RECOVERY AND AVAILABILITY .

A recovery action may last several hours, depending on the length of the runtime which should be recovered. This decreases the availability of the system for the users, especially when the system should be available 24 hours per day and 7 days per week. Partial recover actions may be done on the other configuration but this is not possible for a total recovery. Fortunately those total recoveries are very rare.

Table 1

1980	Hospital 1		Hospital 2		Hospital 3	
	avail.%	MTBI hrs	avail.%	MTBI hrs	avail.%	MTBI hrs
jan.	99,85	14,6	99,71	29,8	99,11	26,6
feb.	99,91	20,5	99,99	31,6	96,60	21,8
mar.	99,88	20,0	99,99	32,3	99,70	31,0
apr.	98,53	18,9	99,99	36,0	99,60	28,8
may	99,99	26,5	99,99	35,4	99,85	31,0
jun.	99,00	14,5	99,98	31,3	99,64	31,3
jul.	99,39	8,2	99,95	31,0	99,60	27,6
aug.	99,90	12,0	99,87	33,8	99,72	28,6
sep.	99,83	10,7	99,98	27,7	97,93	24,0
oct.	99,73	13,2	99,95	27,6	96,77	27,6
nov.	99,89	12,6	99,63	34,3	99,40	30,0
dec.	99,68	20,0	99,55	21,3	99,53	26,6

In table 1 figures are given about the availability of the system in three different hospitals together with the Mean-Time-Between-Interruption (MTBI: the average time a user can have a terminal session without interruption of the service by a "(re)boot" or a system controlled "escape"). The MTBI of hospital 1 differs from the other hospitals. This is explained by the fact that new versions of the operating system are implemented first in this hospital. Errors in the new version which are not detected by testing, cause a number of software dumps. Because the system is started up automatically immediately after the software crash the availability of the system in hospital 1 is not influenced.

In table 2 the number of recover actions and the recovertime in some hospitals
are given for 1980 and 1981 (until sept).

Table 2

Hospital	1980		1981 (until sept.)	
	# of recov. actions	time in minutes	# of recov. actions	time in minutes
1	1	433	1	0
2	2	540	0	0
3	0	0	0	0
4	0	0	2	418

Some case stories which required a partial or a total recovery, which happened in the
past two years are:
- A thesaurus initiation which intentionally should be performed on the test configuration, was performed accidentaly on the production system. This error
  required a copy action of the old diskpacks, a partial recovery of the appropriate
  thesaurus on the back-up system, and a reload via tape in the production thesaurus.
  De production remained running during the recovery but the application which
  required the damaged thesaurus, was not available for about three hours.
- Hardware errors in the dual port electronics of the disc memory caused the situation that during some days intermittent write actions of the test configuration
  were performed on the production databank, and vice versa.
  For this situation it was also necessary to copy the old diskpacks and recover all
  database mutations of the previous runs.
- An exercise of the emergency energy provisions in the hospital crashed the system.
  The diskpower failed but the heads were not drawn in, so they landed on the
  disksurface. As this was early in the morning, not long after the normal copy of
  the disks, there were not very much actions to recover.
  Including the copying of the (old) disks the system was off the air for about
  fifty minutes.

FUTURE DEVELOPMENTS.

At this moment, the mutations in the database description are not yet logged.
The problems that arise from this, are solved by manual interventions. The logging
and recover programs will be adapted,so that all changes in the definition of the
database are also recovered.

In case of a total loss of a computer centre in a hospital, it would be impossible to restore the data because the logtapes and (some) copypacks are possibly lost too. The logging of all input data on a remote location of one of the other participants with a Hospital Information System, will make it possible to recover the data after such accidents. For a reliable recovery, by means of the replay of the input data, it is necessary to log sufficient checkpoints so that the synchronisation problems with programs that are influencing each other, can be solved.

At present, software is being developed for the analysis of logged information for measurement of the system performance and the composition of a workload profile. This will provide information regarding the behaviour of both user and programs and will allow a classification of the workload, which again offers the possibility of a simulation of the system. With such a simulation model, the improvement of strategies and algoritms can be examined and evaluated to increase the performance, even with a increasing workload.

THE USE OF PHONETIC CODE FOR PATIENT IDENTIFICATION

I. Bräuer
Institut für Med. Informatik und Systemforschung
Gesellschaft für Strahlen- und Umweltforschung mbH München
Ingolstädter Landstraße 1
D-8042 Neuherberg

R. Thurmayr, R. Busch, M. Schnabel
Institut für Med. Statistik und Epidemiologie
Technische Universität München
Sternwartstraße 2
D-8000 München 80

Summary

The Cologne Phonetic Code was used for the identification of patient data   This
code clusters names into classes of similarity represented by the code-number
These classes reveal to be appropriate for further selection procedures towards
patient identification.
The paper presents two applications of the Phonetic coding procedure for patient
identification. One in a data collection system for cytological data and the other
in the data base documentation for the Klinikum rechts der Isar of the Technische
Universität München.

1. What is a phonetic code ?

Patient identification in large data bases has to deal with the problem of matching two possibly error afflicted character strings. To realize an effective matching process a measure of closeness between two strings has to be found. This enables the formation of classes where each class contains a correct character string and its incorrect correspondents. Phonetic codes are able to generate these classes. They try to correct errors due to bad pronounciation or bad understanding usually of names. Therefore the actual phonetic coding procedure depends on the linguistic region in which it will be employed. In the anglo-american region the Russell Soundex Code is wide-spread, in the german linguistic region there exist the Cologne Phonetic Code and the Vienna Phonetic Code. Some of the characteristics of the Cologne Phonetic Code will be discussed in the following.

The Cologne Phonetic Code was developed especially for the encoding of persons names. Like the other quoted systems it is based on the linguistic fact that the significance of a word's letters decreases towards its end and that consonants are more significant than vowels. Studies preceeding the development of the Cologne Phonetic Code revealed that personal names consist on the average of nine letters. 63 per cent of these letters are consonants. Considering only the first letter of the names, the amount of consonants rises to 80 per cent (2).

The coding procedure substitutes the 26 letters of the alphabet with the digits 1 to 9. A vowel is suppressed if not the first letter of the word. The following are examples of names placed into the same phonetic class by the Cologne Phonetic Code (3):

Müller	--> 657	Breschnew	--> 17863
Miller	--> 657	Breznev	--> 17863
Moeller	--> 657	Breshnew	--> 17863
Moliere	--> 657	Preczneff	--> 17863
Miehler	--> 657		

The number of members of a phonetic class, using a given set of names, depends on the number of regarded phonetic digits. 4 such digits (in the above example _657 and 1786) allow 5265 possible phonetic classes. Based on a set of 1.000.000 names, the average number of names in a class is 190.

2. The Use of the Cologne Phonetic Code in a data collection system

ZEISIG (Zytologie Erfassungs- und Informationssystem in der Gynäkologie) is a data collection system for cytologic diagnoses resulting from cervix cancer screening. It was developed in the Institute for Medical Informatics and Health Services

Research (medis) of the Society for Radiation and Environmental Research (gsf) in Munich (1). 325.000 patient data records are stored in the underlying data base. The patient data collection module of the system uses an identification procedure that was developed with regard to on-line usage. This procedure consists of an automatic and a manual component. The automatic component tries to find (using a suitable algorithm) a unique association between the input data and one of the patient records of the data base. If not successful, the remaining set of possible corresponding records may be used for manual identification.

The automatic identification algorithm is implemented as a hierarchical process of three levels. At each level, a suitable original set of patient records is derived by a primary search criterion from the data base. Starting from this set, the algorithm tries to find a unique correspondence between the input record and one of the records of the set. This is done restricting the original set by applying further comparisons.

If the algorithm succeeds in finding a unique correspondence on one of the levels, identification is terminated. If the original set at each of the identification levels is empty, it is assumed that no corresponding record in the data base exists. If a unique correspondance cannot be found, a set union of the remaining record sets of all identification levels is built and the resulting set is presented for manual identification. The identification algorithm passes through the three levels in the following order:

1. Primary search by the last sample number,
2. primary search with a search criterion built from the birth name and the birth date,
3. primary search with a search criterion built from the surname and the birth date.

The two search criteria built from the names are computed in the following manner: First, the name is transformed to its phonetic code by the discussed process. The identifier of a phonetic class is the number built from the first four phonetic digits.

Second, the birth date is linearised by counting the number of days since a given starting date (for the presented system this is 1.1.1850).

The two resulting numbers are concatenated to form the search criterion. The refinement of the phonetic classes is done because the number of records in some of the classes is too large to get good response times with an on-line system. This is true especially for classes containing very common names. The reason for the choosen solution is the following:

Refinement can also be achieved by regarding more than four phonetic digits as a class identifier. This is not a good solution. Since the significance of letters decreases at the end of a word, the selectivity of the classification would also decrease. Therefore, the necessary refinement is obtained using the linearised birth date to subdivide the phonetic classes. This tends to be less errorprone, since a birth date can be submitted to stronger plausibility tests than a person's name. Yet any erroneous but plausible birth date leads out of the appropriate original class and the automatic algorithm will qualify the input record as not contained in the data base. Another unknown fact is the impact of the similarity of letters in a hand-written text – over half of the input data originates from hand-written forms. An algorithm covering this topic might be interfered with the phonetic coding approach. This improves the selectivity of an automatic identification procedure.

An earlier implementation of the presented system used the identification number (I-number) recommended by the GMDS as the main identification criterion. This I-number, discussed in more detail in the next section, is constructed using birth date, birth name, mother's birth name, sex and code for twins. Evaluations (5) revealed that for this system the identification number has a very weak selectivity, since mother's birth name and code for twin are not known and all of the patients are women. The first duplicate identification number emerged within 3000 patient records. Identification results had to be improved applying further algorithms regarding similarity between patients names, first names and birth names.

3. Identification in Data Base Documentation Using a Phonetic Code

The Klinikum rechts der Isar carries out data base documentation for six clinics (Surgery, Dermatology, Toxicology, Urology, Orthopaedics and Psychiatry) (4). The patient data base (family name, surname, birthday, birthday-place and sex) and some specific administrational data are collected via the admission dialogue. The medical data base (diagnosis, operations, post-operative complications and risk factors) are collected frome case histories, unstructured or semi-automatically generated physicians reports. The programs were also developed by medis. Until the finish of processing the data base is managed in a current file and then spooled to the archive data base for final storage. During the collection phase the data base is identified by an admission number. The admission number is an eleven digit code comprising a clinic number, a sequential number, admission year and a check digit. It is distributed during the admission dialogue. The data base is stored within the current file by the aid of a hospitalisation number These are sorted according to each patients hospitalisation number. On the other hand the archive data base contains patient oriented files. The I-number is used here for identification purposes. It is a fourteen digit code comprising birthday, sex, a code for twins etc., a code for birth or maiden name, maiden name of the mother, a sequential code for cases of non-unique identification and a check digit. The

I-number is formed during the admission dialogue from the patient data. It is used to search for previously stored data from earlier admissions and match then to the admitted patient in the archive data base.

Since construction of the I-number depends upon correct and exhaustive collection of the corresponding patient data base, which is not always possible, the search in the archive data base cannot be limited to the I-number search alone. Therefore an algorithm was developed which finds patient data bases even in cases where errors exist in the patient data structure. These errors are not only caused by admissions personel but also by sometimes changing information from the patient especially in the case of foreign immigrant workers.

This algorithm consists of a search and a comparison procedure. Our original process was based upon a bytewise comparison of the patient data bases. This however had the disadvantage of finding too many probable matches which had to be subsequently verified manually.

We therfore used the Cologne Phonetic Code for identification purposes. Five digits of this phonetic code are used. A phonetic code is constructed for name, surname, birth-place and street during spooling of the patients data base form the current file to the archive data base. These four phonetic codes are stored for each patient in the archive data base and are addressable. The identification algorithm starts with a search based upon the I-number. If a match is found then the phonetic codes, birthday and sex of the given case are compared to those of the probable match. In the case of correspondence of all checked data this case is classed as a repeater, i.e. the patient has already been treated at least once in the clinic.

If the I-number search and the data comparison do not discover a repeater a search is begun for similar cases. For this purpose cases in the archive data base are selected whose birthday or phonetic code of family name is identical.

In the case where there is a change in family status an identical birthname is searched for. Further the phonetic codes, birthday and sex are compared and if at least five of these seven variables correspond the patient is classed as a repeater. When only four variables correspond the patient ist classed as a probable repeater whose identity has to be checked manually. Probable cases also consist of a correspondence in the variable birthday when only four of the six positions in the variable birthdate are identical. A maximum of three correspondences or less are classed as new admission.

Our data base documentation currently contains 70.000 patients of which 19.2 per cent are repeaters. Of these 77 per cent are found via I-number searches and 23 per cent are clarified using further patient information. Those repeaters must be determined manually from a certain number of probable cases. Using the phonetic code the number of probable cases is reduced to one fourth. Further the search algorithm using the phonetic code is more exact which is proved by the fact, that the phonetic code identification discovered 1 per mille incorrect classified

816

patient data records in the whole data base.

Our next goal will be to include this identification procedure in the admission dialogue after enough experience using the new algorithm has been gathered and the program rewritten to improve speed and reliability.

References:

(1) Bräuer, I.; Keicher, M.; Zock, H.: ZEISIG - Zytologie Erfassungs-
und Informationssystem in der Gynäkologie. In: Tagungsband der 25.
Jahrestagung der GMDS, Erlangen, 15.-17. 9. 1980
(Ed.: L. Horbach). Berlin: Springer(1980)

(2) Postel, H.-J.: Die Kölner Phonetik.
IBM-Nachrichten

(3) Postel, H.-J.: Die besonderen Probleme beim Aufbau eines Informations-
systems für Sicherheitsbehörden (II).
Datenverarbeitung in Steuer, Wirtschaft und Recht, 4(1975), Heft 2/75,
pp. 55-61.

(4) Thurmayr, R.; Schnabel, M.; Thurmayr, G.R.; Laux, S.; Schöffel, J.;
Stieber, J.: Präsentation von Basis- und medizinischen Berichtsdaten.
In: Möhr, J.B.; Köhler, C.O.: Datenpräsentation, Frühjahrstagung,
Heidelberg 1979
Berlin - Heidelberg - New York: Springer, 164 - 176 (1979)

(5) Raimar, W.; Stolley, H.: Probleme der Patientenidentifizierung bei
einem Krebs-Vorsorge-Projekt. In: AMK Berlin: Dokumentation II der
MEDCOMP 77, Berlin (1977)

A DATA BASE PACKAGE FOR A SMALL SYSTEM AND A MEDICAL APPLICATION

William D. Grove

Queensland Radium Institute

Royal Brisbane Hospital

Herston

Australia. 4029

Summary

Mini and micro computer applications can call for data base facilities to save online storage space and the duplication of mostly inefficient programs to handle different data files. A library of callable routines can be linked with a user program. A number of utility programs which create, backup and restore the data base will make up the package. The complexity of the data base definition can be over-come by the use of the data base facilities to manage its own administration. Recursive procedures and Recent Use Pools for data definitions reduce the size of the library. An application to the storage of statistical data at the Queensland Radium Institute is outlined.

1.   INTRODUCTION

The advantages of using a mini computer for the storage of statistical data are firstly, cost savings especially if most of the hardware exists, and secondly, having direct control of the data. This second aspect is important considering the often very sensitive nature of medical data. Data manipulation and retrieval programs can be lengthy and messy. The statistician has many data files and many entry and retrieval programs to administer, so that data base facilites can relieve him of much of this administrative burden. Operating systems for mini computers rarely offer data base facilities. A limited data base facility is proposed for mini and micro systems. Rather than using a data base operating system; a basic scientific or time sharing operating system is employed. The operating systems file handling procedures are used and a data base structure set up within these files. A library of fortran compatible routines is linked with programs to give this facility, and a number of utility programs for creation, copying, backup and restoration of the data base make up the data base package.

The Queensland Radium Institute has a Digital Equipment PDP 11/40 mini-computer which is primarily used for Radiotherapy treatment planning. It runs under RT-11 foreground/background operating system. The package was designed to function in this environment and to be capable of being upgraded to run under RSX-11M a time sharing operating system, or TSX - a time sharing extension of RT-11. The structure of the data base is a network type and the data description and manipulation could be described broadly though not accurately as a subset of CODASYL (1), (2) or DBMS-11.

2.   DEFINITION OF DATA BASE FEATURES AND THEIR METHOD OF IMPLEMENTATION

> Ordering and Addressing of Records
> Variable Length Records
> Sequential Storage of Records
> Data Base Locking
> Access Control of Records
> Duplicates Allowed/Not Allowed
> Activity Logging

For these facilities to work efficiently on a small computer they have to be limited to some extent. At data base generation time, the size and number of records must be defined. The data base may only be extended by full or partial regeneration.

2.1   Ordering of Records

An ordered record is defined at data base generation time. The generation program allows space for ordered pointers. A data base number is a combination of two numbers, the record type number and the record number. (Figure 1). This uniquely defines every record in the data base. The generation program usually allows space for twice the number of pointers as records to accommodate hash addressing. The records themselves are not ordered and are stored sequentially. The pointers are ordered in ascending order. Records are addressed by hashing to these ordered pointers. If the pointers are heavily populated in some areas as can happen with ordered names, the FIND routine detects this and does a binary search rather than a sequential search in this area to reduce the number of disk accesses. The hash routine is the same for all records and it uses the parameters set up at generation time - lowest record value, highest record value and the number of pointers possible.

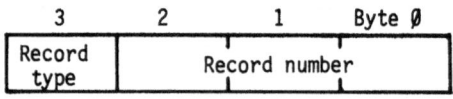

Data base number uniquely defines a record
Figure 1

2.2   Variable Length Records

This facility in data bases usually requires a lot of administration with tables, free space lists etc. The complexity of being able to add, delete, append or modify such a record would be beyond the scope of this limited package. To provide this feature the record is divided into fixed length records-- a base record similar to a fixed length record plus the necessary fixed length extension records. To minimize the waste with this method, the data base generation needs the expected length of the record. Two samples one of names and one of addresses from an existing data file showed that the lengths of these were distributed similarly to a Poisson variable. An iterative program was written to find the best values of the base length b and extension records x for values of   from 4 to 100. It was found that the best value of b was always very close to   and the average waste was not very sensitive to the value of x. For several reasons this was taken to be 12 bytes plus 4 bytes for a pointer. With this method of providing variable length records, delete and modify procedures are very much simplified.

2.3   Sequential Storage of Records

Records are stored sequentially within files managed by the normal file management system. An ordered and/or a variable length record is stored with its list of hashed pointers and/or extension records. A record type must be contained wholly within a file; but a file can contain more than one record type. A file with the data base name is required for the administration records and a log file is required for the storage of alterations to the data base. The advantage of many files comprising the data base is seen when storage facilities are limited. Only files actually accessed need by on the line at any one time. Backup can also be done incrementally or more frequently for the more volatile files.

When a record is deleted, it is removed from all its set occurrences, its pointers nulled to indicate deletion and its data base number is written to the temporary deletion list at the end of the file. At backup, its number is written to the permanent deletion list and it is permanently deleted. Before a new record is written the permanent deletion list is checked for available space.

2.4   Data Base Locking

During any writing procedures such as STORE, MODIFY, INSERT, REMOVE, DELETE; the data base is locked to other write procedures by the use of a dummy device handler. The data base can also be LOCKed and UNLOCKed by the user program prior to and after a section of code.

2.5   Access Control on Records

Each record can be allocated two passwords, the first for total access and the second for read only access. A PASSWORD call must be completed before record access is attempted.

2.6   Duplicates not Allowed

This facility is defined at generation time and returns an error condition at run time if a record of the same value is attempted to be stored. The default is

Duplicates Allowed.

2.7   Activity Logging

Alterations to any records or pointers in the data base are stored in this file. Should a programming or hard disk fault cause the data base to become irrepairable then a new copy can be made of all or part of the data base from the backup files and the log file. Log files are backed-up also and so the data base can be restored from any level of backup. The log file is best kept on another medium to the greater part of the data base.

3.   DEFINITION OF DATA BASE STRUCTURE

The CODASYL features of SUBSCHEMA and AREA have not been supported in this implementation so as to reduce the complexity and because the advantages of these features can be partly realised through the SET feature and the division of the data base into files on various media. The versatility of the SET feature has been extended to cover most relationships between records. This allows the data base to be described more easily and with fewer set types. At the expense of more disk accesses but greater simplicity, keys are not used. The record is its own key.

3.1   Set

A Set is an ordered collection of records. Each set type must have an owner record type and zero or more member record types. The records in each set are linked by cyclic pointers. There are two classes of sets depending on the relationship between records types in the set. Class 1 is an owner related set class. This means that the relationship of each record type is related to the owner. If empty records exist in this class, the circular set pointer points to the next record in the set. Class 2 is a heirarchical related set class. Each record type is related to the previous record. If an empty record exists the next relationship is undefined and the cyclic set pointer points back to the owner record.

A record in a set may have a 1 to 1 relationship or a 1 to many relationship with the owner record (class 1) or with the previous record (class 2). The 1 to many relationship is managed by a repeating record pointer in this record. This pointer cyclically connects all associated records. As well, the relationship can be unique or complex. In a unique relationship the record can be pointed to only once within the set eg. mother - child relationship. In a complex relationship the record can be pointed to any number of times, eg. parent - child relationship. The complex relationship is managed by setting up another record type which holds the intersection data or merely a pointer to the child record. This can be handled manually or automatically by the data base routines. To fully support a many to many complex relationship we need to define two sets; a parent - child set and a child - parent set (3).

3.2   Record

A Record can consist of one or more items. It is the basic unit of the data base
and can be accessed sequentially; by set pointers; or by ordered pointers if it is an
ordered record. The definition of a record contains information about its storage space,
space for ordered pointers, space for extension records, its logical length and length
including pointers, passwords etc.

3.3   Item

An item is defined as a part of a record. The main reason this facility is included is to compress the data by writing in it other than ASCII format. When an item or
record is accessed it is seen not in the storage mode, but in the defined ASCII expansion.

4.   USING THE DATA BASE FACILITIES FOR ITS OWN ADMINISTRATION

The complexity of the definition of a data base tends to limit its use on small
systems; but the data needed in its definition can be stored as data within the data
base. In this case seven record types in four set definitions define the structure of
the data. (Figure 2).

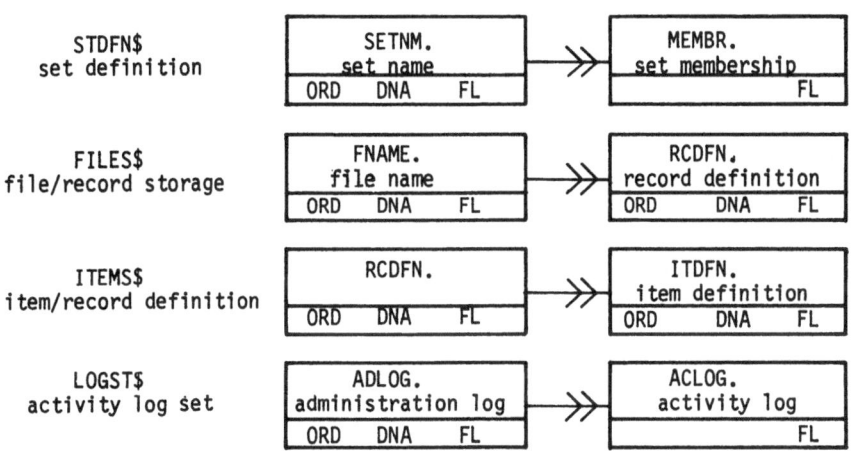

Data base administration data base
Figure 2

Definitions are stored in buffer areas which hold the most recently used definitions plus the system definition. Block ∅ of the data base contains these definitions
which could be called the 'data base bootstrap'. The advantage of this method of storage
is realised in the simplicity of library routines by using recursive procedures. An example of the algorithm for the GET routine is as follows:

GET needs the data base number that has been obtained from the FIND or NEXT

procedure and the program address for the record. It returns the record value starting
at this address.

      1.0 Is the record definition in the record definition pool? If yes go to 1.2

      1.1 GET record definition put it in record definition pool.

      1.2 Test password,exit on failure.

      1.3 Is the record in the record recent use pool? If yes go to 2.0

      1.4 Calculate block address and offset.

      1.5 Is the file record in the file pool? If yes go to 1.7

      1.6 GET file record put it in file pool.

      1.7 Is it a file record? If no go to 1.9

      1.8 Close presently open file in pools(if open). Open a channel for this file.

      1.9 Read Block/s write record to appropriate pool. Exit if deleted/no record.

      2.0 If fixed length go to 2.2

      2.1 Read extension record/s append to base record.

      2.2 Is it an intersection record? if no go to 2.4

      2.3 GET record pointed to by this record. Go to 3.0

      2.4 If address specified write to specified address.

      2.5 Is it itemized? if no go to 3.0

      2.6 GET item record.

      2.7 Expand record.

      2.8 Are there any more items? If yes go to 2.6

      3.0 Return

5.   AN APPLICATION

The application is the storage of data for statistical purposes at the Queensland
Radium Institute. Each patient has personal data plus data referring to a malignancy
which may be more than one. Most of the malignancy sites have a small amount of data
which is specific for each site. As well as this there are several large retrospective
studies concerning various sites. The records and sets are arranged as in Figure **3**.

5.1   The advantages of a data base structure for this application are

5.1.1 <u>Saving of Space</u>. When we have multiple malignancies (especially skin cancer) we
do not have to duplicate the data relating to the patient. The previous name record is
relevant in only about 1% of cases and so only 1/100 the number of name records need to
be allocated for it, and these may be stored with and linked to the present name.

5.1.2 <u>Organizational Ease</u>. Special study data needs to be updated periodically with
follow up data and this can be done by a small program which tests the date seen in the
patient data record. Alternatively this can signal that a study record is due for completion or update. Definitions of terms relating to some part of the data which are

used by entry programs can also be stored within the data base.

5.1.3 <u>Backup</u>. Backing up numerous data files is often incomplete as they are commonly spread around many disks. With the data base, backup procedures are guided and document- ed as they are done.

5.2   The disadvantage over conventional chained records is mainly the loss of speed of storage due to breaking a single record into several records and the added overhead of activity logging.

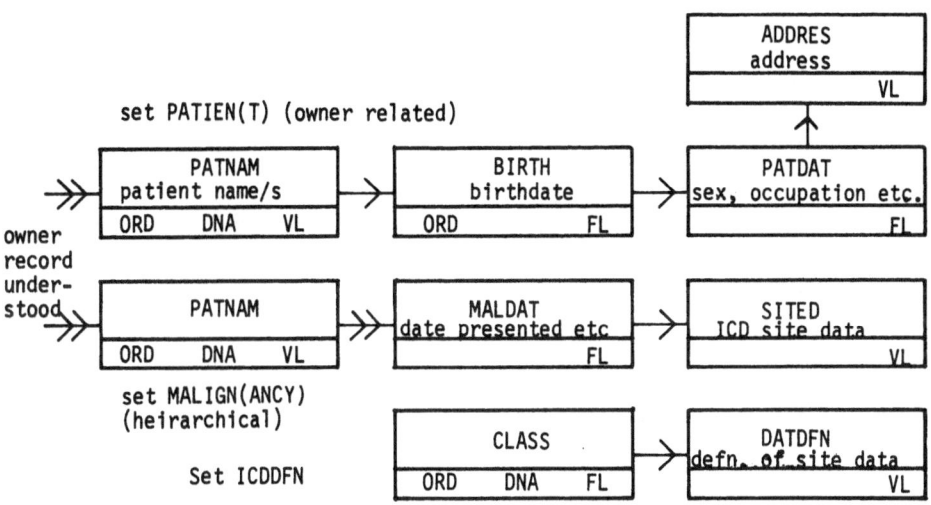

Definition of data at Queensland Radium Institute
Figure 3

References:
 (1) CODASYL Data Description Language Committee: journal of development 1978, Secretariat of the Canadian Government EDP Standards Committee, 1978
 (2) CODASYL FORTRAN data base facility: journal of development Jan. 1, 1977/ Fortran Data Base Manipulation Language Committee of the Conference on Data Systems Languages, Specifications Board Supply and Services Canada, 1977.
 (3) Martin, James, Computer Data Base Organisation, 2nd Ed., New Jersey, Prentice Hall, 1977.

A data model for a personnel information system

H. Simmes

Medical Information Department,

St. Radboud Hospital/University of Nijmegen

Erasmuslaan 17, P.O. Box 9101

6500 HB Nijmegen, the Netherlands

tel. 080-517065/513979

1. Summary

At this moment we distinguish two schools in information analysis
theory. One is primarily interested in the analysis of the information
processes the other accentuates the development of a data model. In
this paper an example is given of the data model approach used for
the development of a personnel information system at the St. Radboud
Hospital.
The development of the data-model facilitates mutual communication
between users and creates an easy transition to, and understanding
of the actual database.

2. Introduction

Designing informationsystems with the help of specific methods is
growing.
More and more systematic approaches are developed to support this
activity. In the information theory we see basically two different
approaches emerging, the information process analysis (e.q. Swedish
school (1)) and the data model approach (2). The first method starts
with a top down analysis of all the information processes in the field
of investigation. After this activity is finished an overall data model
is made by normalizing all the data needed by each of the subprocesses.
The data model approach starts developing a data model from the
beginning. Seen from the point of view of the latter method, the major
difference between the two approaches is that the data model is not
just the automatic result of the normalisation process but an essential
tool for designing an information system from the start.
Especially when there is a wide range of users with a different need
for information from the same system it is important to develop a
mutual language and understanding in the form of a data model as soon
as possible.

In the case of a personnel system with users like heads of departments, the personnal department, the planning department and the salary department this proved to be extremely helpful.

3. The data model approach

In this section the data model approach will be briefly introduced. The approach makes use of the group of models known under different names like entity-type, object-type or relational model. Those models basically consist of the following concepts:

- entity-type
- attributes
- three different types of relations between entity-types

An entity is an abstract or a real 'thing' in our environment which we consider important for our information system, e.q. employees, job descriptions, etc.
An entity-<u>type</u> is a generalization of a set of the same entities. Each entity of the set is uniquely described by the values of attributes like data of birth, salary level, address, etc. The choice of the attributes belonging to an entity-type also depends on the goal of the information system. We distinguish three different types of relations between entity-types.

1:1: One entity of a specific entity-type occurs only with zero or one entity of the other entity-type.
1:n; One entity of a specific entity-type occurs with zero, one <u>or more</u> entities of the other entity-type. The other way around one entity occurs only with zero or one entity of the first entity-type.
n:m; One entity of a specific entity-type occurs with zero, one or more entities of the other entity-type. This is also possible the other way around.

The three types of relations are presented below for the two entity-types MAN and WOMAN.

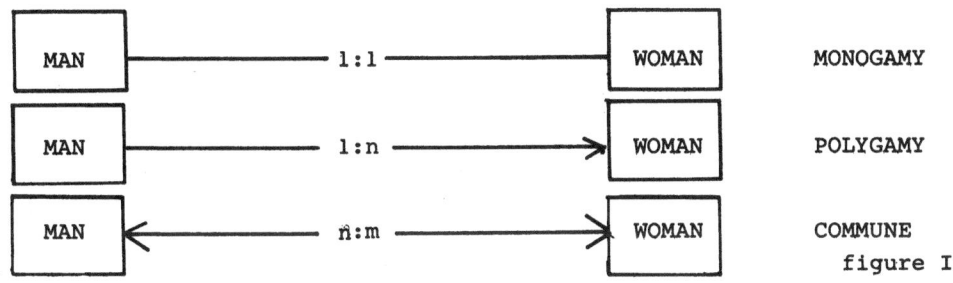

figure I

4. The entity-type model for a personnel information system

Three major steps were required to arrive at the data model. The result will in general depend on the local situation. Therefore, the entity-types are only globally defined for the purpose of illustrating the design process.

4.1. The first step

Entities on first sight important to a personnel system are: employees, positions in the organization, departments and job-types. As we see in the illustration below we have choosen to characterize the position by TYPE OF JOB (job description) rather than the employee. It was also found in our organization that one employee could hold two different positions at the same time. In such case one has to decide if this posibility should also be available in the information system. A lot of minor exceptions were not projected in the model deliberately.

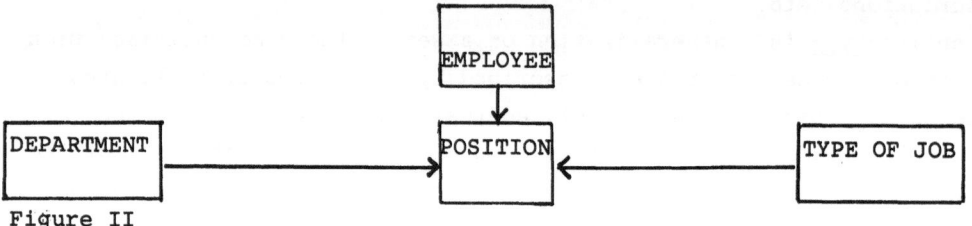

Figure II

4.2. The second step

After discussing this model we found that people of the personnel department and people of the planning and financial departments had quite different views on the same 'reality'.
This resulted in splitting the entity-type POSITION into POSITION and FORMATIONAL POSITION.
POSITION represents the day to day situation in the organization. Every change is immediately updated. FORMATIONAL POSITION represents the concept of position used for personnel and budget planning.
Those plans are updated only once a year and serve as standard during the planning period. This way we developed a measuring instrument, for comparing actual and planned use of personnel. The FORMATION plan represents the organization as it should be, the position plan represents the day to day situation. By comparing these two we can identify problem area's and make decisions which way things have to be adapted.

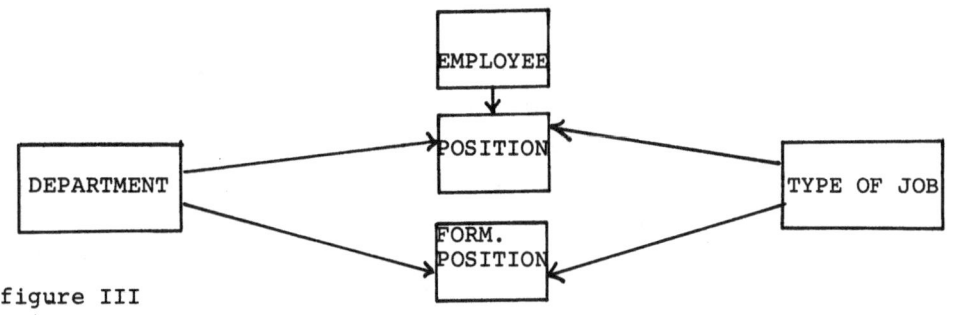

figure III

4.3. The third step

In the first two illustrations we saw the entity-type DEPARTMENT. Also
in this case we discovered a different point of view between the people
of the personnel department and the financial department. From the
financial point of view an employee is working in the department on
whose budget his salary is booked. In reality a lot of employees were
working in totally different departments but paid by other departments
for budgetary reasons. This different point of view had been a source
of misunderstanding over the years.
This discussion ended with defining two new entity-types PERSONNEL
ORGANIZATIONAL UNIT and FINANCIAL ORGANIZATIONAL UNIT and the introduction of the entity-type BUDGET. Check the arrows for all the
implications of this extension.

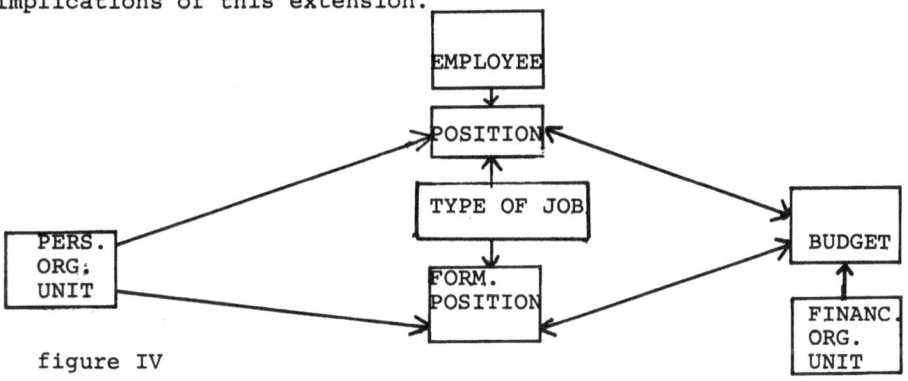

figure IV

The final version of the model still required some minor modifications.
However the step by step development of the data model supported the
creation of a mutually accepted set of definitions and conceptions.
Further specification of the new system using those definitions was
much less frustrated by formerly often ill understood semantical
problems.

5. Conclusions

It is important to develop a commonly accepted data model by a wide range of users as soon as possible. The model helps to clarify all kinds of different views between the users. This model is used (and refined) during the whole information analysis process. Secondly the data model is the basis for the data base design, and what is more important users who are mostly not that interested in data base design found it very easily to understand after they had worked so hard at the data model.

6. References

(1) Mats Lundeberg, Göran Goldkuhl, Anders Nilsson. Systemering.
    ISBN 90/14/03017 7 D 1981/0247/20.
(2) C.J. Date, Introduction to data base systems, Addison - Wesley.

A COMPUTER NETWORK IN A RESEARCH ENVIRONMENT

E.W.Kruyt
Department of Physiology
State University
P.O. box 9604
2300 RC Leiden
Netherlands

SUMMARY

A distributed network of computer systems is operational at the medical faculty of Leiden. Data acquisition, interactive preprocessing and primary data storage is performed on small local systems. For program development, data storage and interactive dataprocessing centralised multiproject computers are used. The computers are interconnected using Decnet. Batch processing is done on mainframes via remote job entry.
In this way advanced facilities are available for many people at moderate costs. For the on-line data processing systems a high level of availability is reached.

1. INTRODUCTION

At the medical faculty of Leiden we started in 1975 to build a distributed computer network. Beside some small dedicated computers an IBM 1800 computer was used at that time as a general purpose computer for both on-line data acquisition, batch oriented program development, image processing and signal analysis. To cope with the increasing demand for on-line signal processing, data storage and computer power the IBM 1800 had to be replaced. We decided to build a network of computers both to bring the computer facilities to the experiments for better interactive on-line signal analysis and to provide centralised facilities for data storage, program development and off-line data processing.
In the course of the years some 25 local and 2 central computers have been installed. These computers are used for different research projects, e.g.:
-study of electrical cel membrane noise
-epidemiological survey of lung function
-analysis of the regulation mechanism of respiration
-circadian rithms in man and animals
-EEG analysis
-metastase detection
-cardiovascular research

This computer network exists independent of the Leiden hospital information system, which is used for patient oriented data processing.

2. DEFINITIONS

In this paper the computer systems are classified as mainframes, multiproject computers, preprocessors and single project computers.
-a mainframe is a large central computer for administrative, general

purpose and database applications
-a multiproject computer (MPC) is used simultaneously for more then
one project. It is primarily suited for interactive program development, image processing, signal analysis and data storage. It forms
the central node in a network of small computers.
-a preprocessor is a small computer used for one project at a time.
During an experiment it may be used stand-alone but for program development and bulk data storage it depends on a MPC.
-a single project computer is a stand-alone configuration, used for
one project at a time. The system is suited for both program development, data acquisition, signal analysis and data storage.

Apart from these computers there are some dedicated (micro-)computers
which often are integrated in the equipment. This paper will concentrate on information processing systems rather then (micro-)computers
used as intelligent logic.
Personal computers like programmable calculators can fit in this
scheme as single project computers.

3.   THE COMPUTER NETWORK

The aim of the computer network is to provide advanced computer facilities to all who want to use them. The facilities that are needed
on-line should be brought to the experiment to facilitate interactive
data acquisition and preprocessing. Capital costs should be kept moderate without duplication of effort. The availability of the on-line
facilities should be high to make sure that the experiments can go on
and no data are lost.
Therefore data acquisition, preprocessing and primary data storage are
done locally on preprocessors, while program development, data storage
and data processing are done on MPC's. Number crunching can be done
on mainframes using batch processing.
In this way expensive resources are shared, advanced programming tools
are available and common libraries can be used. In addition back up
facilities and alternative ways of data storage can be provided. In
combination with a suitable operating system this scheme has the advantage that program development can go on during the experiments.

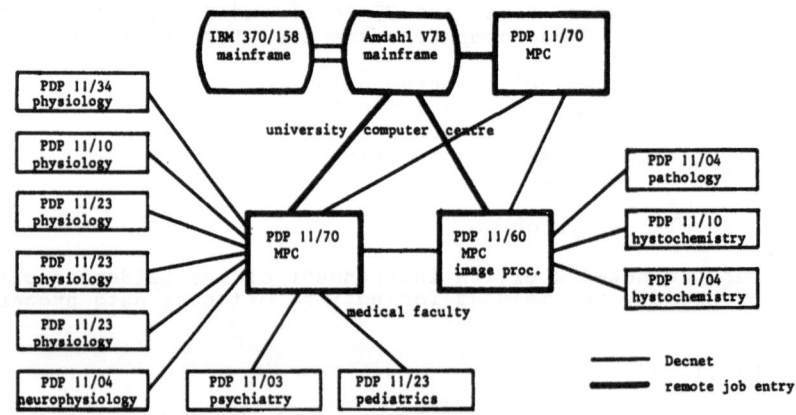

Fig. 1   the computer network

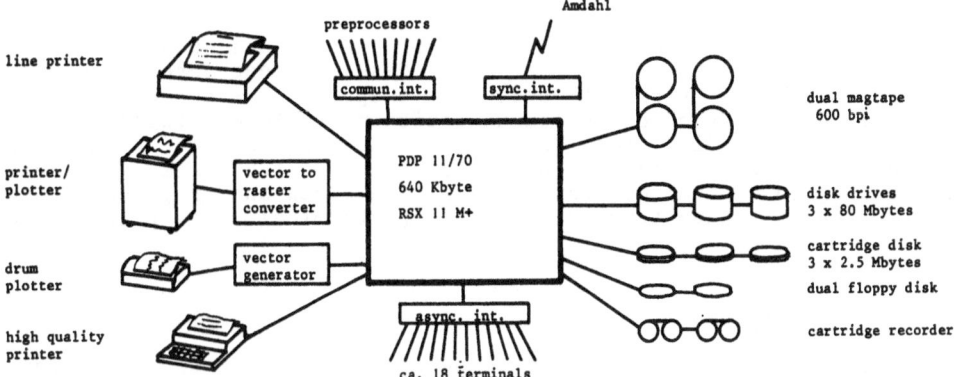

Fig. 2 Multiproject computer

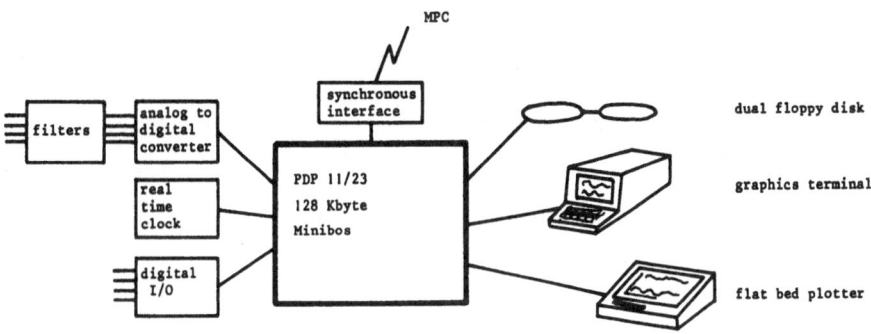

Fig. 3 Preprocessors

4. HARDWARE CONFIGURATION

The multiproject computers (PDP 11/70, PDP 11/60) are powerful midi computers with large memory, large disks, lineprinter, printer plotter, (graphics-) terminals etc. The preprocessors are coupled to the MPC's through synchronous communication multiplexers (DV11). They vary from a naked LSI 11 to a PDP 11/34 with hard disk. A typical preprocessor installation is composed of a processor, memory, floppy disk, analog to digital convertor, real time clock and graphics terminal. Often a video terminal, a hardcopy terminal and a plotter are added.

5. OPERATING SYSTEMS

On the MPC's a timesharing system is needed with good program development tools, extensive file- and graphics systems and data communication facilities.
On the preprocessors on the other hand a small real time system is necessary with nevertheless a simple file system, graphics, multiprocessing and data communication capabilities. The system should be able to function without a disk.
The operating systems on the MPC's and preprocessors must be compatible in some sense, e.g.:
-both systems should have a comparable human interface
-it should be easy to copy files from one system to the other
-the systems must support the same data communication protocol
-it should be possible to prepare tasks for the preprocessors on the MPC's.

Commercially available operating systems are not designed for such an environment.
If members of the same family of operating systems (RSX 11) are chosen for the MPC's and the preprocessors large preprocessors with hard disks are necessary. Such a system is complex to use for real time applications. In addition the licenses, datacommunication software included would become prohibatively expensive.
If different operating systems on the MPC and preprocessors are chosen a simple to use system (RT11) with good real time facilities for the preprocessors is available. The human interface will be different however and no program development tools for the preprocessors on the MPC's will be available.

Though nowadays the choice might be different we decided to implement RSX 11 systems on the MPC's and to develop our own operating system "Minibos" for the preprocessors (1). The need to build Minibos arose from the necessity for multiprocessing for some of the applications.
Minibos has the following characteristics:
-real time, multiprocessing
-RT11 compatible file system
-Decnet datacommunication protocol (DDCMP, NSP, DAP)
-task building under RSX 11
-graphics support (Tektronix 4010-series)

6. PROGRAM DEVELOPMENT

The application software is in general written in Fortran IV. Minibos, the low level real time routines and some of the older applications are written in Macro 11. Because of the many man-years invested in Fortan programs and program libraries we can only start to use e.g. Pascal if existing Fortran routines, I/O included, can be used and if modular program development is supported. These features recently have become available and we will now adapt a Pascal run time library to Minibos.

Editing, compiling and taskbuilding are done on the MPC's. We use terminals directly connected to the MPC's as well as remote access facilities.

By using the remote access facility a preprocessors terminal functions virtually as a MPC terminal. This feature is developed at the Leiden university computer centre. The additional software in the preprocessor takes only 0.5 Kbytes.

Minibos loads tasks in RSX format. In this way we can exploit the advanced taskbuilding features of the RSX task builder such as read-only resident libraries and system commons. This provides for a very efficient usage of the preprocessor's memory in a multiprocess environment. This used to be an important feature because of the 56 Kbyte memory limit of the older minicomputers.

Minibos is booted from local disk, if present, or via Decnet. Tasks are loaded from local disk or Decnet at choice.

Program development for eight bit microprocessors (M6800-series) is also done on the MPC's. The load modules are transferred to the microcomputer or PROM programmer using the existing terminal lines.

7. SOFTWARE SUPPORT

On the MPC's libraries are supported for:
-matrix arithmetic
-graphics
-interactive I/O
-timeseries analysis
-non-linear parameter estimation
-image processing
-statistics
Interactive work is done merely at the MPC's and preprocessors. Utilities are available for text processing and literature retrieval. Batch oriented work is submitted via remote job entry to the mainframes. General database software is only available on the mainframes (IMS).

8. COSTS

The costs of the hardware are not minimised, the installations are "professional". By standardisation of equipment and solutions the software development costs are minimised. Eight bit micro processors are only used as intelligent logic. For the information processing systems LSI 11/PDP 11 processors are used. Large savings on software licences are achieved by the use of MPC's for program development.

The manpower to build and maintain Minibos with data communication software is one man. This is comparable to the costs of the many software licences needed for a commercial operating system.

All installations used to be maintained by the supplier under a fixed maintenance contract. However these costs became too high. Therefore we have bought spare modules to maintain all LSI 11 based systems ourselves. Gradually the older machines will be replaced by LSI 11 systems.

9. CONCLUDING STATEMENTS

The price payed for such a distributed network is high. To keep all software compatible with new releases of operating systems and data communication protocols, implement new devices, maintain the hardware, provide utilities etc. places a high base load on the data processing people. But in this way optimal facilities are available for all kinds of data processing needed.
The medical faculty has a central information processing group for system programming and signal analysis. Application programming however is often done locally by people within the organisation of the projects. The network functions according to the requirements because its structure fits well to the organisation.

10. REFERENCES

(1)Boleij H.F, Hortensius A. Miniboss: an operating system for pre-processors. Proceedings of the Digital Equipment Computer Users Society 1976;3-1:333-336.

Correction of Spelling Errors in Medical Records in a Free-Text-Coding-System of Pathology

Wilfried Raufmann, Peter Ries

Institute of Medical Informatics   Pathologisches Institut
Medical School Hannover   Krankenhaus Wilhelmstrasse 5
Prof.P.L. Reichertz   325 Hameln,Germany

Abstract

Spelling errors cannot be completely avoided during data acquisition for
free-text-coding-systems.   It is possible to classify these errors into
different classes.   In relation to these classes the possibilities to
correct spelling errors are analysed.   The method of correction depends
on the complexity of the error.   The errors can be corrected during data
acquisation if search- and storage-techniques are used fitted to these
error classes.

1.Introduction

A number of free-text-systems have been developed to evaluate the semantic information of medical records, e.g. AURA by Gell (4) REMEDE by de
Heaulme (2), PAS by Kuesel (6), KLAUKON by Sager and Dudeck (8), and the
systems developed by Coles (1) and by Thurmayer (9).   This selection is
incomplete and contains only systems, which were presented during the
conferences of EFMI in the years 1978 - 1980. In all these papers the
correction of spelling errors was not described or the descriptions were
very short. As the error correction of misspellings is very important
for free-text-coding in routine systems,   (especially in those cases in
which the error occurs in words with semantic information), this problem
has been investigated.

2.Recognition of Spelling Errors

In a former publication (6) the algorithms of PAS (Pathologie Auswer-
tungssystem) for text decomposition, for coding using the entry-term
file of the AGK (Arbeitsgemeinschaft Klartextanalyse) thesaurus (7) and
for the standardisation with the standard-term file of the AGK have been
described.   The AGK-Thesaurus is a two file thesaurus with a file for

entry-terms and a descriptor file. All words for which a match cannot
be found during analysis of the report, are stored temporarily into an
error-word file. This means, mispelled words and words not contained
within the entry-term file are treated as errors. This file serves as
input for the correction routines.

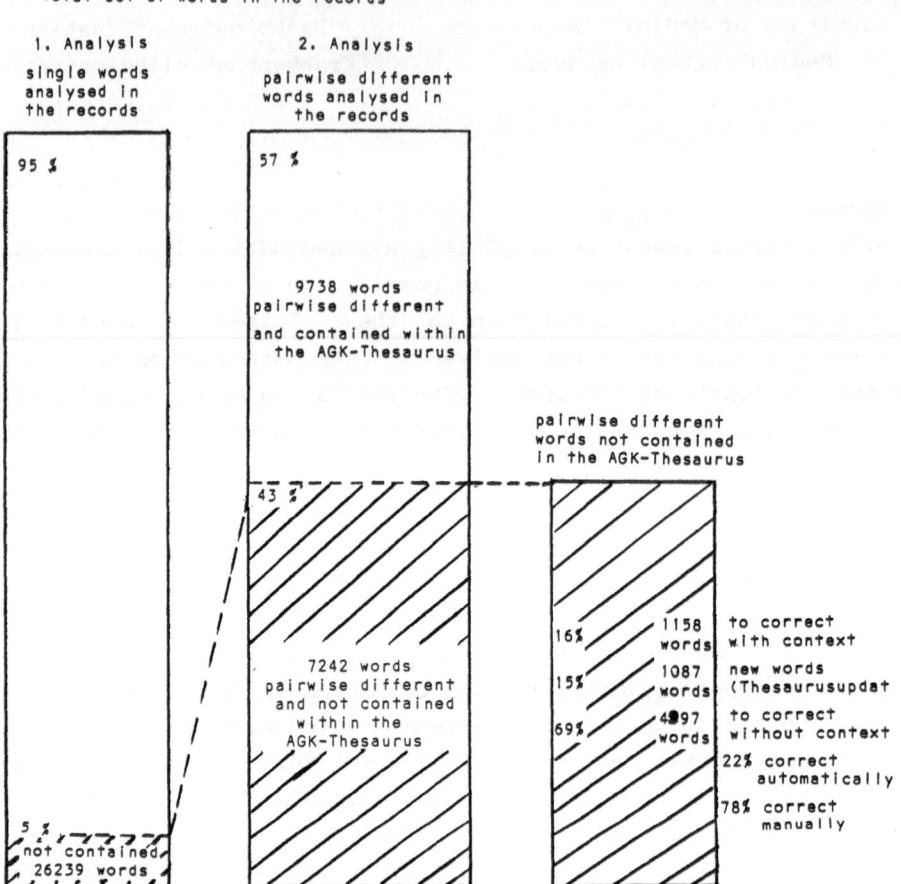

Fig. 1 The different error classes in Pathology records of the year 1979
The distribution is given of the various classes, related to a
total of 500542 words. A set of words contains only pairwise
different words, if each single word is spelled different to all
other words of the set.

Only sixty percent of a total of 500542 words are without any spelling
error. The errors can be divided into different classes. The first
class contains those words, which are spelled wrong but correctly
spelled they are elements of the entry-term file. The second class consists of words, which are spelled correctly but are not represented in

the AGK-Thesaurus. The class of mispelled words is again subdivided. One set contains those words, which meaning can be recognized directly. Those words, which can only be corrected in context with the whole medical utterance are in the second set. The group of semantic errors, which can only be corrected by a second dignosis of the material, that was sent to the Pathology, is smaller than 1% and therefor not considered in this paper. The classes and their volume in percent are shown in Fig. 1.

First it is to be seen that the number of errors is so great that a complete standardisation of the reports is only possible after error correction. If this does not take place the loss of information is too great. Secondly the error correction must correspond to the problems of the class. Otherwise some errors cannot be detected at all, or the correction would be too time consuming.

3. Automatic Error Correction

If one letter is wrong or one letter is missing or too much in a word, the automatic correction is useful. The procedure for this way of correction is that the words of the whole entry-term file are converted into sorted strings together with the length of the word and the two entry letters (Fig. 2) (3,6). For instance the word carcinom is converted in 'accinmor'.

word	letters of the word alphabetic sorted	way of holding in storage
carcinom	accimnor	┌8┐ca┐accimnor┐
carcinome	acceimnor	└9┘ca┘acceimnor┘
mispelled word		length of the word
		first two letters of the word
carcenom	accemnor	
caricnóm	accimnor	letters of the word alphabetic sorted
carcnom	accmnor	

Fig. 2 Preparation of the words for the automatic error correction.
An alphabetically sorted character string is stored for every word of the entry-term file and for the words of the error-file. Together with the length and the first two characters of the word these character strings are stored in a special file for the automatic error correction.

After converting the file with the mispelled words in the same way, the algorithm searches for all words in the entry-file which have the same two entry letters, the same word length or plus / minus one letter. If such a word is found the mispelled word is substituted and a hardcopy with the correction is printed. The hardcopy is verified by a Pathologist, so that incorrect automatic corrections can be detected. Nearly one percent of the automatic corrections are wrong. From Fig. 1 it is to be seen that only 22 percent of mispelled words could be corrected in this way. The remainder must be corrected manually.

4.On-line Error Correction
4.1.Old On-line Concept
Till last year there was a possibility for correcting mispelled words on-line from the error word file. But very soon we recognized that the correction word by word without the context was insufficient. For instance the abbreviation 'ca'. for cancer would lead to an error, because the abbreviation is not in the AGK-Thesaurus. But in the algorithm of the text decomposition the next word after 'ca.' would be treated as first word in a new sentence,because of the period. Therefore it is not sufficient to correct 'ca.' in carcinom but the positions of all words, which follow in the medical report, must be changed accordingly in the error word file. The second reason for giving up the word by word correction is the great multitude of words, which are mispelled in a way that the Pathologist can find out the meaning of the word by knowledge of the whole text of the report. And the third reason for another way of on-line correction is the impossibility to correct such errors like 'ca cinom'. In the error file would be stored 'ca' and 'cinom'. Perhaps the Pathologist would correct 'ca' in 'cancer' and 'cinom' in carcinom. Very seldomly he will notice that the reason for these two error words at the error file is only the omission of a letter in one word.

4.2.New On-line Concept
Corresponding to the different error classes the method for on-line corrections was changed. At the moment the misspelled words are corrected in the record directly. Therefore a hardcopy of the record and of the words which must be corrected in this record are printed. With the support of a Pathologist the error words are corrected in the hardcopy. Then the corrections are carried out within the record at a terminal directly.
This way of correction is not sufficient, because it took nearly two months until the correction of all 17000 records could be made. To find

a solution for a quicker way of correction, we are now trying to correct
one subset of the errors immediately during the data acquisation.

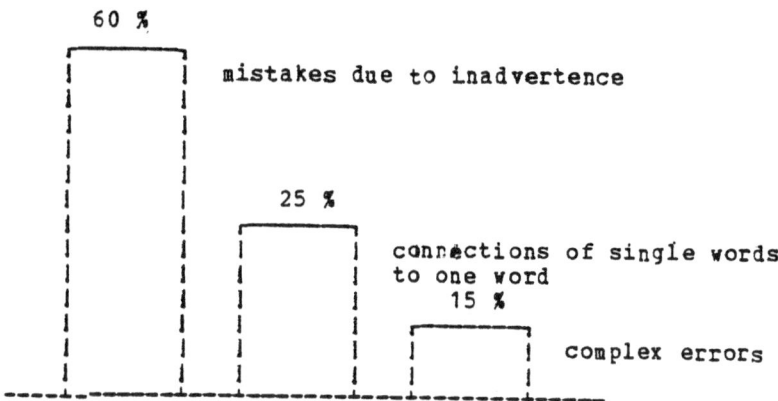

Fig. 3 Frequencies of spelling errors according to the difficulty
        of correction

In figure 3 the set of error words of figure 1 is divided into groups of
different degrees of difficulty for the correction. It is to be seen
that many errors can be corrected at the terminal while entering of
text, e.g. abbriveations and mistakes due to inadvertence. In the test-
set mentioned above these type of mistakes accounts nearly sixty percent
of all errors.   25 percent of spelling errors are caused by a typical
charisteristic of the German language. It is the nearly endless combination of words e.g. the word 'Oberschenkelamputatspraeparat'. The same
semantic information is conveyed when single words are used, e.g 'Prae-
parat eines Amputats des Oberschenkels'.   Approxemately 15 percent of
the error words need a special handling routine for correction.   Therefore we plan on-line interaction when the phrases are entered into the
acquisition system.
In routine use such a system is only successful when the response time
is short. At the moment the system is still in development. By measurements in off-line simulation we obtained response times of 10 - 20 milli
seconds. In this time the medical record is decomposed into single words
and checked against the entry-term file. We hope to obtain satisfactory
values in routine application.   For a good response time it is very

important how the entry file is stored. We chose an ISAM-technique for
our first test. The kind of storage of the entry-term file is to be seen
in Fig 4.

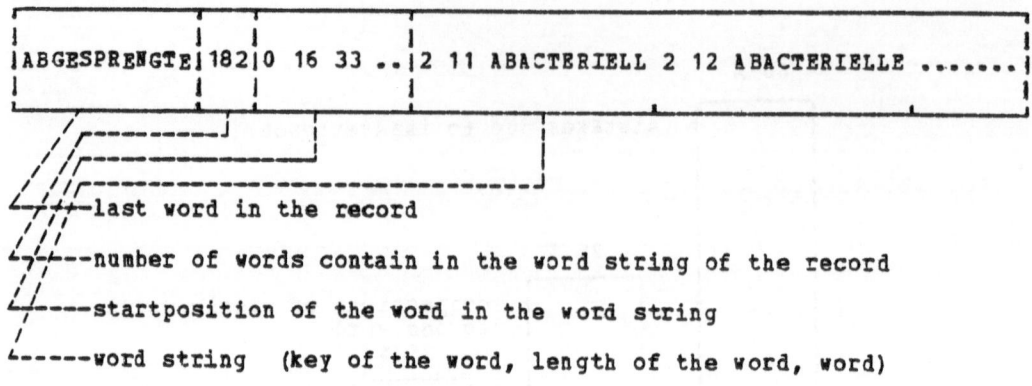

Fig. 4 Structur of the records of the ISAM-file for the direct access
        of the entry-term-file

A small stop word file is checked through before the entry term file is
searched for a word. In this stop word file those words are stored,
which are most frequent in the records.

Conclusion

For the precision of a free text evaluation system the correction of
misspelled words is very important. The correction should be on-line as
the same time as the input of the medical records, because most errors
are mistakes due to inadvertance. Without error correction an evaluation
is incorrect, because most spelling errors are in words, which contain
semantic information. If the error correction will be done not during
the data acquisition, the correction becomes more difficult and increasingly expensive. Also error correction outside context can lead to
semantic errors. By skillful storage of the entry term file it is possible to correct errors on-line without impairing the data input.

References
(1)Coles,E.C.,Stavin,G.:   Experience   of   automatic   Coding   of
Histopathology   Diagnoses.   in   Medical   Informatics   Berlin
1979(Proceedings); 789-796. Springer Verlag, Berlin-Heidelberg-New York
(1979)

(2) de Heaulme,M.: Artificial Medical Languages, a Solution for Clinical Needs in Documentation. Example Using REMEDE System. Medical Informatics Europe 1978; 63-71. Springer Verlag, Berlin-Heidelberg-New York (1978)

(3) Fischer,R.J.: Automatische Schreibfehlerkorrektur in Texten. Medizinische Informatik und Statistik, Vol.17, Springer Verlag, Berlin-Heidelberg-New York (1980)

(4) Gell,G., Sager,W.D.: Evaluation of Documentation and Retrieval Quality in a Free Text Documentation System. in Medical Informatics Europe 1978; 83-89. Springer Verlag, Berlin-Heidelberg-New York (1978)

(5) Hoffmann,E.G., Simon,F.: Ein Verfahren zum fehlerorientierten Vergleich von Worten. in Klartextanalyse: Wingert,F. (Hrsg), Medizinische Informatik und Statistik, Vol(4); 44-50. Springer Verlag, Berlin-Heidelberg-New York (1977)

(6) Kuesel,W. : Klartextverarbeitung in der Pathologie. in Klartextanalyse, Wingert,F. (Hrsg), Medizinische Informatik und Statistik, Vol(4); 137-152. Springer Verlag, Berlin-Heidelberg-New York (1977)

(7) Roettger,P., Wingert,F.: Konzeption und Organisation des AGK-Thesaurus. in: Symposium Klartextanalyse in der Medizin, Wien 1973; 52-60. Siemens, Erlangen (1974)

(8) Sager,W.K.M., Dudeck,J., Kinnling,J.: Klaukon - A microprocessor System for Free Text Acquisation with automatic Error Checking. in Medical Informatics Europe 1978; 73-81. Springer Verlag, Berlin-Heidelberg-New York (1978)

(9) Thurmayer,R., Ohngemach, D., Suppan,M.: Verschluesselung von Basisdaten aus der Urologie unter Einsatz der Klartextanalyse. in Klartextanalyse, Wingert,F. (Hrsg), Medizinische Informatik und Statistik, Vol(4); 94-103. Springer Verlag, Berlin-Heidelberg-New York (1977)

A THRESHOLD METHOD OF APPROXIMATE STRING MATCHING.

Rudolf-Josef Fischer,
Institut für Medizinische Informatik und Biomathematik
der Westfälischen Wilhelms-Universität Münster,
Hüfferstr. 75, D-4400 Münster, Tel. 251/83 5265
(Direktor: Prof. Dr. F. Wingert)

SUMMARY.

A threshold method of approximate string matching is discussed. It is
applied to problems which require both high precision and recall, such
as patient identification retrieval and automated error correction. The
paper presents the calculation of a subdistance matrix omitting serious
constraints required by other algorithms. In addition, strings are
grouped into subsets of strings of equal lengths, stored in a special
tree structure. Furthermore, a threshold frequently allows omitting the
calculation of most of the subdistance matrix without decrease in recall
and precision. Some practical results are presented and discussed.

Zeichenreihen-Identifikation mit gegebener Distanz-Schranke.

Es wird eine Methode zur Berechnung einer Teildistanz-Matrix für zwei
Zeichenreihen beschrieben. Die Vorgabe einer Distanz-Schranke erlaubt,
einen bedeutenden Anteil der Berechnungen zu sparen. Das Vergleichslexi-
kon, aus dem ähnliche Zeichenreihen bestimmt werden sollen, ermöglicht
durch eine spezielle Struktur eine wirksame Vorauswahl. Einschränkungen
aus bisher bekannten Verfahren entfallen. An den Beispielen "Patienten-
identifikation" und "automatische Fehlerkorrektur" werden die Ergebnisse
des Verfahrens denen bisheriger Methoden gegenübergestellt.

Identigo de signovicoj per distanc-baro.

Prezentata estas jen metodo kalkuli subdistancan matricon por du signovicoj. Uzo de donita distanc-baro kaŭzas grandkvantan ŝparon de kalku-
lado. Pro speciala strukturo de la aro de komparendaj signovicoj efika
selektado de similaj elementoj eblas. Limigaj kondiĉoj de ĝisnunaj algoritmoj forfalas. Komparcele prezentataj estas rezultoj de malnovaj
kaj la nova algoritmoj aplikitaj al la taskoj "identigo de pacientaj
datumoj" kaj "aŭtomata korektado de eraroj en tekstoj". Ĉe la aŭtoro
haveblas detalaj priskriboj de la programoj ankaŭ en Esperanto.

1. TWO PROBLEMS OF APPROXIMATE STRING MATCHING.

(i) When a patient is admitted to a hospital, there should be an automated search in a master data file in order to <u>retrieve patient data</u>.
These data should always be found, if the correct patient identification is entered. A small list of candidates should result, with the
first one having the highest probability of being correct.

(ii) During <u>automated off-line error correction</u> the correct word has
to be found in a lexicon and there should be a single candidate.

2. A SOUNDEX METHOD FOR APPROXIMATE STRING MATCHING.

2.1. Definition of the SOUNDEX method used.

SOUNDEX methods for patient identification retrieval (1) and automated
error correction (2) have been reported. The method used here has the
following encoding rules for a given string s:

a) Retain the first character of s.
b) If there are at least two identical characters in adjacent positions,
   then omit all characters but the first one.
c) Drop all vowels, digits, letters H, blanks, and hyphens after the
   first character.
d) Assign the following digits to the remaining characters after the
   first one: 1 to B, F, P, V, and W; 2 to C, G, K, Q, X, and Z; 3 to
   D and T; 4 to J and Y; 5 to L; 6 to M and N; 7 to R; 8 to S; 9 to
   all other.

For patient identification, the first letter of the first name is added
at the beginning of the code string.

2.2. Patient identification retrieval.

A set of 88 patients was collected whose surnames had falsly been entered during admission to an university hospital of Münster, and whose
correct data were already included in the master data file. Then all
surnames of the 75,356 patients were encoded by the algorithm described
above. Table I shows the results after trying to identify the 88 patients
by a varying length code (i.e., breaking off encoding after reaching a defined number
of code bytes). For example, using a surname code of 4 bytes, in 55 cases
a total of 272 candidates was found including the correct one, in 12
cases only the correct one, in 43 cases more than the correct one; in
33 cases the correct candidate was not found, in 20 cases no candidate,
in 4 cases one, and in 9 cases more than one.

	correct candidate					recall	precision
	found		not found				
number of can- didates found	1	>1	0	1	>1		
4 byte surname code	12	43	20	4	9	$\frac{55}{88}$	$\frac{55}{272}$
5 byte surname code	23	27	29	4	5	$\frac{50}{88}$	$\frac{50}{151}$
26 byte surname code	26	21	34	3	4	$\frac{47}{88}$	$\frac{47}{131}$

Table I: Results of patient identification retrieval by a SOUNDEX method.

2.3. Automated error correction.

Automated error correction requires a lexicon of admitted words. For
this example the AGK thesaurus with 33,952 medical words (3) was chosen.
During daily data collection in the university hospitals, 83 false words
were found whose correct versions are in the AGK thesaurus. Using the
SOUNDEX code, described above, there was a search for candidates in the
thesaurus. Table II shows the results depending on the number of bytes
used for the code.

	correct candidate					proportion of successful correc- tion
	found		not found			
number of can- didates found	1	>1	0	1	>1	
4 byte code	2	52	13	3	13	$\frac{2}{83}$
5 byte code	7	41	20	5	10	$\frac{7}{83}$
32 byte code	26	12	39	4	2	$\frac{26}{83}$

Table II: Results of automated error correction by a SOUNDEX method.

2.4. Discussion of the results.

Certainly the results are not statistically proved and depend considerably on the coding rules. But the tendency is obvious: A high portion
of data cannot be identified by a SOUNDEX method, because type and number of errors in a word two often affect the SOUNDEX code more than can

be tolerated. Patient identification retrieval has the best recall using a surname code of 4 bytes, while precision is still tolerable. However, for automated error correction the longest possible code gives the best results, i.e., it gives the highest number of cases, where only the correct candidate is retrieved. All the other cases are not interesting, because the false word cannot be corrected.

In practice, these results are not satisfying, because "having the same code, is an equivalence relation, but the string matching problem ... is a similarity problem" (4).

Patient identification retrieval requires a recall approximating 1, while automated error correction not only should have more than 90 percent of successful correction, but also a very low probability for miscorrecting (just one candidate found, but not the correct one).

These ambitious requirements are met only by a method presented in (5,6) using a DAMERAU LEVENSHTEIN metric (4). This metric is based on a distance function counting the minimum number of some operations required to convert a given string s into a candidate string t taken from a lexicon. The admitted operations include deletion, insertion, and substitution of single characters, and reversal of adjacent characters.

So far, these methods seem to be used only infrequently, because the distance calculation by calculating a subdistance matrix P is rather extensive and time consuming. Some improvements reported in the literature use various techniques such as binary trees to store the lexicon, or grouping methods to select the relevant data rapidly. These improvements, however, have intolerable constraints, e.g., two strings being compared must match in the first character and/or differ in at most one position.

3.   A THRESHOLD METHOD USING A DAMERAU LEVENSHTEIN METRIC.

3.1. A new threshold method.

This paper presents a new threshold method which combines the possible advantages. Strings t of a lexicon are grouped into subsets of strings of equal lengths, stored as a special tree structure.

Furthermore, a threshold M frequently allows omitting the calculation of most of the subdistance matrix without decrease in recall and precision. During search many subtrees may completely be skipped.

The subdistance p_{ij} ($1 \leq i \leq n$, $1 \leq j \leq m$) is the distance between the leading i characters of t and the corresponding j characters of s, i.e.,
the minimum number of operations required to convert the leading i characters of t to the leading j characters of s from left to right. Thus,
p_{nm} yields the distance between s and t.

If a certain subdistance p_{ij} exceeds a threshold M_1, given by a function
of M, n, and m, then the calculation of the subdistance matrix P can
be broken off, because one can prove that the distance will exceed M.

This has to be shown in detail: Let the diagonal of P, containing the
element p_{nm}, be the main diagonal; parallel diagonals may be called
k-th upper or k-th lower diagonal ($k \geq 1$). Then the following propositions can be proved:

In every diagonal containing an element p_{ij} all subdistances $p_{i+\ell, j+\ell}$
($\ell \geq 1$) are at least equal to p_{ij}.
If a subdistance p_{ij} in the k-th upper or lower diagonal exceeds $M_1 = M-k$,
then it can only contribute to a distance p_{nm} exceeding M.
If a subdistance p_{ij} in the k-th lower (upper) diagonal exceeds M-k,
then all elements $p_{i,j-\ell}$ ($p_{i,j+\ell}$) ($\ell \geq 1$) located to its left (right) in
the same row of the matrix P exceed $M-(k+\ell)$.

Therefore, in every i-th row only some elements p_{i,j_1} to p_{i,j_2} have to
be calculated, and there may be less and less elements in the following
rows which have to be considered.

If a subdistance in the main diagonal exceeds the threshold M, then the
distance p_{nm} will also exceed this threshold. Thus, the calculation can
be broken off because the candidate string t cannot match s.

Grouping the lexicon of candidate strings into subsets of strings of
the same lengths has some advantages:

The threshold M permits neglecting all subsets whose strings are of
lengths n with $|m-n| > M$ because these strings cannot match the given
string s of length m.

If a dynamic threshold M is used, it indicates the smallest distance
already found. Therefore, calculation begins with those candidate strings

847

whose lengths are m, subsequently considering those subsets of strings
with a length different from m, because their number will decrease due
to decreasing M.
The thresholds M_1 of a row have to be initialized only once for the whole
subset (as long a M remains constant).

A special storage structure for a subset of candidate strings results
from the following: Given two candidate strings t_1 and t_2. The first
i rows of the subdistance matrix for s and t_1 are the same as for s and
t_2, if the leading i characters of t_1 and t_2 are identical. Therefore,
strings are ordered alphabetically, replacing the first i characters
of t_2 by one byte containing the number i, if they are identical to the
first i characters of the preceding string t_1. This results not only
in low storage requirements but also in a powerful selection strategy:
If during calculation of the i-th row of the subdistance matrix fo s
and t_1 the string t_1 can be proved as not matching, then all following
strings with at least i characters being identical do not match and can
be neglected. Further evaluation of the actual record containing the
candidate strings restarts only with the next byte containing a number
less than i.

3.2. Patient identification retrieval.

Given surname, first name, birth date, and sex of a patient, the simplest method to find matching data in the patient master file is to present all patient data with identical birth date and sex. However, comparison of patient data from two hospitals showed 36 cases (out of 855)
of different sex or birth date, stored for identical patients. Therefore, these data are not always reliable, and, furthermore, they may
miss.

The threshold method searches 10 groups of candidates, each group having
less probably identical candidates than the preceding one.

group number	surname	first name	birth date/sex
1	identical	identical	identical
2	identical	similar	identical
3	identical	identical	similar
4	identical	similar	similar
5	similar	identical	identical
6	similar	similar	identical
7	identical	different	identical
8	similar	different	identical
9	identical	identical	missing
10	identical	similar	missing

Similarity of surnames was defined by a threshold M for the distance depending on the length of the given surname. First names were treated as similar even if one was a substring of the other. "Different" was defined as "not similar".

Out of the 88 patients, mentioned in section 2.2, 87 were successfully identified, 1 was not found. 6 twins with the same sex werde indicated and no other candidates retrieved. So, recall was 98.8 % and precision 93.5 %. To find the candidates out of 75,356 patients required 18 sec CPU time on an average (IBM 3032), but this rate depends considerably on the hardware configuration and the structure of the patient data master file.

3.3. Automated error correction.

There were 80 out of the 83 false words, i.e., 96.5 %, mentioned in section 2.3, successfully corrected; three times two candidates with the same distance were found; no case of miscorrection occurred. Calculating the whole subdistance matrix (5,6) processing time was 864.63 sec CPU time for all words; the threshold method required only 40.37 sec.

4.   STATE OF IMPLEMENTATION.

The threshold method is used off-line to discover misidentifications after admission of patients of 9 university hospitals of Münster. Up to now, it is not used for automated error correction.

5.   BIBLIOGRAPHY.

(1) Greenfield RH. An Experiment to Measure the Performance of Phonetic Key Compression Retrieval Schemes. Meth Inform Med. 1977; 16, 4; 230-33.

(2) Joseph DM, Wong RL. Correction of Misspellings and Typographical Errors in a Free-Text Medical English Information Storage and Retrieval System. Meth Inform Med. 1979; 18, 4: 228-34.

(3) Fischer R-J. Automatische Schreibfehlerkorrektur in Texten. Med Inform u Stat 18, Springer, Berlin-Heidelberg-New York 1980.

(4) Hall PAV, Dowling GR. Approximate String Matching. Com Surv. 1980; 12, 4: 381-402.

(5) Wagner RA, Fischer MJ. The String-to-String Correction Problem. J of the ACM. 1974; 21: 168-73.

(6) Lowrance R, Wagner RA. An Extension of the String-to-String Correction Problem. J of the ACM. 1975; 22: 177-83.

AURA: A CLINICAL DATA BANK BASED ON FREE TEXT

Günther Gell
Universitätsklinik für Radiologie
A-8036 Graz, Austria

SUMMARY: At the Department of Radiology of the University of Graz, radiologic reports are stored in a direct-access data base in clear text. The data-base is used primarily to get immediate information about previous examinations of the patient. It is also used for scientific evaluations and the provision of feedback information. All these functions are available on CRT-devices on or near the examination rooms for 24 hours a day. Data are collected by the normal routine of dictating and typing reports without a need for additional work or coding.

1. INTRODUCTION

At the Department of Radiology of the University of Graz, a free text documentation system, called AURA (Automatic Report Analysis), has been in operation for more than ten years /1,2/. The system, following the example of free text processing in Pathology /3/ started as a pure documentation system with off-line data input and on-line retrieval. The reports were typed in the conventional way on a typewriter and afterwards a shortened version was retyped on a computer terminal. An on line query language allowed for interactive selective retrieval of stored reports. The second step in the evolution of the system was the elimination of the retyping of reports for the computer by the use of an off-line CRT-device with magnetic tape cassette and printer, generating at the same time the printed report and a computer-readable copy on magnetic tape cassette. This solution proved to be very stable and useful because of the independence of the off-line writing function from the availability of the computer. This feature was essential because the hardware did not support multiprogramming. On the other hand such a method cannot provide checks for correctness and completeness of data during input; errors are detected later during computer analysis and then error correction becomes complicated and cumbersome. So, when cheaper and more powerful minicomputers with multiprogramming for uninterrupted on-line service became available we developed an on-line data acquisition method, where the typist enters the reports under the supervision and guidance of the computer who performs an immediate check of the data according to different criteria with the possibility of immediate correction of errors /4/. The computer also supplies default values for some parameters (e.g. the date) and does the formatting of the output and the creation of backup copies on magnetic disc.

We have reported on different occasions about the value, the frequency and the quality of retrieval from the stored data /1,2,5/. However, with increasing experience with the operation of the system it became clear, that besides case retrieval and statistical evaluation, which are undoubtedly important and useful for scientific work, other aspects of communication and documentation which may be summarized under the term feedback, are even more important for the benefit of the patients. Paradoxically enough, Radiology, whose main purpose is the production of information for other departments, has itself a deficit of information. This holds true also for other diagnostic departments and the problem is especially severe in large hospitals like the University and General Hospital of Graz with over 3.000 beds and an understaffed central Department of Radiology. At the moment a radiologist performing an examination gets very little information about previous data on his patient and none at all about further developments and results except if he becomes personally interested in the case and tries to procure himself with such data spending a considerable amount of time and work.

The development of AURA into an on-line data bank was planned to alleviate this situation allowing immediate access to all the data stored about the patient and providing radiologists automatically with feedback information, if data from subsequent examinations become available.

2. THE AURA DATA BASE SYSTEM

2.1. Data acquisition

Data acquisition is performed through the AURA on line report typing system as a result of the routine operation of the department without any need for duplicate work. If the report is keyed into the terminal, it becomes available for the data base. The printed copy is proof-read and signed by the radiologist - if changes are made, they are also corrected by the typist in the computer-stored version. From the legal point of view, we maintain at the moment the position, that only the printed and signed report is legally valid. We do our best to provide an identical computer version, but we cannot guarantee it. It might be a possible development for the future to do proof-reading on the terminal and to sign by typing a personal key.

2.2. Data Organisation

The data base is organised on a PDP 11/34 with the aid of DEC's (Digital Equipment Corporation) record management system RMS11K using two keys. The primary key consists of an examination code (for the type of examination e.g. angiography or computed tomography), the date of the examination and an examination number. A secondary key is built by surname (truncated to 8 digits), Christian name (2 digits) and the date of birth. Each of the keys allows direct access to the stored records. Generic access with incomplete keys is also possible. The secondary key may be used for example to produce an alphabetically ordered list of all patients, the primary key to retrieve all reports of a certain examination in chronological order.

2.3. Patient oriented query and feedback

For the retrieval of patient data from prior examinations we use terminals in the examination rooms, where the secondary key of the patient (or a truncated radix of the key, e.g. only the first letters of the surname) is provided by the radiologist or by a secretary. The computer then displays the results of prior examinations of the patient (any special examination performed within the department) in plain text.

If after the examination additional data from other examinations become available, the physician is informed and again provided with the text of the reports.

This service is very important for the improvement of the quality of the examinations and their interpretation since it enables the radiologist to come back to questionable and difficult cases and to reexamine the whole procedure from the viewpoint of the confirmed final result.

2.4. Case retrieval

With case retrieval we mean a retrieval based on medical criteria - e.g. a retrieval based on a search for occurences of a specific tumor in a certain location. For this purpose, AURA uses a special interactive retrieval language which is described elsewhere /1,2/. The introduction of the on-line data base gives the physician a much more direct access to the medical content. Although the query language was designed from the begin for use by non-programmers, response times were too long because of the sequential search on magnetic tape, and therefore a true interaction could not develop and the physicians usually passed their retrieval requests to the informatics section for processing. With the faster availability of the data through the data base a new possibility has been created which gives the radiologist the opportunity to really "play" with the data and to explore the different aspects of a scientific question.

2.5. Data privacy and access policies

Every medical data base deals with highly confidential data and has to worry about data privacy and protection. In this connection it must be noted that not only the patient's privacy must be protected, but that reporting physicians may also have a legitimate right of protection of privacy. To give an example we might consider a case where several radiologists compete for the leading post in a department - it would certainly be a violation of privacy if one of the candidates could use the data base to retrieve a list of false diagnoses made by a fellow-candidate.

The Austrian law for the protection of data (whose implications are as yet not fully understood, not even by it's authors) states for example, that at the request of an individual erroneous data about this individual must be corrected. This leads to the question whether the data in a radiologic report are data about the patient (and should be corrected) or data about the radiologist's impression about the condition of the patient at a given time (than a 'correction' would be a forgery of a document)?

Apart from those legal intricacies there is the basic issue of protecting data against access from and misuse by unauthorized persons. The problem has two levels: first, one has to decide about a policy who is authorized to access to what data and second, one has to devise measures to enforce the policy decision.

Our basic policy is that every physician within the hospital who treats the patient (including purely diagnostic procedures) should have access to all medical data about the patient. For the moment where only a few departments may be concerned, this policy may suffice. For scientific purposes (i. e. case retrieval according to general medical criteria) each physician has unlimited access to his own data (or data of the section or department he belongs to) own data meaning reports that he (or his section etc.) had produced. To link these data to reports from other sources for scientific purposes needs the consent of all concerned. At least in our hospital such a policy which is designed to protect 'scientific property' is essential for the successful implementation of a interdepartmental data base. Any physician-oriented retrieval (all reports from Dr. X) is only possible with the written consent of the concerned physician and cannot be done from a user terminal.

From the technical point of view data privacy is protected by several measures: the computer room is always locked and only very few people have physical access to the computer or to the storage media (and even if access were possible, a high amount of technical knowledge about our particular system would be required to gain access to data). All terminals outside of the computer section operate in 'slave' mode; they may only be used under the control of certain well defined programs which in turn are protected against misuse by passwords.

2.6. Quantitative data

The reports of the so called special examinations in our department have been collected since more than ten years and a large amount of data (over 100.000 reports) is available for scientific evaluation. For the purpose of the on-line data-base however, it was decided to begin with the reports for one year since in most instances the results of older examinations should have no significance for the present treatment. An exception was made with reports from computed tomography – this section requested that all CT-reports should be accessible on-line, replacing the manual patient index. The whole matter about the optimal size of the on-line data-base is still under review. The easy access case retrieval (2.4.) has created a need for more comprehensive files.

A separate data-base has been set up for neurosurgery reports. Figure 1 gives an idea about the data-base at a certain point in time.

Angiography	2.333	Ultrasound	1.703
Myelography	640	Computed tomography	21.114
Mammography	1.940	Other examinations	1.030
ERCP	746	Neurosurgery	2.354

Figure 1.: content of the AURA on-line data-base as of October 13, 1981 with 29.506 radiologic examinations and 2.354 neurosurgery case histories.

3. CONCLUSION

The development of computer hard- and software has made data-base systems affordable even at the departmental level. The evolution of the AURA system has rendered the medical information more and more accessible, integrating the documentation aspect into the routine work of the department. Free text processing is certainly the most natural way to store and retrieve medical information.
The disadvantages of the use of free text fall into two classes. First, the formulation of medical concepts in free text is less precise and standardized as in the case of structured code according to a classification of findings and diseases. Second, free text needs more storage capacity and higher processing power than structured methods. The first problem is closely connected with the very nature of medical data, which are highly individual and often subjective. The second becomes less and less important with the rapid progress of computer technology.
By the use of free text the computer has been integrated in the information flow of our department and has become an unobtrusive yet indispensable tool for everyday medical work.

Acknowledgements:

This work was supported by the "Österreichische Krebsliga", Sektion Steiermark and by the "Österreichischer Forschungsfonds".

References

1. Gell G, Oser W, Schwarz G: AURA: Automatische
    Befunddokumentation durch Klartextverarbeitung, Fortschr
    Röntgenstr, 1974; 121: 384 - 388.

2. Gell G, Oser W, Schwarz G: Experience with the AURA Free-Text
    Documentation System, Radiology 1976; 119: 105 - 109.

3. Gell G, Becker H: Klartextanalyse pathologischer
    Biopsiebefunde mit Bildschirmabfrage, Meth Inf Med 1973; 12:
    10 - 16.

4. Egger G: DEFASS, Datenerfassungs-, Ausgabe- und
    Speichersystem, Diplomarbeit, Technische Universität Graz,
    1981

5. Gell G, Sager WD: Evaluation of Documentation and Retrieval
    Quality: Free Text versus Coding, In: Gremy F et al (Ed):
    Lecture Notes in Medical Informatics, Springer,
    Berlin-Heidelberg-New York 1981; Vol. 11: 446 - 453.

AN INFORMATION SYSTEM FOR TEXT RETRIEVAL OF MEDICAL RECORDS

D.Köberl, W.Feigl

EDV-Zentrum der Universität Wien, Universitätsstr. 7, A-1010 Wien

Institut für Pathologische Anatomie, Universität Wien
Spitalg. 4, A-1090 Wien, Austria

Summary: The prototype of a text retrieval system for medical records is presented. The thesaurus system and the inverted file are realized by means of the information base management system IMF. The functions of the system are used for the maintenance of the thesaurus and for document retrieval.

1. THE INFORMATION SITUATION

The information flow diagram of Figure 1 depicts the information situation in broad outline. The medical records are acquired with the help of a microprocessorsystem and stored in the data base. By means of a thesaurus system an inverted file is prepared (list of all word occurrences). The inverted file which can be seen as part of the thesaurus is used for the calculation of the search results to Boolean search requests. The maintenance and updating of the thesaurus system is supervised by a thesaurus specialist.

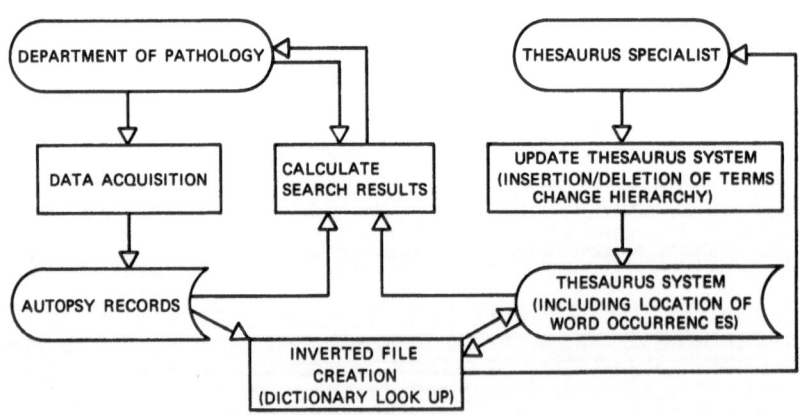

Figure 1: Information flow diagram

2. THE INFORMATION BASE MANAGEMENT SYSTEM IMF /1/

The architecture of the information base management system IMF follows a three schemata approach:

The conceptual schema is derived from a prescriptive grammar for a specific information situation. This conceptual or significational grammar can be viewed as a special case of communication between human beings. It is a set of rules describing which information may reside in the information base and the meaning of the elements of the information base.

Interaction with the information base is possible either using a query/update system or by means of application programs written in FORTRAN 4, FORTRAN 5 or COBOL. The external schema is a description which specifies a subset of a conceptual schema needed for a specific application.

The realization of the conceptual grammar in the information base is called internal schema. It is a set of rules describing how the information of the conceptual information base is physically represented on the storage media and depends on considerations like response time to retrieval interactions.

3. THE THESAURUS SYSTEM

The AGK-Thesaurus is the largest thesaurus of German medical language used in pathology. It was developed empirically by several Departments of Pathology in the Federal Republic of Germany and in Austria. The terms of the thesaurus have been derived from a representative set of documents /2/.

The monumental task of thesaurus construction was started more than ten years ago. The main application of the thesaurus is the support of text retrieval of medical records (autopsy and biopsy) formulated in natural language. For this purpose two types of relations are displayed in the thesaurus:

- Preferential relation: One term out of several entry terms (synonyms, spelling variants, abbreviations) is selected as standard term (descriptor).

- Hierarchical relation: This relation between descriptors is used for the specification of the implied information (= medical knowledge) associated with each descriptor.

There are six different facet classes (or descriptor types):

F finding broader term (186 terms)
f finding narrower term
L localizer broader term (112 terms)
l localizer narrower term
m modifier
v miscellaneous (terms not in one of the other five classes)

The class of finding broader terms with the subgroups "etiology", "morphe" and "function" contains many artificial terms which are important for retrieval (e.g. INFLAM/LOCAL, CIRCULATION/PULMONAL). The concept of the thesaurus and the classification of the broader term classes is such that each diagnostic statement should be made up of at least the information of one finding broader term and one localizer broader term (with the exception of some finding broader terms, which cannot be correlated with any type of localization, e.g. a General Intoxicaton or a Mycosis). The broader term classes are therefore especially important for automatic indexing to enable a general view of the data.

According to the "original indexing" or "stalagmitic" approach of the thesaurus construction process the structure of the thesaurus is a polyhierarchical one. Terms were added to the thesaurus in a rather nonrestrictive way, only the hierarchical relations were formulated with care to improve the recall parameter of retrieval. The dictionary of the thesaurus consists of about 30 000 entry terms (words with different suffixes and inflectional endings are not included in this version), each entry term contains a pointer to one of the 19000 standard terms. More than 51 000 hierarchical relations between the standard terms have been specified.

4. APPLICATION DESCRIPTION

A simplified version of the conceptual grammar for our information situation is shown in Figure 2. The four sentence types of the grammar represent the entry term dictionary, the descriptors (standard terms), the thesaurus hierarchy and the inverted file for retrieval. According to the axioms of G.M.Nijssens approach to information systems /3/ this sentence base grammar describes all the permitted sentence base states and the permitted sentence base transitions. From this conceptual (or significational) grammar a conceptual schema can be derived which supports the defined constraints. The main applications of the information base created from this conceptual schema are:

- Thesaurus maintenance and display

  The thesaurus can be displayed in all necessary ways to show its organization (alphabetic display, display of the terms with the synonyms, cross reference between the standard terms). By the formulation of constraints in the conceptual schema (subset constraint, equality and inequality constraint) the introduction of structural inconsistencies into the data base can be prevented. All update and maintenance functions are supported by the Query/Update System which is part of IMF.

- Retrieval

  Cosets are used for the retrieval of occurrences in a hierarchy of owner and member records. A typical example for cosets are all occurrences of the single descriptors within the document texts. This coset serves as descriptive inverted file. The responses to queries are calculated by IMF appplication programs.

Figure 2: Conceptual grammar

CONCEPTUAL GRAMMAR NAME IS RETRIEVAL-SYSTEM

OBJECT DIVISION

OBJECT TYPE NAME IS TERM   NOTATION CHAR 40
OBJECT TYPE NAME IS NO   NOTATION BINARY
OBJECT TYPE NAME IS LOCATION   NOTATION CHAR 10

ELEMENTARY SENTENCE DIVISION

SENTENCE TYPE NAME IS STANDARD-TERM-SENT
   REFERENCED OBJECT TYPE NAME IS TERM
      ROLE IS STANDARD-TERM
   REFERENCED OBJECT TYPE NAME IS NO
      ROLE IS STANDARD-TERM-NO

SENTENCE TYPE NAME IS ENTRY-TERM-SENT
   REFERENCED OBJECT TYPE NAME IS TERM
      ROLE IS ENTRY-TERM
 REFERENCED OBJECT TYPE NAME IS NO
      ROLE IS STANDARD-TERM-PTR

SENTENCE TYPE NAME IS THESAURUS-REL
   REFERENCED OBJECT TYPE NAME IS NO
      ROLE IS HYPONYM
   REFERENCED OBJECT TYPE NAME IS NO
      ROLE IS HYPERNYM

SENTENCE TYPE NAME IS STANDARD-TERM-NO-LOCATION
   REFERENCED OBJECT TYPE NAME IS NO
      ROLE IS DESCRIPTOR-NO
   REFERENCED OBJECT TYPE NAME IS LOCATION
      ROLE IS DESCRIPTOR-LOCATION

CONSTRAINT DIVISION

CONSTRAINT NAME IS ONE UNIQUE-STANDARD-TERM
   CODE IS C1
   ROLE STANDARD-TERM IN STANDARD-TERM-SENT IS UNIQUE

CONSTRAINT NAME IS UNIQUE-STANDARD-TERM-NO
   CODE IS C2
   ROLE STANDARD-TERM-NO IN STANDARD-TERM-SENT IS UNIQUE

CONSTRAINT NAME IS UNIQUE-ENTRY-TERM
   CODE IS C3
   ROLE ENTRY-TERM IN ENTRY-TERM-SENT IS UNIQUE

CONSTRAINT NAME IS ONE-DESCRIPTOR-PER-LOCATION
   CODE IS C4
   ROLE DESCRIPTOR-LOCATION IN STANDARD-TERM-NO-LOCATION IS UNIQUE

CONSTRAINT NAME IS EXISTING-STANDARD-TERM-TO-ENTRY
   CODE IS C5
   ROLE STANDARD-TERM-PTR IN ENTRY-TERM-SENT IS SUBSET OF
   ROLE STANDARD-TERM-NO IN STANDARD-TERM-SENT

```
CONSTRAINT NAME IS DESCRIPTOR-HYPONYMIE
   CODE IS C6
   ROLE HYPONYM IN THESAURUS-REL IS SUBSET OF
   ROLE STANDARD-TERM-NO IN STANDARD-TERM-SENT

CONSTRAINT NAME IS DESCRIPTOR-HYPERNYMIE
   CODE IS C7
 ` ROLE HYPERNYM IN THESAURUS-REL IS SUBSET OF
   ROLE STANDARD-TERM-NO IN STANDARD-TERM-SENT

CONSTRAINT NAME IS STANDARD-TERM-IN-ENTRY-TERM-LIST
   CODE IS C8
   ROLE STANDARD-TERM IN STANDARD-TERM-SENT IS SUBSET OF
   ROLE ENTRY-TERM IN ENTRY-TERM-SENT

CONSTRAINT NAME IS LOCATION-OF-STANDARD-TERM
   CODE IS C9
   ROLE DESCRIPTOR-NO IN STANDARD-TERM-NO-LOCATION IS SUBSET OF
   ROLE STANDARD-TERM-NO IN STANDARD-TERM-SENT

CONSTRAINT NAME IS. THESAURUS-HIERARCHY
   CODE IS C10
   ROLE HYPONYM,HYPERNYM IN THESAURUS-REL EXCLUDES
   ROLE HYPERNYM,HYPONYM IN THESAURUS-REL

END OF CONCEPTUAL GRAMMAR
```

REFERENCES

/1/ Information Management Facility, Version 1, Schema Defini-
    tions, Reference Manual. Control Data Corporation, Publica-
    tion No. 60484400, 1981.

/2/ D.Köberl, P.Röttger, W.Feigl, Free Text Analysis of Findings
    in Pathology. Proceedings of the MEDINFO 80 - Congress, North
    Holland Publishing Company, 1980.

/3/ G.M.Nijssen, A Framework for Advanced Mass Storage Appli-
    cations. Proceedings of the MEDINFO 80 - Congress, North Hol-
    land Publishing Company, 1980.

FORMAL MEANS FOR THE SEMANTIC REPRESENTATION

OF MEDICAL DATA AND CLINICAL KNOWLEDGE

Dietmar GRAICHEN, Frank DÖRRE, Wolf-Dieter GRIMM

Medizinische Akademie "Carl Gustav Carus"

Dresden, GDR

1. Introduction

In medicine, the ever increasing need to develop subject-oriented
interfaces in a natural language mainly arises from the fact that
- there is a great deal of findings in which the flexibility of a
  specialized natural language cannot be dispensed with;
- communication between the physician and the medical staff and the
  computer cannot be attained by means of artificial languages
  (e. g. advanced programming languages) but requires the use of a
  natural language.

In practice, this involves the problem to convert the content of a
medical text given in natural language (case history, findings etc.)
to a formal logic representation that, with only little loss in
information, allows the evaluation by comparison with other texts.

2. Activities and Results

At the Dresden Medical Academy we have first investigated a rather
simple method for the semantic representation of biopsy findings.
Here substrate evaluation by the pathologist, which includes macroscopic and microscopic descriptions as well as diagnoses, had to be
formalized in computer-internal mode with the aid of thesaurus
elements. The thesaurus used was worked out on the basis of a German
version of SNOP.
Thesaurus-supported indexing in this case comprises a morpheme
analysis of the entered biopsy findings. All morphemes or segments
are compiled in a special segment list which contains references for
all entries in the thesaurus concerning the associated morpheme or
segment. Selection of a descriptor is by looking for morphemes or
segments which coincide with the text and point to the corresponding
descriptor.
The queries for searching medical facts are represented in the same
manner as the findings. Thus the content of each clear text is given
by a sequence of conjunctively linked thesaurus elements. The drawback

of this procedure is that only text elements (words, word groups) can be looked up for which adequate entries exist in the thesaurus. A semantic analysis proves to be possible only on a word level so that syntacmatic and paradigmatic relations cannot be taken into account.

For this reason we have developed a thesaurus-independent method in which a morphosyntactic-semantic analysis serves for converting the medical text to an artificial language (indexing language) which is accessible for evaluation (1). This artificial language represents the syntacmatic and semantic relations of the information on word and phrase levels.

A classified dictionary was used as a reference system which unites the various words or roots subdivided in syntactic/semantic categories. An analysis grammar then recognizes single and multi-term nominal phrase structures as well as simple verbal phrases which, in compliance with transformation rules, are subsequently represented in the so-called indexing languages. A query in natural language can then be answered if the generated "semantic query pattern" of the indexing language is contained in at least one of the medical findings.

But this method still proves to be inadequate for handling more complex queries. Here it will be necessary to generate answers by way of logic deductions according to defined rules on stored clinical knowledge. Besides the complete logic significance representation concerning the text of the finding in the form of a semantic network, it is also required to store in the data bank axiomatic information as background knowledge (2). It is the significance interrelations between the individual medical data (relations) as well as between the relations themselves (relational axioms) that are represented here.

Plotted on the poster is a tentative medical question-answering system which allows the following conclusion:
- In medical fields the production and predicate logical representation of axiomatic background knowledge obviously seems to be possible only in relatively closed special fields (e. g. periodontology) or exactly defined disease groups (glaucoma etc.) of adequate system invariance.
- Questions being of relevance for the physician essentially concern data or content-oriented searches and their statistical evaluation. More complicated queries usually refer to problems related to medical decision support systems and require a rule based system

on a "fact" level with specific assignment relations and functions.

3. Discussion of Results

We think that the presented possibilities of a formal semantic representation of specialized medical texts are a substantial prerequisite to the further development of clinical decision support systems. The still existing barriers between the medical staff on the one hand and the computer on the other hand can be overcome by abandoning the conventional formalized modes of man-machine communication hitherto employed; i. e. by the development of natural language components in medical information systems.

References

(1) Grimm WD, Graichen D, Dörre F.
     Development of a natural linguistic medical indexing language
     based on a syntactic-semantic analysis.
     in: Lindberg DAB, Kaihara S. (eds). MEDINFO 80, North-Holland
     Publ.Comp. 1980, 1295 - 1300

(2) Helbig H.
     Ein Repertoire von Darstellungsmitteln für die semantische
     Repräsentation von Wissen in einem Frage-Antwort-System
     (Forschungsbericht).
     Dresden, VEB Robotron - Zentrum für Forschung und Technik, 1978

THE ROLE OF MODDELLING IN CARE SYSTEM PLANNING AND CARE EVALUATION.

Leif Gustafsson (1,3), Inge Hesselius (2), Alf Lycksell (1), Bengt
Sandblad (1,3) and Werner Schneider (1).
(1) Uppsala University Data Center, Box 2013 S-750 02 Uppsala,SWEDEN.
(2) Uppsala University Hospital, S-850 14 Uppsala, SWEDEN.
(3) Dept. of Automatic Control and Systems Analysis, Inst. of Technology,
    Uppsala University, Box 534, S-751 21 Uppsala, SWEDEN.

ABSTRACT.

The oncological care in the Uppsala health care region of Sweden is
coordinated by a Regional Oncological Center (ROC).   Main tasks for ROC
are development of information systems and evaluation and planning of
the oncological care system.

To fulfil these tasks the structure and dynamic behaviour of the
care process must be understood.   The approach presented here is to
describe this process with a set of simulation models connected within
the same conceptual frame work.

The care process is composed of two interacting subprocesses, the
patient process and the care delivery process.   The main component of
the model describing the logics of the care delivery process is the care
program which controls the actions of this process.   For studies of
the efficacy of health care activities, models of the natural history
of the disease and the patient's response to therapy are crucial.

The description of the oncological care process with a set of
related models is an effective way to relate various kinds of structural
and statistical information and to evaluate their dynamical consequences.
The main problem of this approach is the uneven quality of knowledge and
information available.   A very important result of the modelling process
is the identification of those parts of the system where existing
knowledge is not enough detailed or operational.

W.J. Cleijne,
F.E. Riphagen,

General management of the GG en GD Utrecht
Jaarbeursplein 17,
Postbus 2423, 3500 GK Utrecht.

Title: A model for dataflow in the current Dutch Health Care System.

Summary

Information is necessary for each organization and therefore one needs a good information system.
An information system can be based on the theory that economic processes can be subdivided in the logic process and the management process. Each process can be supported by an information system, respectively the logic information system (L.I.S.) and
the management information system (M.I.S.). Responsible for the informations systems
is the information manager. Applying the theory of organization theory maintains
each organization unit has its own targets and therefore its own information needs
and information system(s). With this theory one can build on information systems
from hospital departments, to hospitals, to regions and so on.

Introduction:

Information is as vital for an organization as blood for a human being.
It is therefore important that every part of the body (=organization) has the just
quality and quantity at its disposal.
A good information system is needed for that purpose when we consider the health
care system.
One of the most important conditions for a good information system is that top-management accepts direct responsibility for its contents.
Information management has become an important part of general management. The following requirements are equally vital:
- The information must be consistent, reliable and related to the organization based
  upon well defined needs.
- The dataflow must be continuous.
After defining information management and after drawing up an informationplan the
various users have to define their information needs, thus providing the whole system with the necessary basic level.

Information systems:

The information system depends on:
- the goals and targets of the organization
- the nature of the primary process
- the scale of the organization
- the economic order
- the available technology

- the current social developments

This leads to some more specific conditions:
- Top-management has to define the goals of the whole system and, secondly, its own information needs.
- Output of the system has to be made suitable for decision making.
- The responsibility for the information process (input, output) must be clear.
- The information must give answers to questions and must be relevant to operations.
- The information has to support the management for decision making and for controlling the organization.
- The system must be economic and efficient.

Last but not least each information system has to be <u>evaluated</u> to check the:
- effectivity of data-management
- suitability of the information
- influence of the data on operation and management
- efficiency and economy of the system

The goal of the information system will remain supporting the organization to reach its goals.

The theory:
Economic processes can be sub-divided as follows (see figure 1)
- the logistic process
- the management process

Each process has to be supported by an information system; the logistic information system (L.I.S.) and the management information system (M.I.S.).

The L.I.S.:
This system provides information needed for the supporting, the planning and the managing of the logistic process. This kind of information is characterized by its standards, forms and periodicity.
Each L.I.S. is controlled by a responsable information manager who has the following tasks:
- To translate and define the information needs.
- To be an intermediary between users and computerstaff.
- To design and maintain the system requirements.
- To design and maintain system procedures.
- The co-ordination with other information systems.
- The training and coaching of the users of the system.

The M.I.S.:
The management process is focussed on the decision making process (renovation, simulation, management). This process must be supported by a "M.I.S.".
The information for this purpose has to be flexible and variable regarding (i.e. not

FIGURE 1

THE ECONOMIC PROCESS

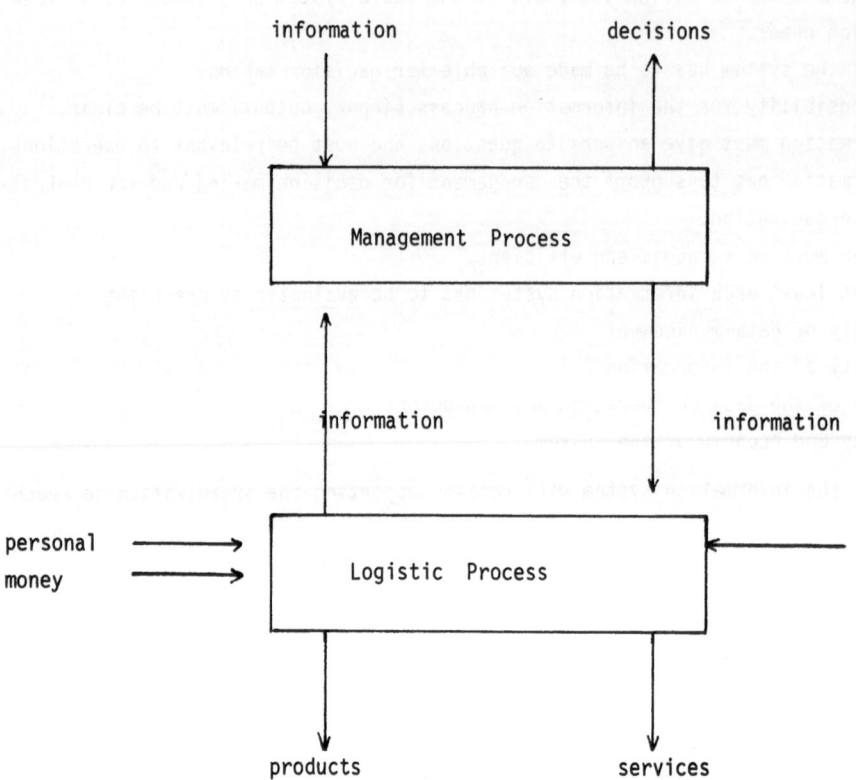

information   decisions

Management   Process

information   information

personal ⟶
money   ⟶   Logistic   Process

products   services

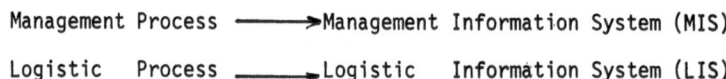

Management Process ⟶Management Information System (MIS)

Logistic   Process ⟶Logistic   Information System (LIS)

869

algoritmic) contents and periodicity.

Responsible for the M.I.S. is another information manager. His most important tasks
are:
- To act as intermediary and co-ordinator between management and information sup-
  pliers.
- To establish the requirements for the M.I.S.
- To design and maintain procedures, standards, rules etc.
- To look for information needs.
- Evaluate and maintain the system concerning efficiency, effectivity and economy.
The main differences between a L.I.S. and a M.I.S. are nature and periodicity of the
information. A L.I.S. has to give standard information at regular intervals. A M.I.S.
has to provide variable information when needed.
Applying the theory of organization theory maintains each organization unit (depart-
ment, hospital, concern and so on) has its own targets.
Thus every organization unit can be considered a configuration of organizations
which are more or less independent.
A hospital composed by different departments can be considered likewise.
A hospital has his own M.I.S. with a responsable information manager.
Each department has its own L.I.S. and its own information or systems manager.
The information is generated on the "basic-departments level" that uses it for its
own logistic processes. Management information is output for the department L.I.S.
and input for the M.I.S. (figure 2).

Extrapolation of this model gives several L.I.S.es and M.I.S.es in each regional
area. The"departments"in this case are for instance the hospitals and the general
practitioners. Information belonging to M.I.S. on hospital level, belongs to L.I.S.
and regional level.
On its turn the various regions can be regarded as "departments" within the national
framework (figure 2).
The national health care system can be compared to an industrial company when information processes are considered.
For example:
Unilever has ± 160.000 employees and a budget of ± 50 milliard guilders.
The dutch health care system has ± 275.000 workers and a budget of 30 milliard dutch
guilders.
The following steps in the construction of a health care information system have to
be taken:
- Appoint information managers for the health care organizations
- Appoint information managers on the same conditions for the different sectors of
  health care ("first line", "second line" and so on)
- Appoint regional information managers on likewise conditions.

FIGURE 2

THE (HOSPITAL) INFORMATION SYSTEM

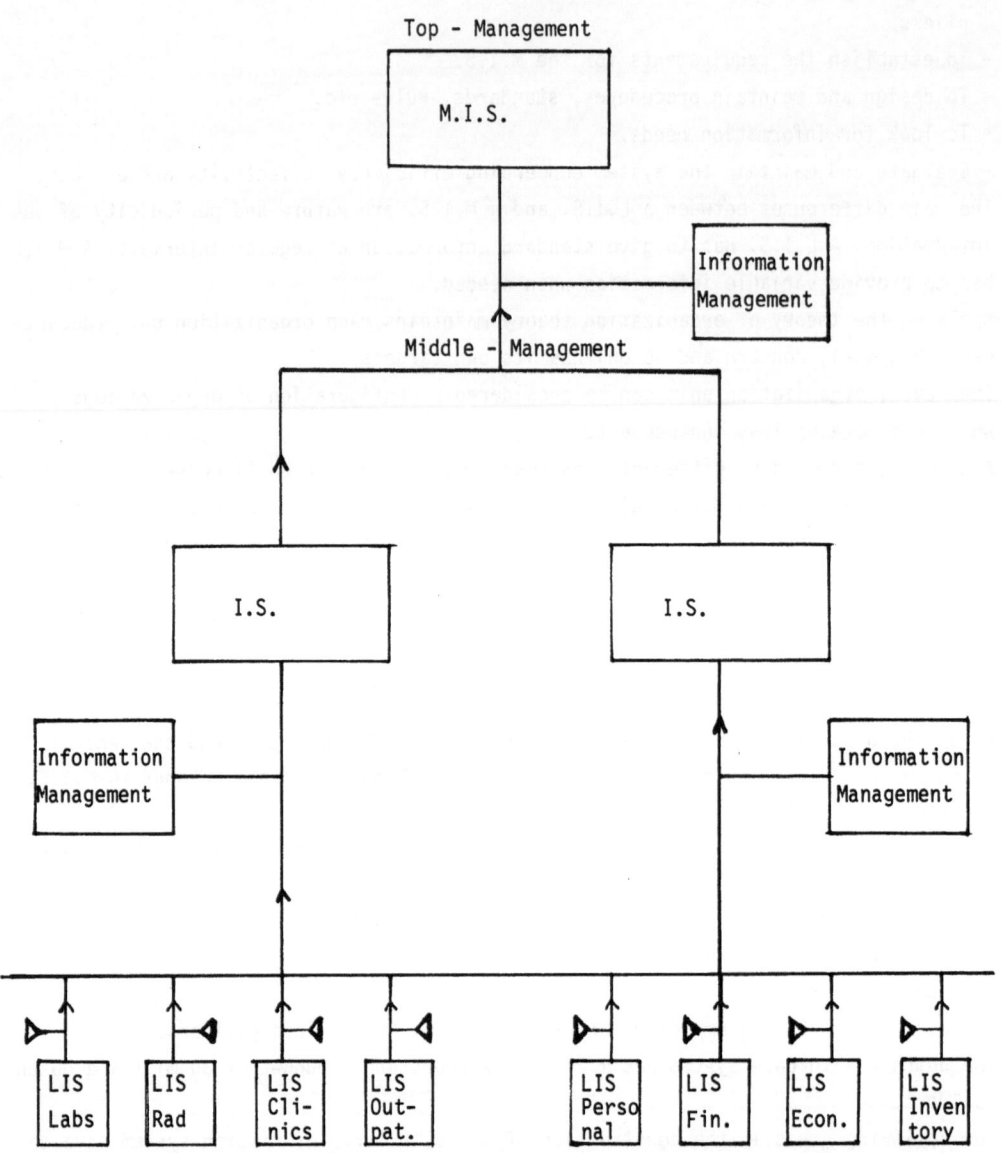

Δ   System Information Management

FIGURE 3

INFORMATION SYSTEM HEALTH CARE

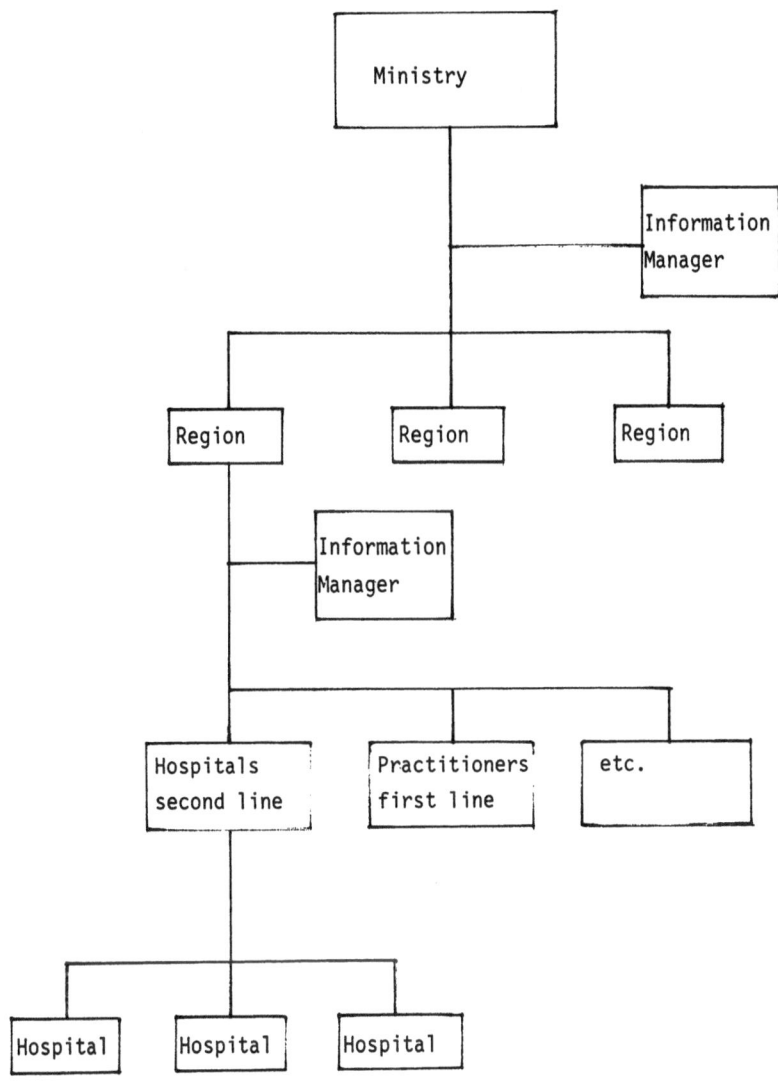

- Appoint an information manager for the national health care system.
- Design the information systems (starting in the departments).
- Introduce (level by level, starting from the basis) the system.

The big mistake of building information systems in the past has been that one started at the bottom by buying a computer, and wrongly, assumed that the remaining steps would follow on their own.

The appointment of information managers can start on every moment and on each level. He has to be a member of the organization unit which uses the information system. Waiting with his appointment until computers are used or replaced is from a practical point of view acceptable but not necessary.

Bibliografy

Brevoord, C.
Informatiebeleid
Leiden, Stenfert Kroese 1971.

Gaag, J. v.d.
De Economie van de gezondheidszorg
E.S.B. 65 (1980) nr. 3270 september.

Rappaport, A.
Information for decision making.
Englewood Cliffs N.I. Prentice-Hall 1975.

Schrode, W.A. and Vorich Jr, D.
Organization and management, basic system.
Irwin Series in management and behavioural sciences 1974.

Tieleman, T.
Management information and information management.
Amsterdam, Agm Elsevier 1974.

Völmar, H.
Systeembeheer.
Informatie 19 (1977) nr. 9 - page 512.

Deployment of Emergency Anaesthetists

Terence Bates, Senior Operational Research Scientist
North East Thames Regional Health Authority
The John Ellicott Centre
Cavell Street, The London Hospital
WHITECHAPEL, London, England

Abstract

Anaesthetists at The London Hospital, Northampton General Hospital and Alder Hey Children's Hospital, Liverpool, requested the Operational Research Unit to undertake a study of the emergency anaesthetic services at the three hospitals. A previous study had been conducted in 1967, but since then the caseload and mix of the work had changed. Throughout a six week sample period anaesthetists recorded the details of each emergency case at the three hospitals. Assorted cross tabulations were produced. A two priority transient queueing theory computer model with a 'goal' seeking capacity was developed to evaluate complex allocation problems. It was found that 'pooling' resources was the most effective way of deploying staff. The 'blocking' effect of low priority emergency work, eg, fractures, was not great enough to justify anaesthetists specialising on particular categories of work.

1. INTRODUCTION

In 1967 anaesthetists at The London Hospital, Northampton General Hospital and Alder Hey Children's Hospital in conjunction with the Operational Research Unit, carried out a study of the emergency anaesthetic services at the three hospitals. The main emphasis of the study was to improve the level of service provided to patients through better manpower planning. The findings of the study were reported in papers by Taylor et-al (1) and Jennings (2).

However, since then the emergency workload of these departments has changed significantly through:-

a)   changes in the effective population served;
b)   the type of work now carried out;
c)   the number of cases seen.

The previous study findings were no longer applicable, as the nature of the work had dramatically changed. Against this background, anaesthetists at the three hospitals, requested the Operational Research Unit to conduct a follow up study with the following objectives:-

a) assess the emergency anaesthetic service of The London Hospital, Northampton
    General Hospital and Alder Hey Children's Hospital, Liverpool;
b) evaluate alternative policy options of deploying manpower in order to improve
    the standard of service.

In this paper the mathematical modelling aspects of the study, together with a comparison of the data with the previous study will be discussed. In a paper by Major et-al
(3), the changes in the emergency anaesthetic services at the three hospitals are
reported in more detail. Further information on the study is available in a Management
Services report, A Study of the Emergency Anaesthetic Service at Three Hospitals (4).

2. DATA COLLECTION

Data was collected over a 6-7 week period during November/December 1978 and January
1979 from the three anaesthetic departments. The date of the survey was chosen to
include the Christmas period so as to assess whether the emergency anaesthetic workload changed significantly over the period.

The following data for each episode was collected by the anaesthetists using self
recording:-

a) hospital code   j) grade of staff, suitable
b) date of request   k) type of work
c) time of request   l) location of anaesthetist when called
d) time arranged for start   m) suspect data?
e) start time   n) other delay?
f) finish time   o) accident?
g) priority stated   p) outside call?
h) priority assessed   q) failure of service?
i) grade of staff, action   r) call rota

Anaesthetists have categorised the cases to a five point priority scale:-

1) Immediate   - requiring service within 3 minutes eg, cardiac arrest.
2) Urgent   - requiring service within 15 minutes eg, foetal distress.
3) Emergency   - requiring service within perhaps 90 minutes eg,
                             perforated appendix.
4) Low Priority Emergency - capable of waiting several hours eg, uncomplicated
                             fracture.
5) Cold Surgery   - done out of hours by someone on call.

The survey covered over twelve hundred emergency anaesthetic cases.

3. ANALYSIS OF DATA AND COMPARISON WITH PREVIOUS STUDY

3.1 Analysis carried out

The data for each hospital group was analysed in a number of different ways in order to:-

a)   produce cross-tabulations for comparison with the previous survey;

b)   produce total time spent on emergency anaesthetic work by type of work, priority and grade;

c)   check the homogeneity of the data;

d)   statistically test the independence of one variable with another;

e)   check the assumptions made in the formulation of the mathematical model;

f)   to provide parameters for mathematical modelling.

3.2 Comparison with previous data

Table I shows the broad changes in emergency anaesthetic work at the three hospitals.

HOSPITAL / AGGREGATE DATA	THE LONDON		NORTHAMPTON		ALDER HEY	
	1978	1967	1978	1967	1978	1967
Cases per day	14.0	7.8	10.0	8.5	5.4	7.0
Average Duration of Case (Mins)	87	63	48	33	50	49
Average Total Time Spent on Case Per Day (Hours)	20.3	8.2	8.0	4.7	4.5	5.7

TABLE I : Overall Changes in Emergency Anaesthetic Cases recorded in the Survey.

The data shows a marked increase in emergency anaesthetic work at The London Hospital and Northampton General Hospital. At The London the amount of time spent on emergency anaesthetic work each day had increased by over a factor of two. At all three hospitals the amount of time spent on ITU work had dramatically increased. At Northampton General and Alder Hey Children's Hospital ITU work had trebled, while at The London Hospital the amount of time spent on ITU work had increased by a factor of thirteen. Much of ITU anaesthetic work is of a priority 2 nature, requiring service within 15 minutes. Table II shows the factor increase/decrease in time spent on priority groups at the hospitals in comparison with the previous study. Time spent on priority 2 work at The London Hospital had increased by a factor of eight, while at Northampton General Hospital and Alder Hey Children's Hospital the work had almost doubled.

HOSPITAL GROUP	STATED PRIORITY GROUP			
	1	2	3	4
The London	0.5	8.0	1.6	2.1
Northampton General	1.3	1.6	2.1	1.4
Alder Hey	0.2	1.8	0.9	0.7

TABLE II : Multiplicative Changes in the Total Time Spent on Priority Group by Day.

These overall changes in the pattern of service ie,

a)   the mix of priority cases
b)   the overall workloads
c)   the average duration of the case

throw doubt on the validity of the previous manpower planning findings.

3.3 Previous Manpower Findings

In the previous study it was assumed that 10 percent of the work would be of priority
1, 10 percent priority 2, 30 percent priority 3 and 50 percent priority 4, and that the
average duration of a case irrespective of priority would be 60 minutes. Priority 5
work was excluded from the calculations. Using a non-transient queueing theory
solution for two priority queues, with the same service time between queues, the model
showed that the best way of deploying anaesthetists, so as to improve the standard of
cover was to segregate the priority 1 and 2 work, from the priority 3 and 4 work. By
doing this, it is argued that the low priority work does not occupy an anaesthetist
when he should be available for an emergency.

3.4 Comparison of 1967 assumptions with 1979 data

The data for The London Hospital showed a marked change in the priority groups; 6 percent of the work was priority 1, 29 percent priority 2, 27 percent priority 3 and 38
percent priority 4. Also there were differences in the services times between priorities 1/2 and priorities 3/4. The priority 1 and 2 work took on average twice as long
to complete, as the lower priority work which took on average 60 minutes to complete.

3.5 Options for Deploying Anaesthetists to Emergency Cases

Anaesthetists can be deployed broadly in one of two ways:-

a)   pooled resources. Here duty anaesthetist(s) can be deployed on any type of work
     as it arrives, subject to priority and suitability;
b)   specialisation on priority groups. Here a duty anaesthetist(s) can be assigned
     to a particular type and/or priority of work.

Anaesthetists sometimes argue that the second method is more effective than the first method, since low priority work does not occupy an anaesthetist when he should be available for high priority cases. Conversely the first option it is argued saves resources due to the 'pooling' effect. The real situation is more complex and depends on the magnitude of the conflicting parameters.

4. MATHEMATICAL MODEL

4.1 Formulation of Model

Analysis of the data revealed that the arrival rates were random (Poisson) within each hour of the day, and the treatment times fitted well to a negative exponential distribution. There is however an overall 24 hour demand pattern throughout the day. Figure 1 shows the distribution of the starting time of emergency anaesthetic cases for The London Hospital by stated priority and grouped by hour.

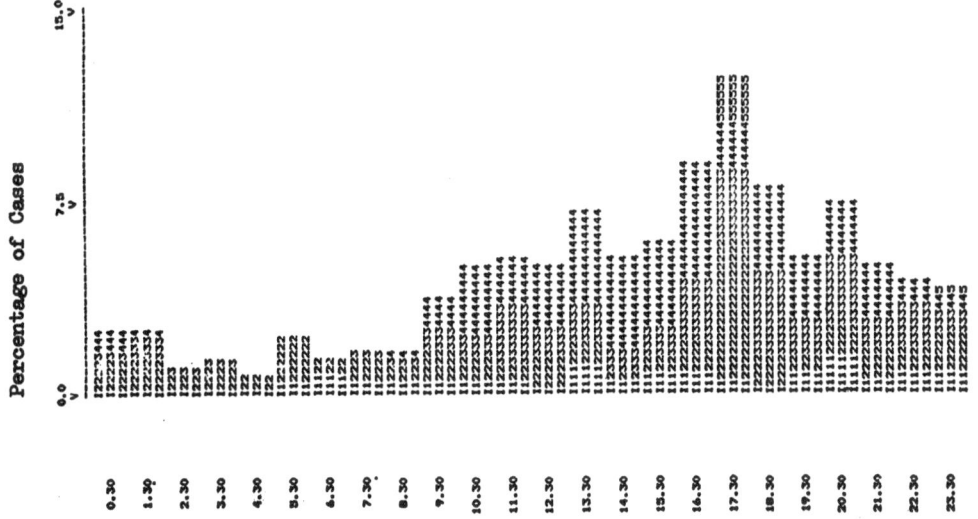

FIGURE 1 : Distribution of Emergency Cases at The London Hospital.

The emergency anaesthetic service can be characterised by a non-preemptive priority queueing mechanism, where cases queue up for service in a number of priority queues, ranging from high priority cases requiring service within 3 minutes to low priority routine work carried out in emergency time by an anaesthetist. For example, the highest priority queue would include cardio-respiratory arrests and intensive therapy cases, while the lowest priority queue would for example cover fracture cases. When an anaesthetist completes a case, the anaesthetist will take the next case from the front of the highest priority queue.

Standard analytic queueing theory solutions (5) do not exist for transient priority queueing systems, with differing service times by priority. Therefore computer sim-

ulation techniques have to be used. Normal discrete simulation has the disadvantage
that long computer runs are required in order to simulate the system for one combination
of variables. Many computer runs are required in order to simulate a number of staffing
arrangements throughout the day. Continuous system simulation of the actual queueing
theory state equations together with a goal seeking procedure, offers in some instances,
savings in computer time and a speedy solution to the problem. Therefore after
experimentation a two priority transient queueing theory model, with a goal seeking
option was developed. Two priority queueing theory can be used to model multi-priority
queues by simply compounding the system into two queues. In essence, the model
computes the staffing levels required over a 24 hour period in order to just satisfy
the service standards measured in terms of the average maximum wait time for service
in each queue. Priority 5 work is included in the model because it is carried out in
emergency time.

4.2 Applying the Model to The London Hospital Service

In the case of The London Hospital, the data showed that with the present 'pooled'
system, up to five anaesthetists had worked concurrently on different emergencies.
With the large increase in ITU work, it is attractive proposition to deploy two teams
of anaesthetists to work on high priority 1 and 2 work and low priority 3, 4 and 5 work.
The model was run, using the arrival time, service time and standards of service times
data for The London Hospital as measured in the survey. The model when run provides
the required 24 hour manning levels in order to just satisfy the standard of service.

4.3 The Present Situation

Under the 'pooled resources' policy (the present situation) the model is run once, with
the queue mechanism reduced to two queues. The model results agreed well with the
recorded data, that up to five anaesthetists would be required to maintain the service
standards.

4.4 Segregation Option

Under the alternative policy of segregating priority 1 and 2 work from priority 3, 4
and 5 work, the model is run twice in order to produce the manning levels for the high
priority and low priority work separately. By addition of the results from the two
separate runs a comparison can be made of the total manning level required under the
segregation policy with the pooled resources policy.

4.5 Comparison of Methods of Deployment

The comparison showed that an additional two to three anaesthetists would be required,
if the segregation policy was adopted. The actual staffing requirements allowing for
shift, leave and sickness would be greater than this.

5. CONCLUSION

5.1 Specific Results

Mathematical analysis, using computer techniques, of alternative manpower deployment options has indicated that the most effective way of deploying existing staff to emergency anaesthetic work at The London Hospital, is by the use of 'pooled' resources.

5.2 Benefits and Limitations of the Mathematical Technique Adopted

The technique of solving the two priority non preemptive queueing theory state equations numerically, using exogenous inputs for arrival rates over a 24 hour period, together with the goal seeking procedure for finding the number of 'servers' to just satisfy given service standards, allowed a rapid solution to the problem. If discrete simulation had been used, the transient patterns of demand would have been difficult to incorporate into the model, while many computer runs would have had to be made, in order to find the optimum number of 'servers' required, subject to given service standards. At present the model will produce solutions for this type of queueing problem, where the traffic density is low eg, for emergency services. For higher traffic densities, the capacity of the region's ICL 1904S in terms of processing power makes the solution of the equations slow. With more modern machines, and the ever increasing power of new machines, this technique will become more applicable and desirable for more general use.

5.3 The Importance of Monitoring

This follow up study also shows the importance of careful monitoring of implemented systems. In this study the 'real world' system had evolved to a point, where the earlier model of the system was no longer applicable.

REFERENCES

(1) Taylor T H, Jennings A M C, Nightingale D A, Barber B, Leivers D, Styles M and Magner J. A Study of Anaesthetic Emergency Work. Paper 1-5. British Journal of Anaesthesia, 1969, 41, 70-83, 167-175, 357-370. London 1969.

(2) Jennings A M C. A Statistical Study of Anaesthetic Emergency Work. Medical Computing, pp 321-331. Ed Abrams D E, Chatto and Windus, London 1970.

(3) Major E, Bates T, Jennings A M C, Nightingale D A, Taylor T H, Booker P D, Evans K R L. Anaesthetic Emergency Service at Three Hospitals - A Decade of Change. To be published March 1982 British Journal of Anaesthesia. London.

(4) Bates T. A Study of the Emergency Anaesthetic Service at Three Hospitals. Management Services Report 998, North East Thames Regional Health Authority, London 1980.

(5) Cox D R, Smith W L. Queues. Methuen and Co Ltd. London 1961.

COMPARISON OF THE COSTS OF TWO ANESTHETIC EQUIPMENTS
(CLOSED CIRCUIT AND SEMI-OPEN SYSTEM)

L. DUSSERRE[+], B. CAILLARD[++], P. d'ATHIS[+], J. RACAMIER-WEILLER[+++],
J. FOISSAC[++], M. WILKENING[+++].

+ *Département d'Informatique médicale du C.H.U. de DIJON (Pr. ag. L. DUSSERRE)
- Hôpital du Bocage, 2 Bd Mal Delattre de Tassigny, 21034 DIJON CEDEX -
Tél. : (80) 65. 81. 23.*

++ *Département d'Anesthésie-Réanimation (Pr. B. CAILLARD) - Hôpital du Bocage,*

+++ *Département d'Anesthésie-Réanimation (Pr. ag. M. WILKENING) - Hôpital Général -*

Key-words : *Health care costs, Anesthetic equipments, Working costs*

Abstract :

  Deux systèmes d'anesthésie générale principalement utilisés actuellement, circuit ouvert et circuit filtre, sont comparés en fonction de leurs coûts : coût d'achat du matériel et coût d'utilisation des mélanges gazeux anesthésiques.

  Les temps moyens d'anesthésie, par année d'activité, ont été estimés dans différents services hospitaliers à partir d'un fichier informatique regroupant les caractéristiques de toutes les interventions effectuées pendant un an, en particulier la durée exacte de chaque intervention. Sont connus aussi le type d'anesthésie et le type de système choisi pour chacune d'elles.

  Les résultats, reposant sur une mesure et non sur des notions théoriques, permettent d'évaluer avec fiabilité les coûts annuels d'exploitation des deux systèmes : une nette différence apparaît alors en faveur du circuit filtre, les économies les plus importantes étant obtenues avec les anesthésies de durée égale ou inférieure à une heure.

INTRODUCTION

  To give a general anesthesia, a specialist has various available equipments in his possession. These equipments have various advantages and drawbacks.

  A computerized medical record set in place in teaching Hospital of DIJON in order to survey the activity of anesthesiologists in operating rooms[+] allowed us to evaluate the cost of two anesthetic equipments : semi-open system and closed circuit.

  So, this study has been achieved not from a theoretical model but from actual measurements collected during a whole year, from 1 st of April 1980 to 31 st of March 1981.

+ *This research is granted by the French "Ministère de la Santé et de la Sécurité Sociale".*

OBJECTS

      Amongst anesthetic equipments, two of them are opposed to each other :
- the semi-open one, easy to handle and cheap in investment ;
- the closed one, more delicate to handle and much more expensive in investment, so
  that it became gradually unused during the sixties.

      But a few years ago, the closed circuit recovered some interest, at first
for reasons of pollution but especially for reasons of cost : medical gas (oxygen,
nitrous oxide and volatile anesthetic agents) have become more expensive as the energy
crisis has been developping.

      This is the economic aspect that is studied here, by comparison of the in-
vestment costs and working costs of the closed circuit with those of the semi-open
system.

      Starting from the assumption that the global costs (investment and working
costs) of the closed circuit, so high they are, the costs of semi-open system might be
in excess of them : it seems interesting to analyse the working conditions of the two
equipments systems to optimize the choice between them.

      Indeed it is sure that, in the closed circuit, the mixture of gas must be
renovated continually, proportionally to the ventilation of the patient and that is
a great expense to the working cost.

      Then this study is dealing with two points :
- investment costs
- working costs

METHODS

I - Investment costs

      They are made up of the prime costs of the equipments and have been given by
firms in specifications dated from January 1981 and drawn in French money.

II - Working costs

      They are made up of :
- depreciation expenses
- operating expenses
- cost of professional training

      As a matter of fact these expenses of professional training have not to be
considered because, in practice, they are non-existent : the handling of the equipments
is a part of usual training of specialists and, moreover it cannot, in any case, increase retributions.

1) Depreciation expenses

The amounts written off for depreciation have been set up according to the customs of a hospital center, that is to say spread over a mean time of nine years.

2) Operating expenses

To calculate these costs, that is to say the expenses due to anesthetic mixture of gas, we must know
- on the one hand, unit prices of each gas or of each volatile substance of anesthetic mixture
- on the other hand, used up doses of each part of the mixture.

a) Unit prices :

They are those of January 1981
. The relevant gas are : oxygen and nitrous oxide. Their prices are following :

Oxygen   : 0.00153 FF per litre, VAT included
Nitrogen suboxide : 0.02728 FF per litre, VAT included

. The used volatile substances are Halothane and Enflurane. They are sold as liquid phases which are invoiced per litre :

Enflurane : 850.00 FF per litre, VAT included
Halothane : 508.00 FF per litre, VAT included

They are turned anesthetic vapors by an evaporator and, as gas and vapor use is given per litre, it is necessary to know the amount of vapor produced by a given volume of the liquid substance :

1 ml of liquid Halothane gives 227 ml of vapor
1 ml of liquid Enflurane gives 198 ml of vapor

in standard conditions of temperature and pressure.

In the case of the closed circuit we must moreover take the use of sodium carbonate of lime into consideration : it costs 2.75 FF per hour of operating, VAT included.

b) Used up quantities :

The yearly quantities used up, given in litre of each component of the gas mixtures, have been calculated with information collected in the computerized medical record of anesthesiologists. Indeed, they are found there :

883

age of the patient

delay of any general anesthesia

volatile substance

method used

surgical unit concerned

Effectively the survey has been performed in the three operating rooms of a hospital which is made of detached buildings and the customs may change from a building to an other one. So the used up quantities depend on some data :

- age of the patient : we have had to discriminate children (less than fifteen) and adults (fifteen and more than fifteen)

- semi-open system or closed circuit (nitrous oxide is never used in closed equipment in the concerned operating rooms)

- delay of induction and delay of maintenance of the anesthesia : we have to discriminate between long delay and short delay of maintenance. The delay of short maintenance is equal or smaller than one hour. The delay of long maintenance is greater than one hour. Indeed these data conditions determine the out put rate of anesthetic mixture. Of course, longer is the delay, less large are the used up quantities of anesthetic vapors.

c) Prices of the anesthetic mixtures

The cost, VAT included, of a gas mixture with x% of oxygen and y% of nitrous oxide is given by the following formula :

$$Z = \frac{0.00153\ x\ +\ 0.02728\ y}{100}\ FF$$

where x = 40% and y = 60% in the semi-open equipment, and where x = 100% and y = 0% in the closed equipment.

So the cost, VAT included, of a litre of gas mixture made of p% of this former mixture and of q% of volatile substance is

$$\frac{p\ Z\ +\ 4.2975\ q}{100}\ FF\ for\ Enflurane$$

$$\frac{p\ Z\ +\ 2.2379\ q}{100}\ FF\ for\ Halothane$$

where, during induction 97.5% ⩽ p ⩽ 98.0% and 2% ⩽ q ⩽ 2.5% for adults, p = 96.5% and q = 3.5% for children, then, during a short delay of maintenance p ⩾ 98.5% and q ⩽ 1.5% for adults, p = 98.5% and q = 1.5% for children and during a long delay of maintenance p = 100% and q = 0%.

RESULTS

The results give :

- The cost per litre of each anesthetic mixture (Table 1) according to the surgical
  unit.
- The cost of each equipment with
        . depreciation expenses
        . operating expenses corresponding to use rate of the substances measured
in each surgical unit, according to the different operating conditions written in
Methods.
        . working expenses which are the sums of the two former ones. (Table 2).

Surgical unit	Induction		Short maintenance		Long maintenance	
	Semi-open	Closed	Semi-open	Closed	Semi-open	Closed
I	0.0725	0.0574	0.0336	0.0183	0.00153	0.00153
II	0.1256	0.1107	0.0623	0.0470	0.00153	0.00153
III (Children)	0.0947	0.0798	0.0503	0.0350	0.00153	0.00153
III (Adults)	0.1256	0.1107	0.0511	0.0526	0.00153	0.00153

- Table 1 -

Costs of volatile anesthetic mixture
for semi-open equipment and closed circuit
(FF/litre)

Unit	Depreciation expenses			Operating expenses					Working expenses	
				Maintenance		Sodium carbonate of lime				
	Semi-open	Closed		Semi-open	Closed	Semi-open	Closed		Semi-open	Closed
I	30.23	394.58	Short	14219.08	525.87	0	14249.31		14249.31	3245.47
			Long	3336.05	172.95				3366.28	2892.55
II	30.23	394.58	Short	19240.43	767.93	0	2325.02		19270.66	3487.53
			Long	3724.67	193.90				3754.90	2913.50
III C	30.23	394.58	Short	21330.96	1047.78	0	2325.02		21361.19	3767.38
			Long	2378.83	174.10				2409.06	2893.70
III A	30.23	394.58	Short	29745.38	1220.42	0	2325.02		29775.61	3940.02
			Long	3257.94					3288.17	2898.42

III C   Children
III A   Adults

- Table 2 -

Annual expenses (FF/year)
corresponding to mean output rates.

COMMENTS

The comparison of the annual costs calculated from a linear depreciation system spread over a mean time of nine years, in constant francs, shows that the difference between the working expenses of the two equipments is very large. This difference is in favour of the closed circuit except for the case of long maintenance anesthesia which are achieved in the surgical unit III (Children). But this former difference is negligeable in consideration of the savings allowed by the anesthesia with a short maintenance.

Such studies has been performed already : they are also in favour of the closed circuit. But all of them were performed from theoretical data. (Ref. 1 and 2)

The results, got from experimental measures of activity, daily collected in computerized files and not theoretically estimated, are reliable enough to give an aid to decision :

When the equipment must be changed, objective economic reasons will be available to prefer closed circuit to semi-open system.

This is specially evident in the operating room where anesthesia with volatile anesthetic agent happen usually as in orthopaedic surgery (Surgical unit III). Whereas in digestive and thoracic surgery (Surgical unit I), intravenous anesthesia is usually preferred and the use of gas is obviously smaller.

References :

(1)   COHEN E.N.
                Low flow and Used system Anesthesia - Reports of Scientific
                Meetings
                Anesthesiology 1978, 49, 6, 442-443.

(2)   DELACOUR J.L.
                Constribution à l'étude du bon usage de l'Enflurane - Thèse de
                Médecine de la Faculté de BESANCON - 1980, n° 112.

REVIEW OF MODELLING AND COMPUTING

IN A CANCER TREATMENT CENTRE

R.R.P. Jackson, B.G. Birkhead & W.M. Gregory

Research Centre for the Mathematical Modelling
of Clinical Trials
University of Warwick
Coventry CV4 7AL
England

Introduction:

The problems of evaluating medical care are well known, and have given
rise to the development and design of randomised clinical trials[1].
However, many situations are not conducive to this approach for a
variety of reasons. Principally, the number of patients required
to provide statistically significant results of a given power imply
constant treatment regimes over time periods too long to be feasible.

It was for this reason that use of Operational Research methods
in the evaluation of a specialist cancer treatment centre was first
made. The problem arose because the Funding Bodies wished to answer
such questions as 'did a Special Centre do better than a District
General Hospital in the treatment of cancer patients?' On the other
hand, the centre itself wanted to know whether their present treatment
regimes were producing better results than their previous ones, or
indeed as good as those obtained at other centres. Such questions
contain many elements which, given the present state of modelling,
are difficult to include in analytical form, and which may be critical
to the outcome - chief of which might be quality of life, although
costs and social benefits might also be considered important.
For these reasons a more restricted problem was tackled. Two
diseases were chosen as exemplars and it was decided to characterise
the effects of patient management at the collaborating centre by
identifying a suitable schematic of patient progress and by the
development of an appropriate mathematical model. In order to calibrate
the model for a particular trial it was necessary to obtain reliable
patient data. The model could then be used as the basis for
comparisons.

Although ostensibly the data was routinely available, it soon became
apparent that to facilitate the research a computerised data-base
was needed. This has now been developed and is extensively used for
research and for storing and analysing clinical information.

Clinical Information System:

The clinical research environment in an oncology unit is such that
patient data comes from several specialist departments (e.g.
Haematology, Radiotherapy) within the hospital. Data is collected
together to form individual patient case notes, which comprise the
clinician's data-base for treatment and research. Missing data and
difficulties of interpretation make the system problematical for the
clinician. The modelling proposed also requires access to complete
and accurate data, and to achieve this it was necessary to develop a
computerised data storage, retrieval and analysis system. A
consultancy was commissioned to develop the rudiments of such a
system which was subsequently also made available to the clinicians
through a commercial bureau. It was initially to be used for patients
with AML and Hodgkin's Disease. After the first year or so of
application it was found that the system was not being fully utilised.
The clinicians had not overcome their apprehension of computers in
general, and the system was slow, cumbersome and contained software
errors. A member of the Operational Research team was therefore
assigned to work on site at the hospital, to adapt the system to the
clinicians' requirements. By being on hand he helped them solve
problems as they arose. This co-operation proved so successful that a
clinician was given special responsibility to work more closely with
the team developing the system. The work progressed well, and soon
expanded to include other diseases. (Data on some 3000 patients
covering some 12 diseases are now stored and readily accessible).
The system is now sufficiently flexible to allow clinicians to adapt
their data-base as they proceed, and analyse their data quickly
and effectively. The system has been converted to other computers,
and working versions are now available on a DEC 2060 in FIV, and on
a PRIME 250 in F77, as well as the developed version on a Honeywell
mainframe in GEISCO Fortran 77. The system is more fully described
in (7).

Mathematical Model:

In developing a mathematical model the first problem to be solved was
to agree a patient progress schematic of meaningful states for the
diseases chosen (Acute Myelogenous Leukaemia and Hodgkin's Disease).
This is shown in Figure (1). Given the schematic and some general
assumptions about the state sojourn times it was possible to write
down a series of equations to predict the probabilities of a
patient being in particular states at a given time after entry to
the trial.

For example,

prob that patient is in remission at time 't' after arrival is

$$P. \int_0^t f_1(x)\{\int_{t-x}^{\infty} f_2(y)\,dy\}dx$$

where p = probability that patient is a remitter

$f_1(t)$ = probability distribution of time to remission for
remitting patients

$f_2(t)$ = probability distribution of time from remission to
relapse.

The schematic and the system of equations constitute the model.

To calibrate a model for a particular trial, it is necessary to make
assumptions about the form of the state sojourn distributions and to
estimate the values of their parameters for the trial data. Details
of the mathematics and some results are given in (2), (3) and (4).
As will be seen, the presentation of the results of a calibration
takes the form of a series of graphs (Figure 2) in which actual (*)
versus predicted (—) numbers are shown. 5% & 95% probability limits
(---), as derived in (2), are also shown. The same kind of display is
used for comparisons, where the question of whether the results of
Series A are appearing different to those of Series B is addressed by
using a calibrated model of patient progress in series A to predict
what would have happened to series B patients had they been treated
in the same way. Using the model in this manner, hypotheses can be
formulated to explain any observed differences, as exemplified in the
detailed applications study reported in (5).

The earliest applied model [2] had in fact comprised just the first
three states of the schematic (Figure 1) under the assumption of random

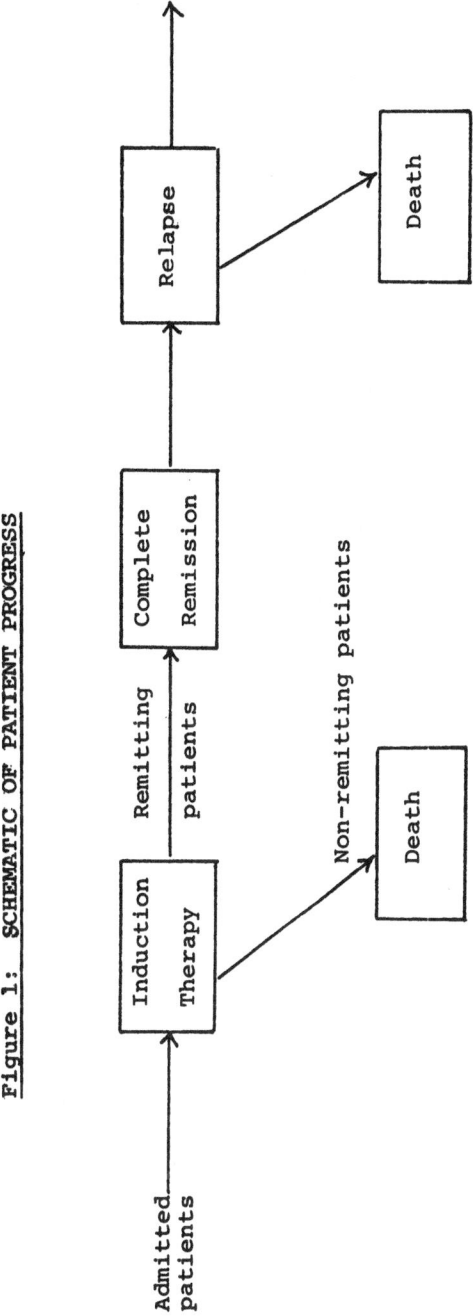

Figure 1: SCHEMATIC OF PATIENT PROGRESS

Figure 2: VALIDATION RUN OF CALIBRATED MODEL

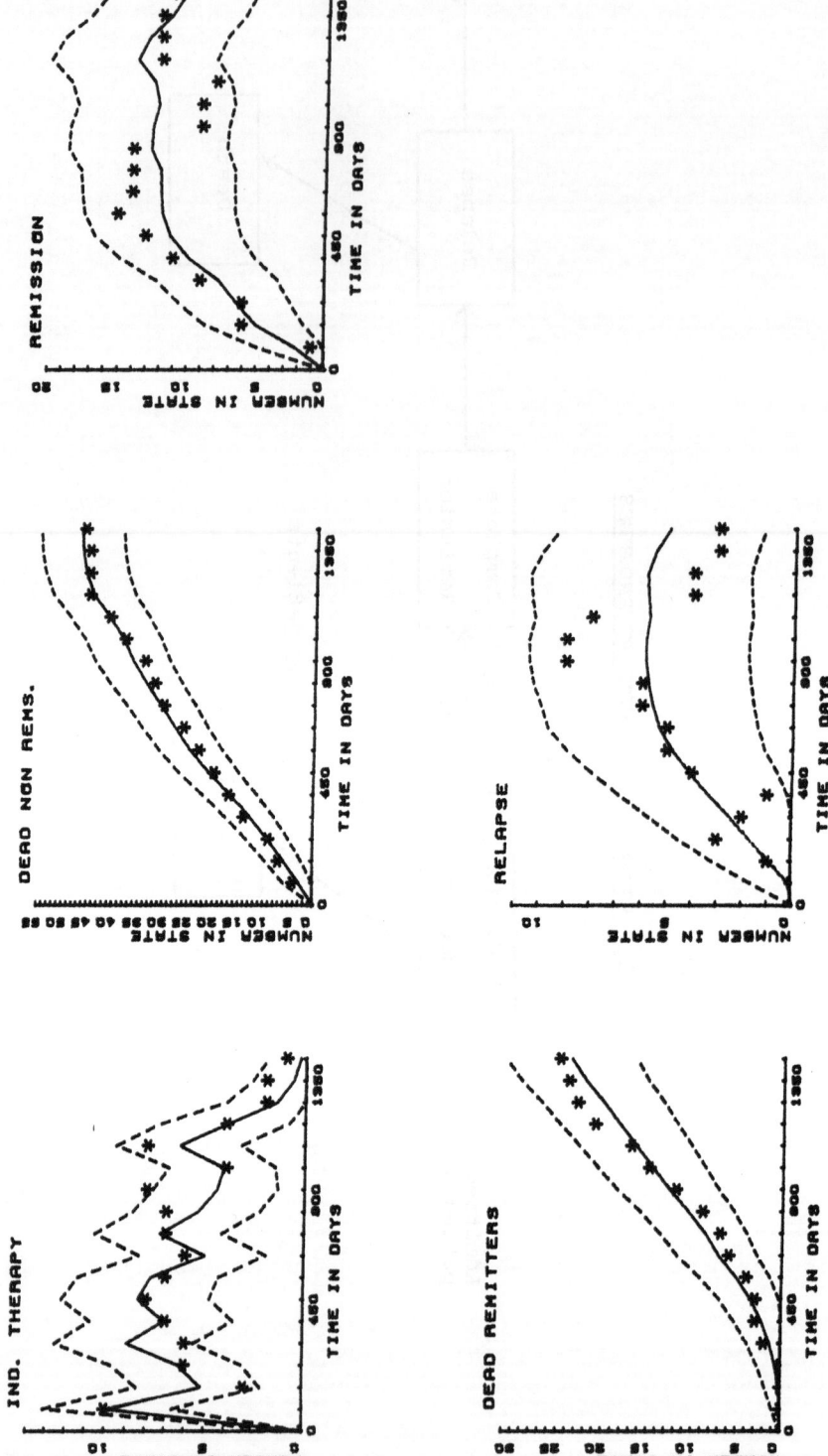

arrival of both remitter and non-remitter streams. Much of the
computation involved in calibration and comparison, together with all
the graphical display work had to be done by hand, and proved to be
both tedious and time-consuming. Since then, with the extension of
the model to include five (sometimes more) states, to replace the
random arrival assumption by the actual patient arrival pattern and
to provide scope for fitting more complex distributions to the state
transition times, the volume of work involved in a single application
has become unmanageable manually. In parallel, therefore, with the
development of the computerised Information System described above,
the modelling process itself has become automated as summarised in
Figure 3.

Model calibration has been streamlined by a facility of the Information
System to produce actuarial survival curves for state sojourn times
and to perform associated standard statistical tests. The main
model comparison monitoring program is written in Fortran IV and
stored on a Burroughs 6700 at the University of Warwick. Input to
this program comprises a file of patient data items relevant to the
modelling, directly accessible on the Information System, a file of
model parameters derived in the calibration process and a file of
run definition instructions controlling such things as patient
selection, the number and length of monitoring intervals and the
output requirements. Output from the program is in the form of
tabulated numerical results (numbers of patients in each state
[predictions and actual], together with 5% and 95% probability limits
at the end of each interval) and a summary plot file which serves as
input to a Tektronix 4052 Graphics Computing System, linked to a
pen plotter which produces the corresponding graphical display.

Conclusion:

It is now seven years since the start of the project reviewed briefly
in this paper. During this time the Clinical Information System has
aroused widespread interest, and proposals for marketing it are now
under consideration. Patient progress models such as that described
for Acute Myelogenous Leukaemia and Hodgkin's Disease have now been
developed in respect of four further diseases, and more detailed
explanatory models of particular states in the schematic have also
produced clinically interesting results[6].

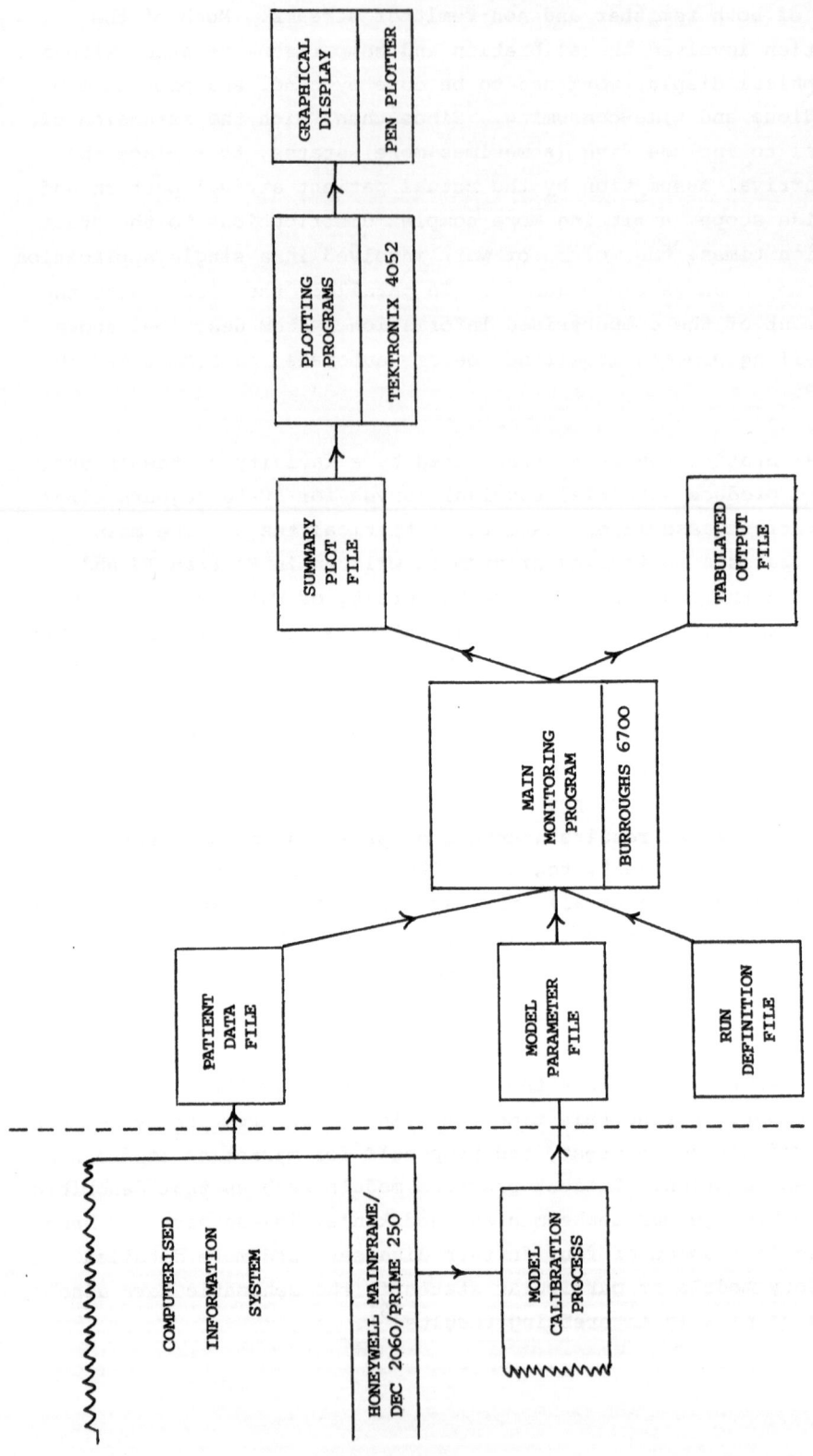

Figure 3: AUTOMATED MODELLING PROCESS

References:

(1) PETO, R., PIKE, M.C., ARMITAGE, P., BRESLOW, N.E., COX, D.R., HOWARD, S.V., MANTEL, N., McPHERSON, K., PETO, R. & SMITH, P.G. Design and Analysis of Randomised Clinical Trials Requiring Prolonged Observations of Each Patient. Br. J. Cancer $\underline{34}$, 585-612 & $\underline{35}$, 1-39.

(2) JACKSON, R.R.P. & ASPDEN, P. Treatment Evaluation - A Modelling Approach with Application to Acute Myeloid Leukaemia. J. Opl. Res. Soc. Vol $\underline{30}$, 1, pp 11-22.

(3) ASPDEN, P., JACKSON, R.R.P. & WHITEHOUSE, J.M.A. A Systems Approach to the Evaluation of Clinical Trials in a Specialist Oncology Centre.

(4) ASPDEN, P., SUTCLIFFE, S.B.J., TIMOTHY, A.R. & JACKSON, R.R.P. An Approach to the Treatment Evaluation of Hodgkin's Disease. Omega. The Int. Jnl. of Mgmt, Sci. Vol. 9, No. 5, pp 537-546.

(5) JACKSON, R.R.P., BIRKHEAD, B.G., BELL, R., LISTER, A. & GREGORY, W.M. Application of Jackson, Aspden Acute Myeloid Leukaemia Model. Accepted for publication. Jnl. Opl. Res. Soc. March 1982.

(6) BIRKHEAD, B.G. A Stochastic Birth-Death Model of Leukaemic Cell Population Growth in the Remission to Relapse Phase of Acute Myelogenous Leukaemia. Submitted for publication.

(7) GREGORY, W., BELL, R. & JACKSON, R.R.P. An Automated Clinical Research and Data Analysis System. Computers and Biomedical Research Vol 14, 472-481. 1981.

MICROCOMPUTER AIDED PSYCHOPHYSIOLOGICAL SYSTEM-ANALYTIC INVESTIGATION METHOD - NEW FACILITIES FOR PREVENTIVE MEDICINE

J. Michel, G.S. Vasadze[+], G.G. Dumbadze[++], H. Cammann, G.-B. Dümde, B. Fleischer, B. Koch, V. Lange

Institute of Medical Physics and Biophysics of the Section of Medicine (Charté) of the Humboldt-University, Berlin - GDR; [+]Dept. of Medical Cybernétics of the Institute for Experimental and Clinical Surgery, Tbilissi and [++]Central Research Laboratory of the State Medical Institute, Tbilissi - USSR

1. INTRODUCTION

The overcoming of the discrepancy between a very extensive knowledge of physiological elementary and partial processes as well as partial causal relationships and extremely scarce knowledge of their connection in the organism as a whole reflected a.o. in the still dominant diagnostics oriented towards organ pathology has to be considered one of the main prerequisites to the further development of preventive medicine. It generally holds for biological systems that not all properties of the organism can be predicted from the sum of properties of their subsystems. By methods allowing a representative characterization of the system behaviour of the human organism under simulated environmental load and finally its diagnostic and prognostic assessment, a.o. the detection of regulatory disturbances as precursors of regulatory diseases appears to be possible. By the modern computer technology such complex cybernetic methods have become realizable.

Based on the present insights into the pathogenesis of most important cardiovascular diseases, esp. ischaemic heart disease (IHD) and hypertension, a respective system-analytic investigation procedure with well-defined psychic load was developed - particularly for the detection of premorbid stages and further elucidation of the pathogenesis of these diseases. The routine application of such procedures becomes practicable by means of microcomputers.

2. METHODS

Essential features of the system-analytic investigation procedure described in detail elsewhere [1], are (cp. Figure 1):
a) Simulation of a quantitatively describable and adequate psychic load in terms of a jump function as input "disturbance value".
b) Program control of the dynamic investigation with continuous acquisition of relevant biosignals and performance parameters (see

Figure 1) as output values under rest- and load conditions.
c) Automated information-exploiting analysis of output values to obtain
   all relevant information on the transmission properties of system
   elements and the interactions between different subsystems.
To ensure a large-scale application of the method developed in practice,
a problem-oriented distributed system of microcomputers is built up for
reliable and economic on-line signal processing as shown in Figure 1.
The microcomputers adapted to the various signals work in parallel and
independently of each other under the control of a master microcomputer.
The relevant characteristics of the system behaviour computed by the
various microcomputers are transferred to the master microcomputer and
are available as effective combination of characteristics for

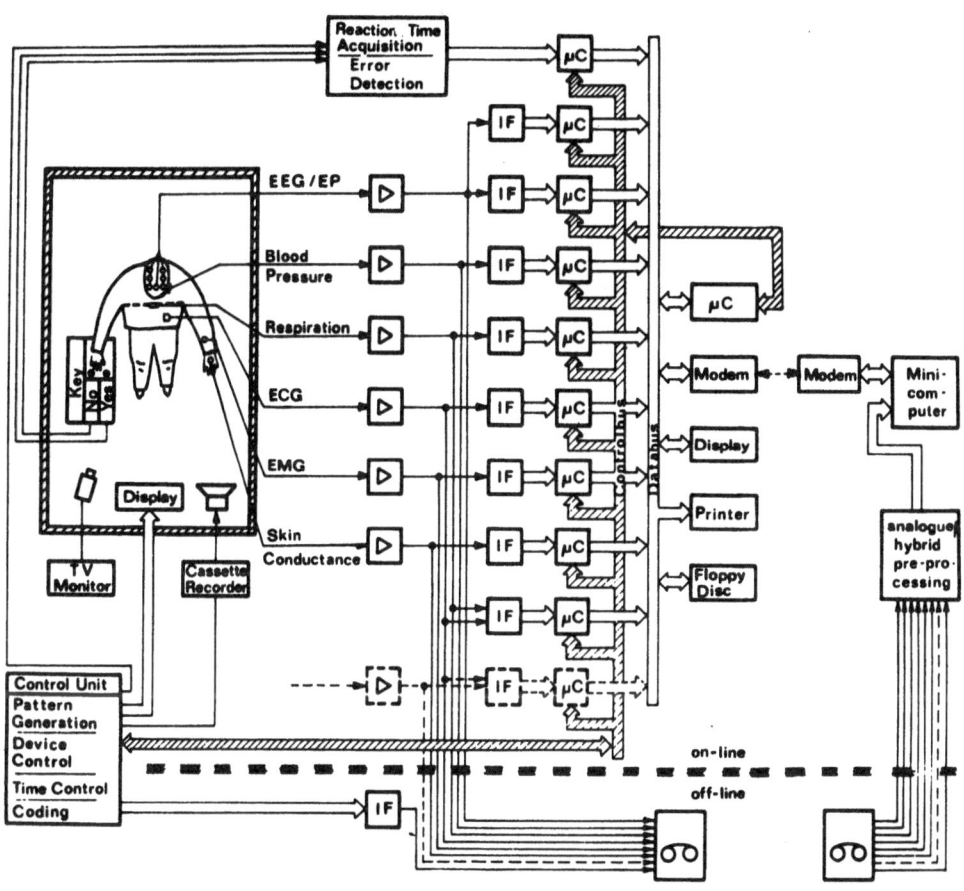

Figure 1: Schematic representation of the setup for microcomputer-
aided psychophysiological system-analytic investigation with on-line
processing of biosignals and performance parameters by a distributed
system of microcomputers (μC). IF = interface.

d) the condensed description and diagnostic and prognostic assessment
   of the psychophysiological system behaviour, so far based on a ma-
   thematical-statistical model (cp. Figure 2).

3. RESULTS AND DISCUSSION

By way of example, Figure 2 shows the results of discrimination of
clinically healthy subjects 46 to 56 years of age (group IIA, 28 men)
and patients of the same age with symptoms of IHD (group IIB, 27 men)
by means of a combination of the behaviour characteristics of the physiological function parameters heart rate, heart rate variability, respiration rate, respiration rate variability, skin conductance, EMG
and EEG. Based on this combination of characteristics of 27 group IIB
subjects, all were correctly re-
classified, while one subject of
group IIA was wrongly reclassified
as group IIB. The first place in
the rank of selectivity in this
combination of characteristics is
taken by an EEG characteristics
reflecting the relaxation after
the load phase of the investigation. The results obtained agree
with the hypothesis on the development of cerebrovisceral regulatory diseases. They show that subjects with and without IHD symptoms
differ in their psychophysiological system behaviour and support
the hypothesis that, after respec-
tive optimization, such system-analytic procedures may attain major
practical importance in preventive medicine.

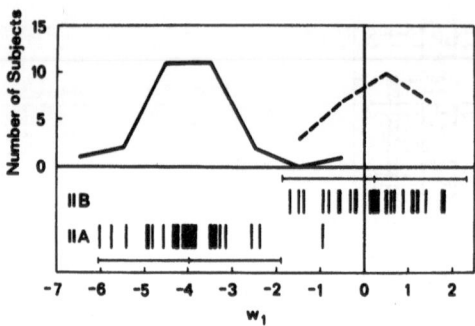

Figure 2: Result of discrimination
of subjects of groups IIA and IIB
by means of 19 physiological characteristics obtained as representatives of system behaviour from
7 functional parameters (for further details see text).

4. REFERENCES

[1] Michel J, Vasadze GS, Dumbadze GG, Cammann H, Lange V,
     Guráth B, Hiller E, Dümde G.-B.   Automated system-analytic in-
     vestigations of the human organism.   MEDINFO 80 Lindberg/Kaihara
     Editors, IFIP Amsterdam: North Holland 1980; 101-105

Dr H.R.A.Townsend
The National Hospital
Queen Square
London

Overview.

In the UK every young doctor on graduation must, before becoming fully registered complete six months practical training in an approved Medical unit and a similar period in an approved Surgical unit. These are paid Pre-Registration House Officer appointments and as such are the responsibility of the Area Health Boards. The posts must have been inspected and approved by the University, which is responsible to the General Medical Council for certifying that students have properly completed their practical training before they can be offered full registration.

There is keen competition, both by students for posts in University hospitals or for posts whose Chief is a well known and respected teacher, and by consultants to get the best students for their units. This competition has in the past led to pressure on students to agree, sometimes even in the pre-clinical years, to take particular posts on graduation. There were consequent frustration, recriminations or both, when they subsequently discovered that their interests had changed or that the student's career would have been better served by a different choice.

The first suggested solution was to arange that all appointments should be made effectively simultaneously just before graduation. All students were asked to provide a telephone number at which they could be contacted on a particular day. On the designated day each consultant telephoned the students to whom he wished to offer a post. Verbal agreements were then made between the parties. Not surprisingly this idea did not prove practical when it was tried!

A computer system was then proposed which assigned preference weights to the choices of both consultants and students. Posts were allocated by an algorithm which aimed to maximise the combined preferences of consultants and students. This system was an improvement, but in a few embarrassing cases particular consultant/student pairs had very low combined preferences and it was not possible to demonstrate in any simple way to the parties involved the justice - or even rationale - of the assignment.

The basic allocation mechanism.

The method eventually adopted is a technique (1) for computing an assignment of partners such that <u>no two individuals find themselves in a position such that each would prefer the other to the partner actually assigned</u>. If such a situation existed then the pair in question would wish to leave their assigned partners and form a new association which would make the situation <u>unstable</u>. Otherwise the assignment is termed <u>stable</u> because none of the participants has a valid reason to wish to alter the status quo.

The stable assignment has the advantage that it is possible to demonstrate to any individual who feels aggrieved that all partners who might have been preferred to the individual allocated are in fact matched with other participants for whom the potential partner has indicated a prior preference.

The algorithm itself is very simple. As implemented for PRAMS we take each of the various units in turn and "offer" a post in the unit to the applicant at the top of the consultant's preference list. The applicant is recorded as "accepting" the post unless s/he has already accepted a post which ranks higher on the applicant's preference list. In this latter case the applicant "rejects" the post which is offered to the next person on the consultant's list, and so on until all the unit's posts have been accepted or the list is exhausted.

Now when an applicant accepts a post and then upon receiving a subsequent better offer accepts a different one, this implies rejection of the previous offer, implying in turn that the post should be offered to the next applicant (if any) on the consultant's list, who may accept it and in the process reject another post, which in turn should be offered, and so on and so on.

This chain reaction must terminate because an applicant always remembers the "best offer so far" and rejects all less desirable offers. Each applicant's "accepted offer" can only be revised in one direction - towards the more preferable jobs at the top of the applicant's preference list.

The version of the algorithm used in this program is iterative. Consultant's lists are arranged in an arbitrary (numerical) order. Offers are made on behalf of each consultant in turn, and the process repeated until a complete scan has been made during which no applicant revises an "accepted offer". At this stage the assignments are STABLE as defined above.

Some consultants have specified that not more than one female resident may hold a post in the unit at any one time. This restriction can be met by not offering a post to a

female student if two female students have already
"accepted" posts in the unit concerned.

Seasonal Allocations

At this stage each applicant will have been allocated a
Medical and a Surgical job. Some students may, of course,
have been unsuccesful in obtaining one or both appointments,
and some may have already arranged an appointment in another
region, but have applied to the scheme for "only a Medical"
or "only a Surgical" job. Similarly a Unit with, say, 2
posts will have had allocated up to 4 student applicants. It
is now necessary to make detailed allocations which will
determine which students take up the posts for the
August-January period and which will take the posts in
Febuary.

This is a fairly simple version of a general problem which
has been extensively (2) studied. Because we are effectively
timetabling some 200 individuals to a similar number of
posts the problem is non-trivial. (It is one of a class of
problems termed "N-P complete", which means that the most
efficient algorithm theoretically possible will probably
need an exponential amount of time). Since in this case we
have a fairly large problem it will not be possible to
obtain an optimal solution.

Our particular version has two interesting characteristics.

In the first place it may prove to be insoluble. For
example if we have two units each with a single post
and sharing an applicant, while the second applicant to
each unit is only available to take up the post in the
August-January period, then the vacancy available to
the shared applicant will be limited to Febuary-July
for both the Medical and the Surgical post - which is
manifestly impossible.

Fortunately however there are, in general a large
number of more or less equivalent solutions which we
can hold to be "acceptable" since the vast majority
will not have any very pressing reason to prefer a
particular season - August or Febuary, so long as they
obtain the best possible Medical and Surgical
experience.

The approach is therefore as follows:-

i) First we allocate all those students who are
only available in a particular season because they
have already arranged another job outside the

900

scheme. It is necessary to check that the
constraints have not been violated at this stage –
we might have two individuals both only available
in August and allocated to the single post in a
particular Unit.

ii) The Units are taken one by one in a convenient
order. Possible allocations of the assigned
applicants to the available August and Febuary
slots are tried until an acceptable arangement is
found.

iii) The next Unit is then taken and the process
repeated until either all the Units have been
succesfully allocated, or until a Unit is found
where, after all possible arrangements have been
tried, no satisfactory allocation has been found.

iv) When this "failure" occurs the program goes
back to an earlier stage, undoing all allocations
performed en-route (this process is called
"backtracking") and starts afresh with a different
allocation at the stage in question. After
backtracking to a particular unit a number of
times all possible arrangements for this unit will
be exhausted, and it will be necesary to backtrack
further, and so on.

Heuristics

In theory it is possible for the program to explore all
possible solutions in this way, and if all possible
arrangements for the first Unit are exhausted the problem
must be declared insoluble. If there are more than two or
three Units, however, it will take an impossibly long time
to carry out an exhaustive search. A little ingenuity (or
elementary "machine intelligence") is required.

If the difficulty is localised (for example the two units
with a shared applicant mentioned above), then by
considering the two Units concerned first and second the
impossibility will be revealed after only a few seconds
computation. A facility is therefore provided to allow the
operator to specify the order in which the first few (or
indeed if necessary all) Units are to be considered. If the
system appears to be having difficulty with one or more
Units, then by promoting these to be considered first the
trouble may be resolved or an unsuspected impossibility
revealed.

I have not been able to devise any cast-iron rules to
determine precisely which Units should be promoted in this
way, and in what order. For this reason the choice is left
to human intuition. Automatic promotion is however applied
to ensure that as far as possible groups of Units sharing

applicants are considered together. In this way potential interactions are revealed as early as possible.

The other choice which needs to be made as the program runs is the order in which the different possible arrangements of the assigned students are considered. This seems to me essentially arbitrary so I have simply arrranged that all possible combinations for students who have indicated "no particular preference" are exhausted before any allocations contrary to the expressed seasonal preferences are tried.

Since allocation of an Applicant to a particular Unit in a given season necessarily involves allocation of the same Applicant to the other assigned Unit in the contrary season, some time is saved by carrying out the associated allocation at the same time and checking that no constraints have been violated.

Observation of the "backtracking" mechanism in action reveals that it is very often grossly inefficient because each time that a new arrangement is tried at a particular level the same subsequent sequence of allocations leads to the same impasse.

This led to the formulation of a 'pruning rule', so called because the operation of the program can be likened to a search of a large tree, and the pruning operation can be likened to cuting off one or more branches – search of which is judged to be unprofitable. The rule states that "If an allocation fails it is necessary to backtrack at least as far as a Unit previously considered which shares an applicant with the failed Unit".

This pruning is generally useful in practice although it may prove to be over-enthusiastic by eliminating branches which do contain an acceptable allocation, because of second or higher order interactions. The rule should properly read " ......which shares an applicant with the failed unit, or shares an applicant with a unit which shares an applicant with the failed unit, or shares an applicant with a unit which shares an applicant with a unit which shares an applicant with the failed unit, or ....etc.etc" (i.e. sharing should be defined recursively).

Preference Lists.

Each student is allowed to apply to a maximum of eight (8) units. The PRAMS registration form requires the applicant to list, in order of preference the Medical, and (separately) Surgical Units to which he or she has applied.

It is essential that students list all and only the units to which they have applied and notify the PRAMS office if, for any reason, it is necessary to withdraw an application from some or all of the units listed.

Any such 'withdrawn' applications are appended at the end of the preference list, but separated from it by a special mark, entered as the dummy number -999, which is printed on listings as a slash (/).

In a similar way consultants will list on their forms in order of preference the numbers of all the applicants for posts in each unit. Any aplicants who are considered unsuitable or not worth considering must be listed at the end separated from the preference list proper by the slash (/ or -999) mark.

The PRAMS programs

There are seven programs in all -

PRAMSJ - used for entering, updating, and editing the main APPS and JOBS files. (PRAMS Jobs & applicants)

PRAMSK - used to carry out the comprehensive crosschecking procedure, which is necessary prior to allocation. (PRAMS Krosscheck)

PRAMSL - used to list records on the printer for sending out to participants for verification, and to keep as a Reference List. (PRAMS Listings)

PRAMSM - the Stage 1 matching procedure - see "The basic allocation mechanism" Section 1.1 above. (PRAMS Matching)

PRAMSN - the Stage 2 assignment procedure - see "Seasonal Allocations" Section 1.2 above. (PRAMS Next stage)

PRAMSO - the results listing program, providing results to be sent to consultants and applicants as well as to employing authorities. (PRAMS Output)

PRAMSP - a program to pick out the unallocated jobs and applicants and to present these in a suitable form for circulation to unsuccessful participants. (PRAMS Pick unallocated)

PRAMSQ - produces a simple statistical summary of the results of the year's allocation.

References

(1) McVitie,D.G., and Wilson,L.B. "The Stable Marriage Problem" Comm ACM, July 1971, 14:7 pp 486-490

(2) Schmidt,G., and Strohlein,T. "Timetable construction - an annotated bibliography" The Computer Journal Nov 1980 23:4 pp 307-316

THE MEDICAL RECORD AS A BASIS FOR DECISION MAKING

Professor J. Anderson,
Department of Medicine,
King's College Hospital
Medical School,
Denmark Hill, London SE5.

Summary.

The theoretical and practical basis of the medical record are discussed to show how decision support may be achieved. The complexity
of the purposes for which the medical record is used indicate that
there will be several different decision support systems ready to
access the record. Data base technology is available to allow such
interaction on a routine or individual query basis. As yet not enough
research has been done to support medical decision making outside
limited diagnostic and therapy areas.

Introduction.

Medical Records are complex patient oriented documents reflecting
medical theory and practice. While medical teaching assumes that a
universal model of a medical record exists, in reality medical records
are adapted to the specialty needs of the doctors as well as to
general medical, surgical and psychological requirements.

The essential theoretical specialty constructs of diagnosis, prognosis, investigation, therapy and patient management are represented
in different parts of the record, but rarely are data matched to
theoretical needs in a direct manner. 1. For example, diagnosis is a
general construct dealing not only with the classification of disease,
but with the application of that classification to a particular
patient in relation to his illness and its evolution. 2. A diagnosis
reached at the first encounter with the patient is a working or provisional diagnosis and may or may not be at the level of a symptom or
sign, a syndrome, or includes some aetiological agent as part of its
formulation. At the patient's bedside the diagnosis is no longer a
theoretical construct, but a guide for individual patient management.
Other types of diagnosis, such as differential diagnosis, are related
to investigations with laboratory and other tests. The final diagnosis is a clinical diagnosis but the recorded administrative diagnosis
relates to a pre-coordinated formulation for epidemiological purposes
and death certificate diagnosis may be coded in a different way.
Pathological and histological diagnosis reflect the special nature of
the statements in relation to structure rather than functions. Thus
these theoretical constructs are themselves complex and are becoming
increasingly so.

Decision making from the medical record occurs at all levels.
First there is the necessity to encode data about the history of the

patient and his life situation in medical language. This not only
reflects convention and medical theory but is related to the expected
output. The formalisation increases if the system is designed to
assist the doctor by providing aids to decision making. In recent
years most assistance has been provided for diagnosis in limited
areas (3) and for therapy guidance (4,5). More recently advice about
drug interaction and side effects has become available and aids
decision are given in a real time mode. The order of investigation
from the simple to the complex and the most costly has not yet been
well researched for many areas in medicine, nor has the ideal mix of
investigation and therapy been devised which is covered by the construct of patient management for common diseases. Much more research
work needs to be done before sophisticated advisory systems for aiding
medical decision will arrive. Nevertheless, these are likely to be
based on new forms of medical records.

2. Medical Record Structure and Definition.

Medical records have grown and developed as long as pen and paper
have existed. Medical theory has continued to grow and develop more
rapidly in the 20th century due to research efforts. At its best the
initial medical record reviews the history of the patient's illness in
medical language for subsequent usage. The record of the patient's
complaints is in lay language for different purposes. His life
situation is recorded, including its physical, social and psychological aspects and note is taken relevant to environmental factors.
Following the record of the physical examination, usually a standardized review of structure and some important functions, the level of
working diagnosis is reached.

Weed sees this part of the record as a data base and formulates
the patient's problems. It is difficult to decide whether this is
the patient's or the doctor's view of them and the 'problem' concept
lacks the sophistication and hypothetico-deductive aspects of the
diagnostic construct. Other different models of diagnosis based on
a systems approach including input, state and output considerations
have also been formulated, which may use different data with a
different emphasis. (6). These new models may have use in relation to
care of the elderly and in chronic disease embodying control concepts
and feedback in relation to clinical 'state'.

The clinical record goes on to deal with both investigation and
treatment of symptoms and also determines the cause of disease.
Initial treatment aims to relieve system failure as effectively as
possible, especially in the critically ill patient. Here well tried
therapy is matched to clinical observation and tests. Advisory
systems have much potential in this area of active decision making
and could ensure optimum care for the seriously ill patient.

Decisions about therapy are largely based on the results of clinical
trials, but also with a view of clinical effects in the individual

patient. Problems arise with the linking of investigations and
therapy which are part of therapeutic clinical management. Clinical
management is difficult and much more research is needed before
advisory systems can be created even for common disorders.

What has become apparent is that the medical record is becoming
more complex and elaborate with increasing definition to support
medical decision. It is no longer organised as a time sequence of
events and tests but needs to be re-organised in other formal ways
for more appropriate usage. Without information systems such complex
re-organisation will not be well achieved. The profession has been
slow to recognise this usage of medical informatics, although it has
jumped on the bandwagon of microprocessors.

3. Medical Record Decision Support Processes.

At present medical record structure reflects historical and
educational processes rather than reflecting the support it gives to
medical decision making. Admittedly, this is only one of the major
uses for medical records though they also have medico-legal purposes
and reflect problems in privacy, confidentiality, medical administration, etc. The development of modern data base technology offers much
to the medical record enabling the user either to use standard algorithms or to use a query language and interrogate the data himself.
So far there is little evidence that doctors would use such technology
although it can be provided. However, there is no doubt that doctors
are going to require more decision support and the use of such informatics technology will undoubtedly become more widespread to meet
this need.

As decision support develops, so medical theory is extended. A
typical example is in relation to prognosis where this now not only
deals with what the patient's future is likely to be but also relies
on a detailed prognosis, in relation to certain disease areas enabling
therapy choices to be made. Thus medical information systems are
pushing medical therapy to develop the decision aiding processes in
relation to prognosis.

Medical administration also received support from medical records
and this is used to document service needs, so that we can make
better provision for a comprehensive health care system. From detailed medical records, data about disease and resource utilisation
can be determined and provide the basis for the necessary improvements to occur.

4. Investigative Decisions.

Investigation of a patient's physical, psychological and social
state is an essential part of determining the effects of the disease
process over time. To do this effectively, the nature, cost and
effectiveness of each investigation has to be taken into account and

linked with the diagnosis. Investigative decision support can be
critical but as yet only a few experiments have been undertaken to
indicate the way forward.

5. Therapy Decisions.

Therapy may be achieved by several other means than drugs, for
example physiotherapy, psychotherapy and physical therapy. In therapy
there are challenges both in relation to risk and result. Surgery
and anaesthesia are important modes of therapy and are by no means
without risk in relation to death, side effects and complications.
But drug therapy too has its side effects and complications both in
the short and long term. As yet long term studies are difficult to
design and carry out and progress is slow. Psychotherapy also has its
difficulties of time scale and cost as well as problems of anticipat-
ing outcome. Thus decision systems which would support therapy are
important. Already there are significant developments for physical
therapy and also for drugs.

6. Patient Management.

This is a complex construct dealing with the relationship of
investigation, therapy and clinical state as revealed by the course of
the patient's illness. Decision support systems so far being investigated are rather theoretical and have to deal with control and
feedback. However, with more research such advisory systems might
well develop and have much practical usage.

7. Conclusions.

For all doctors the medical record is an essential platform for
decision making. It also records the reasons for decisions for
medico-legal purposes as well as providing information for administration and other review and reflects the exploitation of professional and other resources. As yet, the use of an information
system to support the medical record has been slow to arrive. However, advisory systems are now beginning to be based on medical record
data especially in relation to diagnosis and therapy and newer
applications are being developed. It does reflect the importance of
medical theory which interacts with clinical knowledge and practice
so that better care can be given to patients.

REFERENCES

1. Llewelyn, D.E.H., Anderson, J.(1980) Medical Informatics 5, 267-8.

2. Lenoir, P., Charles, G. (1980) Medical Informatics 5, 281.

3. Leaper, D.J., Horrocks, J.C., Staniland, J.R., de Dombal, F.T.
   (1972) Brit. Med. J. 3, 350.

4. Shortcliffe, E.H., Buchanan, B.C., Fiegenbaum, E.A. (1979) Proc.
   3rd Annl.Symp. Comp. Appl. Health Care. IEE, USA.

REFERENCES (cont'd)

5. Shortcliffe, E.H. (1976) Computer based Medical Correlations
   IMYCIN, North Holland New York.

6. Cooper, D.J., Graham, A., Anderson, J. (1976) Medical Data
   Processing. Proceedings Toulouse Conference. Taylor & Francis
   London.

THE CHALLENGE OF MEDICAL INFORMATICS
- DELUSIONS OR NEW PERSPECTIVES? -

Peter L. Reichertz
Institute for Medical Informatics
Medical School Hannover
D 3000 Hannover 61 /Fed. Rep. Germany

1. SUMMARY.

Medical Informatics claims to be the science of the nature, the construction and the application of algorithms in medicine /see 21, 22/.
Interdisciplinary by nature, it developed with a growing number of
applications of information technology in theoretical medicine and all
fields of health care.
This contribution examines the originality of Medical Informatics as a
discipline between medicine and informatics and its 'raison d'etre'.
The question is asked, whether the work, successfully done in many
fields so far, will not eliminate the necessity of an own discipline.
In the light of growing 'peripheralization' and commercially developed
application systems the increasing importance is discussed of applied
system analysis and the methodological expansion into epidemiological
and health care support analysis.   Future possibilities are seen to
lie in decision analysis and support based on the process nature of
medical decision making.   Increasing activities are predicted in the
field of imaging, pattern recognition, robotics and endoprothetics.
New areas are suggested like the application of concepts of informatics to biological processes of control and communication, even down to
the cellular level.   Again the necessity is stressed of a conceptual
approach and to develop respective curricula.

2. DATA PROCESSING AND MEDICAL INFORMATICS.

The development of data processing and the application of information
technology in all sectors of medicine is well known. The present congress reflects in its many sessions the great spectrum and growing
number of methodological approaches and practical applications.

The 'penetration' of information technology into medicine happened in
various areas and was pioneered by individuals with varying back-
grounds /18/. This meant that usually there was a lack of a strate-
gical and methodological approach and that the actual problem was

attacked on the basis of the methods and methodologies available in the particular context. This led to two problems /14/:

1. The methodology used and the theoretical background were often lagging behind the scientific advances in informatics; however, great insight was gained into particular application problems and the specific environmental conditions.

2. The respective teams grew and learned with requirements of the project; i.e. very seldomly a specific education was already present to provide the tools and experiences needed for the solution of the problem.

The consequences were very often ad-hoc-solutions tailored to the particular application with the necessity to design new systems when new problems arose without a satisfactory degree of generalization which could have led to a solution for a multitude of similar problems.

The specific requirements in medicine and the particular constellation of interdisciplinary work, needing a profound knowledge of the theoretical and organizational structure of medicine and health care delivery, favored the contention, that medical informatics is or has to become a medicine-based discipline of its own, requiring particular curricula and, last, but not least, sociological recognition in the medical hierarchies /7, 10, 12, 16, 21/. This concept, however, has been contested especially by informaticians /e.g. 29/, who claimed that informatics is capable of developing a general, meta-methodology which makes it possible to recognize and describe all possible problems in any field and to develop solutions in direct communication with those concerned.

In parallel to these discussions, curricula and educational concepts were developed /e.g. 1, 5, 8, 9, 13/. Provisions for a post-graduate training were made /e.g. 6/ and plans to train auxiliary personnel were developed /e.g. 2, 25/.

Though still discussed controversially, the word 'Medical Informatics' become increasingly used for associations, curricula, journals and general reference to the application of data processing and methodology in medicine.

3. GENERAL DEVELOPMENT.

In the course of the general development, <u>applications</u> could be seen in the following areas /see also 22/:

1. Advanced data analysis

   including the application of analytical software to large or complex sets of data in clinical trials, epidemiology and other areas together with the development of analytical tools for dedicated projects and studies.

2. Logistics of information

   in medicine and health care delivery at large, concerning both medical records and administrative data to provide information systems within regions, hospitals, complex departments and the office of the private physician, and

3. (Bio)Signal analysis

   and direct processing of various types of data derived from the body of the patient, transducers or analytical instruments.

Lately, image-processing techniques have received a growing attention including the development of computer-aided tomography and digital processing of radiographic images. Some applications have been seen in the area of endoprothetics or robotics but have not yet advanced beyond spot-applications or research endeavors.

So far, the mere data processing activities have prevailed. Though of early interest, computer support of the medical decision making has not yet resulted in a general penetration in the various areas of medicine and health care delivery, though recently new efforts can be noted, in particular using methods of artificial intelligence and other advanced techniques /see also 24, 28/.

The <u>background of people</u> dedicating their work completely to Medical Informatics showed a gradual shift from primarily involved medical people to those with training in informatics, engineering, economics and management sciences, though the medical people still are, in most instances, the single major professional groups in the national societies concerned with medical informatics and related fields. To reflect a regional development, a recent survey in the German Society for Informatics (Gesellschaft fuer Informatik, about 2000 members) revealed an interest of approximately 5 % of all members in further education in the application field of medicine. Out of the 41 persons who received the Certificate of a Medical Informatician for respective training and proven leading experience in the field /6/, awarded jointly by the German Society for Informatics (Gesellschaft fuer Informatik) and the Association for Medical Documentation, Informatics and Statistics (GMDS, about 700 members and being the competent scientific society for medical informatics) 23 i.e. 56 % were physicians. The largest single group, however, seeking admission to the GMDS during the last years, were those graduating from a special curriculum of medical informatics (Heidelberg/Heilbronn) or informatics with particular emphasis on medical applications /5/. In times of reduced funds for research projects and theoretical development, the attraction of clinical medicine and general practice for students of medicine or younger doctors still seems not to be entirely detached from financial aspects.

Technologically and in terms of application, there is a growing tendency towards 'peripherilization', i.e. the development of competence in the periphery of hospitals and health care delivery units, away from central computer facilities and based on own personnel and machinery /18, 21/. This tendency, with the inherent danger of decomposition of larger and centrally developed systems, has been largely enhanced by the advent of microcomputers and the decreasing cost for hardware /22/.

Such a peripherilization is not exclusively caused by the technological development. Often the resulting consolidated hardware costs are not necessarily lower than those of a central installation, and the applications developed show a lower degree of performance and the time involvement of the users is greater than when using central services or systems. The self-determination of the various user groups, the feeling of having control of the own system and the independence from central planning is a strong sociological factor which can be observed also outside medical applications as a general trend. Peripheral systems seem to satisfy the sociological and psychological requirements to a much greater extent than performance, though, naturally, the own control of a system and its availability certainly facilitates optimal usage and availability. Also reasons for failure or hardware break-down are easily recognized and, since falling under the own responsibility, explained and accepted. The same is true for errors of the system itself or other deficiencies.

Such a tendency certainly is enhanced by the growing engagement of industry which, after an original and disappointing involvement in hospital information systems and a consequent withdrawal, has increasingly become active both in the field of direct instrumentation as well as in the area of information systems for hospitals, larger departments or general practitioners, not to forget the dynamic area of imaging, including computer-aided tomography, sonography with further developments going on here. By offering dedicated solutions, i.e. for heart-catheterization, clinical laboratories, radiological departments and the like, the development of applications away from central units or plans is prompted or supported. Also, with the availability of these products, a central institution becomes of lesser importance to develop applications and to assist in developments and research projects in the various departments.

4. RESULTING TRENDS.

These developments led to certain consequences for those working in the field of medical informatics and the development of this discipline in general:

1. Replacement by the end-user.

   In the various application areas, the end-user takes over more and more of the duties to maintain and operate the various systems. Even to a certain degree development work is done here using the computer power available and the accessibility of systems, even with low efficiency programming languages and dilettante skills.

2. Decomposition of systems.

   The decomposition of integrally conceived systems receives a particular emphasis in the administrative area, which, more and more, is run directly by administration with a growing tendency towards independence from medical applications. This tendency has always been pertinent in the United States after an initial phase of integral hospital information systems. In several European pilot developments, however, there has been the strong contention that the combination of medical and administrative data yields more

information and possibilities than approaches independent from
each other. However, the separation or isolation of administrative
services from the medical applications removes, in many applications on the European scene, the justification for hardware and
software expenses and for a staff, which can also be used for
other developments and research applications. Only gradually considerations like cost-effectiveness of the medical action or quality assurance regain general interest and need, again, the integration with the financial and administrative applications.

3. Increasing availability of industrial products.
   The availability of commercial products eliminates the necessity
   for dedicated programming and developments, supported by medical
   informaticians, in the hospital or in the research environment.
   These products begin to change the attitude of the user, who
   begins to select such a product according to the features he
   wants. Development work in the respective areas is decreased or,
   as stated above, carried out using the delivered products by the
   own staff.
   Increasingly, for systems of a more complex nature (like hospital
   information systems) software tools are developed, which allow for
   a parametrized approach so that the systems can be adapted to
   local requirements, react to new or varying demands of the users
   and allow for a gradual expansion of services and applications.

5. ASSESSMENT.
As a result of this development, there seems to be a decreasing necessity for the work done so far in the field of medical informatics
respectively in central institutions: the design and construction of
information systems, problem-dedicated projects and central monolithic
approaches. Without doubt is the growing number of applications of
information technology down to the departmental level to a certain
degree the result of the success to develop adaptable systems, to
refine software tools and to develop techniques which allow for general application and adaptation; work done by those working in medical
informatics. Industrial products have only become reality after scientific projects have provided experience and knowledge about the specific environments in medicine and the structure of motivation and
user attitude in the medical field. Thus, the paradox of Medical
Informatics is:

> The more successful the medical informatician is, the more
> he will eliminate the need for his existence.

This principle renders it necessary to examine the present situation and trends in order to find an orientation towards the future.

6. EVALUATION AND CONSEQUENCES.

In some instances, those who have been pioneers in the late sixties and early seventies have gone back to practicing medicine and, though continuing to use computers as a tool for their daily work, have discontinued the development of applications or the experimentation with new approaches or ideas. Others have dedicated their work to the development of medical methodology in the attempt to further the systematization in medicine and the analysis respectively support of decision making and reasoning. Such a medical methodology needs concepts of formalization and advanced tools of mathematical and statistical analysis. Therefore, this approach shows a certain similarity to the developments from biometrical and biostatistical points of departure.

If the paradox stated above is true, the question is whether the only development is the abandonment of medical informatics and the choice between the two principles of attitude as described. This would mean that the development of further tools for the practical use in clinical and theoretical medicine would be left to industry and a few research centers respectively development projects.

However, there seems to be another alternative which has to be considered: reorientation of medical informatics and development of new application areas respectively foci of interest. Such a reorientation and development should, in my opinion, be along the following five main axes:

1. Methodology research and development
2. Systems analysis
3. Tool development
4. Applied research
5. Basic research,

whereby an individual project may be centered around one major axis or may involve several orientations.

6.1. Methodology Research and Development.

The necessity for the development of a methodology will be the topic of a major contribution to this meeting /see also 3, 11, 12/. In this context, medical methodology is to be defined as follows:

> Medical methodology is the approach to the formalization of medical facts and events and the attempt to describe their causal relations. Its goal is the systematization of decision making and medical action where possible.

Medical methodology involves mathematical analytical methods for various purposes, especially, however, for decision making including the analysis of facts in regard to their relevance in the process of clinical decision making and action. Research into decision making involves also experimental studies and prospective research into the discriminating power of the various variables and facts in regard to diagnoses, risks and chances for success of the various actions under scrutiny.

Methodological approaches also should include attempts of a formal description of information flow in theoretical and clinical medicine and research into the process aspects and hierarchical steps of decision making and risk assessment.

In the light of increasing cost in health care delivery the development of methods to optimize the diagnostic and therapeutic strategy in terms of cost and effectiveness will gain importance. Technology is almost unlimited in medicine; methods have to be developed to assess the effectivity of the measures opposed to outcome, risk and cost. Quality and risk assessment of medical decision and medical action together with attempts of optimization of choice and sequence of procedures will be fields for the development of such a medical methodology. Hopefully, the clinical decision will become more transparent and, if formalized to a certain degree, subject of teaching medicine in areas where formerly only the own experience was able to provide and accumulated knowledge and skills.

Clearly, the development of such a methodology involves clinical trials, planned studies and epidemiological research. Here an overlap is apparent with other areas of medical disciplines. However, the essential element of process-orientation of medical informatics and its attempt to contribute to the decision making in medicine in an innovative approach authorizes the direct involvement in clinical medicine. If decision algorithms, based on the findings during a surgical intervention, have to be developed to decide between different operation techniques for certain types of carcinoma /e.g. 4/, studies have to precede to determine the information content of the various symptoms and the outcome of the respective operation methods. The development of decision support modules for general practice e.g. requires the examination of the epidemiological environment, types and mix of diagnostic decisions etc. in general practice.

6.2. System Analysis.

The growing availability of general tools to be used in the various parts of medicine increases the necessity to develop skills and methods for system analysis in order to assess the problem and to formulate solutions or approaches for research projects or routine applications. Even when hospital information systems become available, the various departments have to be analyzed, their requirements have to be assessed and expressed in a way that the system can be adapted using its inherent tools e.g. in parametrization. This system analysis is directed towards 3 levels:

The task-oriented analysis is concerned with the individual task to be implemented, be it in a new experimental design or in the adaptation of generally available software to a specific problem.

The system analysis of a general type is directed towards the behavior of a certain discipline, the requirements of a certain application in a general way, so that rules can be developed to construct e.g. information systems for the general practitioner, a specific department or certain needs for data acquisition in administration.

The macro-analysis, finally, is concerned with the analysis of health care delivery systems as a whole and the inherent aspects of economics, efficiency and health status assessment.

The specific contribution of medical informatics here should be the innovative introduction of new ideas of problem solution beyond adaptive or reactive analysis. To do this, a profound understanding is necessary of the respective clinical process and its ramifications.

The acceptance of systems is highly influenced by the motivation of the end-user to apply the system in his daily work. Little, however, is known about those facts which influence the attitude and therefore the acceptance or rejection of a system. Studies have shown that by Delphi-methods and other techniques a convergence can be reached between the principles of the system designer and the expectations and motivations of the prospective users /17, 20, 23, 26, 27/.

6.3. Tool Development.

The development of general tools has become a major trend in informatics. Also in medical informatics, more and more 'carrier systems', 'interpreters', 'generator systems' etc. have been developed and provide a general methodology to write systems for a class of problems with the possibility to adapt them to individual environmental conditions by the user or the implementation team. The tendency to develop these carrier systems, /18, 21/, i.e. general problem-oriented systems, based either on interpreters, tables, lists or macro-processors, will increase because this is the only way to transport systems from one location to another and to avoid the ad-hoc hard-programming of a certain solution which will soon be out of date or confined to a single location. Industry will use this method more and more in order to develop its products and to market them on a broad basis. Information systems will always have to be adapted to the local requirements, a general purpose and universal system cannot be expected to satisfy all prospective users. Medical informatics will be instrumental in developing the design criteria, application aspects and criteria for usage of these systems in the various areas.

With the increasing peripherilization, there will be a tendency to decompose integral systems into separate units and increasing the amount of administration and the redundancy of data. A possible counteraction to this development is the research into networks in hospitals, dedicated data bases and combination of systems in and between the units of health care delivery between institutions /12, 18, 19, 21/.

Into the category of tool development also falls the provision of an adequate _teaching_ of the skills and techniques necessary for an adequate application of information technology in the periphery of medicine. In the Federal Republic of Germany e.g., a small but nonetheless mandatory curriculum exists to teach basic concepts of informatics to medical students /8, 9, 15/.

The penetration into clinical medicine will, however, only be successful if _support tools_ can be developed to help in the daily decision making process for both diagnostic evaluation and therapeutic action /24/. These tools will require the development of general software systems to handle the various applications as well as the results of methodological research for the recognition of information content of medical data and their relevance for the decision making process. The development of such tools thus encompasses

-   methodological research for the development of pertaining algorithms and the necessary knowledge bases, and

-   the construction of adequate software tools to handle such algorithms and expert knowledge. New developments show a promising potential of methods of artificial intelligence /see e.g. 28/.

Applications of such sort will have to recognize the time constraints of the decision making process in clinical medicine and its hierarchical structure /24/.

Also _simulation tools_ can be developed for therapeutical procedures, disease processes and physiological systems, just to name a few. These simulation tools will be of particular value for risk assessment and training.

6.4. Applied Research.

In the future, medical informatics should seek greater involvement in clinical research. Tools developed as described above can be used for the documentation of the data collected in research projects, in clinical trials, cancer registers, and for any other purposes. Medical informatics can assist in the validation of the documentated items, in

the assessment of the quality of the data entered and can provide the
tools for analysis and evaluation and presentation including graphical
support.   From its methodological standpoint, the clinical questions
addressed can be enlarged by aspects of methodological research into
information content, validity etc. Often only with a few additions a
genuine research interest of medical informatics can be and should be
identified and implemented together with the clinical objectives. This
holds specifically true for the research into the decision making process.   In this way, medical informatics will become a partner in
research and not only a supporting service.

New areas of applied research and those of particular interest in the
next future will be imaging with all its applications of digital picture processing and subsequent pattern recognition.

Furthermore, new storage techniques will appear on the basis of the
optical disk and the like, which might cause considerable new developments in the area of storage of analog and digital data, including
the storage of x-ray images and the manual chart in the hospital.
Combined with videotex techniques, this may open new dimensions of
applications, even in the field of patient and health education.

Recent attempts show encouraging results in the areas of robotics and
endoprothetics, especially in the latter area in the provision of
intelligent implantates for the continuous release of metabolic active
agents such as insulin and in controlled cytostatic therapy in leuce-
mia or cancer.

6.5. Basic Research.

Medical informatics should also try to identify areas, where information theory, net-theory and other instruments may be applied directly
to the communication process both in the nervous system of the body
and the textural control on the cellular level. Control, so far, is
assumed to be mainly effected by a biochemical transmission system in
the cellular growth and the textural structure. There have been some
theories that photones transmit direct signals between cells and that
here disturbancies may result in an uncontrolled growth such as in
cancer or similar disease. Nothing so far has proven to be of clinical
value and the application of Petri-nets e.g. to structures in

organisms has not yet been tested and evaluated.

7.   CONCLUSIONS.

In summary, there seem to be many possibilities for future activities
in the various areas. A certain change in orientation and work style
will become necessary.   The medical informatician may no longer see
himself as being in charge of large computer systems which dominate
the development in a hospital and where he exercises complete control
of what is happening in the field of informatics.   He has to become a
partner in the various areas of application, such as x-ray examinations are made in traumatology, cardiology and other areas than central radiological units. He should remain, however, in charge of the
integration efforts and the development of network systems in units of
health care delivery, such as the hospital. To do so, he has to
develop central competence, mechanisms for integration and has to do
research into the motivation of people to use a combined effort for a
common goal. This, as our daily life teaches us, is not always easy.

On the other side, the medical informatician should turn himself
closer to the clinical areas as such. The described fields of possible
applications and research should demonstrate the potential range of
such an orientation. Computers, programs and tools can be developed by
industry alone. Research has to be carried on by the medical informatician, innovative research,   which is going beyond reactive system
analysis, mere duplication of existing procedures and mapping them
onto computer systems. To do this, specific knowledge in the medical
field is necessary; education has to be one of the major emphases in
the further development of medical informatics.

One danger is inherent. The more successful the medical informatician
is, the more he may render himself superfluous. This paradox has to be
compensated by a clear recognition of the trends and constant adaptation to a changing world.   It must be avoided that the various new
aspects recognized and followed are considered as completely independent of each other, this being reflected in using different names,
seeking different scientific affiliations and justifications. Conceptual work is necessary to combine the aspects into a theoretical
structure.   If this attempt is not successful, information technology
will remain in medicine, but will become only a tool in the various
medical areas. The challenge for medical informatics is to provide an

own spirit of development. The years to come will prove whether such a spirit can be provided. But even if this does not happen, the disappointment of some of us may be compensated by the recognition that at least part of this spirit has been transmitted by many small sparks into numerous fields of theoretical and clinical medicine.

8. REFERENCES.

(1) Anderson J, Gremy F, Pages JC: Education in Informatics of Health Personnel. (Amsterdam, North-Holland, 1974).

(2) Bock G, Glashoff H, Hueper R, Reichertz PL, Rienhoff O, Sauppe, E: Entwurf einer gemeinsamen Diplompruefungsordnung fuer die Studiengaenge Bibliothekswesen, Allgemeine Dokumentation und Biowissenschaftliche Dokumentation der Fachhochschule Hannover. Konzeption und Entwicklung von Studiengaengen im Bereich Bibliothek, Information und Dokumentation, Nr. 5 (Hannover, Institut f. Regionale Bildungsplanung, 1980).

(3) Gremy F: The future of information processing in medicine and public health. IMIA-T.C.4 Meeting and IMIA Inaugural Session, Paris/France, May 11, 1979.

(4) Gunselmann W: Prognosestellung beim Rektumkarzinom mit Hilfe des Cox-Modells. In: Horbach L, Duhme C (Hrsg.): Nachsorge und Krankheitsverlaufsanalyse. Reihe Med. Informatik und Statistik, Bd. 28 (Berlin/Heidelberg/New York, Springer, 1981) 70-76.

(5) Koeppe P, Reichertz PL: Uebersicht ueber Stand und Ausbildung in der medizinischen Informatik. In: Moehr JR, Koehler CO (Hrsg.): Datenpraesentation. Reihe Med. Informatik und Statistik, Bd. 14 (Berlin/Heidelberg/New York, Springer, 1979) 220-231.

(6) Moehr JR (Hrsg.); Bertram HJ, Deussen P, Eickel J, Koehler CO, Koeppe P, Reichertz, PL, Schuster WR, Victor N: Durchfuehrungsrichtlinien zum Zertifikat Medizinischer Informatiker. Schriftenreihe d. Deutschen Gesellschaft f. Med. Dokumentation, Informatik und Statistik, Heft 2, 2. Auflage (Stuttgart/New York, Schattauer, 1979).

(7) Reichertz PL, Holthoff G: Methoden der Informatik in der Medizin. (Heidelberg, Springer, 1975).

(8) Reichertz PL: Education. Computer Programs in Biomedicine 1976; 5: 206-214.

(9) Reichertz PL: Educational requirements to prepare for expanded usage of information and computer science in health. In: Weller C (edit.): Computer Applications in Health Care Delivery. (Miami, Symposium Specialists, 1976) 113-120.

(10)   Reichertz PL: Medizinische Informatik 1975.   Reihe Med. Informatik und Statistik, Bd. 1 (Heidelberg, Springer, 1976).

(11) Reichertz PL: Medical Methodology (Introduction). In: Laudet M, Anderson J, Begon F (eds.): Medical Computing.   Proceedings of an International Symposium, Toulouse, March 22-25, 1977 (London, Taylor and Francis, 1977) 507-510.

(12) Reichertz PL: Towards systematization. Meth. Inform. Med. 1977; 16: 125-130.

(14) Reichertz PL: MIE-News: Presidential Address. Meth. Inform. Med. 1979; 18: 46-47.

(15) Reichertz PL: Present status of education in Medical Informatics in the Federal Republic of Germany. MEDIS'78, International Symposium on Information System, Osaka/Japan, Oct. 2-6, 1978, Workshop 'Education in Medical Informatics',   (published in: Computer Society of Japan, 1978, 10/11) 1-14.

(16) Reichertz PL: Aufgaben,   Ziele und Moeglichkeiten der medizinischen Informatik.   In: Lange HJ, Michaelis J, Ueberla K (Hrsg.):   15 Jahre Med. Statistik u.   Dokumentation, Aspekte eines Fachgebietes. Reihe Med.   Informatik und Statistik, Bd. 9 (Berlin/Heidelberg/New York, Springer, 1978) 143-150.

(17) Reichertz PL, Moehr JR, Schwarz B, Schlatter A, v. Gaertner-Holthoff, G, Filsinger E: Evaluation of a field test of computers for the doctor's office. Meth. Inform. Med. 1979; 18: 61-70.

(18) Reichertz PL: Forecast of hospital information systems. In: Abe H, Inada H et al. (eds.): MEDIS'78, International Symposium on Medical Information System, Osaka/Japan, Oct. 2-6, 1978 (Tokyo/Osaka, The Medical Information System Development Center and the Kansai Institute of Information Systems, 1979) 157-168.

(19) Reichertz PL: Structure and   content of information systems in the hospital environment.   In: Shannon RH (edit.): Hospital Information Systems. IFIP-Working Conference, Cape Town, April, 4-6 1979 (Amsterdam, North-Holland, 1979) 83-98.

(20) Reichertz PL: Evaluation of a field test of computer application in physicians' offices. In: Rienhoff O, Abrams ME (eds.): The Computer in the Doctor's Office.   (Amsterdam, North-Holland,   1980) 227-242.

(21) Reichertz PL: Medical Informatics - Fiction or Reality?   Meth. Inform. Med. 1980; 19: 11-15.

(22) Reichertz PL: Future developments of data processing in health care. National Informatica Congres, Amsterdam/The Netherlands, Nov.

25, 1981. (in press: Meth. Inform. Med.)

(23) Reichertz PL, Schwarz B: Informationsvermittlung aus der Sicht des Informationsvermittlers - eine Delphi-Studie als Begleituntersuchung zum Projekt DIMDINET. Bundesministerium f. Forschung u. Technologie, Forschungsbericht ID 81 - 004 (Karlsruhe, Fachinformationszentrum Energie, Physik, Mathematik, 1981).

(24) Reichertz PL: Wesen und Probleme der Urteilsfindung in der Medizin. In: Brauer, W. (Hrsg.): GI - 11. Jahrestagung. Informatik-Fachberichte, Nr. 50 (Berlin/Heidelberg/New York, Springer, 1981) 549-556.

(25) Rienhoff O: From 'Medicine' to 'Bioscience' - a modified concept for the education of documentation clerks. In: Lindberg DAB, Kaihara, S (eds.): MEDINFO 80. (Amsterdam/New York/Oxford, North-Holland, 1980) 349-352.

(26) Schwarz B: Analysis of physicians' subjective attitudes concerning EDP applications in physicians' practices. In: Rienhoff O, Abrams ME (eds.) The Computer in the Doctor's Office. (Amsterdam, North-Holland, 1980) 87-99.

(27) Schwarz B, Reichertz PL: Computer in doctor's office: system design, physicians' motivation and reaction. In: Lindberg DAB, Kaihara S (eds.): MEDINFO 80. (Amsterdam/New York/Oxford, North-Holland, 1980) 886-890.

(28) Wahlster W: KI-Verfahren zur Unterstuetzung der aerztlichen Urteilsbildung. In: Brauer W (Hrsg.): GI - 11. Jahrestagung. Informatik-Fachberichte Nr. 50 (Berlin/Heidelberg/New York, Springer, 1981) 568-579.

(29) Wedekind H: Quo vadis Informatik? (Editorial). Informatik-Spektrum 1980; 3: 69-70.

Data Bases (continued)
- Data Reliability   791,798
- Design   1, 58,133
-Haemophilia (treatment)   737
- Management Systems   1,45,587,739,784
- Medical Literature   556,567
- Obstetrics   132,143,156
- Package   818
- Radiology (clinical)   851
- Thalassaemia   700
Data Decay   686
Data Dictionaries   755
Data Protection   3,134,686,853
Data Recovery   805,853
Data Validation   30,134,396,534,597, 792,798,836
Decision Making
- General Practice   272,484
- Intensive Care   431
- Medicical Records   895
- Rheumatology   484,495
Delphi Method   581
Diagnosis
- Computer Assisted   470,477,484,489,495
- Infrequent Index   553
- Discharge Letter   44,157
Distributed Systems   7,14,21,28,76,95,394,434,770,777, 830
Documentation   23, 70,366
Drug Information
- Adverse Reaction   372,380
- Clinical Trials   596
- Intravenous Infusion   468
- Pharmacy   355,369
- Toxicology (poisoning)   362
Education
- Medical   663,669,673
- Patient   290
Medical Computing/Informatics
- Community Physicians   662
- Curriculum   656
- Documentalists   680
- Health Care Personnel   348,666,708

...spektiven der Gesundheitssystemforschung. Frühjahrstagung, Wuppertal, 19... ...ausgegeben von W. van Eimeren. V, 171 Seiten. 1978.

Band 11: U. Feldmann, Wachstumskinetik. Mathematische Modelle und Methoden zur Analy altersabhängiger populationskinetischer Prozesse. VIII, 137 Seiten. 1979.

Band 12: Juristische Probleme der Datenverarbeitung in der Medizin. GMDS/GRVI Date schutz-Workshop 1979. Herausgegeben von W. Kilian und A. J. Porth. VIII, 167 Seiten. 19...

Band 13: S. Biefang, W. Köpcke und M. A. Schreiber, Manual für die Planung und Durc führung von Therapiestudien. IV, 92 Seiten. 1979.

Band 14: Datenpräsentation. Frühjahrstagung, Heidelberg 1979. Herausgegeben v J. R. Möhr und C. O. Köhler. XVI, 318 Seiten. 1979.

Band 15: Probleme einer systematischen Früherkennung. 6. Frühjahrstagung, Heidelberg 19... Herausgegeben von W. van Eimeren und A. Neiß. VI, 176 Seiten, 1979.

Band 16: Informationsverarbeitung in der Medizin -Wege und Irrwege-. Herausgegeben v C. Th. Ehlers und R. Klar. XI, 796 Seiten. 1980.

Band 17: Biometrie – heute und morgen. Interregionales Biometrisches Kolloquium 198 Herausgegeben von W. Köpcke und K. Überla. X, 369 Seiten. 1980.

Band 18: R. Fischer, Automatische Schreibfehlerkorrektur in Texten. Anwendung auf ein me zinisches Lexikon. X, 89 Seiten. 1980.

Band 19: H. J. Rath, Peristaltische Strömungen. VIII, 119 Seiten. 1980.

Band 20: Robuste Verfahren. 25. Biometrisches Kolloquium der Deutschen Region der Int nationalen Biometrischen Gesellschaft, Bad Nauheim, März 1979. Herausgegeben v H. Nowak und R. Zentgraf. V, 121 Seiten. 1980.

Band 21: Betriebsärztliche Informationssysteme. Frühjahrstagung, München, 1980. Herau gegeben von J. R. Möhr und C. O. Köhler. XI, 183 Seiten. 1980.

Band 22: Modelle in der Medizin. Theorie und Praxis. Herausgegeben von H. J. Jesdinsky u V. Weidtman. XIX, 786 Seiten. 1980.

Band 23: Th. Kriedel, Effizienzanalysen von Gesundheitsprojekten. Diskussion und Anwendu auf Epilepsieambulanzen. XI, 287 Seiten. 1980.

Band 24: G. K. Wolf, Klinische Forschung mittels verteilungsunabhängiger Methoden. 141 Seiten. 1980.

Band 25: Ausbildung in Medizinischer Dokumentation, Statistik und Datenverarbeitun Herausgegeben von W. Gaus. X, 122 Seiten. 1980.

Band 26: Explorative Datenanalyse. Frühjahrstagung, München, 1980. Herausgegeben v N. Victor, W. Lehmacher und W. van Eimeren. V, 211 Seiten. 1980.

Band 27: Systeme und Signalverarbeitung in der Nuklearmedizin. Proceedings. Herausg geben von S. J. Pöppl und D. P. Pretschner. IX, 317 Seiten. 1981.

Band 28: Nachsorge und Krankheitsverlaufsanalyse. 25. Jahrestagung der GMDS, Erlange September 1980. Herausgegeben von L. Horbach und C. Duhme. XII, 697 Seiten. 1981.

Band 29: Datenquellen für Sozialmedizin und Epidemiologie. Herausgegeben von Ral Brennecke, Eberhard Greiser, Helmut A. Paul und Elisabeth Schach. VIII, 277 Seiten. 198

Medizinische Informatik und Statistik